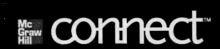
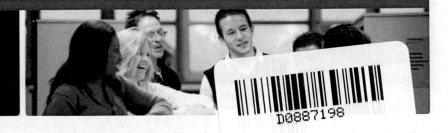

# Student Quick Tips

Use this Student Quick Tips guide for a quick and easy start with McGraw-Hill Connect. You'll get valuable tips on registering, doing assignments, and accessing resources, as well as information about the support center hours.

## Getting Started

**TIP:** To get started in Connect, you will need the following:

- Your instructor's Connect Web Address

> Sample of Connect Web Address:
>
> http://www.mcgrawhillconnect.com/class/instructorname_section_name

- Connect Access Code

**TIP:** If you do not have an access code or have not yet secured your tuition funds, you can click "Free Trial" during registration. This trial will provide temporary Connect access (typically three weeks) and will remind you to purchase online access before the end of your trial.

## Registration and Sign In

1. Go to the Connect Web Address provided by your instructor
2. Click on **Register Now**
3. Enter your email address

**TIP:** If you already have a McGraw-Hill account, you will be asked for your password and will not be required to create a new account.

4. Enter a registration code or choose **Buy Online** to purchase access online

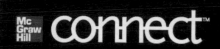
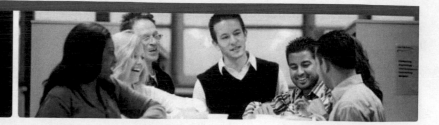

5. Follow the on-screen directions

**TIP:** Please choose your Security Question and Answer carefully. We will ask you for this information if you forget your password.

6. When registration is complete, click on **Go to Connect Now**

7. You are now ready to use **Connect**

## Trouble Logging In?

• Ensure you are using the same email address you used during registration

• If you have forgotten your password, click on the "Forgot Password?" link at your Instructor's Connect Course Web Address

• When logged into Connect, you can update your account information (e.g. email address, password, and security question/answer) by clicking on the *"My Account"* link located at the top-right corner

## Home (Assignments)

**TIP:** If you are unable to begin an assignment, verify the following:

• The assignment is available (start and due dates)

• That you have not exceeded the maximum number of attempts

• That you have not achieved a score of 100%

• If your assignment contains questions that require manual grading, you will not be able to begin your next attempt until your instructor has graded those questions

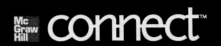 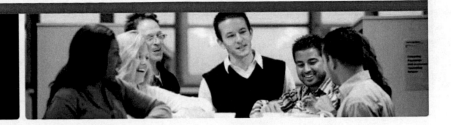

**TIP:** Based on the assignment policy settings established by your Instructor, you may encounter the following limitations when working on your assignment(s):

- Ability to Print Assignment

- Timed assignments – once you begin a "*timed assignment*," the timer will not stop by design

**TIP:** "*Save & Exit*" vs. "*Submit*" button

- If you are unable to complete your assignment in one sitting, utilize the "*Save & Exit*" button to save your work and complete it at a later time

- Once you have completed your assignment, utilize the "*Submit*" button in order for your assignment to be graded

## Library

**TIP:** The *Library* section of your Connect account provides shortcuts to various resources.

- If you purchased ConnectPlus, you will see an *eBook* link, which can also be accessed from the section information widget of the *Home* tab

- *Recorded Lectures* can be accessed if your instructor is using *Tegrity Campus* to capture lectures. You may also access recorded lectures when taking an assignment by clicking on the projector icon in the navigation bar

- Many McGraw-Hill textbooks offer additional resources such as narrated slides and additional problems, which are accessible through the *Student Resources* link

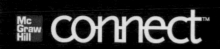 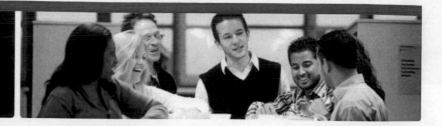

## Reports

**TIP:** Once you submit your assignment, you can view your available results in the *Reports* tab.

• If you see a dash (-) as your score, your instructor has either delayed or restricted your ability to see the assignment feedback

• Your instructor has the ability to limit the amount of information (e.g. questions, answers, scores) you can view for each submitted assignment

## Need More Help?

### CONTACT US ONLINE

Visit us at:

www.mcgrawhillconnect.com/support

Browse our support materials including tutorial videos and our searchable Connect knowledge base. If you cannot find an answer to your question, click on "Contact Us" button to send us an email.

### GIVE US A CALL

Call us at:

1-800-331-5094

Our live support is available:

| | |
|---|---|
| Mon-Thurs: | 8 am – 11 pm CT |
| Friday: | 8 am – 6 pm CT |
| Sunday: | 6 pm – 11 pm CT |

TENTH EDITION

# FIT & WELL

## Core Concepts and Labs in Physical Fitness and Wellness

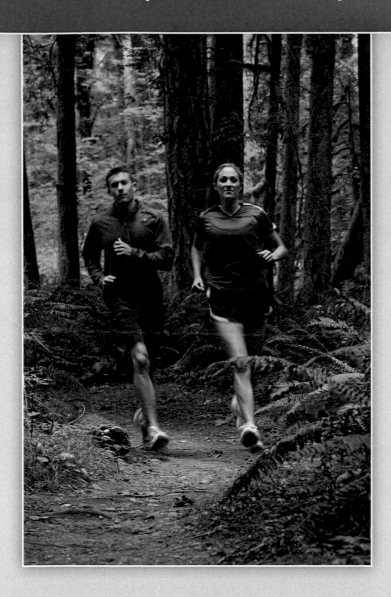

**Thomas D. Fahey**
*California State University, Chico*

**Paul M. Insel**
*Stanford University*

**Walton T. Roth**
*Stanford University*

BELMONT UNIVERSITY

Mc
Graw
Hill
Education

1 2 3 4 5 6 7 8 9 0 GPC GPC 15 14 13

ISBN-13: 978-0-07-811573-8
ISBN-10: 0-07-811573-6

*Learning Solutions Consultant: Judson Harper*
*Associate Project Manager: Alyssa Gantzert*

# BRIEF CONTENTS

**PREFACE** *xiii*

**1** INTRODUCTION TO WELLNESS, FITNESS, AND LIFESTYLE MANAGEMENT *1*

**2** PRINCIPLES OF PHYSICAL FITNESS *29*

**3** CARDIORESPIRATORY ENDURANCE *61*

**4** MUSCULAR STRENGTH AND ENDURANCE *97*

**5** FLEXIBILITY AND LOW-BACK HEALTH *141*

**6** BODY COMPOSITION *175*

**7** PUTTING TOGETHER A COMPLETE FITNESS PROGRAM *199*

**8** NUTRITION *223*

**9** WEIGHT MANAGEMENT *273*

**10** STRESS *301*

**11** CARDIOVASCULAR HEALTH *331*

**12** CANCER *351*

**13** SUBSTANCE USE AND ABUSE *373*

**14** SEXUALLY TRANSMITTED DISEASES *401*

**15** ENVIRONMENTAL HEALTH *421*

**APPENDIX**

**A** INJURY PREVENTION AND PERSONAL SAFETY *A-1*

**B** EXERCISE GUIDELINES FOR PEOPLE WITH SPECIAL HEALTH CONCERNS *B-1*

**C** MONITORING YOUR PROGRESS *C-1*

**BEHAVIOR CHANGE WORKBOOK** *W-1*

**CREDITS** *CR-1*

**INDEX** *I-1*

# CONTENTS

**PREFACE** *xiii*

## 1

## INTRODUCTION TO WELLNESS, FITNESS, AND LIFESTYLE MANAGEMENT 1

**WELLNESS: NEW HEALTH GOALS** 2

The Dimensions of Wellness 2

New Opportunities for Taking Charge 4

The Healthy People Initiative 6

Behaviors That Contribute to Wellness 7

The Role of Other Factors in Wellness 11

**REACHING WELLNESS THROUGH LIFESTYLE MANAGEMENT** 11

Getting Serious About Your Health 12

Building Motivation to Change 13

Enhancing Your Readiness to Change 16

Dealing with Relapse 16

Developing Skills for Change: Creating a Personalized Plan 17

Putting Your Plan into Action 20

Staying with It 20

Being Fit and Well for Life 21

*Tips for Today* 21

*Summary* 22

*For Further Exploration* 22

*Selected Bibliography* 23

**LAB 1.1 Your Wellness Profile** 25

**LAB 1.2 Lifestyle Evaluation** 27

## 2

## PRINCIPLES OF PHYSICAL FITNESS 29

**PHYSICAL ACTIVITY AND EXERCISE FOR HEALTH AND FITNESS** 30

Physical Activity on a Continuum 30

How Much Physical Activity Is Enough? 34

**HEALTH-RELATED COMPONENTS OF PHYSICAL FITNESS** 34

Cardiorespiratory Endurance 35

Muscular Strength 35

Muscular Endurance 36

Flexibility 36

Body Composition 36

Skill (Neuromuscular)-Related Components of Fitness 36

**PRINCIPLES OF PHYSICAL TRAINING: ADAPTATION TO STRESS** 37

Specificity—Adapting to Type of Training 38

Progressive Overload—Adapting to the Amount of Training and the FITT Principle 38

Reversibility—Adapting to a Reduction in Training 40

Individual Differences—Limits on Adaptability 40

**DESIGNING YOUR OWN EXERCISE PROGRAM** 40

Getting Medical Clearance 40

Assessing Yourself 41

Setting Goals 41

Choosing Activities for a Balanced Program 41

Guidelines for Training 44

*Tips for Today* 48

*Summary* 48

*For Further Exploration* 48

*Selected Bibliography* 51

**LAB 2.1 Safety of Exercise Participation** 53

**LAB 2.2 Overcoming Barriers to Being Active** 55

**LAB 2.3 Using a Pedometer to Track Physical Activity** 59

## 3

## CARDIORESPIRATORY ENDURANCE 61

**BASIC PHYSIOLOGY OF CARDIORESPIRATORY ENDURANCE EXERCISE** 62

The Cardiorespiratory System 62

Energy Production 64

Exercise and the Three Energy Systems 64

**BENEFITS OF CARDIORESPIRATORY ENDURANCE EXERCISE** 66

Improved Cardiorespiratory Functioning 66

Improved Cellular Metabolism 68

Reduced Risk of Chronic Disease 68

Better Control of Body Fat 70

Improved Immune Function 70

Improved Psychological and Emotional Well-Being 70

**ASSESSING CARDIORESPIRATORY FITNESS** 71

Choosing an Assessment Test 71

Monitoring Your Heart Rate  72
Interpreting Your Score  72

**DEVELOPING A CARDIORESPIRATORY ENDURANCE PROGRAM**  72
Setting Goals  73
Applying the FITT Equation  74
Warming Up and Cooling Down  77
Building Cardiorespiratory Fitness  77
Maintaining Cardiorespiratory Fitness  78

**EXERCISE SAFETY AND INJURY PREVENTION**  79
Hot Weather and Heat Stress  79
Cold Weather  81
Poor Air Quality  82
Exercise Injuries  82
*Tips for Today*  84
*Summary*  85
*For Further Exploration*  86
*Selected Bibliography*  86

**LAB 3.1  Assessing Your Current Level of Cardiorespiratory Endurance**  89

**LAB 3.2  Developing an Exercise Program for Cardiorespiratory Endurance**  95

**4**

**MUSCULAR STRENGTH AND ENDURANCE**  97

**BASIC MUSCLE PHYSIOLOGY AND THE EFFECTS OF STRENGTH TRAINING**  98
Muscle Fibers  98
Motor Units  99

**BENEFITS OF MUSCULAR STRENGTH AND ENDURANCE**  100
Improved Performance of Physical Activities  101
Injury Prevention  101
Improved Body Composition  101
Enhanced Self-Image and Quality of Life  101
Improved Muscle and Bone Health with Aging  101
Metabolic and Heart Health  102

**ASSESSING MUSCULAR STRENGTH AND ENDURANCE**  102

**CREATING A SUCCESSFUL STRENGTH TRAINING PROGRAM**  103
Static Versus Dynamic Strength Training Exercises  103
Weight Machines Versus Free Weights  105
Other Training Methods and Types of Equipment  106
Applying the FITT Principle: Selecting Exercises and Putting Together a Program  107
The Warm-Up and Cool-Down  109
Getting Started and Making Progress  110
More Advanced Strength Training Programs  110

Weight Training Safety  111
A Caution About Supplements and Drugs  112

**WEIGHT TRAINING EXERCISES**  115
*Tips for Today*  115
*Summary*  126
*For Further Exploration*  126
*Selected Bibliography*  127

**LAB 4.1  Assessing Your Current Level of Muscular Strength**  129

**LAB 4.2  Assessing Your Current Level of Muscular Endurance**  135

**LAB 4.3  Designing and Monitoring a Strength Training Program**  139

**5**

**FLEXIBILITY AND LOW-BACK HEALTH**  141

**TYPES OF FLEXIBILITY**  142

**WHAT DETERMINES FLEXIBILITY?**  142
Joint Structure  142
Muscle Elasticity and Length  142
Nervous System Regulation  143

**BENEFITS OF FLEXIBILITY**  143
Joint Health  144
Prevention of Low-Back Pain and Injuries  145
Additional Potential Benefits  145

**ASSESSING FLEXIBILITY**  145

**CREATING A SUCCESSFUL PROGRAM TO DEVELOP FLEXIBILITY**  145
Applying the FITT Principle  146
Making Progress  148
Exercises to Improve Flexibility: A Sample Program  148

**PREVENTING AND MANAGING LOW-BACK PAIN**  152
Function and Structure of the Spine  152
Core Muscle Fitness  153
Causes of Back Pain  154
Preventing Low-Back Pain  155
Managing Acute Back Pain  155
Managing Chronic Back Pain  156
Exercises for the Prevention and Management of Low-Back Pain  156
*Tips for Today*  158
*Summary*  158
*For Further Exploration*  162
*Selected Bibliography*  163

**LAB 5.1  Assessing Your Current Level of Flexibility**  165

**LAB 5.2  Creating a Personalized Program for Developing Flexibility**  171

**LAB 5.3  Assessing Muscular Endurance for Low-Back Health**  173

## 6

### BODY COMPOSITION 175

**WHAT IS BODY COMPOSITION, AND WHY IS IT IMPORTANT?** 176
Overweight and Obesity Defined 176
Prevalence of Overweight and Obesity Among Americans 178
Excess Body Fat and Wellness 178
Problems Associated with Very Low Levels of Body Fat 179

**ASSESSING BODY MASS INDEX, BODY COMPOSITION, AND BODY FAT DISTRIBUTION** 181
Calculating Body Mass Index 182
Estimating Percent Body Fat 183
Assessing Body Fat Distribution 185

**SETTING BODY COMPOSITION GOALS** 185

**MAKING CHANGES IN BODY COMPOSITION** 186
*Tips for Today* 187
*Summary* 187
*For Further Exploration* 187
*Selected Bibliography* 189
**LAB 6.1 Assessing Body Mass Index and Body Composition** 191
**LAB 6.2 Setting Goals For Target Body Weight** 197

## 7

### PUTTING TOGETHER A COMPLETE FITNESS PROGRAM 199

**DEVELOPING A PERSONAL FITNESS PLAN** 200
1. Set Goals 200
2. Select Activities 200
3. Set a Target Frequency, Intensity, and Time (Duration) for Each Activity 202
4. Set Up a System of Mini-Goals and Rewards 204
5. Include Lifestyle Physical Activity in Your Program 204
6. Develop Tools for Monitoring Your Progress 204
7. Make a Commitment 204

**PUTTING YOUR PLAN INTO ACTION** 205

**EXERCISE GUIDELINES FOR LIFE STAGES** 206
Children and Adolescents 207
Pregnant Women 208
Older Adults 209
*Tips for Today* 209
*Summary* 210
*For Further Exploration* 210
*Selected Bibliography* 210
**LAB 7.1 A Personal Fitness Program Plan and Contract** 219
**LAB 7.2 Getting to Know Your Fitness Facility** 221

## 8

### NUTRITION 223

**NUTRITIONAL REQUIREMENTS: COMPONENTS OF A HEALTHY DIET** 224
Calories 224
Proteins—The Basis of Body Structure 225
Fats—Essential in Small Amounts 227
Carbohydrates—An Ideal Source of Energy 230
Fiber—A Closer Look 232
Vitamins—Organic Micronutrients 233
Minerals—Inorganic Micronutrients 235
Water—Vital but Often Ignored 236
Other Substances in Food 237

**NUTRITIONAL GUIDELINES: PLANNING YOUR DIET** 238
Dietary Reference Intakes (DRIs) 238
Dietary Guidelines for Americans 240
USDA's MyPlate 243
Other Food-Group Plans 246
The Vegetarian Alternative 247
Dietary Challenges for Various Population Groups 248

**NUTRITIONAL PLANNING: MAKING INFORMED CHOICES ABOUT FOOD** 252
Food Labels 252
Dietary Supplements 252
Food Additives 252
Foodborne Illness 252
Irradiated Foods 254
Environmental Contaminants and Organic Foods 256

**A PERSONAL PLAN: APPLYING NUTRITIONAL PRINCIPLES** 258
Assessing and Changing Your Diet 258
Staying Committed to a Healthy Diet 258
*Tips for Today* 258
*Summary* 258
*For Further Exploration* 259
*Selected Bibliography* 262
**LAB 8.1 Your Daily Diet Versus MyPlate** 267
**LAB 8.2 Dietary Analysis** 269
**LAB 8.3 Informed Food Choices** 271

## 9

### WEIGHT MANAGEMENT 273

**HEALTH IMPLICATIONS OF OVERWEIGHT AND OBESITY** 274

**FACTORS CONTRIBUTING TO EXCESS BODY FAT** 275
Genetic Factors 275
Physiological Factors 275
Lifestyle Factors 276

**ADOPTING A HEALTHY LIFESTYLE FOR SUCCESSFUL WEIGHT MANAGEMENT** 277

Diet and Eating Habits 277

**PHYSICAL ACTIVITY AND EXERCISE** 280

**THOUGHTS AND EMOTIONS** 281

Coping Strategies 281

**APPROACHES TO OVERCOMING A WEIGHT PROBLEM** 282

Doing It Yourself 282

Diet Books 283

Dietary Supplements and Diet Aids 285

Weight-Loss Programs 285

Prescription Drugs 287

Surgery 287

Psychological Help 288

**BODY IMAGE** 288

Severe Body Image Problems 288

Acceptance and Change 288

**EATING DISORDERS** 289

Anorexia Nervosa 289

Bulimia Nervosa 290

Binge-Eating Disorder 291

Borderline Disordered Eating 291

Treating Eating Disorders 291

*Tips for Today* 292

*Summary* 292

*For Further Exploration* 293

*Selected Bibliography* 294

**LAB 9.1    Calculating Daily Energy Needs** 295

**LAB 9.2    Identifying Weight-Loss Goals** 297

**LAB 9.3    Checking for Body Image Problems and Eating Disorders** 299

## 10

## STRESS 301

**WHAT IS STRESS?** 302

Physical Responses to Stressors 302

Emotional and Behavioral Responses to Stressors 304

The Stress Experience as a Whole 306

**STRESS AND WELLNESS** 306

The General Adaptation Syndrome 306

Allostatic Load 307

Psychoneuroimmunology 307

Links Between Stress and Specific Conditions 308

**COMMON SOURCES OF STRESS** 309

Major Life Changes 309

Daily Hassles 309

College Stressors 309

Job-Related Stressors 310

Relationships and Stress 310

Other Stressors 311

**MANAGING STRESS** 311

Exercise 311

Nutrition 311

Sleep 312

Social Support 313

Communication 314

Conflict Resolution 315

Striving for Spiritual Wellness 315

Confiding in Yourself Through Writing 315

Time Management 315

Cognitive Techniques 318

Relaxation Techniques 318

Other Stress-Management Techniques 320

**GETTING HELP** 320

Peer Counseling and Support Groups 320

Professional Help 321

Is It Stress or Something More Serious? 321

*Tips for Today* 323

*Summary* 323

*For Further Exploration* 323

*Selected Bibliography* 324

**LAB 10.1    Identifying Your Stress Level and Key Stressors** 325

**LAB 10.2    Stress-Management Techniques** 327

**LAB 10.3    Developing Spiritual Wellness** 329

## 11

## CARDIOVASCULAR HEALTH 331

**RISK FACTORS FOR CARDIOVASCULAR DISEASE** 332

Major Risk Factors That Can Be Changed 332

Contributing Risk Factors That Can Be Changed 336

Major Risk Factors That Can't Be Changed 337

Possible Risk Factors Currently Being Studied 337

**MAJOR FORMS OF CARDIOVASCULAR DISEASE** 339

Atherosclerosis 339

Heart Disease and Heart Attacks 339

Stroke 341

Congestive Heart Failure 342

**PROTECTING YOURSELF AGAINST CARDIOVASCULAR DISEASE** 342

Eat a Heart-Healthy Diet 342

Exercise Regularly 343

Avoid Tobacco 343

Know and Manage Your Blood Pressure 343

Know and Manage Your Cholesterol Levels 344

Develop Ways to Handle Stress and Anger 344

*Tips for Today* 345

*Summary* 345
*For Further Exploration* 345
*Selected Bibliography* 346
**LAB 11.1 Cardiovascular Health** 349

# 12

## CANCER 351

**WHAT IS CANCER?** 352
Tumors 352
Metastasis 352

**COMMON CANCERS** 352
Lung Cancer 353
Colon and Rectal Cancer 354
Breast Cancer 354
Prostate Cancer 355
Cancers of the Female Reproductive Tract 356
Skin Cancer 357
Head and Neck Cancers 358
Testicular Cancer 359

**THE CAUSES OF CANCER** 361
The Role of DNA 362
Tobacco Use 362
Dietary Factors 362
Obesity and Inactivity 364
Carcinogens in the Environment 364

**DETECTING AND TREATING CANCER** 366
Detecting Cancer 366
Treating Cancer 366
*Tips for Today* 368
*Summary* 368
*For Further Exploration* 369
*Selected Bibliography* 370
**LAB 12.1 Cancer Prevention** 371

# 13

## SUBSTANCE USE AND ABUSE 373

**ADDICTIVE BEHAVIOR** 374
What Is Addiction? 374
The Development of Addiction 375
Examples of Addictive Behaviors 375

**PSYCHOACTIVE DRUGS** 375
Drug Use, Abuse, and Dependence 377
Who Uses Drugs? 377
Treatment for Drug Abuse and Dependence 378
Preventing Drug Abuse and Dependence 378
The Role of Drugs in Your Life 379

**ALCOHOL** 380
Chemistry and Metabolism 380
Immediate Effects of Alcohol 380
Drinking and Driving 382
Effects of Chronic Alcohol Abuse 383
Alcohol Abuse 383
Binge Drinking 383
Alcoholism 385
Drinking and Responsibility 385

**TOBACCO** 386
Nicotine Addiction 386
Health Hazards of Cigarette Smoking 386
Other Forms of Tobacco Use 387
Environmental Tobacco Smoke 389
Smoking and Pregnancy 390
Action Against Tobacco 390
Giving Up Tobacco 391
*Tips for Today* 392
*Summary* 392
*For Further Exploration* 393
*Selected Bibliography* 395
**LAB 13.1 Is Alcohol a Problem in Your Life?** 397
**LAB 13.2 For Smokers Only: Why Do You Smoke?** 399

# 14

## SEXUALLY TRANSMITTED DISEASES 401

**THE MAJOR STDs** 402
HIV Infection and AIDS 402
Chlamydia 408
Gonorrhea 410
Pelvic Inflammatory Disease 410
Human Papillomavirus (HPV) 411
Genital Herpes 412
Hepatitis B 412
Syphilis 413
Other STDs 413

**WHAT YOU CAN DO ABOUT STDs** 414
Education 414
Diagnosis and Treatment 414
Prevention 414
*Tips for Today* 415
*Summary* 415
*For Further Exploration* 415
*Selected Bibliography* 416
**LAB 14.1 Behaviors and Attitudes Related to STDs** 419

# 15

## ENVIRONMENTAL HEALTH  *421*

**ENVIRONMENTAL HEALTH DEFINED**  *422*

**POPULATION GROWTH AND CONTROL**  *423*
How Many People Can the World Hold?  *423*
Factors That Contribute to Population Growth  *424*

**AIR QUALITY AND POLLUTION**  *425*
Air Quality and Smog  *425*
The Greenhouse Effect and Global Warming  *426*
Thinning of the Ozone Layer  *428*
Energy Use and Air Pollution  *428*
Indoor Air Pollution  *429*
Preventing Air Pollution  *430*

**WATER QUALITY AND POLLUTION**  *430*
Water Contamination and Treatment  *430*
Water Shortages  *431*
Sewage  *432*
Protecting the Water Supply  *432*

**SOLID WASTE POLLUTION**  *432*
Solid Waste  *433*
Reducing Solid Waste  *435*

**CHEMICAL POLLUTION AND HAZARDOUS WASTE**  *436*
Asbestos  *436*
Lead  *436*
Pesticides  *436*
Mercury  *436*
Other Chemical Pollutants  *437*
Preventing Chemical Pollution  *437*

**RADIATION POLLUTION**  *438*
Nuclear Weapons and Nuclear Energy  *438*
Medical Uses of Radiation  *439*
Radiation in the Home and Workplace  *439*
Avoiding Radiation  *439*
*Tips for Today*  *440*
*Summary*  *440*
*For Further Exploration*  *440*
*Selected Bibliography*  *442*
**LAB 15.1  Environmental Health Checklist**  *443*

## APPENDIX A:

## INJURY PREVENTION AND PERSONAL SAFETY  *A-1*

## APPENDIX B:

## EXERCISE GUIDELINES FOR PEOPLE WITH SPECIAL HEALTH CONCERNS  *B-1*

## APPENDIX C:

## MONITORING YOUR PROGRESS  *C-1*

## BEHAVIOR CHANGE WORKBOOK  *W-1*

## CREDITS  *CR-1*

## INDEX  *I-1*

## BOXES

### TAKE CHARGE
Tips for Moving Forward in the Cycle of Behavior Change  *17*
Vary Your Activities  *46*
Rehabilitation Following a Minor Athletic Injury  *83*
Safe Weight Training  *111*
Safe Stretching  *146*
Stretches to Avoid  *153*
Good Posture and Low-Back Health  *157*
Getting Your Fitness Program Back on Track  *207*
Setting Intake Goals for Protein, Fat, and Carbohydrate  *230*
Choosing More Whole-Grain Foods  *232*
Eating for Healthy Bones  *237*
Reducing the Saturated and Trans Fats in Your Diet  *242*
Judging Portion Sizes  *245*
Eating Strategies for College Students  *249*
Safe Food Handling  *255*
Lifestyle Strategies for Successful Weight Management  *283*
If Someone You Know Has an Eating Disorder . . .  *292*
Overcoming Insomnia  *308*
Building Social Support  *313*
Guidelines for Effective Communication  *314*
Dealing with Anger  *316*
Realistic Self-Talk  *318*
What to Do in Case of a Heart Attack, Stroke, or Cardiac Arrest  *341*
Breast Awareness and Self-Exam  *356*
Testicle Self-Examination  *360*
Dealing with an Alcohol Emergency  *382*
Drinking Behavior and Responsibility  *385*
Using Male Condoms  *409*
Protecting Yourself from STDs  *414*
Compact Fluorescent Lightbulbs  *431*

## CRITICAL CONSUMER

Evaluating Sources of Health Information  13

Choosing a Fitness Center  50

Choosing Exercise Footwear  84

Dietary Supplements: A Consumer Dilemma  112

Using Food Labels  251

Using Dietary Supplement Labels  253

Evaluating Fat and Sugar Substitutes  279

Choosing and Evaluating Mental Health Professionals  322

Evaluating Health News  348

Sunscreens and Sun-Protective Clothing  359

Smoking Cessation Products  391

Getting an HIV Test  407

How to Be a Green Consumer  435

## IN FOCUS

Financial Wellness  5

Wellness Matters for College Students  14

Classifying Activity Levels  33

Exercise and Cardiac Risk  42

Interval Training: Pros and Cons  80

Yoga for Relaxation and Pain Relief  158

Diabetes  180

Choosing Healthy Beverages  208

Counterproductive Strategies for Coping with Stress  311

Breathing for Relaxation  321

Club Drugs  379

Benefits of Quitting Smoking  389

## DIMENSIONS OF DIVERSITY

Wellness Issues for Diverse Populations  8

Fitness and Disability  38

Benefits of Exercise for Older Adults  68

Gender Differences in Muscular Strength  102

The Female Athlete Triad  181

Ethnic Foods  257

Gender, Ethnicity, and Body Image  290

Relaxing Through Meditation  320

Gender, Ethnicity, and CVD  338

Ethnicity, Poverty, and Cancer  361

Gender and Tobacco Use  388

HIV Infection Around the World  405

Poverty and Environmental Health  437

## THE EVIDENCE FOR EXERCISE

Does Being Physically Active Make a Difference in How Long You Live?  10

Is Exercise Good for Your Brain?  31

Why Is It Important to Combine Aerobic Exercise with Strength Training?  69

Does Muscular Strength Reduce the Risk of Premature Death?  100

Does Physical Activity Increase or Decrease the Risk of Bone and Joint Disease?  144

Why Is Physical Activity Important Even if Body Composition Doesn't Change?  177

Can Stability Balls Be Part of a Safe and Effective Fitness Program?  203

Do Athletes Need a Different Diet?  250

What Is the Best Way to Exercise for Weight Loss?  281

Does Exercise Improve Mental Health?  312

How Does Exercise Affect CVD Risk?  344

How Does Exercise Affect Cancer Risk?  364

How Does Exercise Help a Smoker Quit?  393

Does Exercise Help or Harm the Immune System?  403

## PERSONAL CHALLENGE

How Active Are You?  9

Picking Target Behaviors  18

To Work Out. . . Or Not to Work Out?  32

Are You Healthy Enough for Exercise?  41

Staying Active Between Workouts  78

How Strong Are You?  103

Keeping Your Back Pain-Free  156

Tracking Your Weight  186

Tracking Your Junk Food Intake  225

Beating the "Freshman 15"  275

Solving Problems  319

Getting to Know Your Pulse Rate  345

Identifying Your Cancer Risks  366

Tracking Your Drinking  384

Checking Your Environmental "Footprint"  424

## WELLNESS IN THE DIGITAL AGE

Digital Workout Aids  47

Heart Rate Monitors and GPS Devices  73

Improving Your Technique with Video  108

Using BIA at Home  184

Digital Motivation  206

High-Tech Weight Management  284

Digital Tools for Heart Health  333

## BEHAVIOR CHANGE WORKBOOK ACTIVITIES

### PART 1
### DEVELOPING A PLAN FOR BEHAVIOR CHANGE AND COMPLETING A CONTRACT

1. Choosing a Target Behavior   W-1
2. Gathering Information About Your Target Behavior   W-1
3. Monitoring Your Current Patterns of Behavior   W-2
4. Setting Goals   W-3
5. Examining Your Attitudes About Your Target Behavior   W-3
6. Choosing Rewards   W-4
7. Breaking Behavior Chains   W-4
8. Completing a Contract for Behavior Change   W-7

### PART 2
### OVERCOMING OBSTACLES TO BEHAVIOR CHANGE

9. Building Motivation and Commitment   W-8
10. Managing Your Time Successfully   W-9
11. Developing Realistic Self-Talk   W-10
12. Involving the People Around You   W-11
13. Dealing with Feelings   W-12
14. Overcoming Peer Pressure: Communicating Assertively   W-13
15. Maintaining Your Program over Time   W-13

## LABORATORY ACTIVITIES

LAB 1.1   Your Wellness Profile   25
LAB 1.2   Lifestyle Evaluation   27
LAB 2.1   Safety of Exercise Participation   53
LAB 2.2   Overcoming Barriers to Being Active   55
LAB 2.3   Using a Pedometer to Track Physical Activity   59
LAB 3.1   Assessing Your Current Level of Cardiorespiratory Endurance   89
LAB 3.2   Developing an Exercise Program for Cardiorespiratory Endurance   95

LAB 4.1   Assessing Your Current Level of Muscular Strength   129
LAB 4.2   Assessing Your Current Level of Muscular Endurance   135
LAB 4.3   Designing and Monitoring a Strength Training Program   139
LAB 5.1   Assessing Your Current Level of Flexibility   165
LAB 5.2   Creating a Personalized Program for Developing Flexibility   171
LAB 5.3   Assessing Muscular Endurance for Low-Back Health   173
LAB 6.1   Assessing Body Mass Index and Body Composition   191
LAB 6.2   Setting Goals For Target Body Weight   197
LAB 7.1   A Personal Fitness Program Plan and Contract   219
LAB 7.2   Getting to Know Your Fitness Facility   221
LAB 8.1   Your Daily Diet Versus MyPlate   267
LAB 8.2   Dietary Analysis   269
LAB 8.3   Informed Food Choices   271
LAB 9.1   Calculating Daily Energy Needs   295
LAB 9.2   Identifying Weight-Loss Goals   297
LAB 9.3   Checking for Body Image Problems and Eating Disorders   299
LAB 10.1   Identifying Your Stress Level and Key Stressors   325
LAB 10.2   Stress-Management Techniques   327
LAB 10.3   Developing Spiritual Wellness   329
LAB 11.1   Cardiovascular Health   349
LAB 12.1   Cancer Prevention   371
LAB 13.1   Is Alcohol a Problem in Your Life?   397
LAB 13.2   For Smokers Only: Why Do You Smoke?   399
LAB 14.1   Behaviors and Attitudes Related to STDs   419
LAB 15.1   Environmental Health Checklist   443

The Behavior Change Workbook and the laboratory activities are also found in an interactive format in Connect (www.mcgrawhillconnect.com).

# THE **FIT & WELL** LEARNING SYSTEM

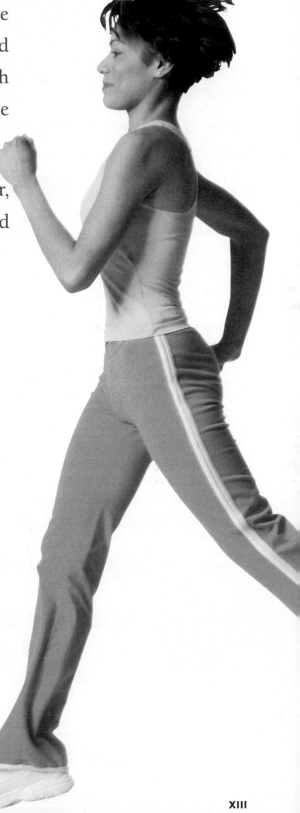

The *Fit & Well* learning system utilizes innovative technologies to personalize the science of fitness and wellness and to motivate students to build research skills, critical thinking skills, and behavior change skills for lifelong wellness.

The new edition of *Fit & Well* is better than ever, thanks to a set of innovative digital teaching and learning tools, including:

- The **LearnSmart adaptive testing program,** which creates individualized study plans for each student, helping to build a strong foundation of knowledge.

- New **College Health Video** activities that discuss topics—like tattoos, tanning salons, DUIs, and stress—relevant to today's students.

- **Connect activities and assessments** that can be seamlessly integrated with your school's course management system.

- The **Tegrity lecture capture system,** which enables instructors to create their own videos and upload them into Connect.

# FIT & WELL WORKS FOR INSTRUCTORS

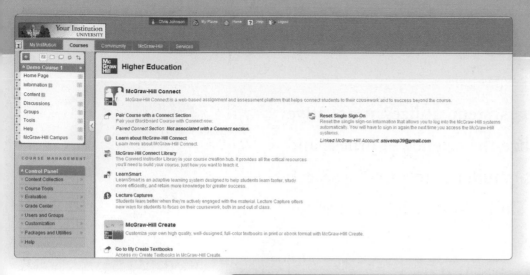

Through McGraw-Hill Campus, *Connect Fit & Well* can be easily integrated with Blackboard or other course management systems. Among other things, this integration enables *Connect* activities, assessments, grades, and other content to appear within your university's system. Setup is fast, easy, and flexible.

New and existing print and digital resources, activities, and assessment in the *Fit & Well* learning system give instructors the tools to challenge students to take small, measurable steps toward achieving a fitness or wellness goal. The result is a program that students can customize to achieve their unique goals.

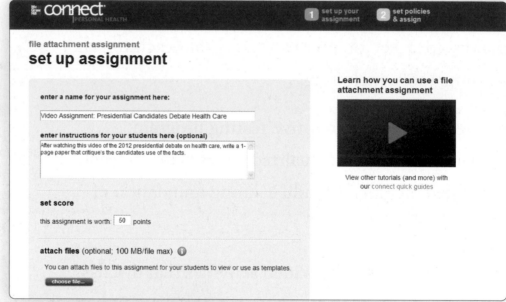

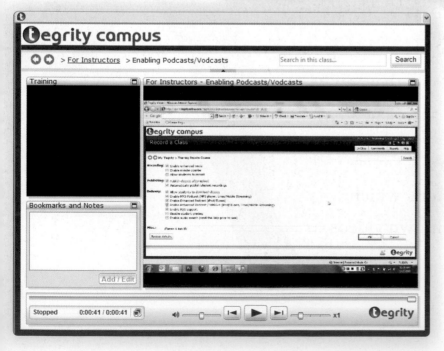

The new Tegrity lecture capture system enables instructors to create and upload into *Connect Fit & Well* their own video lectures.

# FIT & WELL WORKS FOR STUDENTS

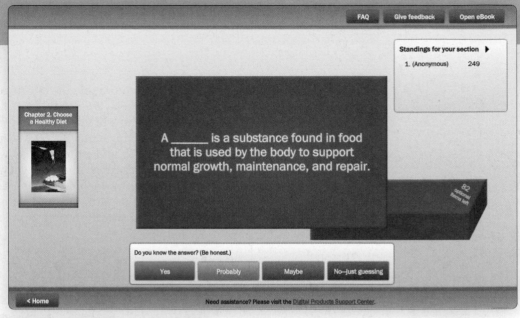

**LearnSmart for Fit & Well:**
*LearnSmart,* an unparalleled adaptive testing program, diagnoses students' knowledge of a subject and then creates an individualized learning path to help them master fitness and wellness concepts. Field studies show that college students who use *LearnSmart* demonstrate a 5% improvement in test scores over students who study without it.

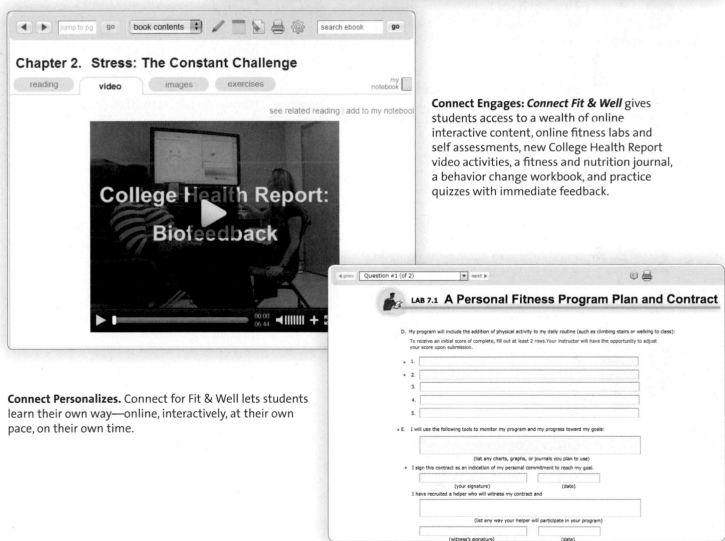

**Connect Engages:** *Connect Fit & Well* gives students access to a wealth of online interactive content, online fitness labs and self assessments, new College Health Report video activities, a fitness and nutrition journal, a behavior change workbook, and practice quizzes with immediate feedback.

**Connect Personalizes.** Connect for Fit & Well lets students learn their own way—online, interactively, at their own pace, on their own time.

# KEY FEATURES AND LEARNING AIDS

The *Fit & Well* learning system continues to provide the information students need to start their journey to fitness and wellness. *Fit & Well*'s authoritative, science-based information is written by experts who work and teach in the field of exercise science, physical education, and health education. *Fit & Well* provides accurate, reliable, current information on key health and fitness topics while also addressing issues related to mind-body health, research, diversity, gender, and consumer health. Text features and interactive activities include self-assessments and fitness labs, videos on timely health topics such as tattooing and tanning beds, exercise demonstration videos, a daily fitness and nutrition log, sample programs, and a wealth of behavior change tools and tips.

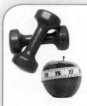 New **Fitness Tips** and **Wellness Tips** catch students' attention and get them thinking—and doing something—about their fitness and wellness.

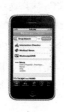 New **Wellness in the Digital Age** sections focus on the many new fitness- and wellness-related devices and applications that are appearing every day, from the Wii Fit system to iPhone apps to digital calorie counters and push-up coaches.

 New **Personal Challenge** activities challenge the student to do something immediately to assess and enhance their fitness or wellness.

 **Evidence for Exercise** sections show students that physical activity and exercise recommendations are based on solid scientific evidence.

 **Critical Consumer** boxes provide reliable consumer information and help students hone their critical thinking and health literacy skills.

 **In Focus** sections explore current trends and topics in fitness and wellness, such as high-interval training and exercising with kettlebells, stability balls, and medicine balls.

 **Hands-on lab activities** give students the opportunity to assess their current level of fitness and wellness and to create their own individualized programs for improvement.

 **Exercise photos and online videos** demonstrate exactly how to perform exercises correctly.

**Behavior change tools** take students through the behavior change process step by step.

**Color Transparency** inserts offer a visually enhanced presentation of key structures and processes, including circulation in the heart and lungs, the deep and superficial muscles, and muscle hypertrophy.

# CHAPTER-BY-CHAPTER CHANGES

## Chapter 1, "Introduction to Wellness, Fitness, and Lifestyle Management"

- The book's key message—that students need to take responsibility for their own fitness and wellness—has been given a new emphasis throughout this chapter, in strong but subtle terms.
- The **In Focus** feature ("Financial Wellness") complements the discussion of the six widely recognized dimensions of wellness and focuses on the importance of mastering basic personal financial skills. The feature has been expanded since the last edition, and includes especially relevant information for students on the dangers of becoming dependent on credit cards.
- The discussions of the Healthy People 2020 and Healthy Campus 2020 initiatives have been refined to focus on the newest round of objectives and the latest statistics on Americans' progress toward meeting those goals.
- All of the chapter's considerable statistical material has been updated to reflect the latest information on morbidity, mortality, and measures of quality of life.

## Chapter 2, "Principles of Physical Fitness"

- Includes the most recent statistics available from the CDC on the physical activity and exercise habits of Americans.
- The **Evidence for Exercise** feature ("Is Exercise Good for Your Brain?") has been revised to make it more relevant to students.
- The discussion of exercise recommendations has been refined to show how the Physical Activity Guidelines for Americans (2008) are in line with recommendations from other agencies.
- Significant new points have been added on the health benefits of weight training, weight training safety, and the effects of weight training on the body's metabolism.

## Chapter 3, "Cardiorespiratory Endurance"

- All statistics have been updated to reflect the latest data from authoritative sources, including the American Heart Association's Heart Disease and Stroke Statistics, 2011.
- New information has been added about the health benefits of combining strength training with aerobic conditioning.
- The chapter presents a wide variety of activities that benefit one's cardiorespiratory health, and challenges students to pick the activity that would best fit with their daily routine.

## Chapter 4, "Muscular Strength and Endurance"

- The chapter presents several basic strength and endurance exercises that students can easily use to assess their fitness level, and challenges them to pick one exercise and set goals for improvement.
- Enumerates more ways than ever to develop muscular strength and endurance without going to the gym.
- Introduces weight training videos and discusses their usefulness.
- Discusses the specific benefits of doing multiple sets of weight-training exercises.

## Chapter 5, "Flexibility and Low-Back Health"

- Reflects the latest recommendations for the minimum and maximum amounts of time to hold a stretch.
- Includes new statistics on the prevalence of osteoporosis, low bone mass.
- Presents a set of basic exercises one can do at home to strengthen the lower back and prevent or alleviate back pain.

## Chapter 6, "Body Composition"

- Makes further distinctions between overweight and obesity.
- Includes newly updated statistics on the prevalence of overweight and obesity in the U.S., from the National Center for Health Statistics.

- Includes new data on the prevalence of metabolic syndrome among Americans, and expands the definition of metabolic syndrome.
- Explains the potential link between obesity and infertility.
- Provides new statistics on the prevalence of all types of diabetes, including prevalence among specific ethnic groups.
- Challenges students to record their weight every day, especially if they are trying to lose weight.

## Chapter 7, "Putting Together a Complete Fitness Program"

- Introduces research indicating that runners may benefit from including stretches in their pre-workout warm-up, contrary to other research indicating stretching should be done after working out.
- Provides new sources and updated data on the benefits and drawbacks of incorporating a stability ball into one's training program.
- Promotes the use of resistance bands as an easy way to incorporate weight training into a total workout program.
- Introduces a variety of motivational programs for use with smart phones, which can help beginning exercisers stick with a program.
- Provides updated research into the benefits and drawbacks of drinking bottled water, and the product's effects on the environment.

## Chapter 8, "Nutrition"

- The overview of nutrients has been expanded and several key terms have been added.
- The entire chapter has been updated, where applicable, to discuss the 2010 Dietary Guidelines for Americans.
- The discussion of sodium intake has been updated to reflect the CDC's latest recommendation that most Americans—not just those with risk factors for heart disease—reduce their sodium intake to 1500 mg per day.
- The discussion of MyPyramid has been re-placed with an introduction to the USDA's new MyPlate program, and explains the program's recommendations.
- The discussion of dietary supplements has been expanded to help students understand when

supplements may be necessary and when they can be most effective.

## Chapter 9, "Weight Management"

- Reiterates the latest statistics on overweight and obesity in the U.S., and breaks down the preva-lence of overweight and obesity by gender and ethnicity.
- Challenges students to examine their own weight, think of reasons they may have gained weight, and list ways they can begin reducing their weight right away.
- Provides new data about the effects of exercise on metabolic rate and resting calorie consumption among college-age men.
- Explains how very simple, small steps—such as cutting back on soda—can have a direct impact on weight loss.
- Discusses high-tech weight management tools and how students can incorporate them into a weight loss program.
- Introduces new data on the impact of psychosocial factors on weight loss among college students.

## Chapter 10, "Stress"

- The definition of "stress" has been clarified and simplified.
- The chapter more clearly defines and differentiates the concepts of "acute stress" and "chronic stress."
- New art illustrates the mechanics of sleep apnea.
- Explains the effects of chronic stress on the body's aging process.
- Expands the discussion of stress's effect on the body's immune system.
- Provides updated statistics on stress from the 2010 Stress in America survey.
- A new section, titled "Relationships and Stress," explores the way our personal and intimate rela-tions with others can be a significant source of stress in our lives.

## Chapter 11, "Cardiovascular Health"

- All statistics have been updated to reflect the lat-est data from authoritative sources, including the American Heart Association's Heart Disease and Stroke Statistics, 2011.

- Introduces easy-to-use and inexpensive digital blood pressure monitors and heart rate monitors that anyone can use at home.
- Provides warnings about the negative effects of weight training on blood pressure.
- Expanded discussions of heart disease risk factors such as C-reactive protein.
- Updated coverage of the benefits of aspirin therapy in some people.
- Instructions for recognizing a heart attack, stroke, and cardiac arrest have been updated to reflect the latest recommendations from the American Heart Association.

### Chapter 12, "Cancer"

- All statistics have been updated to reflect the latest data from authoritative sources, including the American Cancer Society's Cancer Facts and Figures, 2011.
- Discusses the possible links between breast cancer, inactivity, and obesity.
- Provides updated guidelines for Pap tests.
- Outlines new federal regulations of sunscreens and sunscreen labeling.
- A new section, "Detecting and Treating Cancer" focuses on the importance of early detection in successful cancer treatment, and provides more detail than past editions on specific types of cancer treatments.
- The chapter includes all the latest cancer screening guidelines from the American Cancer Society, as well as the ACS's updated guidelines for performing breast self-exams.

### Chapter 13, "Substance Use and Abuse"

- Statistics on drug use and abuse have been updated, based on the latest data from sources such as the Minding the Future Survey, the National Survey on Drug Use and Health, the Youth Risk Behavior Survey, and others.
- The overview of addiction has been revised for clarity and now focuses on addiction in particular and less on habituation.
- Statistics on alcohol use and abuse have been updated, based on the latest data from sources such as the Minding the Future Survey, the National Survey on Drug Use and Health, the Youth Risk Behavior Survey, and others.

- Statistics on alcohol-related accidents, injuries, deaths, and arrests have been updated.
- The new **Personal Challenge** feature challenges students to track their drinking habits daily for two weeks, to get a clear picture of their actual alcohol intake.
- Statistics on tobacco use have been updated, based on the latest data from sources such as the National Survey on Drug Use and Health, the Youth Risk Behavior Survey, the American Cancer Society, and others.
- The Food and Drug Administration's new regulatory authority over tobacco products is described.

### Chapter 14, "Sexually Transmitted Diseases"

- Statistics throughout the chapter have been updated to reflect the latest available information from sources such as the CDC, WHO, Guttmacher Institute, and others.
- The overview of the major STDs, including HIV/AIDS, has been streamlined for easier retention.
- The **Dimensions of Diversity** feature ("HIV/AIDS Around the World") reflects the latest global prevalence estimates from the Joint United Nations Programme on HIV/AIDs.

### Chapter 15, "Environmental Health"

- Current statistics and other information have been gleaned from authoritative sources such as the World Health Organization, World Wildlife Fund, United Nations, and many others.
- The chapter emphasizes ways individuals can take personal responsibility for improving the health of the environment and ensuring that their personal health is not negatively affected by the environment.
- Introduces the concept of sustainability, including sustainable energy and sustainable development, and the potential positive impact of sustainable practices on the environment.
- A **Take Charge** feature on compact fluorescent light bulbs (CFLs) has been expanded to discuss new and prospective state-level legislation regarding their manufacture, use, and disposal.
- The discussion of radiation includes new concerns about cell phone radiation and steps users can take to minimize their exposure.

## FIT & WELL
### in Loose Leaf Format

McGraw-Hill has done a considerable amount of research with college students, not only asking them questions about how they study and use course materials, but also using ethnographic research tools to observe how they study. During the course of this research, students told us they want books and online learning systems that are:

- light and easy to carry
- engaging and relevant to their own lives
- inexpensive
- supported by digital activities that help them learn and succeed in their course

Based on what we heard from students, we are introducing *Fit & Well* in a *three-hole punched, loose leaf* format that is portable, flexible, and cost-effective. *Fit & Well* in loose leaf format offers these advantages:

- Students will need to carry only the portion of the book that's being covered in class with them.
- In addition to the print version of the book, students will receive an integrated multimedia eBook including videos and links to other resources.
- For the same price, students will also receive an access code to *Connect Fit & Well* and *LearnSmart*, providing a number of interactive, multimedia tools that will help them learn.

Would you still like your students to have a bound book? You will be able order one through our *Create* system. While you're at it, we can pull out any of the chapters of the book you don't assign. This ensures that students are purchasing only the content that is being assigned to them, making the book 100% relevant to your course, more affordable for students, and lightweight and portable.

## Mc Graw Hill create
### *Create*, because Customization Matters

Design your ideal course materials with McGraw-Hill's *Create* **www.mcgrawhillcreate.com**! Rearrange or omit chapters, combine material from other sources, and/or upload your syllabus or any other content you have written to make the perfect resource for your students. Search thousands of leading McGraw-Hill textbooks to find the best content for your students, then arrange it to fit your teaching style. You can even personalize your book's appearance by selecting the cover and adding your name, school, and course information. When you order a *Create* book, you receive a complimentary review copy. Get a printed copy in 3 to 5 business days or an electronic copy (eComp) via e-mail in about an hour.

> Register today at **www.mcgrawhillcreate.com**, and craft your course resources to match the way you teach.

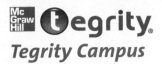

## Tegrity Campus

Tegrity Campus is a service that makes class time available all the time by automatically capturing every lecture in a searchable format for students to review when they study and complete assignments.

With a simple one-click start-and-stop process, you capture all computer screens and corresponding audio. Students replay any part of any class with easy-to-use browser-based viewing on a PC or Mac.

With Tegrity Campus, students quickly recall key moments by using Tegrity Campus's unique search feature. This search helps students efficiently find what they need, when they need it across an entire semester of class recordings.

Help turn all your students' study time into learning moments immediately supported by your lecture.

To learn more about Tegrity watch a 2-minute Flash demo at **http://tegritycampus.mhhe.com**

## McGraw-Hill Campus

McGraw-Hill Campus is the first-of-its-kind institutional service providing faculty with true single sign-on access to all of McGraw-Hill's course content, digital tools, and other high-quality learning resources from any Learning Management System (LMS). This innovative offering allows for secure and deep integration enabling seamless access for faculty and students to any of McGraw-Hill's course solutions such as McGraw-Hill Connect®, McGraw-Hill Create™, McGraw-Hill LearnSmart™, or Tegrity®. McGraw-Hill Campus includes access to McGraw-Hill's entire content library, including eBooks, assessment tools, presentation slides and multimedia content, among other resources, providing faculty open, unlimited access to prepare for class, create tests/quizzes, develop lecture material, integrate interactive content, and more.

## ONLINE LEARNING CENTER

The *Fit & Well* Online Learning Center (**www.mhhe.com/fahey10e**) provides many resources for instructors:

- Course Integrator Guide
- Test bank
- PowerPoint Slides
- Image bank
- Web links

## STUDENT RESOURCES

Resources for student available with *Fit & Well* include the following:

- The Daily Fitness and Nutrition Journal (ISBN 007741179X) is a handy booklet that guides students in planning and tracking their fitness programs. It is available as an optional package with new copies of the text.
- The Health and Fitness Pedometer (ISBN 0077411552) allows students to count their daily steps and track their level of physical activity. The pedometer can also be packaged with new copies of the text.
- NutritionCalc Plus (ISBN 0073328642) is a dietary analysis program that allows users to track their nutrient and food group intakes, energy expenditures, and weight control goals. The ESHA database includes thousands of ethnic foods, supplements, fast foods, and convenience foods; users can also add foods to the database. NutritionCalc Plus is available on CD-ROM (Windows only) or in an Internet version.

# CHAPTER 1

# Introduction to Wellness, Fitness, and Lifestyle Management

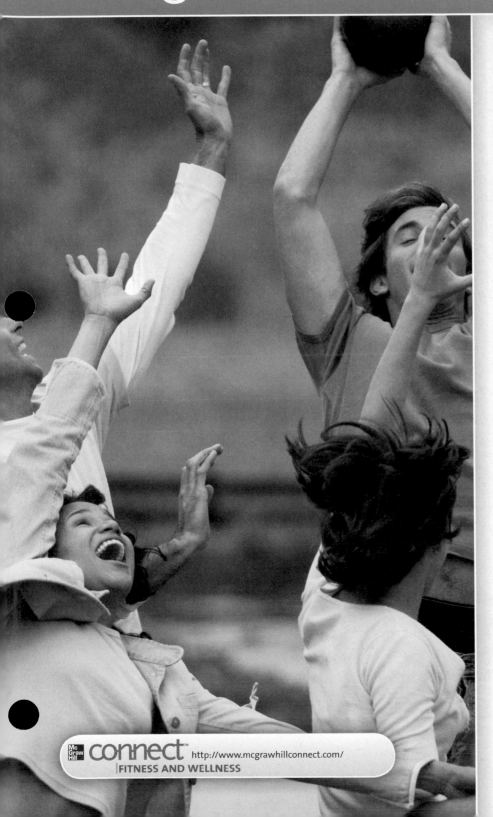

## LOOKING AHEAD. . .

After reading this chapter, you should be able to:

- Describe the dimensions of wellness
- Identify the major health problems in the United States today, and discuss their causes
- Describe the behaviors that are part of a wellness lifestyle
- Explain the steps in creating a behavior management plan to change a wellness-related behavior
- List some of the available sources of wellness information and explain how to think critically about them

## TEST YOUR KNOWLEDGE

1. Which of the following lifestyle factors is the leading preventable cause of death for Americans?
   a. excess alcohol consumption
   b. cigarette smoking
   c. obesity

2. The terms *health* and *wellness* mean the same thing.
   True or false?

3. A person's genetic makeup determines whether he or she will develop certain diseases (such as breast cancer), regardless of that person's health habits.
   True or false?

### ANSWERS

1. **b.** Smoking causes about 440,000 deaths per year. Obesity is responsible for more than 100,000 premature deaths, and alcohol is a factor in as many as 85,000 deaths.
2. **False.** Although the words are used interchangeably, they actually have different meanings. The term *health* refers to the overall condition of the body or mind and to the presence or absence of illness or injury. The term *wellness* refers to optimal health and vitality, encompassing all the dimensions of well-being.
3. **False.** In many cases, behavior can tip the balance toward good health even when heredity or environment is a negative factor.

**A** college sophomore sets the following goals for herself:

- To join new social circles and make new friends whenever possible
- To exercise every day
- To clean up trash and plant trees in blighted neighborhoods in her community

These goals may differ, but they have one thing in common. Each contributes, in its own way, to this student's health and well-being. Not satisfied merely to be free of illness, she wants more. She has decided to live actively and fully—not just to be healthy, but to pursue a state of overall wellness.

## WELLNESS: NEW HEALTH GOALS

Generations of people have viewed health simply as the absence of disease, and that view largely prevails today. The word **health** typically refers to the overall condition of a person's body or mind and to the presence or absence of illness or injury. **Wellness** is a relatively new concept that expands our idea of health to include our ability to achieve optimal health. Beyond the simple presence or absence of disease, wellness refers to optimal health and vitality—to living life to its fullest. Although we use the terms *health* and *wellness* interchangeably, there are two important differences between them:

- Health—or some aspects of it—can be determined or influenced by factors beyond your control, such as your genes, age, and family history. For example, consider

a man with a strong family history of prostate cancer. These factors place this man at a higher-than-average risk for developing prostate cancer himself.

- Wellness is largely determined by the decisions you make about how you live. That same man can reduce his risk of cancer by eating sensibly, exercising, and having regular screening tests. Even if he develops the disease, he may still rise above its effects to live a rich, meaningful life. This means choosing not only to care for himself physically but also to maintain a positive outlook, keep up his relationships with others, challenge himself intellectually, and nurture other aspects of his life.

Enhanced wellness, therefore, involves making conscious decisions to control **risk factors** that contribute to disease or injury. Age and family history are risk factors you cannot control. Behaviors such as choosing not to smoke, exercising, and eating a healthy diet are well within your control.

## The Dimensions of Wellness

Experts have defined six dimensions of wellness:

- Physical
- Emotional
- Intellectual
- Interpersonal
- Spiritual
- Environmental

Each dimension of wellness affects the others. Further, the process of achieving wellness is constant and dynamic (Figure 1.1), involving change and growth. Ignoring any dimension of wellness can have harmful effects on your life. The following sections briefly introduce the dimensions of wellness. Table 1.1 lists some of the specific qualities and behaviors associated with each dimension. Lab 1.1 will help you learn what wellness means to you and where you fall on the wellness continuum.

> **KEY TERMS**
>
> **health** The overall condition of body or mind and the presence or absence of illness or injury.
>
> **wellness** Optimal health and vitality, encompassing all the dimensions of well-being.

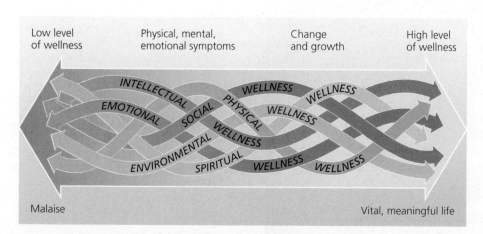

Low level of wellness — Physical, mental, emotional symptoms — Change and growth — High level of wellness

INTELLECTUAL WELLNESS WELLNESS
EMOTIONAL SOCIAL PHYSICAL WELLNESS
ENVIRONMENTAL WELLNESS
SPIRITUAL WELLNESS WELLNESS

Malaise — Vital, meaningful life

**FIGURE 1.1 The wellness continuum.** The concept of wellness includes vitality in six interrelated dimensions, all of which contribute to overall wellness.

| PHYSICAL | EMOTIONAL | INTELLECTUAL | INTERPERSONAL | SPIRITUAL | |
|---|---|---|---|---|---|
| • Eating well | • Optimism | • Openness to new ideas | • Communication skills | • Capacity for l... | |
| • Exercising | • Trust | • Capacity to question | • Capacity for intimacy | • Compassion | |
| • Avoiding harmful habits | • Self-esteem | • Ability to think critically | • Ability to establish and maintain satisfying relationships | • Forgiveness | |
| • Practicing safer sex | • Self-acceptance | • Motivation to master new skills | • Ability to cultivate a support system of friends and family | • Altruism | • Reducing pollution and waste |
| • Recognizing symptoms of disease | • Self-confidence | • Sense of humor | | • Joy | |
| • Getting regular checkups | • Ability to understand and accept one's feelings | • Creativity | | • Fulfillment | |
| • Avoiding injuries | • Ability to share feelings with others | • Curiosity | | • Caring for others | |
| | | • Lifelong learning | | • Sense of meaning and purpose | |
| | | | | • Sense of belonging to something greater than oneself | |

**Physical Wellness** Your physical wellness includes not just your body's overall condition and the absence of disease, but your fitness level and your ability to care for yourself. The higher your fitness level (which is discussed throughout this book), the higher your level of physical wellness will be. Similarly, as you become more able to care for your own physical needs, you ensure greater physical wellness. To achieve optimum physical wellness, you need to make choices that help you avoid illnesses and injuries. The decisions you make now—and the habits you develop over your lifetime—will largely determine the length and quality of your life.

**Emotional Wellness** Your emotional wellness reflects your ability to understand and deal with your feelings. Emotional wellness involves attending to your own thoughts and feelings, monitoring your reactions, and identifying obstacles to emotional stability. Achieving this type of wellness means finding solutions to emotional problems, with professional help if necessary.

**Intellectual Wellness** Those who enjoy intellectual wellness constantly challenge their minds. An active mind is essential to wellness because it detects problems, finds solutions, and directs behavior. People who enjoy intellectual wellness never stop learning; they continue trying to learn new things throughout their lifetime. They seek out and relish new experiences and challenges.

**Interpersonal Wellness** Your interpersonal (or social) wellness is defined by your ability to develop and maintain satisfying and supportive relationships. Such relationships are essential to physical and emotional health. Social wellness requires participating in and contributing to your community and to society.

**Spiritual Wellness** To enjoy spiritual wellness is to possess a set of guiding beliefs, principles, or values that give meaning and purpose to your life, especially in difficult times. The spiritually well person focuses on the positive aspects of life and finds spirituality to be an antidote for negative feelings such as cynicism, anger, and pessimism. Organized religions help many people develop spiritual health. Religion, however, is not the only source or form of spiritual wellness. Many people find meaning and purpose in their lives on their own—through nature, art, meditation, or good works—or with their loved ones.

**Environmental Wellness** Your environmental wellness is defined by the livability of your surroundings. Personal health depends on the health of the planet—from the

> **risk factor** A condition that increases one's chances of disease or injury.

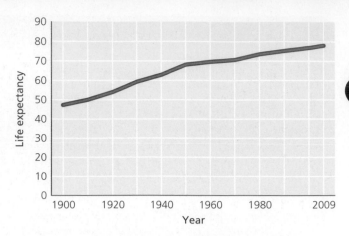

...g one dimension of wellness can have positive
...n others. Joining a meditation group can help
... enhance your spiritual well-being, for example,
...ut can also affect the emotional and interpersonal
dimensions of wellness by enabling you to meet new
people and develop new friendships.

safety of the food supply to the degree of violence in society. Your physical environment either supports your
wellness or diminishes it. To improve your environmental
wellness, you can learn about and protect yourself against
hazards in your surroundings and work to make your
world a cleaner and safer place.

**Other Aspects of Wellness** Many experts consider
occupational wellness and financial wellness to be additional important dimensions of wellness. *Occupational
wellness* refers to the level of happiness and fulfillment
you gain through your work. Although high salaries
and prestigious titles are nice, they alone generally do
not bring about occupational wellness. An occupa-
tionally well person truly likes his or her work, feels a
connection with others in the workplace, and has opportunities to learn and be challenged. Other aspects of
occupational wellness include enjoyable work, job satisfaction, and recognition from managers and colleagues.
An ideal job draws on your interests and passions, as
well as your vocational or professional skills, and allows
you to feel that you are contributing to society in your
everyday work.

To achieve occupational wellness, set career goals that
reflect your personal values. For example, a career in
sales might be a good choice for someone who values
financial security, whereas a career in teaching or nursing might be a good choice for someone who values
service to others.

*Financial wellness* refers to your ability to live within
your means and manage your money in a way that
gives you peace of mind. It includes balancing your
income and expenditures, staying out of debt, saving
for the future, and understanding your emotions about
money. For more on this topic, see the box "Financial
Wellness."

**infectious disease**  A disease that can spread from person to
person; caused by microorganisms such as bacteria and viruses.

**chronic disease**  A disease that develops and continues over a
long period of time, such as heart disease or cancer.

**FIGURE 1.2  Life expectancy of Americans from birth,
1900–2009.**
**SOURCE:** National Center for Health Statistics. 2011. Deaths: Preliminary data for
2009. *National Vital Statistics Reports* 59(4).

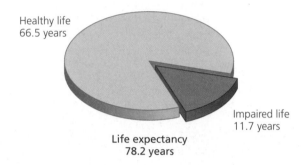

**FIGURE 1.3  Quantity of life versus quality of life.** Years of
healthy life as a proportion of life expectancy in the U.S. population.
**SOURCES:** National Center for Health Statistics. 2011. Deaths: Preliminary data for
2009. *National Vital Statistics Reports.* 59(4); National Center for Health Statistics.
*Healthy People* 2010; Midcourse Review. Hyattsville, Md.: Public Health Service.

## New Opportunities for Taking Charge

Wellness is a fairly new concept. A century ago, Americans
considered themselves lucky just to survive to adulthood
(Figure 1.2). A child born in 1900, for example, could
expect to live only about 47 years. Many people died from
common **infectious diseases** (such as pneumonia, tuberculosis, or diarrhea) and poor environmental conditions
(such as water pollution and poor sanitation).

Since 1900, however, life expectancy has nearly doubled, and as of 2009, the average American's life expectancy was 78.2 years. This increase in life span is due
largely to the development of vaccines and antibiotics to
fight infections, and to public health measures to improve
living conditions. But even though life expectancy has increased, poor health limits most Americans' activities during the last 15% of their lives, resulting in some sort of
impaired life (Figure 1.3). Today, a different set of diseases
has emerged as our major health threat, and heart disease,
cancer, and chronic lower respiratory diseases are now the
three leading causes of death for Americans (Table 1.2).
Treating such **chronic diseases** is costly and difficult.

# Financial Wellness

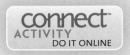

With the news full of stories of home foreclosures, credit card debt, and personal bankruptcies, it has become painfully clear that many Americans do not know how to manage their finances. You can avoid such stress—and gain financial peace of mind—by developing skills that contribute to financial wellness.

Financial wellness means having a healthy relationship with money. It involves knowing how to manage your money, using self-discipline to live within your means, using credit cards wisely, staying out of debt, meeting your financial obligations, having a long-range financial plan, and saving.

## Learn to Budget

Although the word *budget* may conjure up thoughts of deprivation, a budget is really just a way of tracking where your money goes and making sure you're spending it on the things that are most important to you. To start one, list your monthly income and your expenditures. If you aren't sure where you spend your money, track your expenses for a few weeks or a month. Then organize them into categories, such as housing, food, transportation, entertainment, services, personal care, clothes, books and school supplies, health care, credit card and loan payments, and miscellaneous. Use categories that reflect the way you actually spend your money. Knowing where your money goes is the first step in gaining control of it.

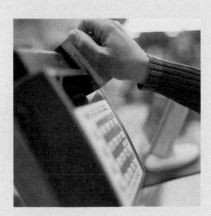

Now total your income and expenditures. Are you taking in more than you spend, or vice versa? Are you surprised by your spending patterns? Use this information to set guidelines and goals for yourself. If your expenses exceed your income, identify ways to make some cuts. If you have both a cell phone and a land line, for example, consider whether you can give one up. If you spend money on movies and restaurants, consider less expensive options like having a weekly game night with friends or organizing an occasional potluck.

## Be Wary of Credit Cards

College students are prime targets for credit card companies, and most undergraduates have at least one card. In fact, many college students use credit cards to live beyond their means, not just for convenience. According a recent report, half of all students have four or more cards, and the average outstanding balance on undergraduate credit cards is over $3000.

The best way to avoid credit card debt is to have just one card, to use it only when necessary, and to pay off the entire balance every month. Make sure you understand terms like *APR* (annual percentage rate—the interest you're charged on your balance), *credit limit* (the maximum amount you can borrow at any one time), *minimum monthly payment* (the smallest payment your creditor will accept each month), *grace period* (the number of days you have to pay your bill before interest or penalties are charged), and *over-the-limit* and *late fees* (the amount you'll be charged if your payment is late or you go over your credit limit).

## Get Out of Debt

If you have credit card debt, stop using your cards and start paying them off. If you can't pay the whole balance, at least try to pay more than the minimum payment each month. It can take a very long time to pay off a loan by making only the minimum payments. For example, to pay off a credit card balance of $2000 at 10% interest with monthly payments of $20 would take 203 months—17 years.

To see for yourself, check out an online credit card calculator like http://www.bankrate.com/calculators/credit-cards/credit-card-payoff-calculator.aspx. And remember: By carrying a balance and incurring finance charges, you are also paying back much more than your initial loan.

## Start Saving

The same miracle of compound interest that locks you into years of credit card debt can work to your benefit if you start saving early (for an online compound interest calculator, visit http://www.moneychimp.com/calculator/compound_interest_calculator.htm). Experts recommend "paying yourself first" every month—that is, putting some money into savings before you start paying your bills, depending on what your budget allows. You may want to save for a large purchase, or you may even be looking ahead to retirement. If you work for a company with a 401(k) retirement plan, contribute as much as you can every pay period.

## Become Financially Literate

Although modern life requires financial literacy, most Americans have not received any kind of basic financial training. Even before the economic meltdown that began in 2008, the U.S. government had established the Financial Literacy and Education Commission (www.MyMoney.gov) to help Americans develop financial literacy and learn how to save, invest, and manage their money better. The consensus is that developing lifelong financial skills should begin in early adulthood, during the college years, if not earlier.

**SOURCES:** Federal Deposit Insurance Corporation. 2010. *Money Smart: A Financial Education Program* (http://www.fdic.gov/consumers/consumer/moneysmart/young.html; retrieved June 23, 2011); Plymouth State University. 2011. *Student Monetary Awareness and Responsibility Today!* (http://www.plymouth.edu/finaid/smart; retrieved June 23, 2011); U.S. Financial Literacy and Education Commission. 2010. *Do You Want to Learn How to Save, Manage, and Invest Your Money Better?* (http://www.mymoney.gov; retrieved June 23, 2011).

**Table 1.2** Leading Causes of Death in the United States, 2009

| RANK | CAUSE OF DEATH | NUMBER OF DEATHS | PERCENTAGE OF TOTAL DEATHS* | DEATH RATE† | LIFESTYLE FACTORS |
|---|---|---|---|---|---|
| | All causes | 2,436,652 | 100.0 | 741.0 | |
| 1 | Heart disease | 598,607 | 24.5 | 179.8 | D I S A |
| 2 | Cancer | 568,668 | 23.3 | 173.6 | D I S A |
| 3 | Chronic lower respiratory diseases | 137,082 | 5.6 | 42.2 | ■ ■ S ■ |
| 4 | Stroke | 128,603 | 5.3 | 38.9 | D I S A |
| 5 | Unintentional injuries (accidents) | 117,176 | 4.8 | 37.0 | D I S A |
| 6 | Alzheimer's disease | 78,889 | 3.2 | 23.4 | |
| 7 | Diabetes mellitus | 68,504 | 2.8 | 20.9 | D I S ■ |
| 8 | Influenza and pneumonia | 53,582 | 2.2 | 16.2 | ■ ■ S ■ |
| 9 | Kidney disease | 48,714 | 2.0 | 14.8 | D I S A |
| 10 | Intentional self-harm (suicide) | 36,547 | 1.5 | 11.7 | ■ ■ ■ A |
| 11 | Septicemia (systemic blood infection) | 35,587 | 1.5 | 10.9 | ■ ■ ■ ■ |
| 12 | Chronic liver disease and cirrhosis | 30,444 | 1.2 | 9.2 | ■ ■ ■ A |
| 13 | Hypertension (high blood pressure) | 25,651 | 1.0 | 7.7 | D I S A |
| 14 | Parkinson's disease | 20,552 | 0.8 | 6.4 | |
| 15 | Assault (homicide) | 16,591 | 0.6 | 5.5 | ■ ■ ■ A |
| | All other causes | 471,455 | | | |

**Key**

D   Diet plays a part      S   Smoking plays a part

I   Inactive lifestyle plays a part      A   Excessive alcohol use plays a part

*Percentages may not total 100% due to rounding.

†Age-adjusted death rate per 100,000 persons.

**NOTE:** Although not among the overall top 15 causes of death, HIV/AIDS is a major killer. In 2009, HIV/AIDS was the twelfth leading cause of death for Americans age 15–24 years and the sixth leading cause of death for those age 25–44 years.

**SOURCE:** National Center for Health Statistics. 2011. Deaths: Preliminary data for 2009. *National Vital Statistics Report* 59(4).

The good news is that people have some control over whether they develop chronic diseases. People make choices every day that increase or decrease their risks for such diseases. These **lifestyle choices** include behaviors such as smoking, diet, exercise, and alcohol use. As Table 1.3 makes clear, lifestyle factors contribute to many deaths in the United States, and people can influence their own health risks. The need to make good choices is especially true for teens and young adults. For Americans age 15–24, for example, the top three causes of death are accidents, homicide, and suicide (Table 1.4).

## The Healthy People Initiative

Wellness is a personal concern, but the U.S. government has financial and humanitarian interests in it, too.

A healthy population is the nation's source of vitality, creativity, and wealth. Poor health drains the nation's resources and raises health care costs for all.

The national Healthy People initiative aims to prevent disease and improve Americans' quality of life. Healthy People reports, published each decade since 1980, set national health goals based on 10-year agendas. The initiative's most recent iteration, *Healthy People 2020,* was developed in 2008–2009 and released to the public in 2010. *Healthy People 2020* envisions "a society in which all people

**KEY TERM**

**lifestyle choice** A conscious behavior that can increase or decrease a person's risk of disease or injury; such behaviors include smoking, exercising, eating a healthy diet, and others.

*Fitness Tip*

In Table 1.2, notice how many causes of death are related to lifestyle. This is an excellent motivator for adopting healthy habits and staying in good condition. Maintaining physical fitness and a healthy diet can lead to a longer life. It's a fact!

## VITAL STATISTICS

### Table 1.3 — Key Contributors to Death Among Americans

|  | NUMBER OF DEATHS PER YEAR | PERCENTAGE OF TOTAL DEATHS PER YEAR |
|---|---|---|
| Tobacco | 440,000 | 18.1 |
| Obesity* | 112,000 | 4.6 |
| Alcohol consumption | 85,000 | 3.5 |
| Microbial agents | 75,000 | 3.1 |
| Toxic agents | 55,000 | 2.3 |
| Motor vehicles | 43,000 | 1.8 |
| Firearms | 29,000 | 1.2 |
| Sexual behavior | 20,000 | 0.8 |
| Illicit drug use | 17,000 | 0.7 |

**NOTE:** The factors listed here are defined as lifestyle and environmental factors that contribute to the leading killers of Americans (health experts often refer to these as the *actual causes of death*). Microbial agents include bacterial and viral infections like influenza and pneumonia; toxic agents include environmental pollutants and chemical agents such as asbestos.

*The number of deaths due to obesity is an area of ongoing controversy and research. Recent estimates have ranged from 112,000 to 365,000.

**SOURCES:** Centers for Disease Control and Prevention. 2005. *Frequently Asked Questions About Calculating Obesity-Related Risk*. Atlanta, Ga.: Centers for Disease Control and Prevention. Mokdad, A. H., et al. 2005. Correction: Actual causes of death in the United States, 2000. *Journal of the American Medical Association* 293(3): 293–294. Mokdad, A. H., et al. 2004. Actual causes of death in the United States, 2000. *Journal of the American Medical Association* 291(10): 1238–1245.

## VITAL STATISTICS

### Table 1.4 — Leading Causes of Death Among Americans Age 15–24, 2008

| RANK | CAUSE OF DEATH | NUMBER OF DEATHS | PERCENTAGE OF TOTAL DEATHS |
|---|---|---|---|
| 1 | Accidents: | 12,351 | 40.8 |
|  | Motor vehicle | 7,648 | 25.2 |
|  | All other accidents | 4,703 | 15.5 |
| 2 | Homicide | 4,820 | 15.9 |
| 3 | Suicide | 4,341 | 14.3 |
| 4 | Cancer | 1,659 | 5.4 |
| 5 | Heart disease | 1,010 | 3.3 |
|  | All causes | 30,252 | 100.0 |

**SOURCE:** National Center for Health Statistics. 2011. Deaths: Preliminary data for 2009. *National Vital Statistics Report* 59(4).

live long, healthy lives" and proposes the eventual achievement of the following broad national health objectives:

• *Eliminate preventable disease, disability, injury, and premature death.* This objective involves activities such as taking more concrete steps to prevent diseases and injuries among individuals and groups, promoting healthy lifestyle choices, improving the nation's preparedness for emergencies, and strengthening the public health infrastructure.

• *Achieve health equity, eliminate disparities, and improve the health of all groups.* This objective involves identifying, measuring, and addressing health differences between individuals or groups that result from a social or economic disadvantage. (See the box "Wellness Issues for Diverse Populations.")

• *Create social and physical environments that promote good health for all.* This objective involves the use of health interventions at many different levels (such as anti-smoking campaigns by schools, workplaces, and local agencies), improving the situation of undereducated and poor Americans by providing a broader array of educational and job opportunities, and actively developing healthier living and natural environments for everyone.

• *Promote healthy development and healthy behaviors across every stage of life.* This goal involves taking a cradle-to-grave approach to health promotion by encouraging disease prevention and healthy behaviors in Americans of all ages.

In a shift from the past, *Healthy People 2020* emphasizes the importance of health determinants—factors that affect the health of individuals, demographic groups, or entire populations. Health determinants are social (including factors such as ethnicity, education level, and economic status) and environmental (including natural and human-made environments). Thus, one goal is to improve living conditions in ways that reduce the impact of negative health determinants.

Examples of individual health promotion goals from *Healthy People 2020,* along with estimates of how well Americans are tracking toward achieving those goals, appear in Table 1.5.

## Behaviors That Contribute to Wellness

A lifestyle based on good choices and healthy behaviors maximizes quality of life. It helps people avoid disease, remain strong and fit, and maintain their physical and mental health as long as they live.

**Be Physically Active** The human body is designed to work best when it is active. It readily adapts to nearly any level of activity and exertion. **Physical fitness** is a set of physical attributes that allow the body to respond or adapt to the demands and stress of physical effort. The more we ask of our bodies, the stronger and more fit they become.

**physical fitness** A set of physical attributes that allows the body to respond or adapt to the demands and stress of physical effort.

**DIMENSIONS OF DIVERSITY**

When it comes to striving for wellness, most differences among people are insignificant. We all need to exercise, eat well, and manage stress. We all need to know how to protect ourselves from disease and injuries.

But some of our differences—both as individuals and as members of groups—have important implications for wellness. Some of us, for example, have grown up with eating habits that increase our risk of obesity or heart disease. Some of us have inherited predispositions for certain health problems, such as osteoporosis or high cholesterol levels. These health-related differences among individuals and groups can be biological (determined genetically) or cultural (acquired as patterns of behavior through daily interactions with family, community, and society). Many health conditions are a function of biology and culture combined.

Every person is an individual with her or his own unique genetic endowment as well as unique experiences in life. However, many of these influences are shared with others of similar genetic and cultural backgrounds. Information about group similarities relating to wellness issues can be useful. For example, it can alert people to areas that may be of special concern for them and their families.

Wellness-related differences among groups can be described along several dimensions, including the following:

● **Gender.** Men and women have different life expectancies and different incidences of many diseases, including heart disease, cancer, and osteoporosis. Men have higher rates of death from injuries, suicide, and homicide, whereas women are at greater risk for Alzheimer's disease and depression. Men and women also differ in body composition and certain aspects of physical performance.

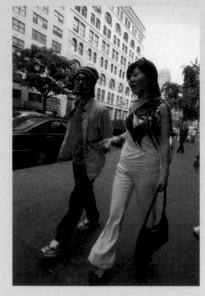

● **Race and ethnicity.** A genetic predisposition for a particular health problem can be linked to race or ethnicity as a result of each group's relatively distinct history. Diabetes is more prevalent among individuals of Native American or Latino heritage, for example, and African Americans have higher rates of hypertension. Racial or ethnic groups may also vary in other ways that relate to wellness: traditional diets; patterns of family and interpersonal relationships; and attitudes toward using tobacco, alcohol, and other drugs, to name just a few.

● **Income and education.** Inequalities in income and education underlie many of the health disparities among Americans. People with low incomes (low *socioeconomic status*, or *SES*) and less education have higher rates of injury and many diseases, are more likely to smoke, and have less access to health care. Poverty and low educational attainment are far more important predictors of poor health than any racial or ethnic factor.

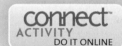

| Table 1.5 | Selected *Healthy People 2020* Objectives | | |
|---|---|---|---|
| **OBJECTIVE** | | **ESTIMATE OF CURRENT STATUS*** | **GOAL*** |
| Reduce the proportion of adults who engage in no leisure-time physical activity | | 36.2 | 32.6 |
| Increase the proportion of adults who are at a healthy weight | | 30.8 | 33.9 |
| Reduce tobacco use (cigarette smoking) among adults | | 20.6 | 12.0 |
| Increase the proportion of adults with mental health disorders who receive treatment | | 58.7 | 64.6 |
| Reduce the proportion of adults with hypertension | | 29.9 | 26.9 |
| Increase the proportion of adults who get sufficient sleep | | 69.6 | 70.9 |
| Reduce the proportion of adults who drank excessively in the previous 30 days | | 28.1 | 25.3 |
| Increase the proportion of persons who use the Internet to communicate with their health care provider | | 13 | 15 |

*Percentage of adult Americans

**SOURCE:** U.S. Department of Health and Human Services. 2011. *Healthy People 2010* (http://www.healthypeople.gov; retrieved April 15, 2011).

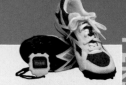
# How Active Are You?

How much of your leisure time do you spend doing nothing? It's easy to figure out: Just keep a simple log (like the one shown here) for a full week. Log the number of minutes of free time you have each day, and list your activities during those times. For our purposes, "free time" means exactly that; it doesn't include time you spend studying.

Day 1: _____    _____
                    (minutes)                              (activities)

Day 2: _____    _____
                    (minutes)                              (activities)

Day 3: _____    _____
                    (minutes)                              (activities)

Day 4: _____    _____
                    (minutes)                              (activities)

Day 5: _____    _____
                    (minutes)                              (activities)

Day 6: _____    _____
                    (minutes)                              (activities)

Day 7: _____    _____
                    (minutes)                              (activities)

Based on this information, do you spend less than 30 minutes of your daily free time engaged in some type of physical activity? If so, look at your log and consider switching some of your current leisure-time activities for moderate-intensity exercise (like a brisk walk or a short bike ride).

Remember: you don't need to exercise for 30 minutes at a time to get the benefits of daily activity. You can break your exercise routine into three 10-minute chunks to make exercise fit your schedule and still enjoy all the health benefits of daily activity.

When our bodies are not kept active, however, they deteriorate. Bones lose their density, joints stiffen, muscles become weak, and cellular energy systems degenerate. To be truly well, human beings must be active.

Unfortunately, a **sedentary** lifestyle is common among Americans. According to recent estmates from the Healthy People program, fewer than one-third of adult Americans regularly engage in some sort of moderate physical activity. A recent study by the National Center for Health Statistics (NCHS) found that nearly 40% of adult Americans get no leisure-time activity at all.

The benefits of physical activity are both physical and mental, immediate and long term (Figure 1.4). In the short term, being physically fit makes it easier to do everyday tasks, such as lifting; it provides reserve strength for emergencies; and it helps people look and feel good. In the long term, being physically fit confers protection against chronic diseases and lowers the risk of dying prematurely. (See the box "Does Being Physically Active Make a Difference in How Long You Live?") Physically active people are less likely to develop or die from heart diease, respiratory disease, high blood pressure, cancer,

- Increased endurance, strength, and flexibility
- Healthier muscles, bones, and joints
- Increased energy (calorie) expenditure
- Improved body composition
- More energy
- Improved ability to cope with stress
- Improved mood, higher self-esteem, and a greater sense of well-being
- Improved ability to fall asleep and sleep well

- Reduced risk of dying prematurely from all causes
- Reduced risk of developing and/or dying from heart disease, diabetes, high blood pressure, and colon cancer
- Reduced risk of becoming obese
- Reduced anxiety, tension, and depression
- Reduced risk of falls and fractures
- Reduced spending for health care

**FIGURE 1.4  Benefits of regular physical activity.**

**KEY TERM**

**sedentary**  Physically inactive; literally, "sitting."

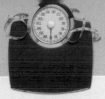

# Does Being Physically Active Make a Difference in How Long You Live?

How can we be sure that physical activity and exercise are good for our health? To answer this question, the U.S. Department of Health and Human Services asked a committee to review scientific literature. The committee's mission was to determine if enough evidence exists to warrant the government making physical activity recommendations to the public. The committee's report, the *Physical Activity Guidelines Advisory Committee Report, 2008*, summarizes the scientific evidence for the health benefits of regular physical activity and the risks of sedentary behavior. The report provides the rationale for the federal government's physical activity guidelines.

The committee started by asking whether physical activity actually helps people live longer. The committee investigated the link between physical activity and all-cause mortality—deaths from all causes—by looking at 73 studies dating from 1995 to 2008. The studies included men and women from all age groups (16 to 65 +) and from different racial and ethnic groups.

The data from these studies strongly support an *inverse relation* between physical activity and all-cause mortality; that is, physically active people were less likely to die during a study's follow-up period (ranging from 10 months to 28 years). The review found that active people have about a 30% lower risk of dying compared with inactive people. These inverse associations were found not just for healthy adults but also for older adults (age 65 and older), for people with coronary artery disease and diabetes, for people with impaired mobility, and for people who were overweight or obese. Poor fitness and low physical activity levels were found to be better predictors of premature death than smoking, diabetes, or obesity. Based on the evidence, the committee determined that about 150 minutes (2.5 hours) of physical activity per week is enough to reduce all-cause mortality (see Chapter 2 for more details). It appears that it is the overall volume of energy expended, no matter what kinds of activities are done, that makes a difference in risk of premature death.

The committee also looked at whether there is a *dose-response* relation between physical activity and all-cause mortality—that is, whether more activity reduces death rates even further. Again, the studies showed an inverse relation between these

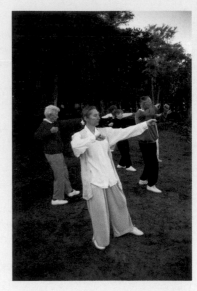

two variables. So, more activity above and beyond 150 minutes per week produces greater benefits. Surprisingly, for inactive people, benefits are seen at levels below 150 minutes per week. In fact, *any* increase in physical activity resulted in reduced risk of death. The committee refers to this as the "some is good; more is better" message. A target of 150 minutes per week is recommended, but any level of activity below the target is encouraged for inactive people.

Looking more closely at this relationship, the committee found that the greatest risk reduction is seen at the lower end of the physical activity spectrum (30 to 90 minutes per week). In fact, sedentary people who become more active have the greatest potential for improving health and reducing the risk of premature death. Additional risk reduction occurs as physical activity increases, but at a slower rate. For example, people who engaged in physical activity 90 minutes per week had a 20% reduction in mortality risk compared with inactive people, and those who were active 150 minutes per week, as noted earlier, had a 30% reduction in risk. But to achieve a 40% reduction in mortality risk, study participants had to be physically active 420 minutes per week (7 hours).

The message from the research is clear: It doesn't matter what activity you choose or even how much time you can devote to it per week, as long as you get moving!

**SOURCE:** Physical Activity Guidelines Advisory Committee. 2008. *Physical Activity Guidelines Advisory Committee Report, 2008*. Washington, D.C.: U.S. Department of Health and Human Services.

---

osteoporosis, and type 2 diabetes (the most common form of diabetes). As they get older, they may be able to avoid weight gain, muscle and bone loss, fatigue, and other problems associated with aging.

**Choose a Healthy Diet** In addition to being sedentary, many Americans have a diet that is too high in calories, unhealthy fats, and added sugars and too low in fiber, complex carbohydrates, fruits, and vegetables. Like physical inactivity, this diet is linked to a number of chronic diseases. A healthy diet provides necessary nutrients and

sufficient energy without also providing too much of the dietary substances linked to diseases.

**Maintain a Healthy Body Weight** Overweight and obesity are associated with a number of disabling and potentially fatal conditions and diseases, including heart disease, cancer, and type 2 diabetes. The Centers for Disease Control and Prevention (CDC) estimates that obesity kills 112,000 Americans each year. Healthy body weight is an important part of wellness—but short-term dieting is not part of fitness or wellness. Maintaining a healthy body weight requires a lifelong commitment to regular exercise, a healthy diet, and effective stress management.

**Manage Stress Effectively** Many people cope with stress by eating, drinking, or smoking too much. Others don't deal with it at all. In the short term, inappropriate stress management can lead to fatigue, sleep disturbances, and other symptoms. Over longer periods of time, poor stress management can lead to less efficient functioning of the immune system and increased susceptibility to disease. Learning to incorporate effective stress management techniques into daily life is an important part of a fit and well lifestyle.

**Avoid Tobacco and Drug Use and Limit Alcohol Consumption** Tobacco use is associated with 8 of the top 10 causes of death in the United States; personal tobacco use and second-hand smoke kill about 440,000 Americans each year, more than any other behavioral or environmental factor. With 21% of adult Americans describing themselves as current smokers as of 2009, lung cancer is the most common cause of cancer death among both men and women and one of the leading causes of death overall. On average, the direct health care costs associated with smoking exceed $100 billion per year. If the cost of lost productivity from sickness, disability, and premature death is included, the total is closer to $193 billion.

Excessive alcohol consumption is linked to 6 of the top 10 causes of death and results in about 85,000 deaths a year in the United States. The social, economic, and medical costs of alcohol abuse are estimated at over $185 billion per year. Alcohol or drug intoxication is an especially notable factor in the death and disability of young people, particularly through **unintentional injuries** (such as drownings and car crashes caused by drunken driving) and violence.

**Protect Yourself from Disease and Injury** The most effective way of dealing with disease and injury is to prevent them. Many of the lifestyle strategies discussed here help protect you against chronic illnesses. In addition, you can take specific steps to avoid infectious diseases, particularly those that are sexually transmitted.

**Take Other Steps Toward Wellness** Other important behaviors contribute to wellness, including these:

- Developing meaningful relationships
- Planning for successful aging
- Learning about the health care system
- Acting responsibly toward the environment

Labs 1.1 and 1.2 will help you evaluate your behaviors as they relate to wellness.

## The Role of Other Factors in Wellness

Heredity, the environment, and adequate health care are other important influences on health and wellness. These factors can interact in ways that raise or lower the quality of a person's life and the risk of developing particular diseases. For example, a sedentary lifestyle combined with a genetic predisposition for diabetes can greatly increase one's risk for developing the disease. If this person also lacks adequate health care, he or she is much more likely to suffer dangerous complications from diabetes.

But in many cases, behavior can tip the balance toward health even if heredity or environment is a negative factor. Breast cancer, for example, can run in families, but it is also associated with overweight and a sedentary lifestyle. A woman with a family history of breast cancer is less likely to die from the disease if she controls her weight, exercises, performs regular breast self-exams, and consults with her physician about mammograms.

## REACHING WELLNESS THROUGH LIFESTYLE MANAGEMENT

As you consider this description of behaviors that contribute to wellness—being physically active, choosing a healthy diet, and so on—you may be doing a mental comparison with your own behaviors. If you are like most young adults, you probably have some healthy habits and some habits that place your health at risk. For example, you may be physically active and have a healthy diet but indulge in binge drinking on weekends. You may be careful to wear your seat belt in your car but smoke cigarettes or use chewing tobacco. Moving in the direction of

**unintentional injury** An injury that occurs without harm being intended.

KEY TERM

wellness means cultivating healthy behaviors and working to overcome unhealthy ones. This approach to lifestyle management is called **behavior change**.

As you may already know from experience, changing an unhealthy habit can be harder than it sounds. When you embark on a behavior change plan, it may seem like too much work at first. But as you make progress, you will gain confidence in your ability to take charge of your life. You will also experience the benefits of wellness—more energy, greater vitality, deeper feelings of appreciation and curiosity, and a higher quality of life.

The rest of this chapter outlines a general process for changing unhealthy behaviors that is backed by research and that has worked for many people. You will also find many specific strategies and tips for change. For additional support, work through the activities in the Behavior Change Workbook at the end of the text.

## Getting Serious About Your Health

Before you can start changing a wellness-related behavior, you have to know that the behavior is problematic and that you *can* change it. To make good decisions, you need information about relevant topics and issues, including what resources are available to help you change.

**Examine Your Current Health Habits** Have you considered how your current lifestyle is affecting your health today and how it will affect your health in the future? Do you know which of your current habits enhance your health and which ones may be harmful? Begin your journey toward wellness with self-assessment: Think about your own behavior, complete the self-assessment in Lab 1.2, and talk with friends and family members about what they've noticed about your lifestyle and your health.

> ### Wellness Tip
>
> When it comes to behavior change, you can win big by starting small, so pick a habit that will be easy to fix. Good examples are drinking more water every day or brushing your teeth for 2 minutes, twice a day. Each time you adopt a healthy new behavior, it's a stepping stone toward a bigger goal.

**Choose a Target Behavior** Changing any behavior can be demanding. This is why it's a good idea to start small, by choosing one behavior you want to change—called a **target behavior**—and working on it until you succeed. Your chances of success will be greater if your first goal is simple, such as resisting the urge to snack between classes. As you change one behavior, make your next goal a little more significant, and build on your success over time.

**Learn About Your Target Behavior** Once you've chosen a target behavior, you need to learn its risks and benefits for you—both now and in the future. Ask these questions:

- How is your target behavior affecting your level of wellness today?
- What diseases or conditions does this behavior place you at risk for?
- What effect would changing your behavior have on your health?

As a starting point, use this text and the resources listed in the For Further Exploration section at the end of

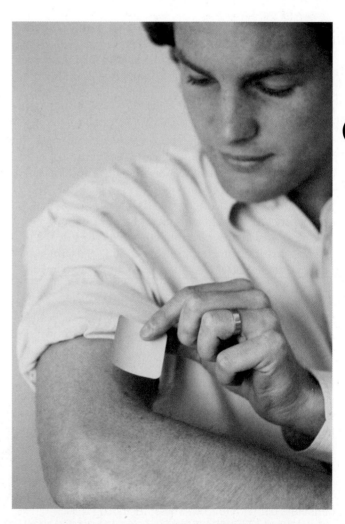

Certain health behaviors are exceptionally difficult to change. Some people can quit smoking on their own; others get help from a smoking cessation program or a nicotine replacement product.

# Evaluating Sources of Health Information

## Believability of Health Information Sources

Surveys indicate that college students are smart about evaluating health information. They trust the health information they receive from health professionals and educators and are skeptical about popular information sources, such as magazine articles and Web sites.

How smart are you about evaluating health information? Here are some tips.

## General Strategies

Whenever you encounter health-related information, take the following steps to make sure it is credible:

● *Go to the original source.* Media reports often simplify the results of medical research. Find out for yourself what a study really reported, and determine whether it was based on good science. What type of study was it? Was it published in a recognized medical journal? Was it an animal study, or did it involve people? Did the study include a large number of people? What did the study's authors actually report?

● *Watch for misleading language.* Reports that tout "breakthroughs" or "dramatic proof" are probably hype. A study may state that a behavior "contributes to" or is "associated with" an outcome, but this does not prove a cause-and-effect relationship.

● *Distinguish between research reports and public health advice.* Do not change your behavior based on the results of a single report or study. If an agency such as the National Cancer Institute urges a behavior change, however, you should follow its advice. Large, publicly funded organizations issue such advice based on many studies, not a single report.

● *Remember that anecdotes are not facts.* A friend may tell you he lost weight on some new diet, but individual success stories do not mean the plan is truly safe or effective. Check with your doctor before making any serious lifestyle changes.

● *Be skeptical.* If a report seems too good to be true, it probably is. Be wary of information contained in advertisements. An ad's goal is to sell a product, even if there is no need for it, and sometimes even if the product has not been proven to be safe or effective.

● *Make choices that are right for you.* Friends and family members can be a great source of ideas and inspiration, but you need to make health-related choices that work best for you.

## Internet Resources

Online information sources pose special challenges. When reviewing a health-related Web site, ask these questions:

● *What is the source of the information?* Web sites maintained by government agencies, professional associations, or established academic or medical institutions are likely to present trustworthy information. Many other groups and individuals post accurate information, but it is important to look at the qualifications of the people who are behind the site. (Check the home page or click the "About Us" link.)

● *How often is the site updated?* Look for sites that are updated frequently. Check the "last modified" date of any Web page.

● *Is the site promotional?* Be wary of information from sites that sell specific products, use testimonials as evidence, appear to have a social or political agenda, or ask for money.

● *What do other sources say about a topic?* Be wary of claims and information that appear at only one site or come from a chat room, bulletin board, or blog.

● *Does the site conform to any set of guidelines or criteria for quality and accuracy?* Look for sites that identify themselves as conforming to some code or set of principles, such as those set forth by the Health on the Net Foundation or the American Medical Association. These codes include criteria such as use of information from respected sources and disclosure of the site's sponsors.

---

each chapter; see the box "Evaluating Sources of Health Information" for additional guidelines.

**Find Help** Have you identified a particularly challenging target behavior or mood—something like alcohol addiction, binge eating, or depression—that interferes with your ability to function or places you at a serious health risk? Help may be needed to change behaviors or conditions that are too deeply rooted or too serious for self-management. Don't be discouraged by the seriousness or extent of the problem; many resources are available to help you solve it. On campus, the student health center or campus counseling center can provide assistance. To

locate community resources, consult the yellow pages, your physician, or the Internet.

## Building Motivation to Change

Knowledge is necessary for behavior change, but it isn't usually enough to make people act. Millions of people have sedentary lifestyles, for example, even though they know it's bad for their health. This is particularly true of young adults, who may not be motivated to change because they feel healthy in spite of their unhealthy behaviors (see the box "Wellness Matters for College Students"). To succeed at behavior change, you need strong motivation.

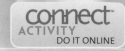

# IN FOCUS

## Wellness Matters for College Students

If you are like most college students, you probably feel pretty good about your health right now. Most college students are in their late teens or early twenties, lead active lives, have plenty of friends, and look forward to a future filled with opportunity. With all these things going for you, why shouldn't you feel good?

### A Closer Look

Although most college-age people look healthy, appearances can be deceiving. Each year, thousands of students lose productive academic time to physical and emotional health problems—some of which can continue to plague them for life.

The following table shows the top 10 health issues affecting students' academic performance, according to the Fall 2010 American College Health Association National College Health Assessment II.

| HEALTH ISSUE | STUDENTS AFFECTED (%) |
|---|---|
| Stress | 25.4 |
| Sleep difficulties | 17.8 |
| Anxiety | 16.4 |
| Cold/flu/sore throat | 13.8 |
| Internet use/computer games | 11.6 |
| Work | 11.4 |
| Concern for a friend/ family member | 10.1 |
| Depression | 10.0 |
| Relationship difficulties | 9.6 |
| Extracurricular activities | 8.8 |

Each of these issues is related to one or more of the six dimensions of wellness, and most can be influenced by choices students make daily. Although some troubles—such as the death of a friend—cannot be controlled, other physical and emotional concerns can be minimized by choosing healthy behaviors. For example, there are many ways to manage stress, the top health issue affecting students. By reducing unhealthy choices (such as using alcohol to relax) and by increasing healthy choices (such as using time management techniques), even busy students can reduce the impact of stress on their life.

The survey also estimated that, based on students' reporting of their height and weight, more than 33% of college students are either overweight or obese. Although heredity plays a role in determining one's weight, lifestyle is also a factor in weight and weight management. In many studies over the past few decades, a large percentage of students have reported behaviors such as these:

- Overeating
- Snacking on junk food
- Frequently eating high-fat foods
- Using alcohol and binge drinking

Clearly, eating behaviors are often a matter of choice. Although students may not see (or feel) the effects of their dietary habits today, the long-term health risks are significant. Overweight and obese persons run a higher-than-normal risk of developing diabetes, heart disease, and cancer later in life. We now know with certainty that improving one's eating habits, even a little, can lead to weight loss and improved overall health.

### Other Choices, Other Problems

Students commonly make other unhealthy choices. Here are some examples from the Fall 2010 National College Health Assessment II:

- About 50% of students reported that they did not use a contraceptive the last time they had vaginal intercourse.

- About 16% of students had 7 or more drinks the last time they partied.

- Almost 15% of students had smoked cigarettes at least once during the past month.

What choices do you make in these situations? Remember: It's never too late to change. The sooner you trade an unhealthy behavior for a healthy one, the longer you'll be around to enjoy the benefits.

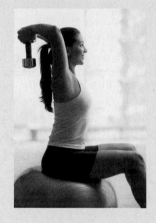

**SOURCE**: American College Health Association. 2011. *American College Health Association National College Health Assessment II: Reference Group Executive Summary Fall 2010*. Linthicum, Md.: American College Health Association.

**Examine the Pros and Cons of Change** Health behaviors have short-term and long-term benefits and costs. Consider the benefits and costs of an inactive lifestyle:

- Short-term, such a lifestyle allows you more time to watch TV and hang out with friends, but it leaves you less physically fit and less able to participate in recreational activities.

- Long-term, it increases the risk of heart disease, cancer, stroke, and premature death.

To successfully change your behavior, you must believe that the benefits of change outweigh the costs.

Carefully examine the pros and cons of continuing your current behavior and of changing to a healthier one. Focus on the effects that are most meaningful to you, including those that are tied to your personal identity and values. For example, if you see yourself as an active person who is a good role model for others, then adopting behaviors such as engaging in regular physical activity and getting adequate sleep will support your personal identity.

If you value independence and control over your life, then quitting smoking will be consistent with your values and goals. To complete your analysis, ask friends and family members about the effects of your behavior on them. For example, a younger sister may tell you that your smoking habit influenced her decision to take up smoking.

The short-term benefits of behavior change can be an important motivating force. Although some people are motivated by long-term goals, such as avoiding a disease that may hit them in 30 years, most are more likely to be moved to action by shorter-term, more personal goals. Feeling better, doing better in school, improving at a sport, reducing stress, and increasing self-esteem are common short-term benefits of health behavior change. Many wellness behaviors are associated with immediate improvements in quality of life. For example, surveys of Americans have found that nonsmokers feel healthy and full of energy more days each month than do smokers, and they report fewer days of sadness and troubled sleep. The same is true when physically active people are compared with sedentary people. Over time, these types of differences add up to a substantially higher quality of life for people who engage in healthy behaviors.

**Boost Self-Efficacy** When you start thinking about changing a health behavior, a big factor in your eventual success is whether you have confidence in yourself and in your ability to change. **Self-efficacy** refers to your belief in your ability to successfully take action and perform a specific task. Strategies for boosting self-efficacy include developing an internal locus of control, using visualization and self-talk, and getting encouragement from supportive people.

**LOCUS OF CONTROL** Who do you believe is controlling your life? Is it your parents, friends, or school? Is it "fate"? Or is it you? **Locus of control** refers to the figurative "place" a person designates as the source of responsibility for the events in his or her life. People who believe they are in control of their own lives are said to have an *internal locus of control*. Those who believe that factors beyond their control determine the course of their lives are said to have an *external locus of control*.

For lifestyle management, an internal locus of control is an advantage because it reinforces motivation and commitment. An external locus of control can sabotage efforts to change behavior. For example, if you believe that you are destined to die of breast cancer because your mother died from the disease, you may view monthly breast self-exams and regular checkups as a waste of time. In contrast, if you believe that you can take action to reduce your risk of breast cancer in spite of hereditary factors, you will be motivated to follow guidelines for early detection of the disease.

If you find yourself attributing too much influence to outside forces, gather more information about your wellness-related behaviors. List all the ways that making lifestyle changes will improve your health. If you believe

you'll succeed, and if you recognize that you are in charge of your life, you're on your way to wellness.

**VISUALIZATION AND SELF-TALK** One of the best ways to boost your confidence and self-efficacy is to visualize yourself successfully engaging in a new, healthier behavior. Imagine yourself going for an afternoon run 3 days a week or no longer smoking cigarettes. Also visualize yourself enjoying all the short-term and long-term benefits that your lifestyle change will bring. Create a new self-image: What will you and your life be like when you become a regular exerciser or a nonsmoker?

You can also use **self-talk,** the internal dialogue you carry on with yourself, to increase your confidence in your ability to change. Counter any self-defeating patterns of thought with more positive or realistic thoughts: "I am a strong, capable person, and I can maintain my commitment to change." See Chapter 10 for more on self-talk.

**ROLE MODELS AND OTHER SUPPORTIVE INDIVIDUALS** Social support can make a big difference in your level of motivation and your chances of success. Perhaps you know people who have reached the goal you are striving for; they could be role models or mentors for you, providing information and support for your efforts. Gain strength from their experiences, and tell yourself, "If they can do it, so can I." In addition, find a buddy who wants to make the same changes you do and who can take an active role in your behavior change program. For example, an exercise buddy can provide companionship and encouragement when you might be tempted to skip your workout.

**Identify and Overcome Barriers to Change** Don't let past failures at behavior change discourage you; they can be a great source of information you can use to boost your chances of future success. Make a list of the problems and challenges you faced in any previous behavior change attempts. To this list, add the short-term costs of behavior change that you identified in your analysis of the pros and cons of change. Once you've listed these key barriers to change, develop a practical plan for overcoming each one. For example, if you always smoke when you're with certain friends, decide in advance how you will turn down the next cigarette you are offered.

## Enhancing Your Readiness to Change

The transtheoretical, or "stages-of-change," model is an effective approach to lifestyle self-management. According to this model, you move through distinct stages as you work to change your target behavior. It is important to determine what stage you are in now so that you can choose appropriate strategies for progressing through the cycle of change. This approach can help you enhance your readiness and intention to change. Read the following sections to determine what stage you are in for your target behavior. For ideas on changing stages, see the box "Tips for Moving Forward in the Cycle of Behavior Change."

**Precontemplation** People at this stage do not think they have a problem and do not intend to change their behavior. They may be unaware of the risks associated with their behavior or may deny them. They may have tried unsuccessfully to change in the past and may now think the situation is hopeless. They may also blame other people or external factors for their problems. People in the precontemplation stage believe that there are more reasons or more important reasons not to change than there are reasons to change.

**Contemplation** People at this stage know they have a problem and intend to take action within 6 months. They acknowledge the benefits of behavior change but are also aware of the costs of changing. To be successful, people must believe that the benefits of change outweigh the costs. People in the contemplation stage wonder about possible courses of action but don't know how to proceed. There may also be specific barriers to change that appear too difficult to overcome.

**Preparation** People at this stage plan to take action within a month or may already have begun to make small changes in their behavior. They may be engaging in their new, healthier behavior but not yet regularly or consistently. They may have created a plan for change but may be worried about failing.

**Action** During the action stage, people outwardly modify their behavior and their environment. The action stage requires the greatest commitment of time and energy, and people in this stage are at risk for reverting to old, unhealthy patterns of behavior.

**Maintenance** People at this stage have maintained their new, healthier lifestyle for at least 6 months. Lapses may have occurred, but people in maintenance have been successful in quickly reestablishing the desired behavior. The maintenance stage can last for months or years.

**Termination** For some behaviors, a person may reach the sixth and final stage of termination. People at this stage have exited the cycle of change and are no longer tempted to lapse back into their old behavior. They have a new self-image and total self-efficacy with regard to their target behavior.

## Dealing with Relapse

People seldom progress through the stages of change in a straightforward, linear way. Rather, they tend to move to a certain stage and then slip back to a previous stage before resuming their forward progress. Research suggests that most people make several attempts before they successfully change a behavior; 4 out of 5 people experience some degree of backsliding. For this reason, the stages of change are best conceptualized as a spiral, in which people cycle back through previous stages but are farther along in the process each time they renew their commitment (Figure 1.5).

If you experience a lapse—a single slip—or a relapse—a return to old habits—don't give up. Relapse can be demoralizing, but it is not the same as failure. Failure means stopping before you reach your goal and never changing your target behavior. During the early stages of

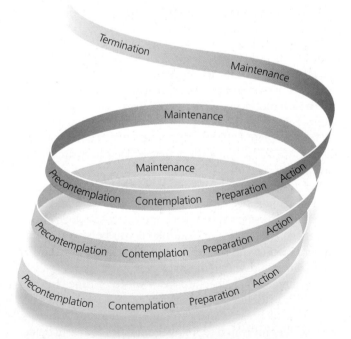

**FIGURE 1.5  The stages of change: A spiral model.**
**SOURCE:** Adapted from Prochaska, J. O., C. C. Diclemente, and J. C. Norcross. 1992. In search of how people change. *American Psychologist* 47(9): 1102–1114. Copyright © 1992 by the American Psychological Association. Reprinted by permission.

# Tips for Moving Forward in the Cycle of Behavior Change

## Precontemplation

- *Raise your awareness.* Research your target behavior and its effects.

- *Be self-aware.* Look at the mechanisms you use to resist change, such as denial or rationalization. Find ways to counteract these mechanisms.

- *Seek social support.* Friends and family members can help you identify target behaviors and understand their impact on the people around you.

- *Identify helpful resources.* These might include exercise classes or stress-management workshops offered by your school.

## Contemplation

- *Keep a journal.* A record of your target behavior and the circumstances that elicit the behavior can help you plan a change program.

- *Do a cost-benefit analysis.* Identify the costs and benefits (both current and future) of maintaining your behavior and of changing it. Costs can be monetary, social, emotional, and so on.

- *Identify barriers to change.* Knowing these obstacles can help you overcome them.

- *Engage your emotions.* Watch movies or read books about people with your target behavior. Imagine what your life will be like if you don't change.

- *Create a new self-image.* Imagine what you'll be like after changing your target behavior. Try to think of yourself in new terms right now.

- *Think before you act.* Learn why you engage in the target behavior. Determine what "sets you off," and train yourself not to act reflexively.

## Preparation

- *Create a plan.* Include a start date, goals, rewards, and specific steps you will take to change your behavior.

- *Make change a priority.* Create and sign a contract with yourself.

- *Practice visualization and self-talk.* These techniques can help prepare you mentally for challenging situations.

- *Take short steps.* Successfully practicing your new behavior for a short time—even a single day—can boost your confidence and motivation.

## Action

- *Monitor your progress.* Keep up with your journal entries.

- *Change your environment.* Make changes that will discourage the target behavior—for example, getting rid of snack foods or not stocking the refrigerator with beer.

- *Find alternatives to your target behavior.* Make a list of things you can do to replace the behavior.

- *Reward yourself.* Rewards should be identified in your change plan. Give yourself lots of praise, and focus on your success.

- *Involve your friends.* Tell them you want to change, and ask for their help.

- *Don't get discouraged.* Real change is difficult.

## Maintenance

- *Keep going.* Continue using the positive strategies that worked in earlier stages.

- *Be prepared for lapses.* Don't let slip-ups set you back.

- *Be a role model.* Once you have successfully changed your behavior, you may be able to help someone else do the same thing.

TAKE CHARGE

the change process, it's a good idea to plan for relapse so you can avoid guilt and self-blame and get back on track quickly. Follow these steps:

1. **Forgive yourself.** A single setback isn't the end of the world, but abandoning your efforts to change could have negative effects on your life.

2. **Give yourself credit for the progress you have already made**. You can use that success as motivation to continue.

3. **Move on.** You can learn from a relapse and use that knowledge to deal with potential setbacks in the future.

If relapses keep occurring or if you can't seem to control them, you may need to return to a previous stage of the behavior change process. If this is necessary, reevaluate your goals and your strategy. A different or less stressful approach may help you avoid setbacks when you try again.

## Developing Skills for Change: Creating a Personalized Plan

Once you are committed to making a change, it's time to put together a plan of action. Your key to success is a well-thought-out plan that sets goals, anticipates problems, and includes rewards.

When starting out on any behavior change plan, the hardest part can be deciding what behavior you want to change. But it doesn't have to be hard; as mentioned in the chapter, you'll probably have the greatest success if you start small. Use the following list to identify five health-related behaviors that you would like to change. List them in order, starting with the behavior you think would be easiest to change and ending with the most difficult.

1. _____
2. _____
3. _____
4. _____
5. _____

The real challenge of this activity is thinking. Examine your lifestyle thoroughly, and consider the things you do (or don't do) every day that may be having a negative effect on your health or wellness. Don't worry if it takes some time to come up with a list, and don't be surprised if you shuffle the items around a few times. The goal is to come up with a list that is doable and realistic for you.

**1. Monitor Your Behavior and Gather Data** Keep a record of your target behavior and the circumstances surrounding it. Record this information for at least a week or two. Keep your notes in a health journal or notebook or on your computer (see the sample journal entries in Figure 1.6). Record each occurrence of your behavior, noting the following:

- What the activity was
- When and where it happened
- What you were doing
- How you felt at that time

If your goal is to start an exercise program, track your activities to determine how to make time for workouts. A blank log is provided in Activity 3 in the Behavior Change Workbook at the end of this text.

**2. Analyze the Data and Identify Patterns** After you have collected data on the behavior, analyze the data to identify patterns. When are you most likely to overeat? What events trigger your appetite? Perhaps you are especially hungry at midmorning or when you put off eating dinner until 9:00 P.M. Perhaps you overindulge in food and drink when you go to a particular restaurant or when you're with certain friends. Note the connections between your feelings and such external cues as time of day, location, situation, and the actions of others around you.

**3. Be "SMART" About Setting Goals** If your goals are too challenging, you will have trouble making steady progress and will be more likely to give up altogether. If, for example, you are in poor physical condition, it will not make

sense to set a goal of being ready to run a marathon within 2 months. If you set goals you can live with, it will be easier to stick with your behavior change plan and be successful.

Experts suggest that your goals meet the "SMART" criteria. That is, your behavior change goals should be:

- *Specific*. Avoid vague goals like "eat more fruits and vegetables." Instead, state your objectives in specific terms, such as "eat 2 cups of fruit and 3 cups of vegetables every day."
- *Measurable*. Recognize that your progress will be easier to track if your goals are quantifiable, so give your goal a number. You might measure your goal in terms of time (such as "walk briskly for 20 minutes a day"), distance ("run 2 miles, 3 days per week"), or some other amount ("drink 8 glasses of water every day").
- *Attainable*. Set goals that are within your physical limits. For example, if you are a poor swimmer, it might not be possible for you to meet a short-term fitness goal by swimming laps. Walking or biking might be better options.
- *Realistic*. Manage your expectations when you set goals. For example, it may not be possible for a long-time smoker to quit cold turkey. A more realistic approach might be to use nicotine replacement patches or gum for several weeks while getting help from a support group.
- *Time frame–specific*. Give yourself a reasonable amount of time to reach your goal, state the time frame in your behavior change plan, and set your agenda to meet the goal within the given time frame.

Using these criteria, a sedentary person who wants to improve his health and build fitness might set a goal of being able to run 3 miles in 30 minutes, to be achieved within a time frame of 6 months. To work toward that goal, he might set a number of smaller, intermediate goals that are easier to achieve. For example, his list of goals might look like this:

| WEEK | FREQUENCY (DAYS/WEEK) | ACTIVITY | DURATION (MINUTES) |
|---|---|---|---|
| 1 | 3 | Walk < 1 mile | 10–15 |
| 2 | 3 | Walk 1 mile | 15–20 |
| 3 | 4 | Walk 1–2 miles | 20–25 |
| 4 | 4 | Walk 2–3 miles | 25–30 |
| 5–7 | 3–4 | Walk/run 1 mile | 15–20 |
| ~ | | | |
| 21–24 | 4–5 | Run 2–3 miles | 25–30 |

Of course, it may not be possible to meet these goals, but you never know until you try. As you work toward meeting your long-term goal, you may find it necessary to adjust your short-term goals. For example, you may find that you can start running sooner than you thought, or you may be able to run farther than you originally estimated. In such cases, it may be reasonable to make your goals more challenging. Otherwise, you may want to make them easier in order to stay motivated.

For some goals and situations, it may make more sense to focus on something other than your outcome goal. If you are in an early stage of change, for example, your goal may be to learn more about the risks associated with your target behavior or to complete a cost-benefit analysis. If your goal involves a long-term lifestyle change, such as reaching a healthy weight, it is better to focus on developing healthy habits than to target a specific weight loss. Your goal in this case might be exercising for 30 minutes every day, reducing portion sizes, or eliminating late-night snacks.

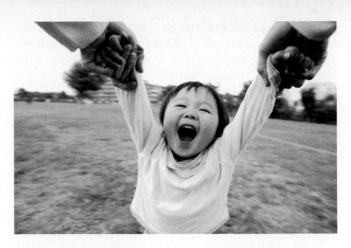

Your environment contains powerful cues for both positive and negative lifestyle choices. The presence of parks and running/bike paths encourages physical activity, even in an urban setting.

**4. Devise a Plan of Action** Develop a strategy that will support your efforts to change. Your plan of action should include the following steps:

- *Get what you need.* Identify resources that can help you. For example, you can join a community walking club or sign up for a smoking cessation program. You may also need to buy some new running shoes or nicotine replacement patches. Get the items you need right away; waiting can delay your progress.
- *Modify your environment.* If there are cues in your environment that trigger your target behavior, try to control them. For example, if you normally have alcohol at home, getting rid of it can help prevent you from indulging. If you usually study with a group of friends in an environment that allows smoking, try moving to a non-smoking area. If you always buy a snack at a certain vending machine, change your route to avoid it.

| Date November 5 | | | | | Day M **TU** W TH F SA SU | | | | | |
|---|---|---|---|---|---|---|---|---|---|---|
| Time of day | M/S | Food eaten | Cals. | H | Where did you eat? | What else were you doing? | How did someone else influence you? | What made you want to eat what you did? | Emotions and feelings? | Thoughts and concerns? |
| 7:30 | M | 1 C Crispix cereal<br>1/2 C skim milk<br>coffee, black<br>1 C orange juice | 110<br>40<br>—<br>120 | 3 | home | reading newspaper | alone | I always eat cereal in the morning | a little keyed up & worried | thinking about quiz in class today |
| 10:30 | S | 1 apple | 90 | 1 | hall outside classroom | studying | alone | felt tired & wanted to wake up | tired | worried about next class |
| 12:30 | M | 1 C chili<br>1 roll<br>1 pat butter<br>1 orange<br>2 oatmeal cookies<br>1 soda | 290<br>120<br>35<br>60<br>120<br>150 | 2 | campus food court | talking | eating w/ friends; we decided to eat at the food court | wanted to be part of group | excited and happy | interested in hearing everyone's plans for the weekend |
| | | M/S = Meal or snack | | | H = Hunger rating (0–3) | | | | | |

**FIGURE 1.6 Sample health journal entries.**

- **Control related habits.** You may have habits that contribute to your target behavior; modifying these habits can help change the behavior. For example, if you usually plop down on the sofa while watching TV, try putting an exercise bike in front of the set so you can burn calories while watching your favorite programs.
- **Reward yourself.** Giving yourself instant, real rewards for good behavior will reinforce your efforts. Plan your rewards; decide in advance what each one will be and how you will earn it. Tie rewards to achieving specific goals or subgoals. For example, you might treat yourself to a movie after a week of avoiding snacks. Make a list of items or events to use as rewards. They should be special to you and preferably unrelated to food or alcohol.
- **Involve the people around you.** Tell family and friends about your plan, and ask them to help. To help them respond appropriately to your needs, create a specific list of dos and don'ts. For example, ask them to support you when you set aside time to exercise or avoid second helpings at dinner.
- **Plan for challenges.** Think about situations and people that might derail your program, and develop ways to cope with them. For example, if you think it will be hard to stick to your usual exercise program during exams, schedule short bouts of physical activity (such as a brisk walk) as stress-reducing study breaks.

**5. Make a Personal Contract** A serious personal contract—one that commits you to your word—can result in a higher chance of follow-through than a casual, offhand promise. Your contract can help prevent procrastination by specifying important dates and can also serve as a reminder of your personal commitment to change.

Your contract should include a statement of your goal and your commitment to reaching it. The contract should also include details, such as the following:

- The date you will start
- The steps you will take to measure your progress
- The strategies you plan to use to promote change
- The date you expect to reach your final goal

Have someone—preferably someone who will be actively helping you with your program—sign your contract as a witness.

Figure 1.7 shows a sample behavior change contract for someone committing to eating more fruit every day. A blank contract is included as Activity 8 in the Behavior Change Workbook at the end of this text.

## Putting Your Plan into Action

The starting date has arrived, and you are ready to put your plan into action. This stage requires commitment, the resolve to stick with the plan no matter what temptations you encounter. Remember all the reasons you have to make the change—and remember that *you* are the boss. Use all

**Behavior Change Contract**

1. I, __Tammy Lau__ , agree to __increase my consumption of fruit from 1 cup per week to 2 cups per day.__
2. I will begin on ____10/5____ and plan to reach my goal of __2 cups of fruit per day__ by __12/7__
3. To reach my final goal, I have devised the following schedule of mini-goals. For each step in my program, I will give myself the reward listed.
   I will begin to have ½ cup of fruit with breakfast __10/5__ __see movie__
   I will begin to have ½ cup of fruit with lunch __10/26__ __new cd__
   I will begin to substitute fruit juice for soda 1 time per day __11/16__ __concert__
   My overall reward for reaching my goal will be __trip to beach__
4. I have gathered and analyzed data on my target behavior and have identified the following strategies for changing my behavior: __Keep the fridge stocked with easy-to-carry fruit. Pack fruit in my backpack every day. Buy lunch at place that serves fruit.__
5. I will use the following tools to monitor my progress toward my final goal: __Chart on fridge door__ __Health journal__

I sign this contract as an indication of my personal commitment to reach my goal: ____Tammy Lau____ __9/28__

I have recruited a helper who will witness my contract and __also increase his consumption of fruit; eat lunch with me twice a week.__
____Eric March____ __9/28__

**FIGURE 1.7   A sample behavior change contract.**

your strategies to make your plan work. Make sure your environment is change-friendly, and get as much support and encouragement from others as possible. Keep track of your progress in your health journal, and give yourself regular rewards. And don't forget to give yourself a pat on the back—congratulate yourself, notice how much better you look or feel, and feel good about how far you've come and how you've gained control of your behavior.

## Staying with It

As you continue with your program, don't be surprised when you run up against obstacles; they're inevitable. In fact, it's a good idea to expect problems and give yourself time to step back, see how you're doing, and make some changes before going on. If your program is grinding to a halt, identify what is blocking your progress. It may come from one of the sources described in the following sections.

**Social Influences** Take a hard look at the reactions of the people you're counting on, and see if they're really supporting you. If they come up short, connect with others who will be more supportive.

A related trap is trying to get your friends or family members to change *their* behaviors. The decision to make a major behavior change is something people come to only after intensive self-examination. You may be able to influence someone by tactfully providing facts or support, but that's all. Focus on yourself. When you succeed, you may become a role model for others.

**Levels of Motivation and Commitment** You won't make real progress until an inner drive leads you to the stage of change at which you are ready to make a personal commitment to the goal. If commitment is your problem, you may need to wait until the behavior you're dealing with makes you unhappier or unhealthier; then your desire to change it will be stronger. Or you may find that changing your goal will inspire you to keep going. For more ideas, refer to Activity 9 in the Behavior Change Workbook.

**Choice of Techniques and Level of Effort** If your plan is not working as well as you thought it would, make changes where you're having the most trouble. If you've lagged on your running schedule, for example, maybe it's because you don't like running. An aerobics class might suit you better. There are many ways to move toward your goal. Or you may not be trying hard enough. You do have to push toward your goal. If it were easy, you wouldn't need a plan.

**Stress Barrier** If you hit a wall in your program, look at the sources of stress in your life. If the stress is temporary, such as catching a cold or having a term paper due, you may want to wait until it passes before strengthening your efforts. If the stress is ongoing, find healthy ways to manage it (see Chapter 10). You may even want to make stress management your highest priority for behavior change.

**Procrastinating, Rationalizing, and Blaming** Be alert to games you might be playing with yourself, so you can stop them. Such games include the following:

• *Procrastinating.* If you tell yourself, "It's Friday already; I might as well wait until Monday to start," you're procrastinating. Break your plan into smaller steps that you can accomplish one day at a time.
• *Rationalizing.* If you tell yourself, "I wanted to go swimming today but wouldn't have had time to wash my hair afterward," you're making excuses.
• *Blaming.* If you tell yourself, "I couldn't exercise because Dave was hogging the elliptical trainer," you're blaming others for your own failure to follow through. Blaming is a way of taking your focus off the real problem and denying responsibility for your own actions.

## Being Fit and Well for Life

Your first attempts at making behavior changes may never go beyond the contemplation or preparation stage. Those that do may not all succeed. But as you experience some success, you'll start to have more positive feelings about yourself. You may discover new physical activities and sports you enjoy, and you may encounter new situations and meet new people. Perhaps you'll surprise yourself by accomplishing things you didn't think were possible— breaking a long-standing nicotine habit, competing in a race, climbing a mountain, or developing a leaner body. Most of all, you'll discover the feeling of empowerment that comes from taking charge of your health. Being healthy takes effort, but the paybacks in energy and vitality are priceless.

Once you've started, don't stop. Assume that health improvement is forever. Take on the easier problems first, and then use what you learn to tackle more difficult problems later. When you feel challenged, remind yourself that you are creating a lifestyle that minimizes your health risks and maximizes your enjoyment of life. You *can* take charge of your health in a dramatic and meaningful way. *Fit and Well* will show you how.

## Ask Yourself

**QUESTIONS FOR CRITICAL THINKING AND REFLECTION**

Think about the last time you made an unhealthy choice instead of a healthy one. How could you have changed the situation, the people in the situation, or your own thoughts, feelings, or intentions to avoid making that choice? What can you do in similar situations in the future to produce a different outcome?

## TIPS FOR TODAY AND THE FUTURE

You are in charge of your health. Many of the decisions you make every day have an impact on the quality of your life, both now and in the future.

**RIGHT NOW YOU CAN**
- Go for a 15-minute walk.
- Have a piece of fruit for a snack.
- Call a friend and arrange for a time to catch up with each other.
- Start thinking about whether you have a health behavior you'd like to change. If you do, consider the elements of a behavior change strategy. For example, begin a mental list of the pros and cons of the behavior, or talk to someone who can support you in your attempts to change.

**IN THE FUTURE YOU CAN**
- Stay current on health- and wellness-related news and issues.
- Participate in health awareness and promotion campaigns in your community—for example, support smoking restrictions in local venues.
- Be a role model for someone else who is working on a health behavior you have successfully changed.

- Wellness is the ability to live life fully, with vitality and meaning. Wellness is dynamic and multidimensional; it incorporates physical, emotional, intellectual, spiritual, interpersonal, and environmental dimensions.

- People today have greater control over and greater responsibility for their health than ever before.

- Behaviors that promote wellness include being physically active, choosing a healthy diet, maintaining a healthy body weight, managing stress effectively, avoiding tobacco and limiting alcohol use, and protecting yourself from disease and injury.

- Although heredity, environment, and health care all play roles in wellness and disease, behavior can mitigate their effects.

- To make lifestyle changes, you need information about yourself, your health habits, and resources available to help you change.

- You can increase your motivation for behavior change by examining the benefits and costs of change, boosting self-efficacy, and identifying and overcoming key barriers to change.

- The stages-of-change model describes six stages that people may move through as they try to change their behavior: precontemplation, contemplation, preparation, action, maintenance, and termination.

- A specific plan for change can be developed by (1) collecting data on your behavior and recording it in a journal; (2) analyzing the recorded data; (3) setting specific goals; (4) devising strategies for modifying the environment, rewarding yourself, and involving others; and (5) making a personal contract.

- To start and maintain a behavior change program, you need commitment, a well-developed and manageable plan, social support, and strong stress-management techniques. It is also important to monitor the progress of your program, revising it as necessary.

## FOR FURTHER EXPLORATION

### BOOKS

American Medical Association. 2006. *American Medical Association Concise Medical Encyclopedia.* New York: Random House. *Includes more than 3000 entries on health and wellness topics, symptoms, conditions, and treatments.*

Claiborn, J., and C. Pedrick. 2009. *The Habit Change Workbook: How to Break Bad Habits and Form Good Ones.* Oakland, Ca.: New Harbinger Publications. *Provides step-by-step instructions for identifying and overcoming a variety of unhealthy behaviors, such as poor eating habits, reluctance to exercise, and addictive behavior.*

Komaroff, A. L., ed. 2005. *Harvard Medical School Family Health Guide.* New York: Free Press. *Provides consumer-oriented advice for the prevention and treatment of common health concerns.*

Krueger, H., et al. 2007. *The Health Impact of Smoking and Obesity and What to Do About It.* Toronto: University of Toronto Press. *Examines the effects of smoking and sedentary lifestyle, the costs to individuals and society, and strategies for overcoming these behaviors.*

Litin, S. C., ed. 2009. *Mayo Clinic Family Health Book,* 4th ed. New York: HarperCollins Publishers. *A complete health reference for every stage of life, covering thousands of conditions, symptoms, and treatments.*

Murat, B., and G. Stewart. 2009. *Do I Need to See the Doctor? The Home-Treatment Encyclopedia—Written by Medical Doctors—That Lets You Decide,* 2nd ed. New York: John Wiley & Sons. *Fully illustrated, easy-to-read guide to hundreds of common symptoms and ailments, designed to help consumers determine whether they can treat themselves or should seek professional medical attention.*

### NEWSLETTERS

*Center for Science in the Public Interest Nutrition Action Health Letter*
   (http://www.cspinet.org/nah/index.htm)
*Consumer Reports on Health (800-274-7596;*
   http://www.consumerreports.org/oh/index.htm)
*Harvard Health Publications (877-649-9457;*
   http://www.health.harvard.edu)
*Harvard Men's Health Watch (877-649-9457)*
*Harvard Women's Health Watch (877-649-9457)*
*Mayo Clinic Health Letter (800-291-1128)*
*Tufts University Health & Nutrition Newsletter*
   (http://www.tuftshealthletter.com)
*University of California at Berkeley Wellness Letter*
   (800-829-9170; http://www.wellnessletter.com)

### ORGANIZATIONS, HOTLINES, AND WEB SITES

The Internet addresses listed here were accurate at the time of publication.

*Centers for Disease Control and Prevention.* Through phone, fax, and the Internet, the CDC provides a wide variety of health information.
   http://www.cdc.gov

*Federal Trade Commission: Consumer Protection—Health.* Includes online brochures about a variety of consumer health topics, including fitness equipment, generic drugs, and fraudulent health claims.
   http://www.ftc.gov/bcp/menus/consumer/health.shtm

*FirstGov for Consumers: Health.* Provides links to online brochures from a variety of government agencies.
   http://consumer.gov/ncpw/category/health

*Healthfinder.* A gateway to online publications, Web sites, support and self-help groups, and agencies and organizations that produce reliable health information.
   http://www.healthfinder.gov

*Healthy Campus.* The American College Health Association's introduction to the Healthy Campus program.
   http://www.acha.org/info_resources/hc2010.cfm

*Healthy People.* Provides information on Healthy People objectives and priority areas.
   http://www.healthypeople.gov

*MedlinePlus.* Provides links to news and reliable information about health from government agencies and professional associations; also includes a health encyclopedia and information on prescription and over-the-counter drugs.
   http://www.medlineplus.gov

*National Health Information Center (NHIC).* Puts consumers in touch with the organizations that are best able to provide answers to health-related questions.

http://www.health.gov/nhic

*National Institutes of Health.* Provides information about all NIH activities as well as consumer publications, hotline information, and an A-to-Z listing of health issues with links to the appropriate NIH institute.

http://www.nih.gov

*National Wellness Institute.* Serves professionals and organizations that promote optimal health and wellness.

http://www.nationalwellness.org

*National Women's Health Information Center.* Provides information and answers to frequently asked questions.

http://www.womenshealth.gov

*Office of Minority Health.* Promotes improved health among racial and ethnic minority populations.

http://minorityhealth.hhs.gov

*Surgeon General.* Includes information on activities of the Surgeon General and the text of many key reports on such topics as tobacco use, physical activity, and mental health.

http://www.surgeongeneral.gov

*World Health Organization (WHO).* Provides information about health topics and issues affecting people around the world.

http://www.who.int

The following are just a few of the many sites that provide consumer-oriented information on a variety of health issues:

*CNN Health:* http://www.cnn.com/health

*FamilyDoctor.Org:* http://familydoctor.org/online/famdocen/home.html

*InteliHealth:* http://www.intelihealth.com

*MayoClinic.com:* http://www.mayoclinic.com

## SELECTED BIBLIOGRAPHY

American Cancer Society. 2011. *Cancer Facts and Figures—2011.* Atlanta: American Cancer Society.

American Heart Association. 2011. *Heart Disease and Stroke Statistics—2011 Update.* Dallas: American Heart Association.

Banks, J., et al. 2006. Disease and disadvantage in the United States and in England. *Journal of the American Medical Association* 295(17): 2037–2045.

Barr, D. A. 2008. *Health Disparities in the United States: Social Class, Race, Ethnicity, and Health.* Baltimore: The Johns Hopkins University Press.

Beckman, M. 2007. Help wanted: In the pursuit of a healthy lifestyle, sheer grit only takes you so far. *Stanford Medicine Magazine* 24(3).

Centers for Disease Control and Prevention. 2008. Racial/Ethnic Disparities in Self-Rated Health Status among Adults with and without Disabilities—United States, 2004–2006. *Morbidity and Mortality Weekly Report* 57(39): 1069–1073.

Centers for Disease Control and Prevention. 2011. *Racial and Ethnic Approaches to Community Health (REACH)* (http://www.cdc.gov/reach; retrieved June 26, 2010).

Finkelstein, E. A., et al. 2008. Do obese persons comprehend their personal health risks? *American Journal of Health Behavior* 32(5): 508–516.

Flegal, K. M., et al. 2005. Excess deaths associated with underweight, overweight, and obesity. *Journal of the American Medical Association* 293(15): 1861–1867.

Flegal, K. M., et al. 2007. Cause-specific excess deaths associated with underweight, overweight, and obesity. *Journal of the American Medical Association* 298(17): 2028–2037.

Flegal, K. M., et al. 2010. Prevalence and Trends in Obesity Among U.S. Adults, 1999–2008. *Journal of the American Medical Association* 303(3): 235–241.

Gorman, B. K., and J. G. Read. 2006. Gender disparities in adult health: An examination of three measures of morbidity. *Journal of Health and Social Behavior* 47(2): 95–110.

Herd, P., et al. 2007. Socioeconomic position and health: The differential effects of education versus income on the onset versus progression of health problems. *Journal of Health and Social Behavior* 48(3): 223–238.

Horneffer-Ginter, K. 2008. Stages of change and possible selves: Two tools for promoting college health. *Journal of American College Health* 56(4): 351–358.

Martin, G., and J. Pear. 2007. *Behaviour Modification: What It Is and How to Do It,* 8th ed. Upper Saddle River, N.J.: Prentice-Hall.

Mokdad, A. H., et al. 2004. Actual causes of death in the United States, 2000. *Journal of the American Medical Association* 291(10): 1238–1245.

Mokdad, A. H., et al. 2005. Correction: Actual causes of death in the United States, 2000. *Journal of the American Medical Association* 293(3): 293–294.

National Center for Health Statistics. 2010. *Health, United States, 2010.* Hyattsville, Md.: National Center for Health Statistics.

National Center for Health Statistics. 2010. Health behaviors of adults: United States, 2005–07. *Vital and Health Statistics* 10(245).

National Center for Health Statistics. 2011. Deaths: Preliminary data for 2009. *National Vital Statistics Report* 59(4).

Nothwehr, F., et al. 2008. Age group differences in diet and physical activity–related behaviors among rural men and women. *Journal of Nutrition, Health and Aging* 12(3): 169–174.

O'Loughlin, J., et al. 2007. Lifestyle risk factors for chronic disease across family origin among adults in multiethnic, low-income, urban neighborhoods. *Ethnicity and Disease* 17(4): 657–663.

Participants at the 6th Global Conference on Health Promotion. The Bangkok Charter for health promotion in a globalized world. Geneva: World Health Organization, August 11, 2005.

Pinkhasov, R. M., et al. 2010. Are men shortchanged on health? Perspective on health care utilization and health risk behavior in men and women in the United States. *International Journal of Clinical Practice* 64(4): 475–487.

Song, J., et al. 2006. Gender differences across race/ethnicity in use of health care among Medicare–aged Americans. *Journal of Women's Health* 15(10): 1205–1213.

U.C. Berkeley. 2010 Update. *Evaluating Web Pages: Techniques to Apply and Questions to Ask* (http://www.lib.berkeley.edu/TeachingLib/Guides/Internet/Evaluate.html; retrieved June 26, 2011).

Walker, B., and C. P. Mouton. 2008. Environmental influences on cardiovascular health. *Journal of the National Medical Association* 100(1): 98–102.

World Health Organization. 2011. *Why Gender and Health?* (http://www.who.int/gender/genderandhealth/en; retrieved June 26, 2011).

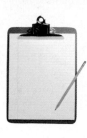

### LAB 1.1  Your Wellness Profile

Consider how your lifestyle, attitudes, and characteristics relate to each of the six dimensions of wellness. Fill in your strengths for each dimension (examples of strengths are listed with each dimension). Once you've completed your lists, choose what you believe are your five most important strengths, and circle them.

**Physical wellness:** To maintain overall physical health and engage in appropriate physical activity (e.g., stamina, strength, flexibility, healthy body composition).

_____

_____

_____

**Emotional wellness:** To have a positive self-concept, deal constructively with your feelings, and develop positive qualities (e.g., optimism, trust, self-confidence, determination).

_____

_____

_____

**Intellectual wellness:** To pursue and retain knowledge, think critically about issues, make sound decisions, identify problems, and find solutions (e.g., common sense, creativity, curiosity).

_____

_____

_____

**Interpersonal/social wellness:** To develop and maintain meaningful relationships with a network of friends and family members, and to contribute to your community (e.g., friendly, good-natured, compassionate, supportive, good listener).

_____

_____

_____

**Spiritual wellness:** To develop a set of beliefs, principles, or values that gives meaning or purpose to your life; to develop faith in something beyond yourself (e.g., religious faith, service to others).

_____

_____

_____

**Environmental wellness:** To protect yourself from environmental hazards and to minimize the negative impact of your behavior on the environment (e.g., carpooling, recycling).

_____

_____

_____

Next, think about where you fall on the wellness continuum for each of the dimensions of wellness. Indicate your placement for each—physical, emotional, intellectual, interpersonal/social, spiritual, and environmental—by placing Xs on the continuum below.

| Low level of wellness | Physical, psychological, emotional symptoms | Change and growth | High level of wellness |

McGraw Hill **connect** http://www.mcgrawhillconnect.com/
**FITNESS AND WELLNESS**

Based on both your current lifestyle and your goals for the future, what do you think your placement on the wellness continuum will be in 10 years? What new health behaviors will you have to adopt to achieve your goals? Which of your current behaviors will you need to change to maintain or improve your level of wellness in the future?

Does the description of wellness given in this chapter encompass everything you believe is part of wellness for you? Write your own definition of wellness, including any additional dimensions that are important to you. Then rate your level of wellness based on your own definition.

## Using Your Results

*How did you score?* Are you satisfied with your current level of wellness—overall and in each dimension? In which dimension(s) would you most like to increase your level of wellness?

*What should you do next?* As you consider possible target behaviors for a behavior change program, choose things that will maintain or increase your level of wellness in one of the dimensions you listed as an area of concern. Remember to consider health behaviors such as smoking or eating a high-fat diet that may threaten your level of wellness in the future. Below, list several possible target behaviors and the wellness dimensions that they influence.

For additional guidance in choosing a target behavior, complete the lifestyle self-assessment in Lab 1.2.

# CHAPTER 2

# Principles of Physical Fitness

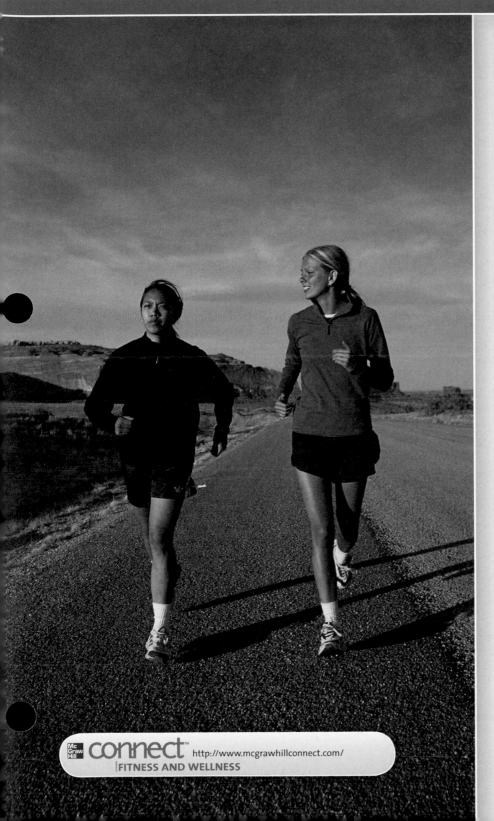

## LOOKING AHEAD...

After reading this chapter, you should be able to:

- Describe how much physical activity is recommended for developing health and fitness
- Identify the components of physical fitness and the way each component affects wellness
- Explain the goal of physical training and the basic principles of training
- Describe the principles involved in designing a well-rounded exercise program
- List the steps that can be taken to make an exercise program safe, effective, and successful

## TEST YOUR KNOWLEDGE

1. To improve your health, you must exercise vigorously for at least 30 minutes straight, 5 or more days per week. True or false?

2. Which of the following activities uses about 150 calories?
   a. washing a car for 45–60 minutes
   b. shooting a basketball for 30 minutes
   c. jumping rope for 15 minutes

3. Regular exercise can make a person smarter. True or false?

### Answers

1. **False.** Experts recommend 150 minutes of moderate-intensity physical activity per week, but activity can be done in short bouts—10-minute sessions, for example—spread out over the course of the day.

2. **All three.** The more intense an activity is, the more calories it burns in a given amount of time. This is one reason that people who exercise vigorously can get the same benefits in less time than people who exercise longer at a moderate intensity.

3. **True.** Regular exercise (even moderate-intensity exercise) benefits the human brain and nervous system in a variety of ways. For example, exercise improves cognitive function—that is, the brain's ability to learn, remember, think, and reason.

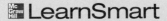

Any list of the benefits of physical activity is impressive. Although people vary greatly in physical fitness and performance ability, the benefits of regular physical activity are available to everyone.

This chapter provides an overview of physical fitness. It explains how both lifestyle physical activity and more formal exercise programs contribute to wellness. It also describes the components of fitness, the basic principles of physical training, and the essential elements of a well-rounded exercise program. Chapters 3–6 provide an in-depth look at each of the elements of a fitness program; Chapter 7 puts these elements together in a complete, personalized program.

## PHYSICAL ACTIVITY AND EXERCISE FOR HEALTH AND FITNESS

Despite the many benefits of an active lifestyle, levels of physical activity remain low for all populations of Americans (Figure 2.1). However, there is some good news. In August 2010, the Centers for Disease Control and Prevention (CDC) reported the following statistics about the physical activity levels of adult Americans:

• About 33% participate in some leisure-time physical activity, 35% engage in leisure-time physical activity on a regular basis, and 28% participate in vigorous leisure-time physical activity lasting at least 10 minutes three or more times per week.

• The percentage of people reporting no leisure-time physical activity decreased by nearly 6% between 1988 and 2009. Physical activity levels decline with age; are higher in men than in women; and are lower in Hispanics, American Indians, and blacks than in whites. Approximately 25% of Americans participate in no leisure-time physical activity—a level that has remained steady for a decade.

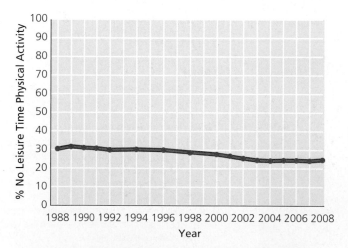

**FIGURE 2.1  Percentage of adult Americans reporting no leisure-time physical activity.**

**SOURCE:** Centers for Disease Control and Prevention. 2010. *Physical Activity Statistics* (http://www.cdc.gov/nccdphp/dnpa/physical/stats/leisure_time.htm; retrieved June 26, 2011).

• People with higher levels of education exercise vigorously more often than people with less education. For example, 78% of high school dropouts never exercise vigorously, compared with 39% of college graduates.

• People living in large urban areas are less active than those living in smaller communities, and those living in the South and Northeast were less active than people living in other areas of the country.

Possible barriers to increased activity include lack of time and resources, social and environmental influences, and—most important—lack of motivation and commitment (see Lab 2.2 for more on barriers). Some people also fear injury. Although physical activity carries some risks, the risks from inactivity are far greater. Increased physical activity may be the single most important lifestyle behavior for promoting health and well-being.

## Physical Activity on a Continuum

**Physical activity** is movement carried out by the skeletal muscles that requires energy. Different types of physical activity can vary by ease or intensity. Standing up or walking down a hallway require little energy or effort. More intense, sustained activities, such as cycling five miles or running in a race, require considerably more.

**Exercise** refers to planned, structured, repetitive movement intended specifically to improve or maintain physical fitness. As discussed in Chapter 1, physical fitness is a set of physical attributes that allows the body to respond or adapt to the demands and stress of physical effort—to perform moderate to vigorous levels of physical activity without becoming overly tired. Levels of fitness depend on such physiological factors as the heart's ability to pump blood and the energy-generating capacity of the cells. These factors depend on genetics—a person's inborn potential for physical fitness—and behavior—getting enough physical activity to stress the body and cause long-term physiological changes.

Physical activity is essential to health and confers wide-ranging health benefits, but exercise is necessary to significantly improve physical fitness. This important distinction between physical activity, which improves health and wellness, and exercise, which improves fitness, is a key concept in understanding the guidelines discussed in this section.

**Increasing Physical Activity to Improve Health and Wellness**  In 2010, the U.S. Surgeon General issued *The Surgeon General's Vision for a Healthy and Fit Nation*, following up the U.S. Department of Health and Human Services' landmark 2008 report, titled *Physical Activity Guidelines for Americans,* which made specific recommendations for promoting exercise and health. (You can read these reports at www.surgeongeneral.gov/library /obesityvision/obesityvision2010.pdf and www.health .gov/paguidelines.) Also, in 2011 the ACSM released its

# Is Exercise Good for Your Brain?

Some scientists are now calling exercise the new "brain food." A variety of studies show that even moderate physical activity can improve brain health and function and may delay the decline in cognitive function that occurs for many people as they age. Recent evidence shows that regular physical activity has the following positive effects on the brain:

- Exercise improves cognitive function—the brain's ability to learn, remember, think, and reason.

- Exercise can help overcome the negative effects of a poor diet on brain health.

- Exercise promotes the creation of new nerve cells (neurons) throughout the nervous system. By promoting this process (called *neurogenesis*), exercise provides protection against injury and degenerative conditions that destroy neurons.

- Exercise enhances the nervous system's *plasticity*—its ability to change and adapt. In the brain, spinal cord, and nerves, this can mean developing new pathways for transmitting sen-

- Exercise appears to have a protective effect on the brain as people age, helping to delay or even prevent the onset of neurodegenerative disorders such as Alzheimer's disease.

Although most people consider brain health to be a concern for the elderly, it is vital to wellness throughout life. For this reason, many studies on exercise and brain health include children as well as older adults. Targeted research has also focused on the impact of exercise on people with disorders such as cerebral palsy, multiple sclerosis, and developmental disabilities. Generally speaking, these studies all reach a similar conclusion: Exercise enhances brain health, at least to some degree, in people of all ages and a wide range of health statuses.

Along with the brain's physical health, mental health is enhanced by exercise. Even modest activity, such as taking a daily

Association, 5.3 million Americans currently suffer from Alzheimer's disease, and the number is increasing at a rate of 70 people per second. People with depression, anxiety, or other mental disorders are more likely to suffer from chronic physical conditions. Taken together, these and other brain-related disorders cost untold millions of dollars in health care costs and lost productivity, as well as thousands of years of productive lifetime lost.

So, for the sake of your brain—as well as your muscles, bones, and heart, start creating your exercise program soon. You'll be healthier, and you may even feel a little smarter.

SOURCES: Garber, C. E., et al. 2011. Quantity and quality of exercise for developing and maintaining cardiorespiratory, musculoskeletal, and neuromotor fitness in apparently healthy adults: guidance for prescribing exercise. *Medicine and Science in Sports and Exercise* 43(7): 1334–1359; Physical Activity Guidelines Advisory Committee. 2008. *Physical Activity Guidelines Advisory Committee Report, 2008.* Washington, D.C.: U.S. Department of Health and Human Services; Stranahan, A. M., and M. P. Mattson. 2011. Bidirectional metabolic regulation of neurocognitive function. *Neurobiology of Learning and Memory* January (epub); Ploughman, M. 2008. Exercise is brain food: The effects of physical activity on cognitive function. *Developmental Neuro-rehabilitation* 11(3): 236–240; van Praag, H. 2009. Exercise and the brain:

mendations from the Surgeon General (2007) the Department of Health and Human Services (2005 and 2008), and the American College of Sports Medicine and American Heart Association (2007). *Physical Activity Guidelines for Americans* and the Surgeon General's

**physical activity** ... muscles that requires energy.

**exercise** Planned, structured, repetitive movement intended to improve or maintain physical fitness.

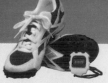

## To Work Out. . . Or Not to Work Out?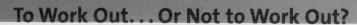

What reasons do you have for not exercising—or not exercising more? Forget about superficial excuses such as "I couldn't run today because a SpongeBob marathon was on." Focus on *real* reasons that consistently interfere with your ability to be physically active. List the top three reasons, in order of significance:

Reason #1: _____

Reason #2: _____

Reason #3: _____

Now, focus on a real solution to each of the three problems. What can you do to prevent these issues from interfering with your ability to exercise in the future? Don't worry about one-time solutions; think about real, permanent solutions that will make these reasons for not exercising go away. List the solutions in the same order as the reasons you listed above:

Solution #1: _____

Solution #2: _____

Solution #3: _____

Think of this as more than just a list. Think of it as a commitment to resolve issues that keep you from meeting your fitness goals. That's the challenging part: Apply your solutions and stay active!

vigorous-intensity aerobic activity. Activity should preferably be spread throughout the week.

- For additional and more extensive health benefits, adults should increase their aerobic physical activity to 300 minutes (5 hours) a week of moderate-intensity activity, or 150 minutes a week of vigorous-intensity activity, or an equivalent combination of moderate- and vigorous-intensity activity. Adults can enjoy additional health benefits by engaging in physical activity beyond this amount.

- Adults should also do muscle-strengthening activities that are moderate or high intensity and involve all major muscle groups on two or more days a week, as these activities provide additional health benefits.

- Everyone should avoid inactivity. Adults, teenagers, and children should spend less time in front of a television or computer screen because it decreases metabolic health and contributes to a sedentary lifestyle and increases the risk of obesity.

The reports state that physical activity benefits people of all ages and of all racial and ethnic groups, including people with disabilities. The reports emphasize that the benefits of activity outweigh the dangers.

These levels of physical activity promote health and wellness by lowering the risk of high blood pressure, stroke, heart disease, type 2 diabetes, colon cancer, and osteoporosis and by reducing feelings of mild to moderate depression and anxiety.

What exactly is moderate physical activity? Activities such as brisk walking, dancing, swimming, cycling, and yard work can all count toward the daily total. A moderate amount of activity uses about 150 calories of energy and causes a noticeable increase in heart rate, such as would occur with a brisk walk. Examples of activities that use about 150 calories are shown in Figure 2.2. You

| Common Activities | Duration (min.) | |
|---|---|---|
| Washing and waxing a car | 45–60 | *Less Vigorous, More Time* |
| Washing windows or floors | 45–60 | |
| Gardening | 30–45 | |
| Wheeling self in wheelchair | 30–40 | |
| Pushing a stroller 1½ miles | 30 | |
| Raking leaves | 30 | |
| Walking 2 miles | 30 (15 min/mile) | |
| Shoveling snow | 15 | |
| Stairwalking | 15 | |
| **Sporting Activities** | | |
| Playing volleyball | 45–60 | |
| Playing touch football | 45 . | |
| Walking 1¾ miles | 35 (20 min/mile) | |
| Basketball (shooting baskets) | 30 | |
| Bicycling 5 miles | 30 | |
| Dancing fast (social) | 30 | |
| Water aerobics | 30 | |
| Swimming laps | 20 | |
| Basketball (playing game) | 15–20 | |
| Bicycling 4 miles | 15 | |
| Jumping rope | 15 | |
| Running 1½ miles | 15 (10 min/mile) | *More Vigorous, Less Time* |

**FIGURE 2.2 Examples of moderate-intensity physical activity.**
Each example uses about 150 calories.
**SOURCE:** National Heart, Lung, and Blood Institute. 2010. *Why Is Exercise Important?* (www.nhlbi.nih.gov/health/public/heart/obesity/lose_wt/physical .htm; retrieved June 26, 2011).

# Classifying Activity Levels

Assessing your physical activity level is easier if you know how to classify different kinds of activities. Fitness experts categorize activities into the following three levels:

- *Light activity* includes the routine tasks associated with typical day-to-day life, such as vacuuming, walking slowly, shopping, or stretching. You probably perform dozens of light activities every day without even thinking about it. You can gain significant health benefits by turning light activities into moderate activities—by walking briskly instead of slowly, for example.

- *Moderate activity*, such as walking at 3–4 miles per hour, causes your breathing and heart rate to accelerate but still allows for comfortable conversation. It is sometimes described as activity that can be performed comfortably for about 45 minutes. Examples of moderate physical activity include brisk walking, social dancing, and cycling moderately on level terrain.

- *Vigorous activity* elevates your heart and breathing rates considerably and has other physical effects that improve your fitness level. Examples include jogging, hiking uphill, swimming laps, and playing most competitive sports.

can burn the same number of calories by doing a lower-intensity activity for a longer time or a higher-intensity activity for a shorter time. College-age people are more likely to participate in physical activities they enjoy, such

The daily total of physical activity can be accumulated in multiple bouts of 10 or more minutes per day—for example, two 10-minute bike rides to and from class and

In contrast to moderate-intensity activity, vigorous physical activity causes rapid breathing and a substantial increase in heart rate, as exemplified by jogging. Physical activity and exercise recommendations for promoting general health, fitness, and weight management are shown in Table 2.1. Examples of light, moderate, and vigorous activities are given in the box "Classifying Activity Levels."

**Fitness Tip**

To make your workouts more effective, find an exercise buddy. You can help each other set goals, stay on track, keep time, and count reps. Exercising with a friend makes working out more enjoyable, too.

| Table 2.1 | Physical Activity and Exercise Recommendations for Promoting General Health, Fitness, and Weight Management |
|---|---|

sources: Garber, C. E., et al. 2011. Quantity and quality of exercise for developing and maintaining cardiorespiratory, musculoskeletal, and neuromotor fitness in apparently health adults: Guidance for prescribing exercise. *Medicine and Science in Sports and Exercise* 43(7): 1334–1359; Physical Activity Guidelines Advisory Committee. 2008. *Physical Activity Guidelines Advisory Committee Report, 2008.* Washington, D.C.: U.S. Department of Health and Human Services; U.S. Department of Health and Human Services. 2010. *The Surgeon General's Vision for a Healthy and Fit Nation.* Rockville, Md: U.S. Department of Health and Human Services, Office of the Surgeon General.

a brisk 10-minute walk to the store. In this lifestyle approach to physical activity, people can choose activities that they find enjoyable and that fit into their daily routine; everyday tasks at school, work, and home can be structured to contribute to the daily activity total. If all Americans who are currently sedentary were to increase their lifestyle physical activity to 30 minutes per day, there would be an enormous benefit to public health and to individual well-being.

### Increasing Physical Activity to Manage Weight

Because two-thirds of Americans are overweight, the U.S. Department of Health and Human Services has also published physical activity guidelines focusing on weight management. These guidelines recognize that for people who need to prevent weight gain, lose weight, or maintain weight loss, 150 minutes per week of physical activity may not be enough. Instead, they recommend up to 90 minutes of physical activity per day.

### Exercising to Improve Physical Fitness
As mentioned earlier, moderate physical activity confers significant health and wellness benefits, especially for those who are currently sedentary and become moderately active. However, people can obtain even greater health and wellness benefits by increasing the duration and intensity of physical activity. With increased activity, they will see more improvements in quality of life and greater reductions in disease and mortality risk.

More vigorous activity, as in a structured, systematic exercise program, is also needed to improve physical fitness; moderate physical activity alone is not enough. Physical fitness requires more intense movement that poses a substantially greater challenge to the body. The American College of Sports Medicine issued guidelines in 2006 and again in 2011 for creating a formal exercise program that will develop physical fitness. These guidelines are described in detail later in the chapter.

## How Much Physical Activity Is Enough?

Some experts feel that people get most of the health benefits of physical activity simply by becoming more active over the course of the day; the amount of activity needed depends on an individual's health status and goals. Other experts feel that leisure-time physical activity is not enough; they argue that people should exercise long enough and intensely enough to improve the body's capacity for exercise—that is, to improve physical fitness. There is probably some truth in both of these positions.

Regular physical activity, regardless of the intensity, makes you healthier and can help protect you from many chronic diseases. Although you get many of the health benefits of exercise simply by being more active, you obtain even more benefits when you are physically fit. In addition to long-term health benefits, fitness also contributes significantly to quality of life. Fitness can give you

freedom to move your body the way you want. Fit people have more energy and better body control. They can enjoy a more active lifestyle than their more sedentary counterparts. Even if you don't like sports, you need physical energy and stamina in your daily life and for many nonsport leisure activities such as visiting museums, playing with children, gardening, and so on.

Where does this leave you? Most experts agree that some physical activity is better than none, but that more—as long as it does not result in injury—is better than some. To set a personal goal for physical activity and exercise, consider your current activity level, your health status, and your overall goals. At the very least, strive to become more active and do 30 minutes of moderate-intensity activity at least 5 days per week. Choose to be active whenever you can. If weight management is a concern for you, begin by achieving the goal of 30 minutes of activity per day and then try to raise your activity level further, to 60–90 minutes per day or more. For even better health and well-being, participate in a structured exercise program that develops physical fitness. Any increase in physical activity will contribute to your health and well-being, now and in the future.

## HEALTH-RELATED COMPONENTS OF PHYSICAL FITNESS

Some components of fitness are related to specific activities, and others relate to general health. **Health-related fitness** includes the following components:

- Cardiorespiratory endurance
- Muscular strength

## Fitness Tip

Very few activities build all the health-related components of fitness at the same time. This is why variety is important. Create a routine that lets you build one or two fitness components every day. Variety also keeps your workouts enjoyable.

- Muscular endurance
- Flexibility
- Body composition

Health-related fitness helps you withstand physical challenges and protects you from diseases.

## Cardiorespiratory Endurance

**Cardiorespiratory endurance** is the ability to perform

ability of the lungs to deliver oxygen from the environment to the bloodstream, the capacity of the heart to pump blood, the ability of the nervous system and blood vessels to regulate blood flow, and the capability of the cells' chemical systems to use oxygen and process fuels for exercise.

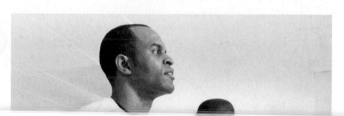

When cardiorespiratory fitness is low, the heart has to work hard during normal daily activities and may not be able to work hard enough to sustain high-intensity physical activity in an emergency. As cardiorespiratory fitness improves, related physical functions also improve. For example:

- The heart pumps more blood per heartbeat.
- Resting heart rate slows.
- Blood volume increases.
- Blood supply to tissues improves.
- The body can cool itself better.
- Resting blood pressure decreases.
- Metabolism in skeletal muscle is enhanced, which improves fuel use.
- Resistance and aerobic training increases the level of antioxidant chemicals in the body and lowers oxidative stress.

A healthy heart can better withstand the strains of everyday life, the stress of occasional emergencies, and

Endurance training the body's chemical systems, particularly in the muscles and liver. These changes enhance the body's ability to derive energy from food, allow the body to perform more exercise with less effort, increase sensitivity to insulin, and prevent type 2 diabetes.

Cardiorespiratory endurance is a central component of health-related fitness because heart and lung function is so essential to overall good health. A person can't live very long or very well without a healthy heart. Poor cardiorespiratory fitness is linked with heart disease, type 2 diabetes, colon cancer, stroke, depression, and anxiety. A moderate level of cardiorespiratory fitness can help com-

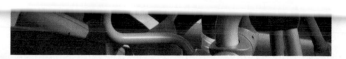

Cardiorespiratory endurance is a key component of health-related fitness.

**cardiorespiratory endurance** The ability of the body to perform prolonged, large-muscle, dynamic exercise at moderate to high levels of intensity.

**muscular strength** The amount of force a muscle can produce with a single maximum effort.

such factors as the size of muscle cells and the ability of nerves to activate muscle cells. Strong muscles are important for everyday activities, such as climbing stairs, as well as for emergency situations. They help keep the skeleton in proper alignment, preventing back and leg pain and providing the support necessary for good posture. Muscular strength has obvious importance in recreational activities. Strong people can hit a tennis ball harder, kick a soccer ball farther, and ride a bicycle uphill more easily.

Muscle tissue is an important element of overall body composition. Greater muscle mass means a higher rate of **metabolism** and faster energy use. Greater muscle mass reduces markers of oxidative stress and maintains mitochondria (the "powerhouses" of the cell), both of which are important for metabolic health and longevity. Training to build muscular strength can also help people manage stress and boost their self-confidence.

Maintaining strength and muscle mass is vital for healthy aging. Older people tend to experience a decrease in both number and size of muscle cells, a condition called *sarcopenia*. Many of the remaining muscle cells become slower, and some become nonfunctional because they lose their attachment to the nervous system. Strength training (also known as *resistance training* or *weight training*) increases antioxidant enzymes and lowers oxidative stress. It also helps maintain muscle mass and function and possibly helps decrease the risk of osteoporosis (bone loss) in older people, which greatly enhances their quality of life and prevents life-threatening injuries.

## Muscular Endurance

**Muscular endurance** is the ability to resist fatigue and sustain a given level of muscle tension—that is, to hold a muscle contraction for a long time or to contract a muscle over and over again. It depends on such factors as the size of muscle cells, the ability of muscles to store fuel, and the blood supply to muscles.

Muscular endurance is important for good posture and for injury prevention. For example, if abdominal and back muscles cannot support the spine correctly when sitting or standing for long periods, the chances of low-back pain and back injury are increased. Good muscular endurance in the trunk muscles is more important than muscular strength for preventing back pain. Muscular endurance helps people cope with daily physical demands and enhances performance in sports and work.

## Flexibility

**Flexibility** is the ability to move the joints through their full range of motion. It depends on joint structure, the length and elasticity of connective tissue, and nervous system activity. Flexible, pain-free joints are important for good health and well-being. Inactivity causes the joints to become stiffer with age. Stiffness, in turn, often causes

people to assume unnatural body postures that can stress joints and muscles. Stretching exercises can help ensure a healthy range of motion for all major joints.

## Body Composition

**Body composition** refers to the proportion of fat and **fat-free mass** (muscle, bone, and water) in the body. Healthy body composition involves a high proportion of fat-free mass and an acceptably low level of body fat, adjusted for age and gender. A person with excessive body fat—especially excess fat in the abdomen—is more likely to experience health problems, including heart disease, insulin resistance, high blood pressure, stroke, joint problems, type 2 diabetes, gallbladder disease, blood vessel inflammation, some types of cancer, back pain, and premature death.

The best way to lose fat is through a lifestyle that includes a sensible diet and exercise. The best way to add muscle mass is through strength training. Large changes in body composition are not necessary to improve health; even a small increase in physical activity and a small decrease in body fat can lead to substantial health improvements.

## Skill (Neuromuscular)-Related Components of Fitness

In addition to the five health-related components of physical fitness, the ability to perform a particular sport or activity may depend on **skill (neuromuscular)-related fitness** components such as the following:

- *Speed*—the ability to perform a movement in a short period of time
- *Power*—the ability to exert force rapidly, based on a combination of strength and speed
- *Agility*—the ability to change the position of the body quickly and accurately
- *Balance*—the ability to maintain equilibrium while moving or while stationary
- *Coordination*—the ability to perform motor tasks accurately and smoothly using body movements and the senses
- *Reaction and movement time*—the ability to respond and react quickly to a stimulus

Skill-related fitness tends to be sport-specific and is best developed through practice. For example, the speed, coordination, and agility needed to play basketball can be developed by playing basketball. These activities are particularly important for older adults for preventing life-threatening falls. Participating in sports is fun, can help you build fitness, and contributes to other areas of wellness. Young adults often find it easier to exercise regularly when they participate in sports and activities they enjoy, such as dancing, tennis, snowboarding, or basketball.

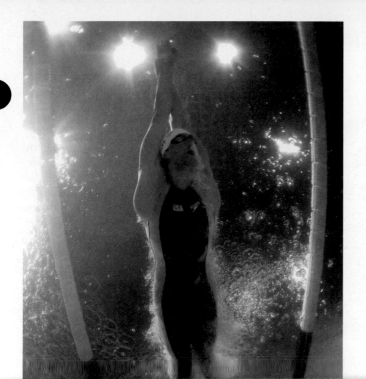

The words "over time" are key to realizing the benefits of physical activity. If you get in the habit of being active, you'll notice the benefits over time. After a few workouts, you'll breathe with less effort and recover faster, feel stronger and more flexible. In a few weeks your clothes will fit differently, and you'll notice changes in the mirror. Practice patience and watch the rewards pile up!

heart rate increase during exercise, for example, the heart gradually develops the ability to pump more blood with each beat. Then, during exercise, it doesn't have to beat as fast to meet the cells' demands for oxygen. The goal of **physical training** is to produce these long-term changes and improvements in the body's functioning. Although people differ in the maximum levels of physical fitness and performance they can achieve through training, the wellness benefits of exercise are available to everyone (see the box "Fitness and Disability").

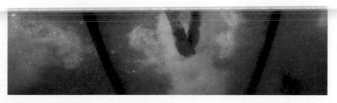

Elite athletes demonstrate sport-specific skills such as speed, power, agility, coordination, and reaction time.

Older adults can develop balance by practicing exercises such as yoga and tai chi.

...lective in developing the various components of fitness. To put together an effective exercise program, you should first understand the basic principles of physical training, including the following:

- Specificity
- Progressive overload
- Reversibility
- Individual differences

All of these rest on the larger principle of adaptation.

or two of the five components of health-related fitness, such as muscular strength or body composition? If so, where do you think your ideas come from? What role do the media play in shaping your ideas about fitness?

and gait.

**physical training** The performance of different types of activities that cause the body to adapt and improve its level of fitness.

**DIMENSIONS OF DIVERSITY**

Physical fitness and athletic achievement are not limited to the able-bodied. People with disabilities can also attain high levels of fitness and performance, as shown by the elite athletes who compete in the Paralympics. The premier event for athletes with disabilities, the Paralympics are held in the same year and city as the Olympics. The performance of these skilled athletes makes it clear that people with disabilities can be active, healthy, and extraordinarily fit. Just like able-bodied athletes, athletes with disabilities strive for excellence and can serve as role models.

According to the U.S. Census Bureau, about 54 million Americans have some type of chronic disability. Some disabilities are the result of injury, such as spinal cord injuries sustained in car crashes or war. Other disabilities result from illness, such as the blindness that sometimes occurs as a complication of diabetes or the joint stiffness that accompanies arthritis. And some disabilities are present at birth, as in the case of congenital limb deformities or cerebral palsy.

Exercise and physical activity are as important for people with disabilities as for able-bodied individuals—if not *more* important. Being active helps prevent secondary conditions that may

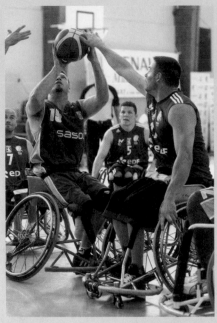

result from prolonged inactivity, such as circulatory or muscular problems. Currently, about 19% of people with disabilities engage in regular moderate-intensity activity.

People with disabilities don't have to be elite athletes to participate in sports and lead an active life. Some health clubs, fitness centers, city recreation centers, and universities offer activities

and events geared for people of all ages and types of disabilities. They may have modified aerobics classes, special weight training machines, classes involving mild exercise in warm water, and other activities adapted for people with disabilities. Popular sports and recreational activities include adapted horseback riding, golf, swimming, and skiing. Competitive sports are also available—for example, there are wheelchair versions of billiards, tennis, weight lifting, hockey, and basketball, as well as sports for people with hearing, visual, or mental impairments. For those who prefer to get their exercise at home, special videos are available geared to individuals who use wheelchairs or who have arthritis, hearing impairments, metabolic diseases, or many other disabilities.

If you have a disability and want to be more active, check with your physician about what's appropriate for you. Call your local community center, university, YMCA/YWCA, hospital, independent living center, or fitness center to locate facilities. Look for a facility with experienced personnel and appropriate adaptive equipment. For specialized videos, check with hospitals and health associations that are geared to specific disabilities, such as the Arthritis Foundation.

## Specificity—Adapting to Type of Training

To develop a particular fitness component, you must perform exercises designed specifically for that component. This is the principle of **specificity**. Weight training, for example, develops muscular strength but is less effective for developing cardiorespiratory endurance or flexibility. Specificity also applies to the skill-related fitness components (to improve at tennis, you must practice tennis) and to the different parts of the body (to develop stronger arms, you must exercise your arms). A well-rounded exercise program includes exercises geared to each component of fitness, to different parts of the body, and to specific activities or sports.

## Progressive Overload—Adapting to the Amount of Training and the FITT Principle

The body adapts to the demands of exercise by improving its functioning. When the amount of exercise (also called

*overload* or *stress* ) is increased progressively, fitness continues to improve. This is the principle of **progressive overload**.

The amount of overload is important. Too little exercise will have no effect on fitness (although it may improve health); too much may cause injury and problems with the body's immune or endocrine (hormone) systems. The point at which exercise becomes excessive is highly individual; it occurs at a much higher level in an Olympic athlete than in a sedentary person. For every type of exercise, there is a training threshold at which fitness benefits begin to occur, a zone within which maximum fitness benefits occur, and an upper limit of safe training.

The amount of exercise needed depends on the individual's current level of fitness, the person's genetically determined capacity to adapt to training, his or her fitness goals, and the component being developed. A novice, for example, might experience fitness benefits from jogging a mile in 10 minutes, but this level of exercise would cause no physical adaptations in a trained distance runner. Beginners should start at the lower end of the fitness benefit zone; fitter individuals will make more rapid gains by exercising at the higher end of the fitness benefit zone. Progression is critical because fitness increases only if the volume and intensity of workouts increase. Exercising at the same intensity every training session will maintain fitness but will not increase it, because the training stress is below the threshold required to produce adaptation.

The amount of overload needed to maintain or improve a particular level of fitness for a particular fitness component is determined through four dimensions, represented by the acronym FITT:

- *Frequency*—how often
- *Intensity*—how hard
- *Time*—how long (duration)
- *Type*—mode of activity

Chapters 3, 4, and 5 show you how to apply the FITT principle to exercise programs for cardiorespiratory endurance, muscular strength and endurance, and flexibility, respectively.

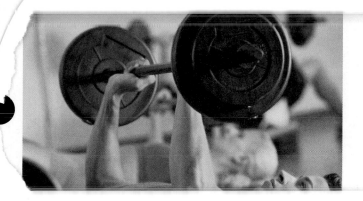

**Frequency** Developing fitness requires regular exercise. Optimum exercise frequency, expressed in number of days per week, varies with the component being developed and the individual's fitness goals. For most people, a frequency of 3–5 days per week for cardiorespiratory endurance exercise and 2 or more days per week for resistance and flexibility training is appropriate for a general fitness program.

An important consideration in determining appropriate exercise frequency is recovery time, which is also highly individual and depends on factors such as training experience, age, and intensity of training. For example, 24 hours of rest between highly intense workouts involving heavy weights or track sprints is not enough recovery time for safe and effective training. Intense workouts need to be spaced out during the week to allow for sufficient recovery time. On the other hand, you can exercise every day if your program consists of moderate-intensity walking or cycling. Learn to "listen to your body" to get enough rest between workouts. Chapters 3–5 provide more detailed information about training techniques and recovery periods for workouts focused on different

**Intensity** Fitness benefits occur when a person exercises harder than his or her normal level of activity. The appropriate exercise intensity varies with each fitness component. To develop cardiorespiratory endurance, for example, you must raise your heart rate above normal. To develop muscular strength, you must lift a heavier weight than normal. To develop flexibility, you must stretch muscles beyond their normal length.

**Time (Duration)** Fitness benefits occur when you exercise for an extended period of time. For cardiorespiratory

Progressive overload is important because fitness increases only when the volume and intensity of exercise increase. The body adapts to overload by becoming more fit.

particular type and amount of stress placed on it.

**progressive overload** The training principle that placing increasing amounts of stress on the body causes adaptations that improve fitness.

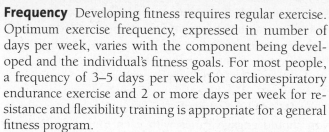

specific number of repetitions of particular exercises. For resistance training, for example, a recommended program includes one or more sets of 8–12 repetitions of 8–10 different exercises that work the major muscle groups. Older adults should do 10–15 repetitions per set.

**Type (Mode of Activity)** The type of exercise in which you should engage varies with each fitness component and with your personal fitness goals. To develop cardiorespiratory endurance, you need to engage in continuous activities involving large-muscle groups—walking, jogging, cycling, or swimming, for example. Resistance exercises develop muscular strength and endurance, while stretching exercises build flexibility. The frequency, intensity, and time of the exercise will be different for each type of activity. (See pp. 41–44 for more on choosing appropriate activities for your fitness program.)

## Reversibility—Adapting to a Reduction in Training

Fitness is a reversible adaptation. The body adjusts to lower levels of physical activity the same way it adjusts to higher levels. This is the principle of **reversibility**. When a person stops exercising, up to 50% of fitness improvements are lost within 2 months. However, not all fitness levels reverse at the same rate. Strength fitness is very resilient, so a person can maintain strength fitness by doing resistance exercise as infrequently as once a week. On the other hand, cardiovascular and cellular fitness reverse themselves more quickly—sometimes within just a few days or weeks. If you must temporarily curtail your training, you can maintain your fitness improvements by keeping the intensity of your workouts constant while reducing their frequency or duration.

## Individual Differences—Limits on Adaptability

Anyone watching the Olympics can see that, from a physical standpoint, we are not all created equal. There are large individual differences in our ability to improve fitness, achieve a desirable body composition, and learn and perform sports skills. Some people are able to run longer distances, or lift more weight, or kick a soccer ball more skillfully than others will ever be able to, no matter how much they train. People respond to training at different rates, so a program that works for one person may not be right for another person.

There are limits on the adaptability—the potential for improvement—of any human body. The body's ability to transport and use oxygen, for example, can be improved by only about 5–30% through training. An endurance athlete must therefore inherit a large metabolic capacity in order to reach competitive performance levels. In the past few years, scientists have identified specific genes

*Fitness Tip*

At the gym, it can be intimidating to find yourself surrounded by people who seem to be in better shape than you are. But remember: They got in shape by focusing on themselves, not by worrying about what other people thought about them. You can avoid feeling intimidated by doing the same thing. Focus on *you*, and let others worry about themselves.

## Ask Yourself

**QUESTIONS FOR CRITICAL THINKING AND REFLECTION**

Many people who play sports have had the experience of realizing that they are not as physically gifted as a teammate or that they are never going to be in the Olympics. What can you say to encourage someone who is discouraged by this realization? What benefits of physical activity, exercise, and sports might you point out?

that influence body fat, strength, and endurance. For example, they have identified more than 800 genes associated with endurance performance, and 100 of those determine individual differences in exercise capacity. However, physical training improves fitness regardless of heredity. For the average person, the body's adaptability is enough to achieve reasonable fitness goals.

## DESIGNING YOUR OWN EXERCISE PROGRAM

Physical training works best when you have a plan. A plan helps you make gradual but steady progress toward your goals. Once you've determined that exercise is safe for you, planning for physical fitness consists of assessing how fit you are now, determining where you want to be, and choosing the right activities to help you get there.

## Getting Medical Clearance

People of any age who are not at high risk for serious health problems can safely exercise at a moderate intensity (60% or less of maximum heart rate) without a prior medical evaluation (see Chapter 3 for a discussion of maximum heart rate). Likewise, if you are male and under 40 or female and under 50 and in good health, exercise is probably safe for you. If you do not fit into these age groups, or if you have health problems—especially high blood pressure, heart disease, muscle or joint problems,

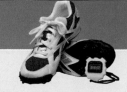

# Are You Healthy Enough for Exercise?

Heart disease and diabetes aren't the only reasons to get a doctor's approval before starting an exercise program. If you are severely overweight, have a family history of some chronic disease, or have just never exercised before, it could be advisable to talk to your doctor before becoming physically active.

Think about your current health status and your family history. If you think of any issues that might interfere with being physically active—or that might make exercise dangerous for you—list them below:

_____

_____

_____

_____

_____

If you write down anything, even *one* thing, make an appointment to see your doctor as soon as possible. Ask your doctor for an overall health evaluation, review your family history, and make sure the doctor knows you want to start being physically active on a regular basis. Then address the specific issues you listed above.

If your physician offers any specific advice, follow it. But if you can be physically active, even with some restrictions, make a commitment and get started on your exercise plan. And see your doctor regularly to make sure physical activity is working for you.

or obesity—see your physician before starting a vigorous exercise program. The Canadian Society for Exercise Physiology has developed the Physical Activity Readiness Questionnaire (PAR-Q) to help evaluate exercise safety; it is included in Lab 2.1. Completing it should alert you to any potential problems you may have. If a physician isn't sure whether exercise is safe for you, she or he may recommend an **exercise stress test** or a **graded exercise test (GXT)** to see whether you show symptoms of heart disease during exercise. For most people, however, it's far safer to exercise than to remain sedentary. For more information, see the box "Exercise and Cardiac Risk."

## Assessing Yourself

The first step in creating a successful fitness program is to assess your current level of physical activity and fitness for each of the five health-related fitness components. The results of the assessment tests will help you set specific fitness goals and plan your fitness program. Lab 2.3 gives you the opportunity to assess your current overall level of activity and determine if it is appropriate. Assessment tests in Chapters 3–6 will help you evaluate your cardiorespiratory endurance, muscular strength, muscular endurance, flexibility, and body composition.

## Setting Goals

The ultimate general goal of every health-related fitness program is the same—wellness that lasts a lifetime.

Whatever your specific goals, they must be important enough to you to keep you motivated. Most sports psychologists believe that setting and achieving goals is the most effective way to stay motivated about exercise. (Refer to Chapter 1 for more on goal setting, as well as Common Questions Answered at the end of this chapter.) After you complete the assessment tests in Chapters 3–6, you will be able to set goals directly related to each fitness component, such as working toward a 3-mile jog or doing 20 push-ups. First, though, think carefully about your overall goals, and be clear about why you are starting a program.

## Choosing Activities for a Balanced Program

An ideal fitness program combines a physically active lifestyle with a systematic exercise program to develop and maintain physical fitness. This overall program is

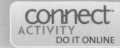

# IN FOCUS

## Exercise and Cardiac Risk

Participating in exercise and sports is usually a wonderful experience that improves wellness in both the short and long term. In rare instances, however, vigorous exertion is associated with sudden death. It may seem difficult to understand that although regular exercise protects people from heart disease, it also increases the risk of sudden death.

Congenital heart defects (heart abnormalities present at birth) are the most common cause of exercise-related sudden death in people under 35. In nearly all other cases, coronary artery disease is responsible. In this condition, fat and other substances build up in the arteries that supply blood to the heart. Death can result if an artery becomes blocked or if the heart's rhythm and pumping action are disrupted. Exercise, particularly intense exercise, may trigger a heart attack in someone with underlying heart disease.

A study of jogging deaths in Rhode Island found that there was one death per 396,000 hours of jogging, or about one death per 7620 joggers per year—an extremely low risk for each individual jogger. Another study of men involved in a variety of physical activities found one death per 1.51 million hours of exercise. This 12-year study of more than 21,000 men found that those who didn't exercise vigorously were 74 times more likely to die suddenly from cardiac arrest during or shortly after exercise. It is also important to note that people are much safer exercising than engaging in many other common activities, including driving a car.

Although quite small, the risk does exist and may lead some people to wonder why exercise is considered such an important part of a wellness lifestyle. Exercise causes many positive changes in the body—in healthy people as well as those with heart disease—that more than make up for the slightly increased short-term risk of sudden death. Training slows or reverses the fatty buildup in arteries, helps protect people from deadly heart rhythm abnormalities, and enhances blood sugar regulation. People who exercise regularly have an overall risk of sudden death only about two-thirds that of nonexercisers. Active people who stop exercising can expect their heart attack risk to increase by 300%.

Obviously, someone with underlying coronary artery disease is at greater risk than someone who is free from the condition. However, many cases of heart disease go undiagnosed. The riskiest scenario may involve the middle-aged or older individual who suddenly begins participating in a vigorous sport or activity after being sedentary for a long time. This finding provides strong evidence for the recommendation that people increase their level of physical activity gradually and engage in regular, rather than sporadic, activity. Fortunately, the risk of heart-related

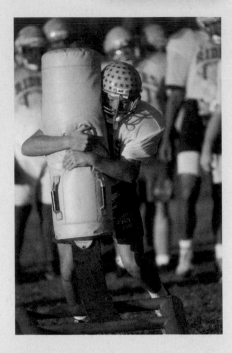

sudden death in middle-aged and older adults is least in people who exercise approximately 150 minutes per week—the activity level recommended by the U.S. Department of Health and Human Services.

SOURCES: Fahey, T. D., and G. D. Swanson. 2008. A model for defining the optimal amount of exercise contributing to health and avoiding sudden cardiac death. *Medicina Sportiva* 12(4): 124–128; Albert, C. M., et al. 2000. Trigger of sudden death from cardiac causes by vigorous exertion. *New England Journal of Medicine* 343(19): 1355–1361.

---

shown in the physical activity pyramid in Figure 2.3. If you are currently sedentary, your goal should be to focus on activities at the bottom of the pyramid and gradually increase the amount of moderate-intensity physical activity in your daily life. Appropriate activities include walking briskly, climbing stairs, doing yard work, and washing your car. You don't have to exercise vigorously, but you should experience a moderate increase in your heart and breathing rates. As described earlier, your activity time can be broken up into small blocks over the course of a day.

The next two levels of the pyramid illustrate parts of a formal exercise program. The principles of this program are consistent with those of the American College of Sports Medicine (ACSM), the professional organization for people involved in sports medicine and exercise

science. The ACSM has established guidelines for creating an exercise program that will develop physical fitness (Table 2.2). A balanced program includes activities to develop all the health-related components of fitness:

- *Cardiorespiratory endurance* is developed by continuous rhythmic movements of large-muscle groups in activities such as walking, jogging, cycling, swimming, and aerobic dance and other forms of group exercise. Choose activities that you enjoy and that are convenient. Other popular choices are in-line skating, dancing, and backpacking. Start-and-stop activities such as tennis, racquetball, and soccer can also develop cardiorespiratory endurance if your skill level is sufficient to enable periods of continuous play. Training for cardiorespiratory endurance is discussed in Chapter 3.

**Sedentary Activities**
*Do infrequently*
Watching television, surfing the Internet, talking on the telephone

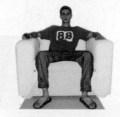

**Strength Training**
*2–3 nonconsecutive days per week (all major muscle groups)*
Bicep curls, push-ups, abdominal curls, bench press, calf raises

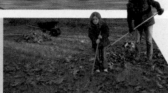

**Flexibility Training**
*At least 2–3 days per week, ideally 5–7 days per week (all major joints)*
Calf stretch, side lunge, step stretch, hurdler stretch

**Cardiorespiratory Endurance Exercise**
*3–5 days per week (20–60 minutes per day)*

Walking, jogging, bicycling, swimming, aerobic dancing, in-line skating, cross-country skiing, dancing, basketball

**Moderate-Intensity Physical Activity**
*150 minutes per week; for weight loss or prevention of weight regain following weight loss, 60–90 minutes per day*

Walking to the store or bank, washing windows or your car, climbing stairs, working in your yard, walking your dog, cleaning your room

**FIGURE 2.3  Physical activity pyramid.**

| Table 2.2 | ACSM Exercise Recommendations for Fitness Development in Healthy Adults |
|---|---|

**EXERCISE TO DEVELOP AND MAINTAIN CARDIORESPIRATORY ENDURANCE AND BODY COMPOSITION**

| | |
|---|---|
| Frequency of training | 3–5 days per week. |
| Intensity of training | 55/65–90% of maximum heart rate or 40/50–85% of heart rate reserve or maximum oxygen uptake reserve.* The lower-intensity values (55–64% of maximum heart rate and 40–49% of heart rate reserve) are most applicable to unfit individuals. For average individuals, intensities of 70–85% of maximum heart rate or 60–80% of heart rate reserve are appropriate. |
| Time (duration) of training | 20–60 total minutes per day of continuous or intermittent (in sessions lasting 10 or more minutes) aerobic activity. Duration depends on the intensity of activity; thus, low-intensity activity should be conducted over a longer period of time (30 minutes or more). Low to moderate-intensity activity of longer duration is recommended for nonathletic adults. |
| Type (mode) of activity | Any activity that uses large-muscle groups, can be maintained continuously, and is rhythmic and aerobic in nature—for example, walking-hiking, running-jogging, bicycling, cross-country skiing, aerobic dancing and other forms of group exercise, rope skipping, rowing, stair climbing, swimming, skating, and endurance game activities. |

**EXERCISE TO DEVELOP AND MAINTAIN MUSCULAR STRENGTH AND ENDURANCE, FLEXIBILITY, AND BODY COMPOSITION**

| | |
|---|---|
| Resistance training | One set of 8–10 exercises that condition the major muscle groups, performed at least 2 days per week. Most people should complete 8–12 repetitions of each exercise to the point of fatigue; practicing other repetition ranges (for example, 3–5 or 12–15) also builds strength and endurance; for older and frailer people (approximately 50–60 and older), 10–15 repetitions with a lighter weight may be more appropriate. Multiple-set regimens will provide greater benefits if time allows. Any mode of exercise that is comfortable throughout the full range of motion is appropriate (for example, free weights, elastic bands, or machines). |
| Flexibility training | Static stretches, performed for the major muscle groups at least 2–3 days per week, ideally 5–7 days per week. Stretch to the point of tightness, holding each stretch for 10–30 seconds; perform 2–4 repetitions of each stretch. |

*Instructions for calculating target heart rate intensity for cardiorespiratory endurance exercise are presented in Chapter 3.

**SOURCE:** Adapted from American College of Sports Medicine. 2009. *ACSM's Guidelines for Exercise Testing and Prescription*, 8th ed. Philadelphia: Lippincott Williams and Wilkins; Garber, C. E., et al. 2011. Quantity and quality of exercise for developing and maintaining cardiorespiratory, musculoskeletal, and neuromotor fitness in apparently healthy adults: guidance for prescribing exercise. *Medicine and Science in Sports and Exercise* 43(7): 1334–1359.

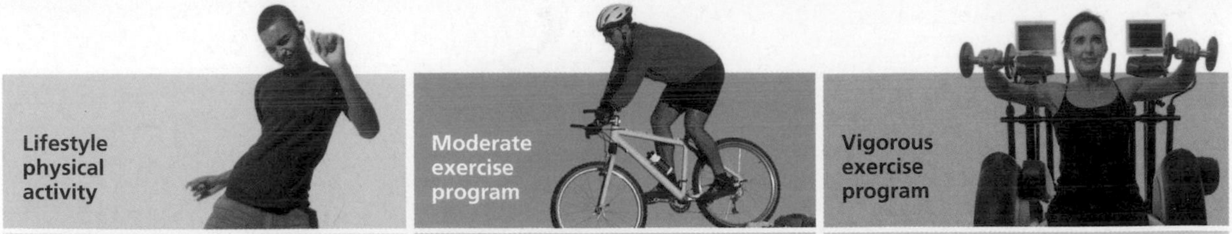

| | Lifestyle physical activity | Moderate exercise program | Vigorous exercise program |
|---|---|---|---|
| **Description** | Moderate physical activity (150 minutes per week; muscle-strengthening exercises 2 or more days per week) | Cardiorespiratory endurance exercise (20–60 minutes, 3–5 days per week); strength training (2–3 nonconsecutive days per week); and stretching exercises (2 or more days per week) | Cardiorespiratory endurance exercise (20–60 minutes, 3–5 days per week); interval training; strength training (3–4 nonconsecutive days per week); and stretching exercises (5–7 days per week) |
| **Sample activities or program** | • Walking to and from work, 15 minutes each way <br> • Cycling to and from class, 10 minutes each way <br> • Doing yard work for 30 minutes <br> • Dancing (fast) for 30 minutes <br> • Playing basketball for 20 minutes <br> • Muscle exercises such as push-ups, squats, or back exercises | • Jogging for 30 minutes, 3 days per week <br> • Weight training, 1 set of 8 exercises, 2 days per week <br> • Stretching exercises, 3 days per week | • Running for 45 minutes, 3 days per week <br> • Intervals, running 400 m at high effort, 4 sets, 2 days per week <br> • Weight training, 3 sets of 10 exercises, 3 days per week <br> • Stretching exercises, 6 days per week |
| **Health and fitness benefits** | Better blood cholesterol levels, reduced body fat, better control of blood pressure, improved metabolic health, and enhanced glucose metabolism; improved quality of life; reduced risk of some chronic diseases <br><br> Greater amounts of activity can help prevent weight gain and promote weight loss | All the benefits of lifestyle physical activity, plus improved physical fitness (increased cardiorespiratory endurance, muscular strength and endurance, and flexibility) and even greater improvements in health and quality of life and reductions in chronic disease risk | All the benefits of lifestyle physical activity and a moderate exercise program, with greater increases in fitness and somewhat greater reductions in chronic disease risk <br><br> Participating in a vigorous exercise program may increase risk of injury and overtraining |

**FIGURE 2.4   Health and fitness benefits of different amounts of physical activity and exercise.**

• *Muscular strength and endurance* can be developed through resistance training—training with weights or performing calisthenic exercises such as push-ups and curl-ups. Training for muscular strength and endurance is discussed in Chapter 4.

• *Flexibility* is developed by stretching the major muscle groups regularly and with proper technique. Flexibility is discussed in Chapter 5.

• *Healthy body composition* can be developed through a sensible diet and a program of regular exercise. Cardiorespiratory endurance exercise is best for reducing body fat; resistance training builds muscle mass, which, to a small extent, helps increase metabolism. Body composition is discussed in Chapter 6.

Chapter 7 contains guidelines to help you choose activities and put together a complete exercise program that will suit your goals and preferences. (Refer to Figure 2.4 for a summary of the health and fitness benefits of different levels of physical activity.)

What about the tip of the activity pyramid? Although sedentary activities are often unavoidable—attending class, studying, working in an office, and so on—many people choose inactivity over activity during their leisure time. Change sedentary patterns by becoming more active whenever you can. Move more and sit less.

## Guidelines for Training

The following guidelines will make your exercise program more effective and successful.

**Train the Way You Want Your Body to Change** Stress your body so it adapts in the desired manner. To have a more muscular build, lift weights. To be more flexible, do stretching exercises. To improve performance in a particular sport, practice that sport or its movements.

**Train Regularly** Consistency is the key to improving fitness. Fitness improvements are lost if too much time passes between exercise sessions.

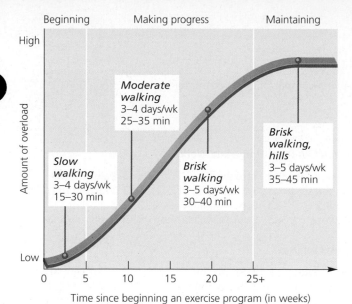

**FIGURE 2.5 Progression of an exercise program.**
This figure shows how the amount of overload is increased gradually over time in a sample walking program. Regardless of the activity chosen, it is important that an exercise program begin slowly and progress gradually. Once you achieve the desired level of fitness, you can maintain it by exercising 3–5 days a week.

**SOURCE:** Progression data from American College of Sports Medicine. 2009. *ACSM's Guidelines for Exercise Testing and Prescription*, 8th ed. Philadelphia: Lippincott Williams and Wilkins.

**Start Slowly, and Get in Shape Gradually** As Figure 2.5 shows, an exercise program can be divided into three phases:

- *Beginning phase.* The body adjusts to the new type and level of activity.
- *Progress phase.* Fitness increases.
- *Maintenance phase.* The targeted level of fitness is sustained over the long term.

When beginning a program, start slowly to give your body time to adapt to the stress of exercise. Choose activities carefully according to your fitness status. If you have been sedentary or are overweight, try an activity such as walking or swimming that won't jar the body or strain the joints.

As you progress, increase duration and frequency before increasing intensity. If you train too much or too intensely, you are more likely to suffer injuries or become **overtrained**, a condition characterized by lack of energy, aching muscles and joints, and decreased physical performance. Injuries and overtraining slow down an exercise program and impede motivation. The goal is not to get in shape as quickly as possible but to gradually become and then remain physically fit.

**Warm Up Before Exercise** Warming up can decrease your chances of injury by helping your body gradually progress from rest to activity. A good warm-up can increase muscle temperature, reduce joint stiffness, bathe

the joint surfaces in lubricating fluid, and increase blood flow to the muscles, including the heart. Some studies suggest that warming up may also enhance muscle metabolism and mentally prepare you for a workout.

A warm-up should include low-intensity, whole-body movements similar to those used in the activity that will follow. For example, runners may walk and jog slowly prior to running at full speed. A tennis player might hit forehands and backhands at a low intensity before playing a vigorous set of tennis. A warm-up is not the same as a stretching workout. For safety and effectiveness, it is best to stretch *after* an endurance or strength training workout, when muscles are warm—and not as part of a warm-up. (Appropriate and effective warm-ups are discussed in greater detail in Chapters 3–5.)

**Cool Down After Exercise** During exercise, as much as 90% of circulating blood is directed to the muscles and skin, up from as little as 20% during rest. If you suddenly stop moving after exercise, the amount of blood returning to your heart and brain may be insufficient, and you may experience dizziness, a drop in blood pressure, or other problems. Cooling down at the end of a workout helps safely restore circulation to its normal resting condition. So, after you exercise, cool down before you sit or lie down or jump into the shower. Cool down by continuing to move at a slow pace—walking for 5–10 minutes, for example, as your heart and breathing rate and blood pressure slowly return to normal. At the end of the cool-down period, do stretching exercises while your muscles are still warm. Cool down longer after intense exercise sessions.

**Exercise Safely** Physical activity can cause injury or even death if you don't consider safety. For example, you should always:

- Wear a helmet when biking, skiing, or rock climbing.
- Wear eye protection when playing racquetball or squash.

**overtraining** A condition caused by training too much or too intensely, characterized by lack of energy, decreased physical performance, and aching muscles and joints. **KEY TERM**

## Vary Your Activities

Do you have a hard time thinking of new activities to try? Check the boxes next to the activities listed here that interest you. Then look for resources and facilities on your campus or in your community.

**Outdoor Exercises**

- ❏ Walking
- ❏ In-line skating
- ❏ Hiking
- ❏ Running
- ❏ Skateboarding
- ❏ Backpacking
- ❏ Cycling
- ❏ Rowing
- ❏ Ice skating
- ❏ Swimming
- ❏ Horseback riding
- ❏ Fly fishing

**Sports and Games**

- ❏ Basketball
- ❏ Softball
- ❏ Bowling
- ❏ Tennis
- ❏ Water skiing
- ❏ Surfing
- ❏ Volleyball
- ❏ Windsurfing
- ❏ Dancing
- ❏ Golf
- ❏ Badminton
- ❏ Snow skiing
- ❏ Soccer
- ❏ Ultimate Frisbee
- ❏ Gymnastics

**Exercises You Can Do at Home and Work**

- ❏ Desk exercises
- ❏ Yard work
- ❏ Painting walls
- ❏ Calisthenics
- ❏ Sweeping
- ❏ Walking the dog
- ❏ Gardening
- ❏ Exploring on foot
- ❏ Shopping
- ❏ Housework
- ❏ Doing a walk-a-thon
- ❏ Doing errands

**Health Club Exercises**

- ❏ Weight training
- ❏ Ski machine
- ❏ Elliptical trainer
- ❏ Circuit training
- ❏ Supine bike
- ❏ Medicine ball
- ❏ Group exercise
- ❏ Rowing machine
- ❏ Rope skipping
- ❏ Treadmill
- ❏ Plyometrics
- ❏ Punching bag
- ❏ Stationary bike
- ❏ Water aerobics
- ❏ Racquetball

---

- Wear bright clothing when exercising on a public street.
- Walk or run with a partner on a deserted track or in a park.
- Give vehicles plenty of leeway, even when you have the right of way.
- In the weight room, be aware of people exercising near you, and use spotters when appropriate.

Overloading your muscles and joints can lead to serious injury, so train within your capacity. Use high-quality equipment and keep it in good repair. Report broken gym equipment to the health club manager. (See Appendix A for more information on personal safety.)

**Listen to Your Body and Get Adequate Rest** Rest can be as important as exercise for improving fitness. Fitness reflects an adaptation to the stress of exercise. Building fitness involves a series of exercise stresses, recuperation, and adaptation leading to improved fitness, followed by further stresses. Build rest into your training program, and don't exercise if it doesn't feel right. Sometimes you need a few days of rest to recover enough to train with the intensity required for improving fitness. Getting enough sleep is an important part of the recovery process. On the other hand, you can't train sporadically, either. If you listen to your body and it always tells you to rest, you won't make any progress.

**Cycle the Volume and Intensity of Your Workouts** To add enjoyment and variety to your program and to further improve fitness, don't train at the same intensity during every workout. Train intensely on some days and train lightly on others. Proper management of workout intensity is a key to improving physical fitness. Use cycle training, also known as *periodization,* to provide enough recovery for intense training: By training lightly one workout, you can train harder the next. However, take care to increase the volume and intensity of your program gradually—never more than 10% per week.

**Vary Your Activities** Change your exercise program from time to time to keep things fresh and help develop a higher degree of fitness. The body adapts quickly to an exercise stress, such as walking, cycling, or swimming. Gains in fitness in a particular activity become more difficult with time. Varying the exercises in your program allows you to adapt to many types of exercise and develops fitness in a variety of activities (see the box "Vary Your Activities"). Changing activities may also help reduce your risk of injury.

**Train with a Partner** Training partners can motivate and encourage each other through rough spots and help each other develop proper exercise techniques. Training with a partner can make exercising seem easier and more fun. It can also help you keep motivated and on track. A commitment to a friend is a powerful motivator. If you can afford it, you may benefit from a personal trainer who can give you instruction in exercise techniques and help provide motivation.

**Train Your Mind** Becoming fit requires commitment, discipline, and patience. These qualities come from understanding the importance of exercise and having clear and reachable goals. Use the lifestyle management

## Digital Workout Aids

When you're just starting to get physically active, you can wind up with a lot of questions. How many miles did I walk? How many sit-ups did I do? How many minutes did I run? When your mind is completely focused on just *doing* an activity, it's easy to lose count of time, distance, and reps. But it's important to keep track of these things: Move too little and you won't see any progress; move too much and you run the risk of injury or burnout. Either outcome is bad news for your exercise program.

Luckily, we live in a digital age, and the fitness industry is providing an ever-growing array of tools that can track your progress for you. If you like to walk or run, digital pedometers can track your distance and the number of steps you take. Advanced trackers can even record any hills you encounter during your workout. If calisthenics are your choice, there are gaming systems and smartphone apps that work for specific exercises to count reps, assess your form, and challenge you to push yourself harder.

You can track more than just your exercise habits with digital assistance. Electronic devices and smart programs are available to help with many aspects of wellness, including the following:

- Dietary habits
- Calories consumed and burned
- Stress management
- Meditation and spirituality
- Heart rate and respiration
- Menstrual cycles
- Family medical history
- Journaling

And that's just to name a few. We'll introduce a variety of these digital devices and apps in later chapters, in the new "Wellness in the Digital Age" feature box like this one. You may find one or more digital apps (many of which are free) that appeal to you and can help you make progress toward your own fitness and wellness goals.

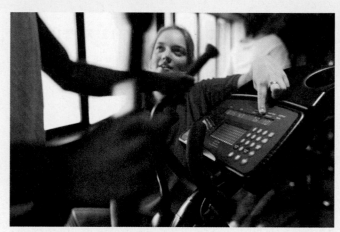

---

techniques discussed in Chapter 1 to keep your program on track.

**Fuel Your Activity Appropriately** Good nutrition, including rehydration and resynthesis of liver and muscle carbohydrate stores, is part of optimal recuperation from exercise. Consume enough calories to support your exercise program without gaining body fat. Many studies show that consuming carbohydrates and protein before or after exercise promotes restoration of stored fuels and helps heal injured tissues so that you can exercise intensely again shortly. Nutrition for exercise is discussed in greater detail in Chapters 3 and 8.

**Have Fun** You are more likely to stick with an exercise program if it's fun. Choose a variety of activities that you enjoy. Some people like to play competitive sports, such as tennis, golf, or volleyball. Competition can boost motivation, but remember: Sports are competitive, whereas training for fitness is not. Other people like more solitary activities, such as jogging, walking, or swimming. Still others like high-skill individual sports, such as skiing, surfing, or skateboarding. Many activities can help you get fit, so choose the ones you enjoy. You can also boost your enjoyment and build your social support network by exercising with friends and family.

**Track Your Progress** Monitoring the progress of your program can help keep you motivated and on track. Depending on the activities you've included in your program, you may track different measures of your program—minutes of jogging, miles of cycling, laps of swimming, number of push-ups, amount of weight lifted, and so on. If your program focuses on increasing daily physical activity, consider using an inexpensive pedometer to monitor the number of steps you take each day. (See Lab 2.3 for more information on setting goals and monitoring activity with a pedometer; see the box "Digital Workout Aids" for an introduction to products and apps that can help you track your progress.) Specific examples of program monitoring can be found in the labs for Chapters 3–5.

**Keep Your Exercise Program in Perspective** As important as physical fitness is, it is only part of a well-rounded life. You need time for work and school, family and friends, relaxation and hobbies. Some people become overinvolved in exercise and neglect other parts of their lives. They think of themselves as runners, dancers,

If you were to start planning a program, what would be your three most important long-term goals? What would you set as short-term goals? What rewards would be meaningful to you?

swimmers, or triathletes rather than as people who participate in those activities. Balance and moderation are the key ingredients of a fit and well life.

## TIPS FOR TODAY AND THE FUTURE

Physical activity and exercise offer benefits in nearly every area of wellness. Even a low to moderate level of activity provides valuable health benefits. The important thing is to get moving!

### RIGHT NOW YOU CAN

- Look at your calendar for the rest of the week and write in some physical activity—such as walking, running, biking, skating, swimming, hiking, or playing Frisbee—on as many days as you can. Schedule the activity for a specific time and stick to it.
- Call a friend and invite her or him to start planning a regular exercise program with you.

### IN THE FUTURE YOU CAN

- Schedule a session with a qualified personal trainer who can evaluate your current fitness level and help you set personalized fitness goals.
- Create seasonal workout programs for the spring, summer, fall, and winter. Develop programs that are varied but consistent with your overall fitness goals.

## SUMMARY

- Moderate daily physical activity contributes substantially to good health. Even without a formal, vigorous exercise program, you can get many of the same health benefits by becoming more physically active.

- If you are already active, you benefit even more by increasing the intensity or duration of your activities.

- The five components of physical fitness most important for health are cardiorespiratory endurance, muscular strength, muscular endurance, flexibility, and body composition.

- Physical training is the process of producing long-term improvements in the body's functioning through exercise.

All training is based on the fact that the body adapts to physical stress.

- According to the principle of specificity, bodies change specifically in response to the type of training received.

- Bodies also adapt to progressive overload. When you progressively increase the frequency, intensity, and time (duration) of the right type of exercise, you become increasingly fit.

- Bodies adjust to lower levels of activity by losing fitness, a principle known as reversibility. To counter the effects of reversibility, it's important to keep training at the same intensity, even if you have to reduce the number or length of sessions.

- According to the principle of individual differences, people vary in the maximum level of fitness they can achieve and in the rate of change they can expect from an exercise program.

- When designing an exercise program, determine if medical clearance is needed, assess your current level of fitness, set realistic goals, and choose activities that develop all the components of fitness.

- Train regularly, get in shape gradually, warm up and cool down, maintain a structured but flexible program, exercise safely, consider training with a partner or personal trainer, train your mind, have fun, and keep exercise in perspective.

## FOR FURTHER EXPLORATION

### BOOKS

American College of Sports Medicine. 2009. *ACSM's Guidelines for Exercise Testing and Prescription,* 8th ed. Philadelphia: Lippincott Williams and Wilkins. *Includes the ACSM guidelines for safety of exercising, a basic discussion of exercise physiology, and information about fitness testing and prescription.*

Earle, R. W., and T. R. Baechle, eds. 2008. *NSCA's Essentials of Personal Training,* 3rd ed. Champaign, Ill.: Human Kinetics. *Comprehensive discussions of fitness testing, exercise and disease, nutrition and physical performance, and exercise prescription.*

Marcus, B. H., and L. A. Forsyth. 2009. *Motivating People to Be Physically Active,* 2nd ed. Champaign, Ill.: Human Kinetics. *Describes methods for helping people increase physical activity levels.*

Page, P. 2011. *Pilates Illustrated.* Champaign, Ill.: Human Kinetics. *A guide to improving muscle fitness, while improving posture, flexibility, and balance.*

### JOURNALS

*ACSM Health and Fitness Journal* (401 West Michigan Street, Indianapolis, In. 46202;
http://journals.lww.com/acsm-healthfitness/pages/default.aspx)
*Physician and Sportsmedicine* (1235 Westlakes Drive, Suite 220, Berwyn, Pa. 19312;
https://physsportsmed.com)

**Q I have asthma. Is it OK for me to start an exercise program?**

**A** Probably, but you should see your doctor before you start exercising, especially if you have been sedentary up to this point. Your personal physician can advise you on the type of exercise program that is best for you, given the severity of your condition, and how to avoid suffering exercise-related asthma attacks.

**Q What should my fitness goals be?**

**A** Begin by thinking about your general overall goals—the benefits you want to obtain by increasing your activity level and/or beginning a formal exercise program. Examples of long-term goals include reducing your risk of chronic diseases, increasing your energy level, and maintaining a healthy body weight.

To help shape your fitness program, you need to set specific, short-term goals based on measurable factors. These specific goals should be an extension of your overall goals—the specific changes to your current activity and exercise habits needed to achieve your general goals. In setting short-term goals, be sure to use the SMART criteria described in Chapter 1. As noted there, your goals should be Specific, Measurable, Attainable, Realistic, and Time frame–specific (SMART).

You need information about your current levels of physical activity and physical fitness in order to set appropriate goals. The labs in this chapter will help you determine your physical activity level—for example, how many minutes per day you engage in moderate or vigorous activity or how many daily steps you take. Using this information, you can set goals for lifestyle physical activity to help you meet your overall goals. For example, if your general long-term goals are to reduce the risk of chronic disease and prevent weight gain, the Dietary Guidelines recommend 60 minutes of moderate physical activity daily.

If you currently engage in 30 minutes of moderate activity daily, then your behavior change goal would be to add 30 minutes of daily physical activity (or an equivalent number of additional daily steps—about 3500–4000); your time frame for the change might be 8–12 weeks.

Labs in Chapters 3–6 provide opportunities to assess your fitness status for all the health-related components of fitness. The results of these assessments can guide you in setting specific fitness goals. For instance, if the labs in Chapter 4 indicate that you have good muscular strength and endurance in your lower body but poor strength and endurance in your upper body, then setting a specific goal for improving upper-body muscle fitness would be an appropriate goal—increasing the number of push-ups you can do from 22 to 30, for example. Chapters 3–6 include additional advice for setting appropriate goals.

Once you start your behavior change program, you may discover that your goals aren't quite appropriate; perhaps you were overly optimistic, or maybe you set the bar too low. There are limits to the amount of fitness you can achieve, but within the limits of your genes, health status, and motivation, you can make significant improvements in fitness. Adjust your goals as needed.

**Q How can I fit a workout into my day?**

**A** Good time management is an important skill in creating and maintaining an exercise program. Choose a regular time to exercise, preferably the same time every day. Don't tell yourself you'll exercise "sometime during the day when you have free time." That free time may never come. Schedule your workout, and make it a priority. Include alternative plans in your program to account for circumstances like bad weather or vacations.

**Q Where can I get help and advice about exercise?**

**A** One of the best places to get help is an exercise class. If you join a health club or fitness center, follow the guidelines in the box "Choosing a Fitness Center." There, expert instructors can help you learn the basics of training and answer your questions. Make sure the instructor is certified by a recognized professional organization and/or has formal training in exercise physiology. Read articles by credible experts in fitness magazines (such as *Fitness Rx for Women* and *Fitness Rx for Men*). Many of these magazines include articles by leading experts in exercise science written at a layperson's level.

A qualified personal trainer can also help you get started in an exercise program or a new form of training. Make sure this person has proper qualifications, such as certification by the ACSM, National Strength and Conditioning Association (NSCA), or International Sports Sciences Association (ISSA). Don't seek out a person for advice simply because he or she looks fit. UCLA researchers found that 60% of the personal trainers in their study couldn't pass a basic exam on training methods, exercise physiology, or biomechanics. Trainers who performed best had college degrees in exercise physiology, physical education, or physical therapy. So choose your trainer carefully and don't get caught up with fads or appearances.

**Q Should I follow my exercise program if I'm sick?**

**A** If you have a mild head cold or feel one coming on, it is probably OK to exercise moderately. Just begin slowly and see how you feel. However, if you have symptoms of a more serious illness—fever, swollen glands, nausea, extreme tiredness, muscle aches—wait until you have recovered fully before resuming your exercise program. Continuing to exercise while suffering from an illness more serious than a cold can compromise your recovery and may even be dangerous.

*For more Common Questions Answered about fitness, visit the Online Learning Center at www.mhhe.com/fahey.*

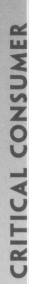
# Choosing a Fitness Center

Fitness centers can provide you with many benefits—motivation and companionship are among the most important. A fitness center may also offer expert instruction and supervision as well as access to better equipment than you could afford on your own. All fitness centers, however, are not of the same overall quality, and every fitness center is not for every person. If you're thinking of joining a fitness center, here are some guidelines to help you choose a club that's right for you.

## Convenience

● Look for an established facility that's within 10–15 minutes of your home or work. If it's farther away, your chances of sticking to an exercise regimen start to diminish.

● Visit the facility at the time you would normally exercise. Is there adequate parking? Will you have easy access to equipment and classes at that time?

● What child care services are available, and how are they supervised?

## Atmosphere

● Look around to see if there are other members who are your age and at about your fitness level. Some clubs cater to a certain age group or lifestyle, such as hard-core bodybuilders.

● Observe how the members dress. Will you fit in, or will you be uncomfortable?

● Observe the staff. Are they easy to identify? Are they friendly, professional, and helpful?

● Check to see that the facility is clean, including showers and lockers. Make sure the facility is climate controlled, well ventilated, and well lit.

## Safety

● Find out if the facility offers some type of preactivity screening as well as basic fitness testing that includes cardiovascular screening.

● Determine if personnel are trained in CPR and if there is emergency equipment such as automated external defibrillators (AEDs) on the premises. An AED can help someone who has a cardiac arrest.

● Ask if at least one staff member on each shift is trained in first aid.

## Trained Personnel

● Determine if the personal trainers and fitness instructors are certified by a recognized professional association such as the American College of Sports Medicine (ACSM), Aerobics and Fitness Association of America (AFAA), National Strength and Conditioning Association (NSCA), or International Sports Sciences Association (ISSA). All personal trainers are not equal; more than 100 organizations certify trainers, and few of these require much formal training.

● Find out if the club has a trained exercise physiologist on staff, such as someone with a degree in exercise physiology, kinesiology, or exercise science. If the facility offers nutritional counseling, it should employ someone who is a registered dietitian (RD) or has similar formal training.

● Ask how much experience the instructors have. Ideally, trainers should have both academic preparation and practical experience.

## Cost

● Buy only what you need and can afford. If you want to use only workout equipment, you may not need a club that has racquetball courts and saunas.

● Check the contract. Choose the one that covers the shortest period of time possible, especially if it's your first fitness club experience. Don't feel pressured to sign a long-term contract.

● Make sure the contract permits you to extend your membership if you have a prolonged illness or go on vacation. Some clubs have exchange agreements that allow you to train in other cities while on vacation or business.

● Try out the club. Ask for a free trial workout, or a 1-day pass, or an inexpensive 1- or 2-week trial membership.

● Find out whether there is an extra charge for the particular services you want. Get any special offers in writing.

## Effectiveness

● Tour the facility. Does it offer what the brochure says it does? Does it offer the activities and equipment you want?

● Check the equipment. A good club will have treadmills, bikes, stair-climbers, resistance machines, and weights. Make sure these machines are up to date and well maintained.

● Find out if new members get a formal orientation and instruction on how to safely use the equipment. Will a staff member help you develop a program that is appropriate for your current fitness level and goals?

● Make sure the facility is certified. Look for the displayed names American College of Sports Medicine (ACSM), American Council on Exercise (ACE), Aerobics and Fitness Association of America (AFAA), or International Health, Racquet, and Sports club Association (IHRSA).

## ORGANIZATIONS, HOTLINES, AND WEB SITES

*American Alliance for Health, Physical Education, Recreation, and Dance (AAHPERD).* A professional organization dedicated to promoting quality health and physical education programs.

http://www.aahperd.org

*American College of Sports Medicine (ACSM).* The principal professional organization for sports medicine and exercise science. Provides brochures, publications, and audio- and videotapes.

http://www.acsm.org

*American Council on Exercise (ACE).* Promotes exercise and fitness; the Web site features fact sheets on many consumer topics, including choosing shoes, cross-training, and steroids.

http://www.acefitness.org

*American Heart Association: Start! Walking for a Healthier Lifestyle.* Provides practical advice for people of all fitness levels plus an online fitness diary.

http://startwalkingnow.org

*CDC Physical Activity Information.* Provides information on the benefits of physical activity and suggestions for incorporating moderate physical activity into daily life.

http://www.cdc.gov/physicalactivity

*Disabled Sports USA.* Provides sports and recreation services to people with physical or mobility disorders.

http://www.dsusa.org

*International Health, Racquet, and Sportsclub Association (IHRSA): Health Clubs.* Provides guidelines for choosing a health or fitness facility and links to clubs that belong to IHRSA.

http://www.healthclubs.com

*International Sports Sciences Association (ISSA).* Trains and certifies personal trainers.

http://www.issaonline.com

*MedlinePlus: Exercise and Physical Fitness.* Provides links to news and reliable information about fitness and exercise from government agencies and professional associations.

http://www.nlm.nih.gov/medlineplus/exerciseandphysicalfitness.html

*President's Council on Fitness, Sports and Nutrition.* Provides information on programs and publications, including fitness guides and fact sheets.

http://www.fitness.gov
http://www.presidentschallenge.org

*Shape Up America!* A nonprofit organization that provides information and resources on exercise, nutrition, and weight loss.

http://www.shapeup.org

*SmallStep.Gov.* Provides resources for increasing activity and improving diet through small changes in daily habits.

http://www.smallstep.gov

## SELECTED BIBLIOGRAPHY

Alzheimer's Association. 2011. *Generation Alzheimer's: The Defining Disease of the Baby Boomers.* Chicago: Alzheimer's Association.

American College of Sports Medicine. 1998. The recommended quantity and quality of exercise for developing and maintaining cardiorespiratory and muscular fitness, and flexibility in healthy adults. ACSM position paper. *Medicine and Science in Sports and Exercise* 30(6): 975–991.

American College of Sports Medicine. 2007. *ACSM's Health/Fitness Facility Standards and Guidelines,* 3rd ed. Champaign, Ill.: Human Kinetics.

American College of Sports Medicine. 2009. *ACSM's Guidelines for Exercise Testing and Prescription,* 8th ed. Philadelphia: Lippincott Williams and Wilkins.

American College of Sports Medicine. 2009. *ACSM's Resource Manual for Guidelines for Exercise Testing and Prescription,* 6th ed. Philadelphia: Lippincott Williams and Wilkins.

American Heart Association. 2007. Resistance exercise in individuals with and without cardiovascular disease, 2007 update: A scientific statement from the American Heart Association Council on Clinical Cardiology and Council on Nutrition, Physical Activity, and Metabolism. *Circulation* 116(5): 572–584.

Ascensao, A., et al. 2011. Mitochondria as a target for exercise-induced cardioprotection. *Current Drug Targets* 12(6): 860–871.

Bouchard, C., et al. 2007. *Physical Activity and Health.* Champaign, Ill.: Human Kinetics.

Centers for Disease Control and Prevention. 2008. Prevalence of self-reported physically active adults—United States, 2007. *Morbidity and Mortality Weekly Report* 57(48): 1297–1300.

Dietary Guidelines Advisory Committee. 2011. *Report of the Dietary Guidelines Advisory Committee on the Dietary Guidelines for Americans, 2010, to the Secretary of Agriculture and the Secretary of Health and Human Services.* Washington, D.C.: U.S. Department of Agriculture, Agricultural Research Service.

Cooper, K. H. 2010. The benefits of exercise in promoting long and healthy lives—my observations. *Methodist DeBakey Cardiovascular Journal* 6(4): 10–12.

Courneya, K. S., and C. M. Friedenreich. 2011. Physical activity and cancer: an introduction. *Recent Results Cancer Research* 186: 1–10.

Donnelly, J. E., et al. 2009. Appropriate physical activity intervention strategies for weight loss and prevention of weight regain for adults (ACSM position stand). *Medicine and Science in Sports and Exercise.* 41(2): 459–471.

Duke University Medical Health News. 2010. Exercise! The anti-aging weapon. 4 new studies affirm the multiple benefits of exercise—at any age, even starting in midlife. *Duke Medical Health News* 16(5): 5–6.

Garber, C. E., et al. 2011. Quantity and quality of exercise for developing and maintaining cardiorespiratory, musculoskeletal, and neuromotor fitness in apparently healthy adults: Guidance for prescribing exercise. *Medicine and Science in Sports and Exercise* 43(7): 1334–1359.

Haskell, W. L., et al. 2007. Physical activity and public health: Updated recommendation for adults from the American College of Sports Medicine and the American Heart Association. *Medicine and Science in Sports and Exercise* 39(8): 1423–1434.

Hobson, K. 2010. How exercise can boost longevity. *US News World Report* 147(2): 30.

Hughes, E., et al. 2010. Surveillance for Certain Health Behaviors Among States and Selected Local Areas — United States, 2008. *Morbidity and Mortality Weekly Report* 597(ss1044): 1203–1205.

Keller, P., et al. 2011. A transcriptional map of the impact of endurance exercise training on skeletal muscle phenotype. *Journal of Applied Physiology* 110(1): 46–59.

Kushi, L. H., et al. 2006. American Cancer Society guidelines on nutrition and physical activity for cancer prevention: Reducing the risk of cancer with healthy food choices and physical activity. *Cancer Journal for Clinicians* 56(5): 254–281.

Lanza, I. R., and K. S. Nair. 2010. Mitochondrial function as a determinant of life span. *Pflugers Archives* 459(2): 277–289.

Masley, S., et al. 2009. Aerobic exercise enhances cognitive flexibility. *Journal Clinical Psychology in Medical Settings* 16(2): 186–193.

Muscari, A., et al. 2010. Chronic endurance exercise training prevents aging-related cognitive decline in healthy older adults: a randomized controlled trial. *International Journal of Geriatric Psychiatry* 25(10): 1055–1064.

National Center for Health Statistics. 2010. *Summary Health Statistics for U.S. Adults: National Health Interview Survey, 2009.* Series 10 (249). Hyattsville, Md.: National Center for Health Statistics.

Nelson, M. E., et al. 2007. Physical activity and public health in older adults: Recommendation from the American College of Sports Medicine and the American Heart Association. *Medicine and Science in Sports and Exercise* 39(8): 1435–1445.

Physical Activity Guidelines Advisory Committee. 2008. *Physical Activity Guidelines Advisory Committee Report, 2008*. Washington, D.C.: U.S. Department of Health and Human Services.

Rhyu, I. J., et al. 2010. Effects of aerobic exercise training on cognitive function and cortical vascularity in monkeys. *Neuroscience* 167(4): 1239–1248.

Richardson, C. R., et al. 2008. A meta-analysis of pedometer-based walking interventions and weight loss. *Annals of Family Medicine* 6(1): 69–77.

Sailors, M. H., et al. 2010. Exposing college students to exercise: the Training Interventions and Genetics of Exercise Response (TIGER) study. *Journal American College of Health* 59(1): 13–20.

Smith, J. K. 2010. Exercise and cardiovascular disease. *Cardiovascular Hematologic Disorders Drug Targets* 10(4): 269–272.

Stranahan, A. M., and M. P. Mattson. 2011. Bidirectional metabolic regulation of neurocognitive function. *Neurobiology Learning Memory*. Published online January 11, 2011.

Tarnopolsky, M. A. 2009. Mitochondrial DNA shifting in older adults following resistance exercise training. *Applied Physiology, Nutrition, and Metabolism* 34(3): 348–354.

Teixeira-Lemos, E., et al. 2011. Regular physical exercise training assists in preventing type 2 diabetes development: focus on its antioxidant and anti-inflammatory properties. *Cardiovascular Diabetology* 10(1): 12.

U.S. Department of Health and Human Services. 1996. *Physical Activity and Health: A Report of the Surgeon General*. Atlanta: U.S. Department of Health and Human Services.

U.S. Department of Health and Human Services. 2008. *Physical Activity Guidelines for Americans*. Washington, D.C.: U.S. Department of Health and Human Services.

U.S. Department of Health and Human Services. 2010. *The Surgeon General's Vision for a Healthy and Fit Nation*. Rockville, Md.: U.S. Department of Health and Human Services, Office of the Surgeon General.

World Health Organization. 2010. *World Health Statistics 2010*. Geneva: World Health Organization.

Name _____  Section _____  Date _____

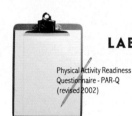

**LAB 2.1** **Safety of Exercise Participation**

Physical Activity Readiness
Questionnaire - PAR-Q
(revised 2002)

# PAR-Q & YOU

**(A Questionnaire for People Aged 15 to 69)**

Regular physical activity is fun and healthy, and increasingly more people are starting to become more active every day. Being more active is very safe for most people. However, some people should check with their doctor before they start becoming much more physically active.

If you are planning to become much more physically active than you are now, start by answering the seven questions in the box below. If you are between the ages of 15 and 69, the PAR-Q will tell you if you should check with your doctor before you start. If you are over 69 years of age, and you are not used to being very active, check with your doctor.

Common sense is your best guide when you answer these questions. Please read the questions carefully and answer each one honestly: check YES or NO.

| YES | NO | | |
|---|---|---|---|
| ☐ | ☒ | 1. | **Has your doctor ever said that you have a heart condition <u>and</u> that you should only do physical activity recommended by a doctor?** |
| ☐ | ☒ | 2. | **Do you feel pain in your chest when you do physical activity?** |
| ☐ | ☒ | 3. | **In the past month, have you had chest pain when you were not doing physical activity?** |
| ☐ | ☒ | 4. | **Do you lose your balance because of dizziness or do you ever lose consciousness?** |
| ☐ | ☒ | 5. | **Do you have a bone or joint problem (for example, back, knee or hip) that could be made worse by a change in your physical activity?** |
| ☐ | ☒ | 6. | **Is your doctor currently prescribing drugs (for example, water pills) for your blood pressure or heart condition?** |
| ☐ | ☒ | 7. | **Do you know of <u>any other reason</u> why you should not do physical activity?** |

**If**

**you**

**answered**

## YES to one or more questions

Talk with your doctor by phone or in person BEFORE you start becoming much more physically active or BEFORE you have a fitness appraisal. Tell your doctor about the PAR-Q and which questions you answered YES.

- You may be able to do any activity you want — as long as you start slowly and build up gradually. Or, you may need to restrict your activities to those which are safe for you. Talk with your doctor about the kinds of activities you wish to participate in and follow his/her advice.
- Find out which community programs are safe and helpful for you.

## NO to all questions

If you answered NO honestly to <u>all</u> PAR-Q questions, you can be reasonably sure that you can:
- start becoming much more physically active — begin slowly and build up gradually. This is the safest and easiest way to go.
- take part in a fitness appraisal — this is an excellent way to determine your basic fitness so that you can plan the best way for you to live actively. It is also highly recommended that you have your blood pressure evaluated. If your reading is over 144/94, talk with your doctor before you start becoming much more physically active.

**DELAY BECOMING MUCH MORE ACTIVE:**
- if you are not feeling well because of a temporary illness such as a cold or a fever — wait until you feel better; or
- if you are or may be pregnant — talk to your doctor before you start becoming more active.

**PLEASE NOTE:** If your health changes so that you then answer YES to any of the above questions, tell your fitness or health professional. Ask whether you should change your physical activity plan.

<u>Informed Use of the PAR-Q</u>: The Canadian Society for Exercise Physiology, Health Canada, and their agents assume no liability for persons who undertake physical activity, and if in doubt after completing this questionnaire, consult your doctor prior to physical activity.

**No changes permitted. You are encouraged to photocopy the PAR-Q but only if you use the entire form.**

NOTE: If the PAR-Q is being given to a person before he or she participates in a physical activity program or a fitness appraisal, this section may be used for legal or administrative purposes.

"I have read, understood and completed this questionnaire. Any questions I had were answered to my full satisfaction."

NAME _____

SIGNATURE _____  DATE _____

SIGNATURE OF PARENT _____  WITNESS _____
or GUARDIAN (for participants under the age of majority)

**Note:** This physical activity clearance is valid for a maximum of 12 months from the date it is completed and becomes invalid if your condition changes so that you would answer YES to any of the seven questions.

 © Canadian Society for Exercise Physiology    Supported by:  Health   Santé
Canada  Canada

Physical Activity Readiness Questionnaire (PAR-Q) © 2002. Reprinted with permission from the Canadian Society for Exercise Physiology. http://www.csep.ca/forms.asp.

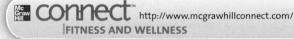
Mc Graw Hill connect™  http://www.mcgrawhillconnect.com/
FITNESS AND WELLNESS

## General Health Profile

To help further assess the safety of exercise for you, complete as much of this health profile as possible.

### General Information

Age: _23_          Total cholesterol: _____          Blood pressure: _____ / _____

Height: _____          HDL: _____          Triglycerides: _____

Weight: _____          LDL: _____          Blood glucose: _____

Are you currently trying to _____ gain or _____ lose weight? (check one if appropriate)

### Medical Conditions/Treatments

Check any of the following that apply to you, and add any other conditions that might affect your ability to exercise safely.

_____ heart disease          _____ depression, anxiety, or other          _____ other injury to joint problem: _____

_____ lung disease          psychological disorder          _____ substance abuse problem

_____ diabetes          _____ eating disorder          _____ other: _____

__X__ allegies          _____ back pain          _____ other: _____

_____ asthma          _____ arthritis          _____ other: _____

_____ Do you have a family history of cardiovascular disease (CVD) (a parent, sibling, or child who had a heart attack or stroke before age 55 for men or 65 for women)?

List any medications or supplements you are taking or any medical treatments you are undergoing. Include the name of the substance or treatment and its purpose. Include both prescription and over-the-counter drugs and supplements.

_____          _____

_____          _____

## Lifestyle Information

Check any of the following that is true for you, and fill in the requested information.

_____ I usually eat high-fat foods (fatty meats, cheese, fried foods, butter, full-fat dairy products) every day.

_____ I consume fewer than 5 servings of fruits and vegetables on most days.

_____ I smoke cigarettes or use other tobacco products. If true, describe your use of tobacco (type and frequency): _____

_____ I regularly drink alcohol. If true, describe your typical weekly consumption pattern: _____

_____ I often feel as if I need more sleep. (I need about ____ hours per day; I get about ____ hours per day.)

_____ I feel as though stress has adversely affected my level of wellness during the past year.

Describe your current activity pattern. What types of moderate physical activity do you engage in on a daily basis? Are you involved in a formal exercise program, or do you regularly participate in sports or recreational activities?

_____

_____

## Using Your Results

*How did you score?* Did the PAR-Q indicate that exercise is likely to be safe for you? Is there anything in your health profile that you think may affect your ability to exercise safely? Have you had any problems with exercise in the past?

*What should you do next?* If the assessments in this lab indicate that you should see your physician before beginning an exercise program, or if you have any questions about the safety of exercise for you, make an appointment to talk with your health care provider to address your concerns.

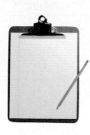

## LAB 2.2 Overcoming Barriers to Being Active

### Barriers to Being Active Quiz

**Directions:** Listed below are reasons that people give to describe why they do not get as much physical activity as they think they should. Please read each statement and indicate how likely you are to say each of the following statements.

| How likely are you to say this? | Very likely | Somewhat likely | Somewhat unlikely | Very unlikely |
|---|---|---|---|---|
| 1. My day is so busy now, I just don't think I can make the time to include physical activity in my regular schedule. | 3 | 2 | 1 | 0 |
| 2. None of my family members or friends like to do anything active, so I don't have a chance to exercise. | 3 | 2 | 1 | 0 |
| 3. I'm just too tired after work to get any exercise. | 3 | 2 | 1 | 0 |
| 4. I've been thinking about getting more exercise, but I just can't seem to get started. | 3 | 2 | 1 | 0 |
| 5. I'm getting older so exercise can be risky. | 3 | 2 | 1 | 0 |
| 6. I don't get enough exercise because I have never learned the skills for any sport. | 3 | 2 | 1 | 0 |
| 7. I don't have access to jogging trails, swimming pools, bike paths, etc. | 3 | 2 | 1 | 0 |
| 8. Physical activity takes too much time away from other commitments—like work, family, etc. | 3 | 2 | 1 | 0 |
| 9. I'm embarrassed about how I will look when I exercise with others. | 3 | 2 | 1 | 0 |
| 10. I don't get enough sleep as it is. I just couldn't get up early or stay up late to get some exercise. | 3 | 2 | 1 | 0 |
| 11. It's easier for me to find excuses not to exercise than to go out and do something. | 3 | 2 | 1 | 0 |
| 12. I know of too many people who have hurt themselves by overdoing it with exercise. | 3 | 2 | 1 | 0 |
| 13. I really can't see learning a new sport at my age. | 3 | 2 | 1 | 0 |
| 14. It's just too expensive. You have to take a class or join a club or buy the right equipment. | 3 | 2 | 1 | 0 |
| 15. My free times during the day are too short to include exercise. | 3 | 2 | 1 | 0 |
| 16. My usual social activities with family or friends do not include physical activity. | 3 | 2 | 1 | 0 |
| 17. I'm too tired during the week and I need the weekend to catch up on my rest. | 3 | 2 | 1 | 0 |

McGraw Hill **connect** http://www.mcgrawhillconnect.com/
|FITNESS AND WELLNESS

| How likely are you to say this? | Very likely | Somewhat likely | Somewhat unlikely | Very unlikely |
|---|---|---|---|---|
| 18. I want to get more exercise, but I just can't seem to make myself stick to anything. | 3 | 2 | 1 | 0 |
| 19. I'm afraid I might injure myself or have a heart attack. | 3 | 2 | 1 | 0 |
| 20. I'm not good enough at any physical activity to make it fun. | 3 | 2 | 1 | 0 |
| 21. If we had exercise facilities and showers at work, then I would be more likely to exercise. | 3 | 2 | 1 | 0 |

## Scoring

- Enter the circled numbers in the spaces provided, putting the number for statement 1 on line 1, statement 2 on line 2, and so on.
- Add the three scores on each line. Your barriers to physical activity fall into one or more of seven categories: lack of time, social influences, lack of energy, lack of willpower, fear of injury, lack of skill, and lack of resources. A score of 5 or above in any category shows that this is an important barrier for you to overcome.

$$\frac{\quad}{1} + \frac{\quad}{8} + \frac{\quad}{15} = \frac{\quad}{\text{Lack of time}}$$

$$\frac{\quad}{2} + \frac{\quad}{9} + \frac{\quad}{16} = \frac{\quad}{\text{Social influences}}$$

$$\frac{\quad}{3} + \frac{\quad}{10} + \frac{\quad}{17} = \frac{\quad}{\text{Lack of energy}}$$

$$\frac{\quad}{4} + \frac{\quad}{11} + \frac{\quad}{18} = \frac{\quad}{\text{Lack of willpower}}$$

$$\frac{\quad}{5} + \frac{\quad}{12} + \frac{\quad}{19} = \frac{\quad}{\text{Fear of injury}}$$

$$\frac{\quad}{6} + \frac{\quad}{13} + \frac{\quad}{20} = \frac{\quad}{\text{Lack of skill}}$$

$$\frac{\quad}{7} + \frac{\quad}{14} + \frac{\quad}{21} = \frac{\quad}{\text{Lack of resources}}$$

## Using Your Results

*How did you score?* How many key barriers did you identify? Are they what you expected?

*What should you do next?* For your key barriers, try the strategies listed on the following pages and/or develop additional strategies that work for you. Check off any strategy that you try.

# Suggestions for Overcoming Physical Activity Barriers

## Lack of Time

_____ Identify available time slots. Monitor your daily activities for 1 week. Identify at least three 30-minute time slots you could use for physical activity.

_____ Add physical activity to your daily routine. For example, walk or ride your bike to work or shopping, organize social activities around physical activity, walk the dog, exercise while you watch TV, park farther from your destination, etc.

_____ Make time for physical activity. For example, walk, jog, or swim during your lunch hour, or take fitness breaks instead of coffee breaks.

_____ Select activities requiring minimal time, such as walking, jogging, or stair climbing.

_____ Other: _____

## Social Influences

_____ Explain your interest in physical activity to friends and family. Ask them to support your efforts.

_____ Invite friends and family members to exercise with you. Plan social activities involving exercise.

_____ Develop new friendships with physically active people. Join a group, such as the YMCA or a hiking club.

_____ Other: _____

## Lack of Energy

_____ Schedule physical activity for times in the day or week when you feel energetic.

_____ Convince yourself that if you give it a chance, exercise will increase your energy level. Then try it.

_____ Other: _____

## Lack of Willpower

_____ Plan ahead. Make physical activity a regular part of your daily or weekly schedule and write it on your calendar.

_____ Invite a friend to exercise with you on a regular basis and write it on *both* your calendars.

_____ Join an exercise group or class.

_____ Other: _____

## Fear of Injury

_____ Learn how to warm up and cool down to prevent injury.

_____ Learn how to exercise appropriately considering your age, fitness level, skill level, and health status.

_____ Choose activities involving minimal risk.

_____ Other: _____

## Lack of Skill

_____ Select activities requiring no new skills, such as walking, jogging, or stair climbing.

_____ Exercise with friends who are at the same skill level as you are.

_____ Find a friend who is willing to teach you some new skills.

_____ Take a class to develop new skills.

_____ Other: _____

## Lack of Resources

_____ Select activities that require minimal facilities or equipment, such as walking, jogging, jumping rope, or calisthenics.

_____ Identify inexpensive, convenient resources available in your community (community education programs, park and recreation programs, worksite programs, etc.).

_____ Other: _____

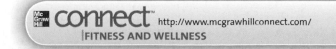

Are any of the following additional barriers important for you? If so, try some of the strategies listed here or invent your own.

## Weather Conditions

_____ Develop a set of regular activities that are always available regardless of weather (indoor cycling, aerobic dance, indoor swimming, calisthenics, stair climbing, rope skipping, mall walking, dancing, gymnasium games, etc.).

_____ Look on outdoor activities that depend on weather conditions (cross-country skiing, outdoor swimming, outdoor tennis, etc.) as "bonuses"—extra activities possible when weather and circumstances permit.

_____ Other: _____

## Travel

_____ Put a jump rope in your suitcase and jump rope.

_____ Walk the halls and climb the stairs in hotels.

_____ Stay in places with swimming pools or exercise facilities.

_____ Join the YMCA or YWCA (ask about reciprocal membership agreements).

_____ Visit the local shopping mall and walk for half an hour or more.

_____ Bring a personal music player loaded with your favorite workout music.

_____ Other: _____

## Family Obligations

_____ Trade babysitting time with a friend, neighbor, or family member who also has small children.

_____ Exercise _with_ the kids—go for a walk together, play tag or other running games, or get an aerobic dance or exercise DVD for kids (there are several on the market) and exercise together. You can spend time together and still get your exercise.

_____ Hire a babysitter and look at the cost as a worthwhile investment in your physical and mental health.

_____ Jump rope, do calisthenics, ride a stationary bicycle, or use other home gymnasium equipment while the kids watch TV or when they are sleeping.

_____ Try to exercise when the kids are not around (e.g., during school hours or their nap time).

_____ Other: _____

## Retirement Years

_____ Look on your retirement as an opportunity to become more active instead of less. Spend more time gardening, walking the dog, and playing with your grandchildren. Children with short legs and grandparents with slower gaits are often great walking partners.

_____ Learn a new skill you've always been interested in, such as ballroom dancing, square dancing, or swimming.

_____ Now that you have the time, make regular physical activity a part of every day. Go for a walk every morning or every evening before dinner. Treat yourself to an exercycle and ride every day during a favorite TV show.

_____ Other: _____

SOURCE: Adapted from CDC Division of Nutrition and Physical Activity. 1999. _Promoting Physical Activity: A Guide for Community Action._ Champaign, Ill.: Human Kinetics.

## LAB 2.3  Using a Pedometer to Track Physical Activity

How physically active are you? Would you be more motivated to increase daily physical activity if you had an easy way to monitor your level of activity? If so, consider wearing a pedometer to track the number of steps you take each day—a rough but easily obtainable reflection of daily physical activity.

### Determine Your Baseline

Wear the pedometer for a week to obtain a baseline average daily number of steps.

|  | M | T | W | Th | F | Sa | Su | Average |
|---|---|---|---|---|---|---|---|---|
| Steps |  |  |  |  |  |  |  |  |

### Set Goals

Set an appropriate goal for increasing steps. The goal of 10,000 steps per day is widely recommended, but your personal goal should reflect your baseline level of steps. For example, if your current daily steps are far below 10,000, a goal of walking 2000 additional steps each day might be appropriate. If you are already close to 10,000 steps per day, choose a higher goal. Also consider the following guidelines from health experts:

- To reduce the risk of chronic disease, aim to accumulate at least 150 minutes of moderate physical activity per week.

- To help manage body weight and prevent gradual, unhealthy weight gain, engage in 60 minutes of moderate to vigorous-intensity activity on most days of the week.

- To sustain weight loss, engage daily in at least 60–90 minutes of moderate-intensity physical activity.

To help gauge how close you are to meeting these time-based physical activity goals, you might walk for 10–15 minutes while wearing your pedometer to determine how many steps correspond with the time-based goals.

Once you have set your overall goal, break it down into several steps. For example, if your goal is to increase daily steps by 2000, set mini-goals of increasing daily steps by 500, allowing 2 weeks to reach each mini-goal. Smaller goals are easier to achieve and can help keep you motivated and on track. Having several interim goals also gives you the opportunity to reward yourself more frequently. Note your goals below:

Mini-goal 1: _____ Target date: _____ Reward: _____
Mini-goal 2: _____ Target date: _____ Reward: _____
Mini-goal 3: _____ Target date: _____ Reward: _____
Overall goal: _____ Target date: _____ Reward: _____

### Develop Strategies for Increasing Steps

What can you do to become more active? The possibilities include walking when you do errands, getting off one stop from your destination on public transportation, parking an extra block or two away from your destination, and doing at least one chore every day that requires physical activity. If weather or neighborhood safety is an issue, look for alternative locations to walk. For example, find an indoor gym or shopping mall or even a long hallway. Check out locations that are near or on the way to your campus, workplace, or residence. If you think walking indoors will be dull, walk with friends or family members or wear headphones (if safe) and listen to music or audiobooks.

Are there any days of the week for which your baseline steps are particularly low and/or it will be especially difficult because of your schedule to increase your number of steps? Be sure to develop specific strategies for difficult situations.

Below, list at least five strategies for increasing daily steps:

_____     _____

_____     _____

_____

Mc Graw Hill connect™  http://www.mcgrawhillconnect.com/
FITNESS AND WELLNESS

## Track Your Progress

Based on the goals you set, fill in your goal portion of the progress chart with your target average daily steps for each week. Then wear your pedometer every day and note your total daily steps. Track your progress toward each mini-goal and your final goal. Every few weeks, stop and evaluate your progress. If needed, adjust your plan and develop additional strategies for increasing steps. In addition to the chart in this worksheet, you might also want to graph your daily steps to provide a visual reminder of how you are progressing toward your goals. Make as many copies of this chart as you need.

| Week | Goal | M | Tu | W | Th | F | Sa | Su | Average |
|---|---|---|---|---|---|---|---|---|---|
| 1 | | | | | | | | | |
| 2 | | | | | | | | | |
| 3 | | | | | | | | | |
| 4 | | | | | | | | | |

## Progress Checkup

How close are you to meeting your goal? How do you feel about your program and your progress?

If needed, describe changes to your plan and additional strategies for increasing steps:

| Week | Goal | M | Tu | W | Th | F | Sa | Su | Average |
|---|---|---|---|---|---|---|---|---|---|
| 5 | | | | | | | | | |
| 6 | | | | | | | | | |
| 7 | | | | | | | | | |
| 8 | | | | | | | | | |

## Progress Checkup

How close are you to meeting your goal? How do you feel about your program and your progress?

If needed, describe changes to your plan and additional strategies for increasing steps:

| Week | Goal | M | Tu | W | Th | F | Sa | Su | Average |
|---|---|---|---|---|---|---|---|---|---|
| 9 | | | | | | | | | |
| 10 | | | | | | | | | |
| 11 | | | | | | | | | |
| 12 | | | | | | | | | |

## Progress Checkup

How close are you to meeting your goal? How do you feel about your program and your progress?

If needed, describe changes to your plan and additional strategies for increasing steps in the space below.

# CHAPTER 3

# Cardiorespiratory Endurance

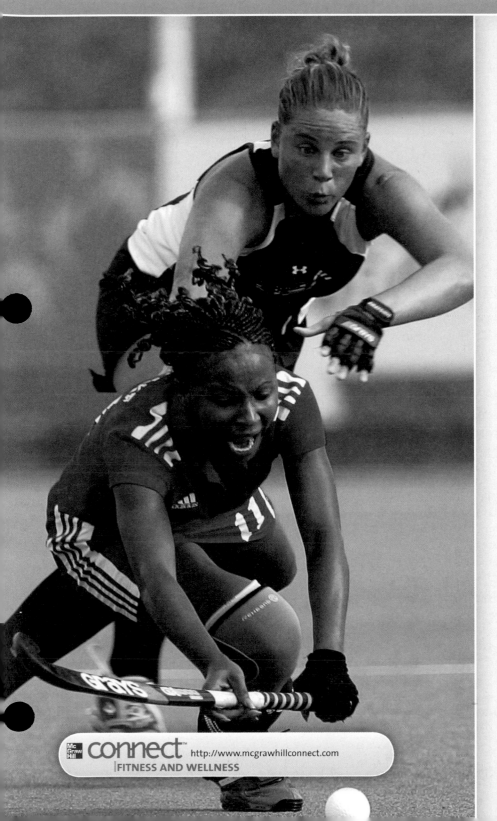

## LOOKING AHEAD...

After reading this chapter, you should be able to:

- Describe how the body produces the energy it needs for exercise
- List the major effects and benefits of cardiorespiratory endurance exercise
- Explain how cardiorespiratory endurance is measured and assessed
- Describe how frequency, intensity, time (duration), and type of exercise affect the development of cardiorespiratory endurance
- Explain the best ways to prevent and treat common exercise injuries

## TEST YOUR KNOWLEDGE

1. Compared to sedentary people, those who engage in regular moderate endurance exercise are likely to
   a. have fewer colds.
   b. be less anxious and depressed.
   c. fall asleep more quickly and sleep better.
   d. be more alert and creative.

2. About how much blood does the heart pump each minute during aerobic exercise?
   a. 5 quarts
   b. 10 quarts
   c. 20 quarts

3. During an effective 30-minute cardiorespiratory endurance workout, you should lose 1–2 pounds. True or false?

**Answers**

1. **All four.** Endurance exercise has many immediate benefits that affect all the dimensions of wellness and improve overall quality of life.
2. **c.** During exercise, cardiac output increases to 20 or more quarts per minute, compared to about 5 quarts per minute at rest.
3. **False.** Any weight loss during an exercise session is due to fluid loss that needs to be replaced to prevent dehydration and enhance performance. It is best to drink enough during exercise to match fluid lost as sweat; weigh yourself before and after a workout to make sure you are drinking enough.

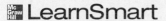

Cardiorespiratory endurance—the ability of the body to perform prolonged, large-muscle, dynamic exercise at moderate to high levels of intensity—is a key health-related component of fitness. As explained in Chapter 2, a healthy cardiorespiratory system is essential to high levels of fitness and wellness.

This chapter reviews the short- and long-term effects and benefits of cardiorespiratory endurance exercise. It then describes several tests that are commonly used to assess cardiorespiratory fitness. Finally, it provides guidelines for creating your own cardiorespiratory endurance training program—one that is geared to your current level of fitness and built around activities you enjoy.

## BASIC PHYSIOLOGY OF CARDIORESPIRATORY ENDURANCE EXERCISE

A basic understanding of the body processes involved in cardiorespiratory endurance exercise can help you design a safe and effective fitness program.

### The Cardiorespiratory System

The **cardiorespiratory system** consists of the heart, the blood vessels, and the respiratory system. (See page T3-2 of the color transparency insert "Touring the Cardiorespiratory System" in this chapter.) The cardiorespiratory system circulates blood through the body, transporting oxygen, nutrients, and other key substances to the organs and tissues that need them. It also carries away waste products so they can be used or expelled.

**The Heart** The heart is a four-chambered, fist-sized muscle located just beneath the sternum (breastbone) (Figure 3.1). It pumps deoxygenated (oxygen-poor) blood to the lungs and delivers oxygenated (oxygen-rich) blood to the rest of the body. Blood actually travels through two separate circulatory systems: The right side of the heart pumps blood to the lungs in what is called **pulmonary circulation**, and the left side pumps blood through the rest of the body in **systemic circulation**.

The path of blood flow through the heart and cardiorespiratory system is illustrated on page T3-3 of the color transparency insert "Touring the Cardiorespiratory System" in this chapter. Refer to that illustration as you trace these steps:

1. Waste-laden, oxygen-poor blood travels through large vessels, called **venae cavae**, into the heart's right upper chamber, or **atrium**.

2. After the right atrium fills, it contracts and pumps blood into the heart's right lower chamber, or **ventricle**.

3. When the right ventricle is full, it contracts and pumps blood through the pulmonary artery into the lungs.

4. In the lungs, blood picks up oxygen and discards carbon dioxide.

5. The cleaned, oxygenated blood flows from the lungs through the pulmonary veins into the heart's left atrium.

6. After the left atrium fills, it contracts and pumps blood into the left ventricle.

7. When the left ventricle is full, it pumps blood through the **aorta**—the body's largest artery—for distribution to the rest of the body's blood vessels.

The period of the heart's contraction is called **systole**; the period of relaxation is called **diastole**. During systole, the atria contract first, pumping blood into the ventricles. A fraction of a second later, the ventricles contract, pumping blood to the lungs and the body. During diastole, blood flows into the heart.

**Blood pressure**, the force exerted by blood on the walls of the blood vessels, is created by the pumping action of the heart. Blood pressure is greater during systole than during diastole. A person weighing 150 pounds has about 5 quarts of blood, which are circulated about once every minute.

The heartbeat—the split-second sequence of contractions of the heart's four chambers—is controlled by nerve impulses. These signals originate in a bundle of specialized cells in the right atrium called the *pacemaker*, or *sinoatrial (SA) node*. Unless it is speeded up or slowed down by the brain in response to such stimuli as danger or the tissues' need for more oxygen, the heart produces nerve impulses at a steady rate.

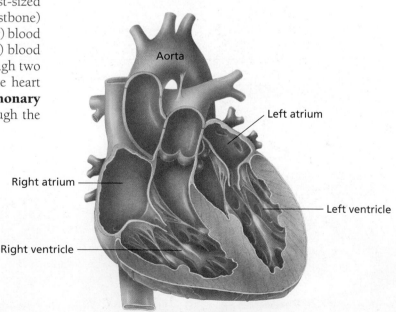

**FIGURE 3.1  Chambers of the heart.**

**The Blood Vessels** Blood vessels are classified by size and function. **Veins** carry blood to the heart. **Arteries** carry it away from the heart. Veins have thin walls, but arteries have thick elastic walls that enable them to expand and relax with the volume of blood being pumped through them.

After leaving the heart, the aorta branches into smaller and smaller vessels. The smallest arteries branch still further into **capillaries,** tiny vessels only one cell thick. The capillaries deliver oxygen and nutrient-rich blood to the tissues and pick up oxygen-poor, waste-laden blood. From the capillaries, this blood empties into small veins (*venules*) and then into larger veins that return it to the heart to repeat the cycle.

Blood pumped through the heart doesn't reach the heart's own cells, so the organ has its own network of blood vessels. Two large vessels, the right and left **coronary arteries,** branch off the aorta and supply the heart muscle with oxygenated blood. The coronary arteries are shown on page T3-3 of the color transparency insert "Touring the Cardiorespiratory System" in this chapter.

**The Respiratory System** The **respiratory system** supplies oxygen to the body, carries off carbon dioxide—a waste product of body processes—and helps regulate acid produced during metabolism. Air passes in and out of the lungs as a result of pressure changes brought about by the contraction and relaxation of the diaphragm and rib muscles. As air is inhaled, it passes through the nasal passages, throat, larynx, trachea (windpipe), and bronchi into the lungs. The lungs consist of many branching tubes that end in tiny, thin-walled air sacs called **alveoli.**

Carbon dioxide and oxygen are exchanged between alveoli and capillaries in the lungs. Carbon dioxide passes from blood cells into the alveoli, where it is carried up and out of the lungs (exhaled). Oxygen from inhaled air is passed from the alveoli into blood cells; these oxygen-rich blood cells then return to the heart and are pumped throughout the body. Oxygen is an important component of the body's energy-producing system, so the cardiorespiratory system's ability to pick up and deliver oxygen is critical for the functioning of the body.

**The Cardiorespiratory System at Rest and During Exercise** At rest and during light activity, the cardiorespiratory system functions at a fairly steady pace. Your heart beats at a rate of about 50–90 beats per minute, and you take about 12–20 breaths per minute. A typical resting blood pressure in a healthy adult, measured in millimeters of mercury, is 120 systolic and 80 diastolic (120/80).

During exercise, the demands on the cardiorespiratory system increase. Body cells, particularly working muscles, need to obtain more oxygen and fuel and to eliminate more waste products. To meet these demands, your body makes the following changes:

- Heart rate increases, up to 170–210 beats per minute during intense exercise.
- The heart's **stroke volume** increases, meaning that the heart pumps out more blood with each beat.
- The heart pumps and circulates more blood per minute as a result of the faster heart rate and greater

**KEY TERMS**

**cardiorespiratory system** The system that circulates blood through the body; consists of the heart, blood vessels, and respiratory system.

**pulmonary circulation** The part of the circulatory system that moves blood between the heart and lungs; controlled by the right side of the heart.

**systemic circulation** The part of the circulatory system that moves blood between the heart and the rest of the body; controlled by the left side of the heart.

**venae cavae** The large veins through which blood is returned to the right atrium of the heart.

**atrium** One of the two upper chambers of the heart in which blood collects before passing to the ventricles (pl. *atria*).

**ventricle** One of the two lower chambers of the heart, from which blood flows through arteries to the lungs and other parts of the body.

**aorta** The body's largest artery; receives blood from the left ventricle and distributes it to the body.

**systole** Contraction of the heart.

**diastole** Relaxation of the heart.

**blood pressure** The force exerted by the blood on the walls of the blood vessels; created by the pumping action of the heart.

**veins** Vessels that carry blood to the heart.

**arteries** Vessels that carry blood away from the heart.

**capillaries** Very small blood vessels that distribute blood to all parts of the body.

**coronary arteries** A pair of large blood vessels that branch off the aorta and supply the heart muscle with oxygenated blood.

**respiratory system** The lungs, air passages, and breathing muscles; supplies oxygen to the body and removes carbon dioxide.

**alveoli** Tiny air sacs in the lungs that allow the exchange of oxygen and carbon dioxide between the lungs and blood.

**stroke volume** The amount of blood the heart pumps with each beat.

stroke volume. During exercise, this **cardiac output** increases to 20 or more quarts per minute, compared to about 5 quarts per minute at rest.

- Blood flow changes, so as much as 85–90% of the blood may be delivered to working muscles. At rest, about 15–20% of blood is distributed to the skeletal muscles.
- Systolic blood pressure increases, while diastolic blood pressure holds steady or declines slightly. A typical exercise blood pressure might be 175/65.
- To oxygenate this increased blood flow, you take deeper breaths and breathe faster, up to 40–60 breaths per minute.

All of these changes are controlled and coordinated by special centers in the brain, which use the nervous system and chemical messengers to control the process.

## Energy Production

*Metabolism* is the sum of all the chemical processes necessary to maintain the body. Energy is required to fuel vital body functions—to build and break down tissue, contract muscles, conduct nerve impulses, regulate body temperature, and so on.

The rate at which your body uses energy—its **metabolic rate**—depends on your level of activity. At rest, you have a low metabolic rate; if you begin to walk, your metabolic rate increases. If you jog, your metabolic rate may increase more than 800% above its resting level. Olympic-caliber distance runners can increase their metabolic rate by 2000% or more.

**Energy from Food** The body converts chemical energy from food into substances that cells can use as fuel. These fuels can be used immediately or stored for later use. The body's ability to store fuel is critical, because if all the energy from food were released immediately, much of it would be wasted.

The three classes of energy-containing nutrients in food are carbohydrates, fats, and proteins. During digestion, most carbohydrates are broken down into the simple sugar **glucose.** Some glucose remains circulating in the blood ("blood sugar"), where it can be used as a quick source of fuel to produce energy. Glucose may also be converted to **glycogen** and stored in the liver, muscles, and kidneys. If glycogen stores are full and the body's immediate need for energy is met, the remaining glucose is converted to fat and stored in the body's fatty tissues. Excess energy from dietary fat is also stored as body fat. Protein in the diet is used primarily to build new tissue, but it can be broken down for energy or incorporated into fat stores. Glucose, glycogen, and fat are important fuels for the production of energy in the cells; protein is a significant energy source only when other fuels are lacking. (See Chapter 8 for more on the roles of carbohydrate, fat, and protein in the body.)

**ATP: The Energy "Currency" of Cells** The basic form of energy used by cells is **adenosine triphosphate**, or ATP. When a cell needs energy, it breaks down ATP, a process that releases energy in the only form the cell can use directly. Cells store a small amount of ATP; when they need more, they create it through chemical reactions that utilize the body's stored fuels—glucose, glycogen, and fat. When you exercise, your cells need to produce more energy. Consequently, your body mobilizes its stores of fuel to increase ATP production.

## Exercise and the Three Energy Systems

The muscles in your body use three energy systems to create ATP and fuel cellular activity. These systems use different fuels and chemical processes and perform different, specific functions during exercise (Table 3.1).

| Table 3.1 | Characteristics of the Body's Energy Systems | | |
|---|---|---|---|
| | ENERGY SYSTEM* | | |
| | IMMEDIATE | NONOXIDATIVE | OXIDATIVE |
| DURATION OF ACTIVITY FOR WHICH SYSTEM PREDOMINATES | 0–10 seconds | 10 seconds–2 minutes | >2 minutes |
| INTENSITY OF ACTIVITY FOR WHICH SYSTEM PREDOMINATES | High | High | Low to moderately high |
| RATE OF ATP PRODUCTION | Immediate, very rapid | Rapid | Slower, but prolonged |
| FUEL | Adenosine triphosphate (ATP), creatine phosphate (CP) | Muscle stores of glucose and glycogen | Body stores of glycogen, glucose, fat, and protein |
| OXYGEN USED? | No | No | Yes |
| SAMPLE ACTIVITIES | Weight lifting, picking up a bag of groceries | 400-meter run, running up several flights of stairs | 1500-meter run, 30-minute walk, standing in line for a long time |

*For most activities, all three systems contribute to energy production; the duration and intensity of the activity determine which system predominates.

**SOURCE:** Adapted from Brooks, G. A., et al. 2005. *Exercise Physiology: Human Bioenergetics and Its Applications,* 4th ed. New York: McGraw-Hill. Copyright © 2005 The McGraw-Hill Companies. Reproduced with permission of The McGraw-Hill Companies.

**The Immediate Energy System** The **immediate ("explosive") energy system** provides energy rapidly but for only a short period of time. It is used to fuel activities that last for about 10 or fewer seconds—examples in sports include weight lifting and shot-putting; examples in daily life include rising from a chair or picking up a bag of groceries. The components of this energy system include existing cellular ATP stores and creatine phosphate (CP), a chemical that cells can use to make ATP. CP levels are depleted rapidly during exercise, so the maximum capacity of this energy system is reached within a few seconds. Cells must then switch to the other energy systems to restore levels of ATP and CP. (Without adequate ATP, muscles will stiffen and become unusable.)

**The Nonoxidative Energy System** The **nonoxidative (anaerobic) energy system** is used at the start of an exercise session and for high-intensity activities lasting for about 10 seconds to 2 minutes, such as the 400-meter run. During daily activities, this system may be called on to help you run to catch a bus or dash up several flights of stairs. The nonoxidative energy system creates ATP by breaking down glucose and glycogen. This system doesn't require oxygen, which is why it is sometimes referred to as the **anaerobic** system. This system's capacity to produce energy is limited, but it can generate a great deal of ATP in a short period of time. For this reason, it is the most important energy system for very intense exercise.

There are two key limitations to the nonoxidative energy system. First, the body's supply of glucose and glycogen is limited. If these are depleted, a person may experience fatigue and dizziness, and judgment may be impaired. (The brain and nervous system rely on carbohydrates as fuel.) Second, increases in hydrogen and potassium ions (which are thought to interfere with metabolism and muscle contraction) cause fatigue. During heavy exercise, such as sprinting, large increases in hydrogen and potassium ions cause muscles to fatigue rapidly.

The anaerobic energy system also creates metabolic acids. Fortunately, exercise training increases the body's ability to cope with metabolic acid. Improved fitness allows you to exercise at higher intensities before the abrupt buildup of metabolic acids—a point that scientists call the *lactate threshold*. One metabolic acid, called **lactic acid** (lactate), is often linked to fatigue during intense exercise. However, lactic acid is an important fuel at rest and during exercise.

**The Oxidative Energy System** The **oxidative (aerobic) energy system** is used during any physical activity that lasts longer than about 2 minutes, such as distance running, swimming, hiking, or even standing in line. The oxidative system requires oxygen to generate ATP, which is why it is considered an **aerobic** system. The oxidative system cannot produce energy as quickly as the other two systems, but it can supply energy for much longer periods of time. It provides energy during most daily activities.

In the oxidative energy system, ATP production takes place in cellular structures called **mitochondria**. Because mitochondria can use carbohydrates (glucose and glycogen) or fats to produce ATP, the body's stores of fuel for this system are much greater than those for the other two energy systems. The actual fuel used depends on the intensity and duration of exercise and on the fitness status of the individual. Carbohydrates are favored during more intense exercise (over 65% of maximum capacity); fats are used for mild, low-intensity activities. During a prolonged exercise session, carbohydrates are the predominant fuel at the start of the workout, but fat utilization increases over time. Fit individuals use a greater proportion of fat as fuel because increased fitness allows people to do activities at lower intensities. This is an important adaptation because glycogen depletion is one of the limiting factors for the oxidative energy system. Thus, by being able to use more fat as fuel, a fit individual can exercise for a longer time before glycogen is depleted and muscles become fatigued.

Oxygen is another limiting factor. The oxygen requirement of this energy system is proportional to the intensity of exercise. As intensity increases, so does oxygen

**KEY TERMS**

**cardiac output** The amount of blood pumped by the heart each minute; a function of heart rate and stroke volume.

**metabolic rate** The rate at which the body uses energy.

**glucose** A simple sugar that circulates in the blood and can be used by cells to fuel adenosine triphosphate (ATP) production.

**glycogen** A complex carbohydrate stored principally in the liver and skeletal muscles; the major fuel source during most forms of intense exercise. Glycogen is the storage form of glucose.

**adenosine triphosphate (ATP)** The energy source for cellular processes.

**immediate ("explosive") energy system** The system that supplies energy to muscle cells through the breakdown of cellular stores of ATP and creatine phosphate (CP).

**nonoxidative (anaerobic) energy system** The system that supplies energy to muscle cells through the breakdown of muscle stores of glucose and glycogen; also called the *anaerobic system* or the *lactic acid system* because chemical reactions take place without oxygen and produce lactic acid.

**anaerobic** Occurring in the absence of oxygen.

**lactic acid** A metabolic acid resulting from the metabolism of glucose and glycogen.

**oxidative (aerobic) energy system** The system that supplies energy to cells through the breakdown of glucose, glycogen, and fats; also called the *aerobic system* because its chemical reactions require oxygen.

**aerobic** Dependent on the presence of oxygen.

**mitochondria** Cell structures that convert the energy in food to a form the body can use.

consumption. The body's ability to increase oxygen use is limited; this limit is referred to as **maximal oxygen consumption**, or $\dot{V}O_{2max}$. $\dot{V}O_{2max}$ determines how intensely a person can perform endurance exercise and for how long, and it is considered the best overall measure of the capacity of the cardiorespiratory system. (The assessment tests described later in the chapter are designed to help you evaluate your $\dot{V}O_{2max}$.)

**The Energy Systems in Combination** Your body typically uses all three energy systems when you exercise. The intensity and duration of the activity determine which system predominates. For example, when you play tennis, you use the immediate energy system when hitting the ball, but you replenish cellular energy stores by using the nonoxidative and oxidative systems. When cycling, the oxidative system predominates. However, if you must suddenly exercise intensely—by riding up a steep hill, for example—the other systems become important because the oxidative system is unable to supply ATP fast enough to sustain high-intensity effort.

**Physical Fitness and Energy Production** Physically fit people can increase their metabolic rate substantially, generating the energy needed for powerful or sustained exercise. People who are not fit cannot respond to exercise in the same way. Their bodies are less capable of delivering oxygen and fuel to exercising muscles, they can't burn as many calories during or after exercise, and they are less able to cope with lactic acid and other substances produced during intense physical activity that contribute to fatigue. Because of this, they become fatigued more rapidly; their legs hurt and they breathe heavily walking up a flight of stairs, for example. Regular physical training can substantially improve the body's ability to produce energy and meet the challenges of increased physical activity.

## Wellness Tip

Feeling tired? Try taking a brisk walk instead of a nap. The more physically active you are, the more energetic you'll feel over the long run.

## Ask Yourself

### QUESTIONS FOR CRITICAL THINKING AND REFLECTION

When you think about the types of physical activity you engage in during your typical day or week, which ones use the immediate energy system? The nonoxidative energy system? The oxidative energy system? How can you increase activities that use the oxidative energy system?

In designing an exercise program, focus on the energy system most important to your goals. Because improving the functioning of the cardiorespiratory system is critical to overall wellness, endurance exercise that utilizes the oxidative energy system—activities performed at moderate to high intensities for a prolonged duration—is a key component of any health-related fitness program.

## BENEFITS OF CARDIORESPIRATORY ENDURANCE EXERCISE

Cardiorespiratory endurance exercise helps the body become more efficient and better able to cope with physical challenges. It also lowers risk for many chronic diseases.

### Improved Cardiorespiratory Functioning

Earlier, this chapter described some of the major changes that occur in the cardiorespiratory system when you exercise, such as increases in cardiac output and blood

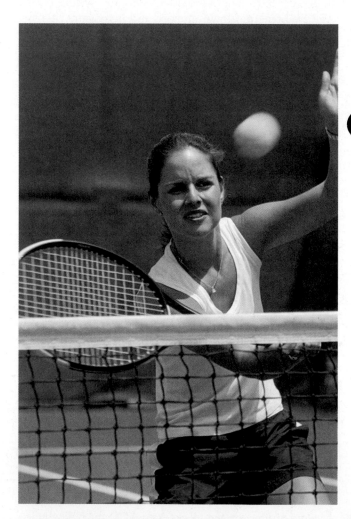

Exercise offers both long-term health benefits and immediate pleasures. Many popular sports and activities develop cardiorespiratory endurance.

**Immediate effects**

Increased levels of neurotransmitters; constant or slightly increased blood flow to the brain.

Increased heart rate and stroke volume (amount of blood pumped per beat).

Increased pulmonary ventilation (amount of air breathed into the body per minute). More air is taken into the lungs with each breath and breathing rate increases.

Reduced blood flow to the stomach, intestines, liver, and kidneys, resulting in less activity in the digestive tract and less urine output.

Increased energy (ATP) production.

Increased blood flow to the skin and increased sweating to help maintain a safe body temperature.

Increased systolic blood pressure; increased blood flow and oxygen transport to working skeletal muscles and the heart; increased oxygen consumption. As exercise intensity increases, blood levels of lactic acid increase.

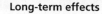

**Long-term effects**

Improved self-image, cognitive functioning, and ability to manage stress; enhanced learning, memory, energy level, and sleep; decreased depression, anxiety, and risk for stroke.

Increased heart size and resting stroke volume; lower resting heart rate. Risk of heart disease and heart attack reduced significantly.

Improved ability to extract oxygen from air during exercise. Reduced risk of colds and upper respiratory tract infections.

Increased sweat rate and earlier onset of sweating, helping to cool the body.

Decreased body fat.

Reduced risk of colon cancer and certain other forms of cancer.

Increased number and size of mitochondria in muscle cells; increased amount of stored glycogen; improved ability to use lactic acid and fats as fuel. All of these changes allow for greater energy production and power output. Insulin sensitivity remains constant or improves, helping to prevent type 2 diabetes. Fat-free mass may also increase somewhat.

Increased density and breaking strength of bones, ligaments, and tendons; reduced risk for low-back pain, injuries, and osteoporosis.

Increased blood volume and capillary density; higher levels of high-density lipoproteins (HDL) and lower levels of triglycerides; lower resting blood pressure; increased ability of blood vessels to secrete nitric oxide; and reduced platelet stickiness (a factor in coronary artery disease).

**FIGURE 3.2    Immediate and long-term effects of regular cardiorespiratory endurance exercise.**
When endurance exercise is performed regularly, short-term changes in the body develop into more permanent adaptations; these include improved ability to exercise, reduced risk of many chronic diseases, and improved psychological and emotional well-being.

pressure, breathing rate, and blood flow to the skeletal muscles. In the short term, all these changes help the body respond to the challenge of exercise. When performed regularly, endurance exercise also leads to permanent adaptations in the cardiorespiratory system (Figure 3.2). These improvements reduce the effort required to perform everyday tasks and make the body better able to respond to physical challenges. This, in a nutshell, is what it means to be physically fit.

Endurance exercise enhances the heart's health by:

• Maintaining or increasing the heart's own blood and oxygen supply.

• Improving the heart muscle's function, so it pumps more blood per beat. This improved function keeps the heart rate lower both at rest and during exercise. The resting heart rate of a fit person is often

10–20 beats per minute lower than that of an unfit person. This translates into as many as 10 million fewer beats in the course of a year.

• Strengthening the heart's contractions.

• Increasing the heart's cavity size (in young adults).

• Increasing blood volume so the heart pushes more blood into the circulatory system during each contraction (larger stroke volume).

• Reducing blood pressure.

**maximal oxygen consumption** ($\dot{V}O_{2max}$) The highest rate of oxygen consumption an individual is capable of during maximum physical effort, reflecting the body's ability to transport and use oxygen; measured in milliliters of oxygen used per minute per kilogram of body weight.

## Benefits of Exercise for Older Adults

Research has shown that most aspects of physiological functioning peak when people are about 30 years old, then decline at a rate of about 0.5–1.0% per year. This decline in physical capacity is characterized by a decrease in maximal oxygen consumption, cardiac output, muscular strength, fat-free mass, joint mobility, and other factors. However, regular exercise can substantially alter the rate of decline in functional status, and it is associated with both longevity and improved quality of life.

Regular endurance exercise can improve maximal oxygen consumption in older adults by up to 15–30%—the same degree of improvement seen in younger adults. In fact, studies have shown that Masters athletes in their seventies have $\dot{V}O_{2max}$ values equivalent to those of sedentary 20-year-olds. At any age, endurance training can improve cardiorespiratory functioning, cellular metabolism, body composition, and psychological and emotional well-being. Older adults who exercise regularly have better balance and greater

bone density and are less likely than their sedentary peers to suffer injuries as a result of falls. Regular endurance training also substantially reduces the risk of many chronic and disabling diseases, including heart disease, cancer, diabetes, osteoporosis, and dementia.

Other forms of exercise training are also beneficial for older adults. Resistance training is a safe and effective way to build strength and fat-free mass and can help people remain independent as they age. Lifting weights has also been shown to boost spirits in older people, perhaps because improvements in strength appear quickly and are easily applied to everyday tasks such as climbing stairs and carrying groceries. Flexibility exercises can improve the range of motion in joints and also help people maintain functional independence as they age.

It's never too late to start exercising. Even in people over 80, beginning an exercise program can improve physical functioning and quality of life. Most older adults can participate in moderate walking and strengthening and stretching

exercises, and modified programs can be created for people with chronic conditions and other special health concerns. The wellness benefits of exercise are available to people of all ages and levels of ability.

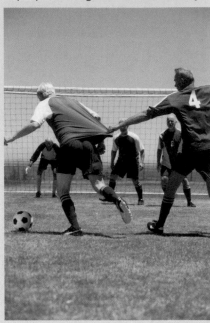

## Improved Cellular Metabolism

Regular endurance exercise improves the body's metabolism, down to the cellular level, enhancing your ability to produce and use energy efficiently. Cardiorespiratory training improves metabolism by doing the following:

- Increasing the number of capillaries in the muscles. Additional capillaries supply the muscles with more fuel and oxygen and more quickly eliminate waste products. Greater capillary density also helps heal injuries and reduce muscle aches.
- Training muscles to make the most of oxygen and fuel so they work more efficiently.
- Increasing the size of and number of mitochondria in muscle cells, increasing cells' energy capacity.
- Preventing glycogen depletion and increasing the muscles' ability to use lactate and fat as fuels.

Regular exercise may also help protect cells from chemical damage caused by agents called *free radicals*. (See Chapter 8 for details on free radicals and special enzymes the body uses to fight them.)

Fitness programs that best develop metabolic efficiency include both long-duration, moderately intense endurance exercise and brief periods of more intense effort. For example, climbing a small hill while jogging or

cycling introduces the kind of intense exercise that leads to more efficient use of lactate and fats.

## Reduced Risk of Chronic Disease

Regular endurance exercise lowers your risk of many chronic, disabling diseases. It can also help people with those diseases improve their health (see the box "Benefits of Exercise for Older Adults"). The most significant health benefits occur when someone who is sedentary becomes moderately active.

**Cardiovascular Diseases** Sedentary living is a key contributor to cardiovascular disease (CVD). CVD is a general category that encompasses several diseases of the heart and blood vessels, including coronary heart disease (which can cause heart attacks), stroke, and high blood pressure (see the box "Why Is It Important to Combine Aerobic Exercise with Strength Training?"). Sedentary people are significantly more likely to die of CVD than are fit individuals.

Cardiorespiratory endurance exercise lowers your risk of CVD by doing the following:

- Promoting a healthy balance of fats in the blood. High concentrations of blood fats such as cholesterol and triglycerides are linked to CVD. Exercise raises levels

# Why Is It Important to Combine Aerobic Exercise with Strength Training?

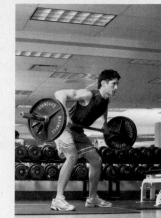

For a variety of reasons, many people choose to focus on only one aspect of physical wellness or fitness. For example, many women concentrate on cardiorespiratory and flexibility exercises but ignore weight training for fear of developing bulky muscles. Many men, conversely, focus exclusively on resistance training in the hope of developing large, strong muscles. They often avoid cardio or flexibility workouts, fearing such exercises will result in loss of hard-earned muscle mass. The fact remains, however, that it is best to include activities that develop all components of health-related fitness.

Emphasizing one aspect of fitness at the expense of others may be a special concern for weight trainers who don't do enough cardiorespiratory conditioning. Although exercise experts universally agree that resistance training is beneficial for a variety of reasons (as detailed in Chapter 4), it also has a downside.

A number of studies conducted around the world have tracked the impact of weight-training exercises on the cardiovascular system, to determine whether resistance training is helpful or harmful to the heart and blood vessels. These studies have shown that strength training poses short- and long-term risks to cardiovascular health and especially to arterial health. Aside from the risk of injury, lifting weights has been shown to have the following adverse effects on the cardiovascular system:

- Weight training promotes short-term stiffness of the blood vessels, which could promote hypertension (high blood pressure) over time and increase the load on the heart.

- Lifting weights (especially heavy weights) causes extreme short-term boosts in blood pressure; a Canadian study revealed that blood pressure can reach 480/350 mm Hg during heavy lifting. Over the long term, sharp elevations in blood pressure can damage arteries, even if each pressure increase lasts only a few seconds.

- Weight training places stress on the endothelial cells that line blood vessels. Because these cells secrete nitric oxide (a chemical messenger involved in a variety of bodily functions), this stress can contribute to a wide range of negative effects, from erectile dysfunction to heart disease.

A variety of studies have shown that the best way to offset cardiovascular stress caused by strength training is to do cardiorespiratory endurance exercise (such as brisk walking or using an elliptical machine) immediately after a weight-training session. Ground-breaking Japanese research showed that following resistance training with aerobic exercise prevents the stiffening of blood vessels and its associated damage. In this 8-week study, participants did aerobics before lifting weights, after lifting weights, or not at all. The group that did aerobics after weight training saw the greatest positive impact on arterial health; participants who did aerobics before lifting weights did not see any improvement in the health of their blood vessels.

Strength training also promotes endurance fitness by improving nervous control of the muscles, increasing type IIa motor units (muscle fibers have a blend of strength and endurance capacity), and increasing tendon stiffness. These changes increase muscle strength and the rate of force development, enhance the economy of movement, and increase the speed that blood cells travel through the muscles.

The bottom line of all this research? Resistance training and cardiorespiratory exercise are both good for you, if you do them in the right order. So, when you plan your workouts, be sure to do 15–60 minutes of aerobic exercise after each weight-training session.

**SOURCES:** Aagaard, P., and J. L. Andersen. 2010. Effects of strength training on endurance capacity in top-level endurance athletes. *Scandinavian Journal Medicine Science Sports.* 20(supplement 2): 39–47; Okamoto, T., M. Masuhara, and K. Ikuta. 2006. Effects of eccentric and concentric resistance training on arterial stiffness. *Journal of Human Hypertension* 20(5): 348–354; Okamoto, T., M. Masuhara, and K. Ikuta. 2007. Combined aerobic and resistance training and vascular function: Effect of aerobic exercise before and after resistance training. *Journal of Applied Physiology* 103(5): 1655–1661; Physical Activity Guidelines Advisory Committee. 2008. *Physical Activity Guidelines Advisory Committee Report, 2008.* Washington, D.C.: U.S. Department of Health and Human Services.

---

of "good cholesterol" (high-density lipoproteins, or HDL) and may lower levels of "bad cholesterol" (low-density lipoproteins, or LDL).

- Reducing high blood pressure, which is a contributing factor to several kinds of CVD.
- Enhancing the function of the cells that line the arteries (endothelial cells).
- Reducing inflammation.
- Preventing obesity and type 2 diabetes, both of which contribute to CVD.

Details on various types of CVD, their associated risk factors, and lifestyle factors that can reduce your risk for developing CVD are discussed in Chapter 11. To learn more about atherosclerosis, the underlying disease process in CVD, see page T3-4 of the color transparency insert "Touring the Cardiorespiratory System" in this chapter.

**Cancer** Although the findings are not conclusive, some studies have shown a relationship between increased physical activity and a reduction in a person's risk of cancer. Exercise reduces the risk of colon cancer, and it may reduce the risk of cancers of the breast and reproductive organs. Physical activity during the high school and college years may be particularly important for preventing breast cancer later in life. Exercise may also reduce the risk of lung cancer, endometrial cancer, pancreatic cancer, and prostate cancer. (See Chapter 12 for more information on various types of cancer.)

**Type 2 Diabetes** Regular exercise helps prevent the development of type 2 diabetes, the most common form of diabetes. Exercise metabolizes (burns) excess sugar and makes cells more sensitive to the hormone insulin, which is involved in the regulation of blood sugar levels. Obesity is a key risk factor for diabetes, and exercise helps keep body fat at healthy levels. But even without fat loss, exercise improves control of blood sugar levels in many people with diabetes, and physical activity is an important part of treatment. (See Chapter 6 for more on diabetes and insulin resistance.)

**Osteoporosis** A special benefit of exercise, especially for women, is protection against osteoporosis, a disease that results in loss of bone density and strength. Weight-bearing exercise—particularly weight training—helps build bone during the teens and twenties. People with denser bones can better endure the bone loss that occurs with aging. With stronger bones and muscles and better balance, fit people are less likely to experience debilitating falls and bone fractures. (See Chapter 8 for more on osteoporosis.)

**Deaths from All Causes** Physically active people have a reduced risk of dying prematurely from all causes, with the greatest benefits found for people with the highest levels of physical activity (Figure 3.3). Physical inactivity is a predictor of premature death and is as important a risk factor as smoking, high blood pressure, obesity, and diabetes.

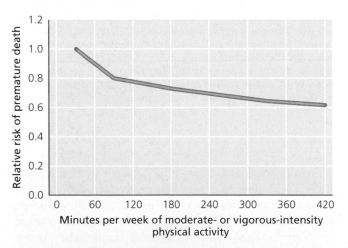

**FIGURE 3.3 Doing only 150 minutes of moderate-intensity physical activity per week provides significant health benefits. As you exercise longer or more intensely, you reduce your risk of dying prematurely from a variety of causes.**
SOURCE: Physical Activity Guidelines Advisory Committee. 2008. *Physical Activity Guidelines Advisory Committee Report, 2008.* Washington, D.C.: U. S. Department of Health and Human Services.

## Better Control of Body Fat

Too much body fat is linked to a variety of health problems, including CVD, cancer, and type 2 diabetes. Healthy body composition can be difficult to achieve and maintain—especially for someone who is sedentary—because a diet that contains all essential nutrients can be relatively high in calories. Excess calories are stored in the body as fat. Regular exercise increases daily calorie expenditure so that a healthy diet is less likely to lead to weight gain. Endurance exercise burns calories directly and, if intense enough, continues to do so by raising resting metabolic rate for several hours following an exercise session. A higher metabolic rate makes it easier for a person to maintain a healthy weight or to lose weight. However, exercise alone cannot ensure a healthy body composition. As described in Chapters 6 and 9, you will lose more weight more rapidly and keep it off longer if you decrease your calorie intake and boost your calorie expenditure through exercise.

## Improved Immune Function

Exercise can have either positive or negative effects on the immune system, the physiological processes that protect us from diseases such as colds, bacterial infections, and even cancer. Moderate endurance exercise boosts immune function, whereas overtraining (excessive training) depresses it, at least temporarily. Physically fit people get fewer colds and upper respiratory tract infections than people who are not fit. Exercise affects immune function by influencing levels of specialized cells and chemicals involved in the immune response. In addition to getting regular moderate exercise, you can further strengthen your immune system by eating a well-balanced diet, managing stress, and getting 7–8 hours of sleep every night.

## Improved Psychological and Emotional Well-Being

Most people who participate in regular endurance exercise experience social, psychological, and emotional benefits. Performing physical activities provides proof of skill mastery and self-control, thus enhancing self-image. Recreational sports provide an opportunity to socialize, have fun, and strive to excel. Endurance exercise lessens

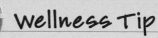

## Wellness Tip

If you have trouble sleeping, exercise could be the cure. Regular physical activity helps people fall asleep more easily; it also improves the quality of sleep.

## Ask Yourself

### QUESTIONS FOR CRITICAL THINKING AND REFLECTION

If you already follow an exercise program, how could you modify it to help improve your cellular metabolism? What specific activities (or changes to existing ones) could you incorporate into your program for this purpose?

anxiety, depression, stress, anger, and hostility, thereby improving mood and boosting cardiovascular health. Regular exercise also improves sleep.

## ASSESSING CARDIORESPIRATORY FITNESS

The body's ability to maintain a level of exertion (exercise) for an extended time is a direct reflection of cardiorespiratory fitness. One's level of fitness is determined by the body's ability to take up, distribute, and use oxygen during physical activity. As explained earlier, the best quantitative measure of cardiorespiratory endurance is maximal oxygen consumption, expressed as $\dot{V}O_{2max}$, the amount of oxygen the body uses when a person reaches his or her maximum ability to supply oxygen during exercise (measured in milliliters of oxygen used per minute for each kilogram of body weight). Maximal oxygen consumption can be measured

pecisely in an exercise physiology laboratory through analysis of the air a person inhales and exhales when exercising to a level of exhaustion (maximum intensity). This procedure can be expensive and time-consuming, however, making it impractical for the average person.

## Choosing an Assessment Test

Fortunately, several simple assessment tests provide reasonably good estimates of maximal oxygen consumption (within 10–15% of the results of a laboratory test). Three commonly used assessments are the following:

- **The 1-mile walk test.** This estimates your level of cardiorespiratory fitness (maximal oxygen consumption) based on the amount of time it takes you to complete 1 mile of brisk walking and your heart rate at the end of your walk. A fast time and a low heart rate indicate a high level of cardiorespiratory endurance.

- **The 3-minute step test.** The rate at which the pulse returns to normal after exercise is also a good measure of cardiorespiratory capacity; heart rate remains lower and recovers faster in people who are more physically fit. For the step test, you step continually at a steady rate and then monitor your heart rate during recovery.

- **The 1.5-mile run-walk test.** Oxygen consumption increases with speed in distance running, so a fast time on this test indicates high maximal oxygen consumption.

Lab 3.1 provides detailed instructions for each of these tests. An additional assessment, the 12-minute swim test, is also provided. To assess yourself, choose one of these methods based on your access to equipment, your current physical condition, and your own preference. Don't take any of these tests without checking with your physician if you are ill or have any of the risk factors for exercise discussed in Chapter 2 and Lab 2.1. Table 3.2 lists the fitness prerequisites and cautions recommended for each test.

| Table 3.2 | Fitness Prerequisites and Cautions for the Cardiorespiratory Endurance Assessment Tests |
|---|---|
| **TEST** | **FITNESS PREREQUISITES/CAUTIONS** |
| 1-mile walk test | Recommended for anyone who meets the criteria for safe exercise. This test can be used by individuals who cannot perform other tests because of low fitness level or injury. |
| 3-minute step test | If you suffer from joint problems in your ankles, knees, or hips or are significantly overweight, check with your physician before taking this test. People with balance problems or for whom a fall would be particularly dangerous, including older adults and pregnant women, should use special caution or avoid this test. |
| 1.5-mile run-walk test | Recommended for people who are healthy and at least moderately active. If you have been sedentary, you should participate in a 4- to 8-week walk-run program before taking the test. Don't take this test in extremely hot or cold weather if you aren't used to exercising under those conditions. |

**NOTE:** The conditions for exercise safety given in Chapter 2 apply to all fitness assessment tests. If you answered yes to any question on the PAR-Q in Lab 2.1, see your physician before taking any assessment test. If you experience any unusual symptoms while taking a test, stop exercising and discuss your condition with your instructor.

## Monitoring Your Heart Rate

Each time your heart beats, it pumps blood into your arteries; this surge of blood causes a pulse that you can feel by holding your fingers against an artery. Counting your pulse to determine your exercise heart rate is a key part of most assessment tests for maximal oxygen consumption. Heart rate can also be used to monitor exercise intensity during a workout. (Intensity is described in more detail in the next section.)

The two most common sites for monitoring heart rate are the carotid artery in the neck and the radial artery in the wrist (Figure 3.4). To take your pulse, press your index and middle fingers gently on the correct site. You may have to shift position several times to find the best place to feel your pulse. Don't use your thumb to check your pulse; it has a pulse of its own that can confuse your count. (Use your middle and ring finger if you have a strong pulse in your index finger.) Be careful not to push too hard, particularly when taking your pulse in the

### Ask Yourself

QUESTIONS FOR CRITICAL THINKING AND REFLECTION

Why do you think a relatively slow resting pulse rate is a sign of good cardiorespiratory fitness? What physical conditions or attributes are reflected in your pulse rate?

carotid artery (strong pressure on this artery may cause a reflex that slows the heart rate).

Heart rates are usually assessed in beats per minute (bpm). But counting your pulse for an entire minute isn't practical when you're exercising. And because heart rate slows rapidly when you stop exercising, a full minute's worth of counting can give inaccurate results. It's best to do a shorter count—10 seconds—and then multiply the result by 6 to get your heart rate in beats per minute. (You can also use a heart rate monitor to check your pulse. See the box "Heart Rate Monitors and GPS Devices" for more information.)

## Interpreting Your Score

Once you've completed one or more of the assessment tests, use the table under "Rating Your Cardiovascular Fitness" in Lab 3.1 to determine your current level of cardiorespiratory fitness. As you interpret your score, remember that field tests of cardiorespiratory fitness are not precise scientific measurements and have up to a 10–15% margin of error.

You can use the assessment tests to monitor the progress of your fitness program by retesting yourself from time to time. Always compare scores for the *same* test: Your scores on different tests may vary considerably because of differences in skill and motivation and weaknesses in the tests themselves.

## DEVELOPING A CARDIORESPIRATORY ENDURANCE PROGRAM

Cardiorespiratory endurance exercises are best for developing the type of fitness associated with good health, so they should serve as the focus of your exercise program. To create a successful endurance exercise program, follow these guidelines:

- Set realistic goals.
- Set your starting frequency, intensity, and duration of exercise at appropriate levels.
- Choose suitable activities.
- Warm up and cool down.
- Adjust your program as your fitness improves.

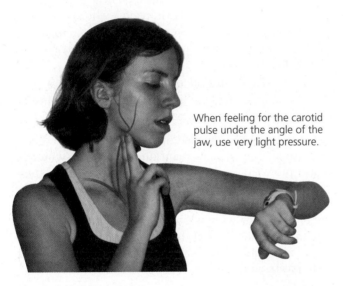

When feeling for the carotid pulse under the angle of the jaw, use very light pressure.

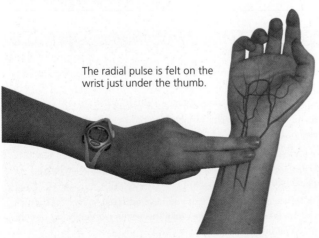

The radial pulse is felt on the wrist just under the thumb.

**FIGURE 3.4  Checking your pulse.**
The pulse can be taken at the carotid artery in the neck (top) or at the radial artery in the wrist (bottom).

# Heart Rate Monitors and GPS Devices

A heart rate monitor is an electronic device that checks the user's pulse, either continuously or on demand. These devices make it easy to monitor your heart rate before, during, and after exercise. Some include global positioning system (GPS) receivers that help you track the distance you walk, run, or bike.

## Wearable Monitors

Most consumer-grade monitors have two pieces—a strap that wraps around the user's chest and a wrist strap. The chest strap contains one or more small electrodes, which detect changes in the heart's electrical voltage. A transmitter in the chest strap sends this data to a receiver in the wrist strap. A small computer in the wrist strap calculates the wearer's heart rate and displays it on a small screen.

In a few low-cost monitors, the chest and wrist straps are connected together by a wire, but the most popular monitors use wireless technology to transmit data between the straps. In advanced wireless monitors, data is encoded so that it cannot be read by other monitors that may be nearby, as is often the case in a crowded gym. A one-piece (or "strapless") heart rate monitor does not include a chest strap; the wrist-worn device contains sensors that detect a pulse in the wearer's hand.

## Monitors in Gym Equipment

Many pieces of workout equipment—including newer-model treadmills, stationary bikes, and elliptical trainers—feature built-in heart rate monitors. The monitor is usually mounted into the device's handles. To check your heart rate at any time while working out, simply grip the handles in the appropriate place; within a few seconds, your current heart rate will appear on the device's console.

## Other Features

Heart rate monitors can do more than just check your pulse. For example, most monitors can tell you the following kinds of information:

- Highest and lowest heart rate during a session
- Average heart rate
- Target heart range, based on your age, weight, and other factors
- Time spent within the target range
- Number of calories burned during a session

Some monitors can upload their data to a computer, so information can be stored and analyzed. The analytical software can help you track your progress over a period of time or a number of workouts. Monitors with GPS provide an accurate estimate of distance traveled during a workout or over an entire day.

## Advantages

Heart rate monitors are useful if very close tracking of heart rate is important in your program. They offer several advantages:

- They are accurate, and they reduce the risk of mistakes when checking your own pulse. (Note: Chest-strap monitors are considered more accurate than strapless models. If you use a monitor built into gym equipment, its accuracy will depend on how well the device is maintained.)
- They are easy to use, although a sophisticated, multifunction monitor may take some time to master.
- They do the monitoring for you, so you don't have to worry about checking your own pulse.

When shopping for a heart rate or exercise GPS monitor, do your homework. Quality, reliability, and warranties vary. Ask personal trainers in your area for their recommendations, and look for product reviews in consumer magazines or online.

# Setting Goals

You can use the results of cardiorespiratory fitness assessment tests to set a specific oxygen consumption goal for your cardiorespiratory endurance program. Your goal should be high enough to ensure a healthy cardiorespiratory system, but not so high that it will be impossible to achieve. Scores in the fair and good ranges for maximal oxygen consumption suggest good fitness; scores in the excellent and superior ranges indicate a high standard of physical performance.

Through endurance training, an individual may be able to improve maximal oxygen consumption ($\dot{V}O_{2max}$) by about 10–30%. The amount of improvement possible depends on genetics, age, health status, and initial fitness level. People who start at a very low fitness level can improve by a greater percentage than elite athletes because the latter are already at a much higher fitness level, one that may approach their genetic physical limits. If you are tracking $\dot{V}O_{2max}$ by using the field tests described in this chapter, you may be able to increase your score by more than 30% due to improvements in other physical factors, such as muscle power, which can affect your performance on the tests.

Another physical factor you can track to monitor progress is resting heart rate—your heart rate at complete rest, measured in the morning before you get out of bed and move around. Resting heart rate may decrease by as much as 10–15 beats per minute in response to endurance training. Changes in resting heart rate may be noticeable after only about 4–6 weeks of training.

You may want to set other types of goals for your fitness program. For example, if you walk, jog, or cycle as part of your fitness program, you may want to set a time or distance goal—working up to walking 5 miles in one session, completing a 4-mile run in 28 minutes, or cycling a total of 35 miles per week. A more modest goal might be to achieve the U.S. Department of Health and Human Services and ACSM's recommendation of 150 minutes per week of moderate-intensity physical activity. Although it's best to base your program on "SMART" goals, you may also want to set more qualitative goals, such as becoming more energetic, sleeping better, and improving the fit of your clothes.

## Applying the FITT Equation

As described in Chapter 2, you can use the acronym FITT to remember key parameters of your fitness program: Frequency, Intensity, Time (duration), and Type of activity.

**Frequency of Training** Accumulating at least 150 minutes per week of moderate-intensity physical activity (or at least 75 minutes per week of vigorous physical activity) is enough to promote health. Most experts recommend that people exercise 3 to 5 days per week to build cardiorespiratory endurance. Training more than 5 days per week can lead to injury and isn't necessary for the typical person on an exercise program designed to promote wellness. It is safe to do moderate-intensity activity such as walking and gardening every day. Training fewer than 3 days per week makes it difficult to improve your fitness (unless exercise intensity is very high) or to use exercise to lose weight. Remember, however, that some exercise is better than none.

**Intensity of Training** Intensity is the most important factor for increasing aerobic fitness. You must exercise intensely enough to stress your body so that fitness improves. Four methods of monitoring exercise intensity are described in the following sections; choose the method that works best for you. Be sure to make adjustments in your intensity levels for environmental or individual factors. For example, on a hot and humid day or on your first day back to your program after an illness, you should decrease your intensity level.

### Fitness Tip

Listen to fast-paced music for a better workout! In a British study, students rode a stationary bike while listening to music at different tempos. The subjects rode harder when listening to faster music and performed less exercise in response to slower music.

**TARGET HEART RATE ZONE** One of the best ways to monitor the intensity of cardiorespiratory endurance exercise is to measure your heart rate. It isn't necessary to exercise at your maximum heart rate to improve maximal oxygen consumption. Fitness adaptations occur at lower heart rates with a much lower risk of injury.

According to the American College of Sports Medicine, your **target heart rate zone**—rates at which you should exercise to experience cardiorespiratory benefits—is between 65% and 90% of your maximum heart rate. To calculate your target heart rate zone, follow these steps:

1. Estimate your maximum heart rate (MHR) by subtracting your age from 220, or have it measured precisely by undergoing an exercise stress test in a doctor's office, hospital, or sports medicine lab. (*Note:* The formula to estimate MHR carries an error of about $\pm 10-15$ beats per minute and can be very inaccurate for some people, particularly older adults and young children. If your exercise heart rate seems inaccurate—that is, exercise within your target zone seems either too easy or too difficult—then use the perceived exertion method described in the next section, or have your maximum heart rate measured precisely.)

2. Multiply your MHR by 65% and 90% to calculate your target heart rate zone. (*Note:* Very unfit people should use 55% of MHR for their training threshold.)

For example, a 19-year-old would calculate her target heart rate zone as follows:

MHR $= 220 - 19 = 201$

65% training intensity $= 0.65 \times 201 = 131$ bpm

90% training intensity $= 0.90 \times 201 = 181$ bpm

To gain fitness benefits, the young woman in our example would have to exercise at an intensity that raises her heart rate to between 131 and 181 bpm.

An alternative method for calculating target heart rate range uses **heart rate reserve**, the difference between maximum heart rate and resting heart rate. Using this method, target heart rate is equal to resting heart rate plus between 50% (40% for very unfit people) and 85% of heart rate reserve. Although some people (particularly those with very low levels of fitness) will obtain more accurate results using this more complex method, both methods provide reasonable estimates of an appropriate target heart rate zone. Formulas for both methods of calculating target heart rate are given in Lab 3.2.

If you have been sedentary, start by exercising at the lower end of your target heart rate range (65% of maximum heart rate or 50% of heart rate reserve) for at least 4–6 weeks. Fast and significant gains in maximal oxygen consumption can be made by exercising closer to the top of the range, but you may increase your risk of injury and overtraining. You *can* achieve significant health benefits by exercising at the bottom of your target range, so don't feel pressure to exercise at an unnecessarily intense level. If you exercise at a

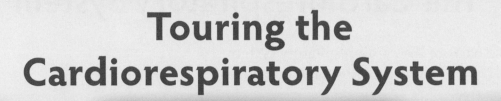

# Touring the Cardiorespiratory System

**The Cardiorespiratory System**

**The Heart and Lungs**

**Atherosclerosis: The Process of Cardiovascular Disease**

**Diabetes: A Disorder of Metabolism**

## GOALS OF THE TOUR

1. **The Cardiorespiratory System.** You will be able to identify the parts of the cardiorespiratory system and the pattern of blood flow through the body.

2. **The Heart and Lungs.** You will be able to identify the chambers of the heart and describe the flow of blood through the right side of the heart to the lungs (pulmonary circulation) and through the left side of the heart to the body (systemic circulation).

3. **Atherosclerosis.** You will be able to explain the process of cardiovascular disease and compare and contrast the outcomes affecting the heart and the brain.

4. **Diabetes.** You will be able to describe how the body uses digested food for energy and growth and how this process is disrupted when a person has diabetes.

# The Cardiorespiratory System

Identify the parts of the cardiorespiratory system and the pattern of blood flow through the body.

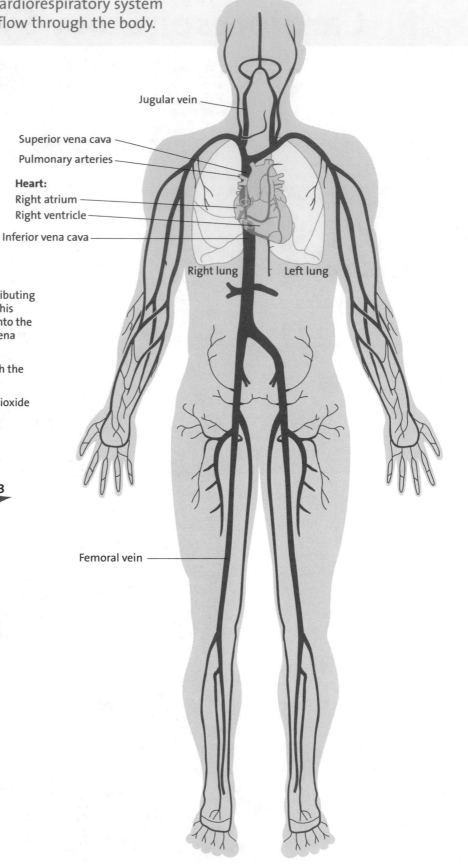

Jugular vein

Superior vena cava

Pulmonary arteries

**Heart:**
Right atrium
Right ventricle

Inferior vena cava

Right lung          Left lung

Femoral vein

## Return of deoxygenated blood to the heart

**1.** Blood travels through the body, distributing oxygen and picking up carbon dioxide. This waste-laden, oxygen-poor blood flows into the right side of the heart via the superior vena cava and the inferior vena cava.

**2.** From there, blood is pumped through the pulmonary arteries into the lungs.

**3.** In the lungs, blood discards carbon dioxide and picks up oxygen.

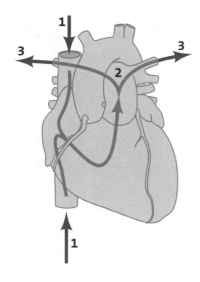

# The Heart and Lungs

Identify the chambers of the heart and describe the flow of blood through the right side of the heart to the lungs (pulmonary circulation) and through the left side of the heart to the body (systemic circulation).

Blood is supplied to the heart muscle by the right and left coronary arteries, which branch off the aorta.

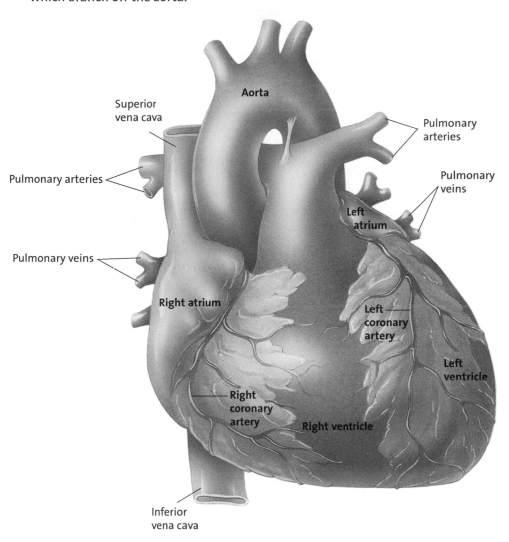

Aorta

Superior vena cava

Pulmonary arteries

Pulmonary arteries

Pulmonary veins

Pulmonary veins

Left atrium

Right atrium

Left coronary artery

Left ventricle

Right coronary artery

Right ventricle

Inferior vena cava

# Atherosclerosis: The Process of Cardiovascular Disease

**3** Explain the process of cardiovascular disease and compare and contrast the outcomes affecting the heart and the brain.

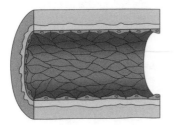

**1.** A healthy artery allows blood to flow through freely.

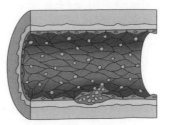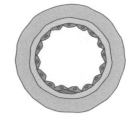

**2.** Plaque buildup begins when endothelial cells lining the arteries are damaged by smoking, high blood pressure, oxidized LDL cholesterol, and other causes. Excess cholesterol particles collect beneath these cells.

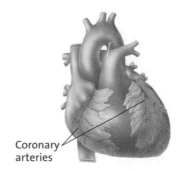

Coronary arteries

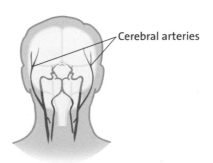

Cerebral arteries

# Diabetes: A Disorder of Metabolism

Describe how the body uses digested food for energy and growth and how this process is disrupted when a person has diabetes.

## Normal metabolism

**1.** When a meal is consumed, food is broken down into nutrients that the body can use to produce energy and build and nourish cells. Carbohydrates are broken down into glucose, which is the body's primary source of energy.

**2.** When glucose enters the bloodstream, the pancreas secretes the hormone insulin, which allows glucose to enter body cells.

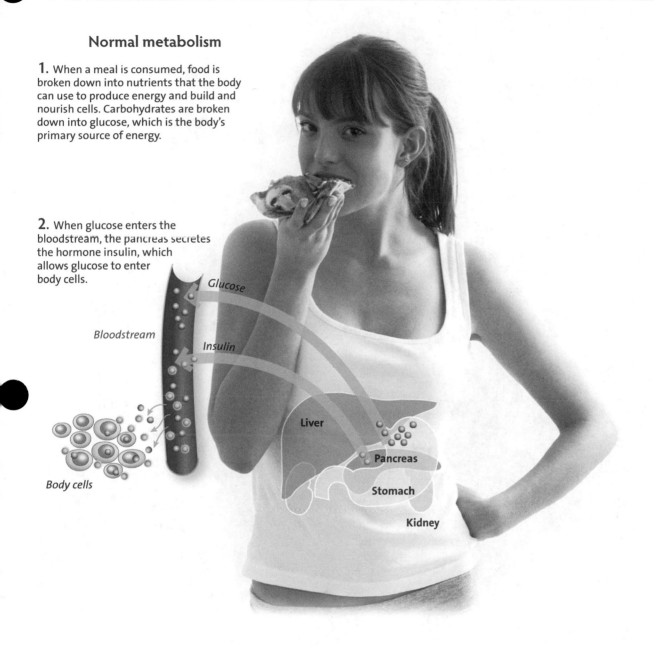

Glucose

Bloodstream

Insulin

Liver

Pancreas

Stomach

Kidney

Body cells

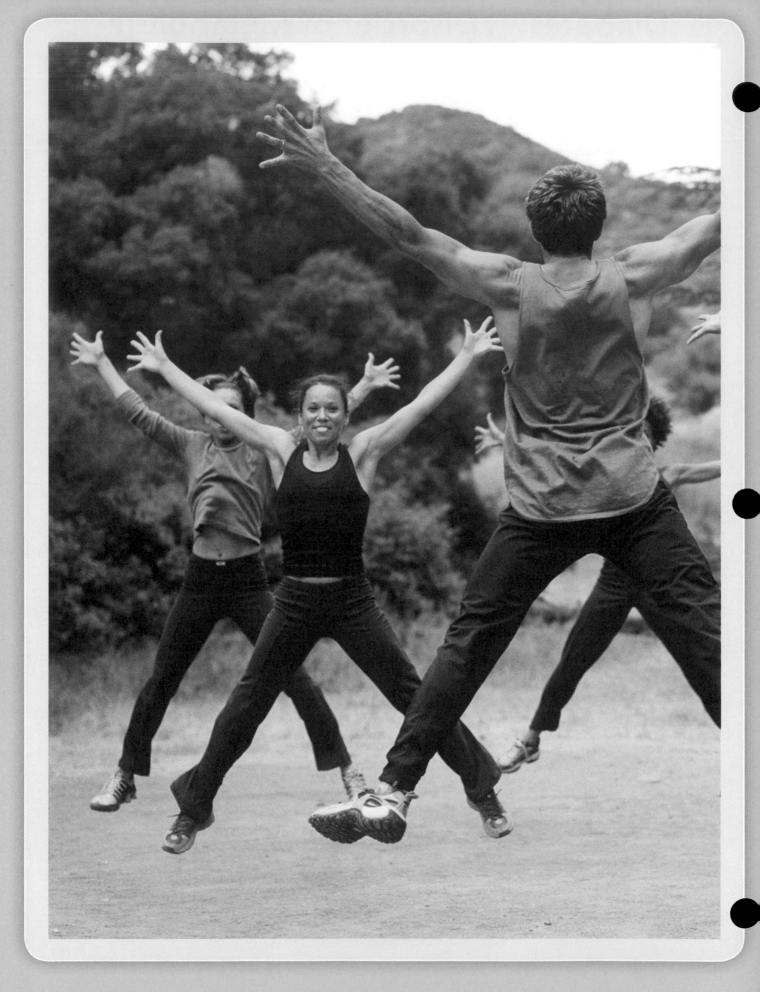

lower intensity, you can increase the duration or frequency of training to obtain as much benefit to your health, as long as you are above the 65% training threshold. For people with a very low initial level of fitness, a lower training intensity of 55–64% of maximum heart rate or 40–49% of heart rate reserve may be sufficient to achieve improvements in maximal oxygen consumption, especially at the start of an exercise program. Intensities of 70–85% of maximum heart rate are appropriate for average individuals.

By monitoring your heart rate, you will always know if you are working hard enough to improve, not hard enough, or too hard. As your program progresses and your fitness improves, you will need to jog, cycle, or walk faster in order to reach your target heart rate zone. To monitor your heart rate during exercise, count your pulse while you're still moving or immediately after you stop exercising. Count beats for 10 seconds, then multiply that number by 6 to see if your heart rate is in your target zone. Table 3.3 shows target heart rate ranges and 10-second counts based on the maximum heart rate formula.

**METS** One way scientists describe fitness is in terms of the capacity to increase metabolism (energy usage level) above rest. Scientists use METs to measure the metabolic cost of an exercise. One **MET** represents the body's resting metabolic rate—that is, the energy or calorie requirement of the body at rest. Exercise intensity is expressed in multiples of resting metabolic rate. For example, an exercise intensity of 2 METs is twice the resting metabolic rate.

METs are used to describe exercise intensities for occupational activities and exercise programs. Exercise intensities of less than 3–4 METs are considered low. Household chores and most industrial jobs fall into this category.

| Table 3.4 | Approximate MET and Caloric Costs of Selected Activities for a 154-Pound Person | |
|---|---|---|
| ACTIVITY | METS | CALORIC EXPENDITURE (kilocalories/min) |
| Rest | 1 | 1.2 |
| Light housework | 2–4 | 2.4–4.8 |
| Bowling | 2–4 | 2.5–5 |
| Walking | 2–7 | 2.5–8.5 |
| Archery | 3–4 | 3.7–5 |
| Dancing | 3–7 | 3.7–8.5 |
| Hiking | 3–7 | 3.7–8.5 |
| Horseback riding | 3–8 | 3.7–10 |
| Cycling | 3–8 | 3.7–10 |
| Basketball (recreational) | 3–9 | 3.7–11 |
| Swimming | 4–8 | 5–10 |
| Tennis | 4–9 | 5–11 |
| Fishing (fly, stream) | 5–6 | 6–7.5 |
| In-line skating | 5–8 | 6–10 |
| Skiing (downhill) | 5–8 | 6–10 |
| Rock climbing | 5–10 | 6–12 |
| Scuba diving | 5–10 | 6–12 |
| Skiing (cross-country) | 6–12 | 7.5–15 |
| Jogging | 8–12 | 10–15 |

**NOTE:** Intensity varies greatly with effort, skill, and motivation.

**SOURCE:** Adapted from American College of Sports Medicine. 2009. *ACSM's Guidelines for Exercise Testing and Prescription*, 8th ed. Philadelphia: Lippincott Williams and Wilkins.

Exercise at these intensities does not improve fitness for most people, but it will improve fitness for people with low physical capacities. Activities that increase metabolism by 6–8 METs are classified as moderate-intensity exercises and are suitable for most people beginning an exercise program. Vigorous exercise increases metabolic rate by more than 10 METs. Fast running or cycling, as well as intense play in sports like racquetball, can place people in this category. Table 3.4 lists the MET ratings for various activities.

METs are intended to be only an approximation of exercise intensity. Skill, body weight, body fat, and environment affect the accuracy of METs. As a practical matter, however, these limitations can be disregarded. METs are

| Table 3.3 | Target Heart Rate Range and 10-Second Counts | |
|---|---|---|
| AGE (years) | TARGET HEART RATE RANGE (bpm)* | 10-SECOND COUNT (beats) |
| 20–24 | 127–180 | 21–30 |
| 25–29 | 124–176 | 20–29 |
| 30–34 | 121–171 | 20–28 |
| 35–39 | 118–167 | 19–27 |
| 40–44 | 114–162 | 19–27 |
| 45–49 | 111–158 | 18–26 |
| 50–54 | 108–153 | 18–25 |
| 55–59 | 105–149 | 17–24 |
| 60–64 | 101–144 | 16–24 |
| 65+ | 97–140 | 16–23 |

*Target heart rates lower than those shown here are appropriate for individuals with a very low initial level of fitness. Ranges are based on the following formula: target heart rate = 0.65 to 0.90 of maximum heart rate, assuming maximum heart rate = 220 − age. The heart rate range values shown here correspond to ratings of perceived exertion (rpe) values of about 12–18.

**KEY TERMS**

**target heart rate zone** The range of heart rates that should be reached and maintained during cardiorespiratory endurance exercise to obtain training effects.

**heart rate reserve** The difference between maximum heart rate and resting heart rate; used in one method for calculating target heart rate range.

**MET** A unit of measure that represents the body's resting metabolic rate—that is, the energy requirement of the body at rest.

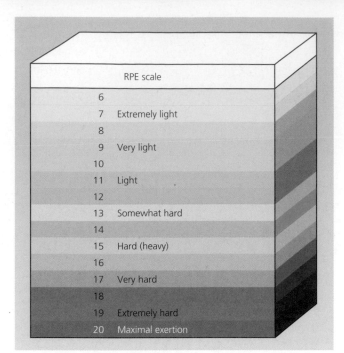

RPE scale

| 6 | |
|---|---|
| 7 | Extremely light |
| 8 | |
| 9 | Very light |
| 10 | |
| 11 | Light |
| 12 | |
| 13 | Somewhat hard |
| 14 | |
| 15 | Hard (heavy) |
| 16 | |
| 17 | Very hard |
| 18 | |
| 19 | Extremely hard |
| 20 | Maximal exertion |

**FIGURE 3.5  Ratings of perceived exertion (RPE).**
Experienced exercisers may use this subjective scale to estimate how near they are to their target heart rate zone.

SOURCE: *Psychology from Research to Practice* (1978), ed. H. L. Pick. Kluwer Academic/Plenum Publishing Corporation. With kind permission of Springer Science and Business Media and the author.

a good way to express exercise intensity because this system is easy for people to remember and apply.

**RATINGS OF PERCEIVED EXERTION**  Another way to monitor intensity is to monitor your perceived level of exertion. Repeated pulse counting during exercise can become a nuisance if it interferes with the activity. As your exercise program progresses, you will probably become familiar with the amount of exertion required to raise your heart rate to target levels. In other words, you will know how you feel when you have exercised intensely enough. If this is the case, you can use the scale of **ratings of perceived exertion (RPE)** shown in Figure 3.5 to monitor the intensity of your exercise session without checking your pulse.

To use the RPE scale, select a rating that corresponds to your subjective perception of how hard you are exercising when you are training in your target heart rate zone. If your target zone is about 135–155 bpm, exercise intensely enough to raise your heart rate to that level, and then associate a rating—for example, "somewhat hard" or "hard" (14 or 15)—with how hard you feel you are working. To reach and maintain a similar intensity in future workouts, exercise hard enough to reach what you feel is the same level of exertion. You should periodically check your RPE against

**ratings of perceived exertion (RPE)**  A system of monitoring exercise intensity by assigning a number to the subjective perception of target intensity.

**KEY TERM**

### Table 3.5  Estimating Exercise Intensity

| METHOD | MODERATE INTENSITY | VIGOROUS INTENSITY |
|---|---|---|
| Percentage of maximum heart rate | 55–69% | 70–90% |
| Heart rate reserve | 40–59% | 60–85% |
| Rating of perceived exertion | 12–13 (somewhat hard) | 14–16 (hard) |
| Talk test | Speech with some difficulty | Speech limited to short phrases |

your target heart rate zone to make sure it's correct. RPE is an accurate means of monitoring exercise intensity, and you may find it easier and more convenient than pulse counting.

**TALK TEST**  Another easy method of monitoring exercise exertion—in particular, to prevent overly intense exercise—is the talk test. Although your breathing rate will increase during moderate-intensity cardiorespiratory endurance exercise, you should not work out so intensely that you cannot speak comfortably. Speech is limited to short phrases during vigorous-intensity exercise. The talk test is an effective gauge of intensity for many types of activities.

Table 3.5 provides a quick reference to each of the four methods of estimating exercise intensity discussed here.

**Time (Duration) of Training**  A total duration of 20–60 minutes per day is recommended; exercise can take place in a single session or in multiple sessions lasting 10 or more minutes. The total duration of exercise depends on its intensity. To improve cardiorespiratory endurance during a low- to moderate-intensity activity such as walking or slow swimming, you should exercise for 30–60 minutes. For high-intensity exercise performed at the top of your target heart rate zone, a duration of 20 minutes is sufficient.

Some studies have shown that 5–10 minutes of extremely intense exercise (greater than 90% of maximal oxygen consumption) improves cardiorespiratory endurance. However, training at high intensity, particularly during high-impact activities, increases the risk of injury. Also, because of the discomfort of high-intensity exercise, you are more likely to discontinue your exercise program. Longer-duration, low- to moderate-intensity activities generally result in more gradual gains in maximal oxygen consumption. In planning your program, start with less vigorous activities and gradually increase intensity.

**Type of Activity**  Cardiorespiratory endurance exercises include activities that involve the rhythmic use of large-muscle groups for an extended period of time, such as jogging, walking, cycling, aerobic dancing and other forms of group exercise, cross-country skiing, and swimming. Start-and-stop sports, such as tennis and racquetball, also qualify if you have enough skill to play continuously and intensely enough to raise your heart rate to target levels.

Other important considerations are access to facilities, expense, equipment, and the time required to achieve an adequate skill level and workout.

## Warming Up and Cooling Down

It's important to warm up before every session of cardiorespiratory endurance exercise and to cool down afterward. Because the body's muscles work better when their temperature is slightly above resting level, warming up enhances performance and decreases the chance of injury. It gives the body time to redirect blood to active muscles and the heart time to adapt to increased demands. Warming up also helps spread protective fluid throughout the joints, preventing injury to their surfaces.

A warm-up session should include low-intensity, whole-body movements similar to those in the activity that will follow, such as walking slowly before beginning a brisk walk. An active warm-up of 5–10 minutes is adequate for most types of exercise. However, warm-up time will depend on your level of fitness, experience, and individual preferences.

Do not use stretching as part of your preexercise warm-up. Warm-up stretches do not prevent injury and have little or no effect on postexercise muscle soreness. Stretching before exercise can increase the energy cost of your workout and adversely affect strength, power, balance, reaction time, and movement time. Stretching interferes with muscle and joint receptors that are vital to performance of sport and movement skills. For these reasons, it is best to stretch at the end of your workout, while your muscles are still warm and your joints are lubricated. (See Chapter 5 for a detailed discussion of stretching and flexibility exercises.)

Cooling down after exercise is important for returning the body to a nonexercising state. A cool-down helps maintain blood flow to the heart and brain and redirects blood from working muscles to other areas of the body. This helps prevent a large drop in blood pressure, dizziness, and other potential cardiovascular complications. A cool-down, consisting of 5–10 minutes of reduced activity, should follow every workout to allow heart rate, breathing, and circulation to return to normal. Decrease the intensity of exercise gradually during your cool-down. For example, following a running workout, begin your cool-down by jogging at half speed for 30 seconds to a minute; then do several minutes of walking, reducing your speed slowly. A good rule of thumb is to cool down at least until your heart rate drops below 100 beats per minute.

### Fitness Tip

Always make warming up and cooling down a part of your exercise routine! Doing so helps the body adapt to being more active, protects from certain injuries, and may make the health benefits of exercise last longer.

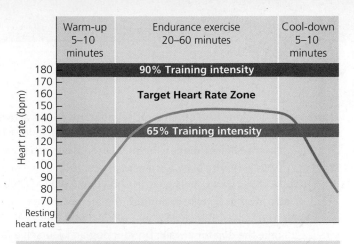

**Frequency: 3–5 days per week**

**Intensity:** 55/65–90% of maximum heart rate, 40/50–85% of heart rate reserve plus resting heart rate, or an RPE rating of about 12–18 (lower intensities—55–64% of maximum heart rate and 40–49% of heart rate reserve—are applicable to people who are quite unfit; for average individuals, intensities of 70–85% of maximum heart rate are appropriate)

**Time (duration):** 20–60 minutes (one session or multiple sessions lasting 10 or more minutes)

**Type of activity:** Cardiorespiratory endurance exercises, such as walking, jogging, biking, swimming, cross-country skiing, and rope skipping

**FIGURE 3.6   The FITT principle for a cardiorespiratory endurance workout.**
Longer-duration exercise at lower intensities can often be as beneficial for promoting health as shorter-duration, high-intensity exercise.

The general pattern of a safe and successful workout for cardiorespiratory fitness is illustrated in Figure 3.6.

## Building Cardiorespiratory Fitness

Building fitness is as much an art as a science. Your fitness improves when you overload your body. However, you must increase the intensity, frequency, and duration of exercise carefully to avoid injury and overtraining.

For the initial stage of your program, which may last anywhere from 3 to 6 weeks, exercise at the low end of your target heart rate zone. Begin with a frequency of 3–4 days per week, and choose a duration appropriate for your fitness level: 12–15 minutes if you are very unfit, 20 minutes if you are sedentary but otherwise healthy, and 30–40 minutes if you are an experienced exerciser. Use this stage of your program to allow both your body and your schedule to adjust to your new exercise routine. Once you can exercise at the upper levels of frequency (4–5 days per week) and duration (30–40 minutes) without excessive fatigue or muscle soreness, you are ready to progress.

The next phase of your program is the improvement stage, lasting from 4 to 6 months. During this phase, slowly and gradually increase the amount of overload until you reach your target level of fitness (see the sample

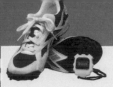

## Staying Active between Workouts

Many people who practice formal exercise programs do less activity during the rest of the day, which partially defeats the purpose of the exercise program. Below are some ideas for becoming more active during the day. Check which one you can work into your lifestyle:

1. _____ **Exercise before dinner:** Pre-meal exercise decreases appetite and promotes a feeling of fullness.

2. _____ **Enter a charity walk-a-thon:** Many charities make money by getting people to sign up as sponsors in walk-a-thons and fun runs. These events help charities and make you look better in a bikini.

3. _____ **Do errands by bike or on foot:** You are not chained to your car. Buy a grocery cart and walk to the store. Carts are small, so you won't buy as much food and will increase fitness at the same time.

4. _____ **Take the dog for a walk:** Do your dog and yourself a favor and go for a walk together.

5. _____ **Hit softballs or baseballs at the batting cage:** Hitting balls is a great way to get ready for springtime softball games and is a terrific total body exercise.

6. _____ **Hit a bucket of balls at the golf course:** Many people think golf is a wimpy sport. Hit a couple of hundred balls at the driving range and see how you feel the next day. This is a great way to burn calories and improve your game.

7. _____ **Do aerobics 30 to 90 minutes a day:** People who walk only 30 minutes, 5 times per week will lose an average of 5 pounds in 6 to 12 months—without dieting, watching what they eat, or exercising intensely.

8. _____ **Do calisthenics first thing in the morning:** Calisthenics are resistive exercises that use body weight as resistance. These are excellent for a person who wants to develop muscle strength but is unwilling to join a health club or devote too much time to the activity. Examples include push-ups, squats, curl-ups, chair dips, crunches, and jumping jacks.

9. _____ **Exercise in the housework gym:** A vacuum cleaner is actually a lunge machine. Use a little creativity and you can turn simple household chores into a weight and aerobics workout. Try wearing a weighted vest while you sweep or mop the floor. Don't walk up the stairs— run. Jog in place as you wash the dishes. Stretch while putting away the dishes.

10. _____ **Active shopping:** Go on a window-shopping hike. Walk through the mall and check out every single shop. If you live in a small town, check out each store twice. If you live near the Mall of America, cover the stores in four days.

11. _____ **Trim the hedge:** Go to the hardware store and purchase hand hedge trimmers. This garden chore burns calories and builds chest, shoulder, leg, and core muscles.

12. _____ **Sweep the walkway:** Try interval sweeping: Pick a 10-yard strip of cement and sweep as fast and as hard as you can. Also, try lunge sweeping: Do a lunge every time you sweep the broom—first your left leg, then your right.

By themselves, few of these methods will make you physically fit. But combining two or three of these techniques gives you powerful tools that will help you build fitness and keep the fat off.

---

training progression in Table 3.6). Take care not to increase overload too quickly. It is usually best to avoid increasing intensity and duration during the same session or all three training variables in one week. Increasing duration in increments of 5–10 minutes every 2–3 weeks is usually appropriate. Signs that you are increasing overload too quickly include muscle aches and pains, lack of usual interest in exercise, extreme fatigue, and inability to complete a workout. Keep an exercise log or training diary to monitor your workouts and progress.

## Maintaining Cardiorespiratory Fitness

You will not improve your fitness indefinitely. The more fit you become, the harder you must work to improve (see the box "Interval Training: Pros and Cons"). There are limits to the level of fitness you can achieve, and if you increase intensity and duration indefinitely, you are likely to become injured or overtrained. After an improvement stage of 4–6 months, you may reach your goal of an acceptable level of fitness. You can then maintain fitness by continuing to exercise at the same intensity at least 3 nonconsecutive days every week. If you stop exercising, you lose your gains in fitness fairly rapidly. If you take time off for any reason, start your program again at a lower level and rebuild your fitness in a slow and systematic way.

### Fitness Tip

A 40-meter running track, found in almost any high school or college, is a great place to do interval training. Start by striding the straight-a-ways and walking the turns. Begin with just one lap and increase the number of laps until you can do 4 to 8 (1 to 2 miles).

| Table 3.6 | Sample Progression for an Endurance Program | | |
|---|---|---|---|
| STAGE/WEEK | FREQUENCY (days/week) | INTENSITY* (beats/minute) | TIME (duration in minutes) |
| Initial stage | | | |
| 1 | 3 | 120–130 | 15–20 |
| 2 | 3 | 120–130 | 20–25 |
| 3 | 4 | 130–145 | 20–25 |
| 4 | 4 | 130–145 | 25–30 |
| Improvement stage | | | |
| 5–7 | 3–4 | 145–160 | 25–30 |
| 8–10 | 3–4 | 145–160 | 30–35 |
| 11–13 | 3–4 | 150–165 | 30–35 |
| 14–16 | 4–5 | 150–165 | 30–35 |
| 17–20 | 4–5 | 160–180 | 35–40 |
| 21–24 | 4–5 | 160–180 | 35–40 |
| Maintenance stage | | | |
| 25+ | 3–5 | 160–180 | 20–60 |

*The target heart rates shown here are based on calculations for a healthy 20-year-old with a resting heart rate of 60 beats per minute; the program progresses from an initial target heart rate of 50% to a maintenance range of 70–85% of heart rate reserve.

**SOURCE:** Adapted from American College of Sports Medicine. 2009. *ACSM's Guidelines for Exercise Testing and Prescription*, 8th ed. Philadelphia: Lippincott Williams and Wilkins. Reprinted with permission from the publisher.

When you reach the maintenance stage, you may want to set new goals for your program and make some adjustments to maintain your motivation. Adding variety to your program can be a helpful strategy. Engaging in multiple types of endurance activities, an approach known as **cross-training**, can help boost enjoyment and prevent some types of injuries. For example, someone who has been jogging 5 days a week may change her program so that she jogs 3 days a week, plays tennis 1 day a week, and goes for a bike ride 1 day a week.

## ? Ask Yourself

### QUESTIONS FOR CRITICAL THINKING AND REFLECTION

Suppose you want to start a new cardiorespiratory exercise program. How do your age, health status, and current level of fitness affect the kind of program you design for yourself? For the first few weeks, how often would you exercise, at what intensity (heart rate), and for how long?

# EXERCISE SAFETY AND INJURY PREVENTION

Exercising safely and preventing injuries are two important challenges for people who engage in cardiorespiratory endurance exercise. This section provides basic safety guidelines that can be applied to a variety of fitness activities. Chapters 4 and 5 include additional advice specific to strength training and flexibility training.

## Hot Weather and Heat Stress

Human beings require a relatively constant body temperature to survive. A change of just a few degrees in body temperature can quickly lead to distress and even death. If you lose too much water or if your body temperature gets too high, you may suffer from heat stress. Problems associated with heat stress include dehydration, heat cramps, heat exhaustion, and heatstroke.

In a high-temperature environment, exercise safety depends on the body's ability to dissipate heat and maintain blood flow to active muscles. The body releases heat from exercise through the evaporation of sweat. This process cools the skin and the blood circulating near the body's surface. Sweating is an efficient process as long as the air is relatively dry. As humidity increases, however, the sweating mechanism becomes less efficient because extra moisture in the air inhibits the evaporation of sweat from the skin. This is why it takes longer to cool down in humid weather than in dry weather.

You can avoid significant heat stress by staying fit, avoiding overly intense or prolonged exercise for which you are not prepared, drinking adequate fluids before and during exercise, and wearing clothes that allow heat to dissipate.

**Dehydration** Your body needs water to carry out many chemical reactions and to regulate body temperature. Sweating during exercise depletes your body's water supply and can lead to **dehydration** if fluids aren't replaced. Although dehydration is most common in hot weather, it can occur even in comfortable temperatures if fluid intake is insufficient.

Dehydration increases body temperature and decreases sweat rate, plasma volume, cardiac output, maximal oxygen consumption, exercise capacity, muscular strength, and stores of liver glycogen. You may begin to feel thirsty when you have a fluid deficit of about 1% of total body weight.

Drinking fluids before and during exercise is important to prevent dehydration and enhance performance. Thirst receptors in the brain make you want to drink fluids, but during heavy or prolonged exercise or exercise

---

**cross-training** Alternating two or more activities to improve a single component of fitness.

**dehydration** Excessive loss of body fluid.

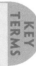 KEY TERMS

# Interval Training: Pros and Cons

Few exercise techniques are more effective at improving fitness rapidly than *high-intensity interval training (HIT)*—a series of very brief, high-intensity exercise sessions interspersed with short rest periods. The four components of interval training are distance, repetition, intensity, and rest, defined as follows:

- *Distance* refers to either the distance or the time of the exercise interval.
- *Repetition* is the number of times the exercise is repeated.
- *Intensity* is the speed at which the exercise is performed.
- *Rest* is the time spent recovering between exercises.

Canadian researchers found that 6 sessions of high-intensity interval training on a stationary bike increased muscle oxidative capacity by almost 50%, muscle glycogen by 20%, and cycle endurance capacity by 100%. The subjects made these amazing improvements by exercising only 15 minutes in 2 weeks. Each workout consisted of 4–7 repetitions of high-intensity exercise (each repetition consisted of 30 seconds at near maximum effort) on a stationary bike. A follow-up study of moderately active women using the same training method showed that interval training increased the body's capacity for burning fat during exercise. These studies (and more than 20 others) showed the value of high-intensity training for building aerobic capacity and endurance.

You can use interval training in your favorite aerobic exercises. In fact, the type of exercise you select is not important as long as you exercise at a high intensity. HIT training can even be used to help develop sports skills. For example, a runner might do 4 to 8 repetitions of 200-meter sprints at near-maximum effort. A tennis player might practice volleys against a wall as fast as possible for 4 to 8 repetitions lasting 30 seconds each. A swimmer might swim 4 to 8 repetitions of 50 meters at 100% effort. It is important to rest from 3 to 5 minutes between repetitions, regardless of the type of exercise being performed.

If you add HIT to your exercise program, do not practice interval training more than 3 days per week. Intervals are exhausting and easily lead to injury. Let your body tell you how many days you can tolerate. If you become overly tired after doing interval training 3 days per week, cut back to 2 days. If you feel good, try increasing the intensity or volume of intervals (but not the number of days per week) and see what happens. As with any kind of exercise program, begin HIT training slowly and progress conservatively. Although the Canadian studies showed that HIT training produced substantial fitness improvements by themselves, it is best to integrate HIT into your total exercise program.

High-intensity interval training appears to be safe and effective in the short term, but there are concerns about the long-term safety and effectiveness of this type of training, so consider the following issues:

- Maximal-intensity training could be dangerous for some people. A physician might be reluctant to give certain patients the green light for this type of exercise.
- Always warm up with several minutes of low-intensity exercise before practicing HIT. Maximal-intensity exercise without a warm-up can cause cardiac arrhythmias (abnormal heart rhythms) even in healthy people.
- HIT might trigger overuse injuries in unfit people. For this reason, it is essential to start gradually, especially for someone at a low level of fitness. Exercise at sub-maximal intensities for at least 4 to 6 weeks before starting high-intensity interval training. Cut back on interval training or rest if you feel overly fatigued or develop overly sore joints or muscles.

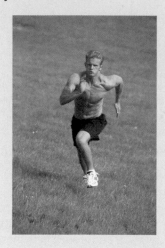

in hot weather, thirst alone isn't a good indicator of how much you need to drink. As a rule of thumb, drink at least 2 cups (16 ounces) of fluid 2 hours before exercise, and then drink enough during exercise to match fluid loss in sweat. Drink at least 1 cup of fluid every 20–30 minutes during exercise, more in hot weather or if you sweat heavily. To determine if you're drinking enough fluid, weigh yourself before and after an exercise session; any weight loss is due to fluid loss that needs to be replaced.

Very rarely, active people consume too much water and develop **hyponatremia,** a condition characterized by lung congestion, muscle weakness, and nervous system problems. Following the guidelines presented here can help prevent this condition.

Bring a water bottle when you exercise so you can replace your fluids when they're being depleted. For exercise

sessions lasting less than 60–90 minutes, cool water is an excellent fluid replacement. For longer workouts, choose a sports drink that contains water and small amounts of electrolytes (sodium, potassium, and magnesium) and simple carbohydrates ("sugar," usually in the form of sucrose, glucose, lactate, or glucose polymers). Electrolytes, which are lost from the body in sweat, are important because they help regulate the balance of fluids in body cells and the bloodstream. The carbohydrates in typical sports drinks are rapidly digestible and can thus help maintain blood glucose levels. Choose a beverage with no more than 8 grams of simple carbohydrate per 100 milliliters. Nonfat milk or chocolate milk, for those who can tolerate dairy products, are excellent fluid replacement beverages because they promote long-term hydration. See Chapter 8 for more on diet and fluid recommendations for active people.

**Heat Cramps** Involuntary cramping and spasms in the muscle groups used during exercise are sometimes called **heat cramps**. Although depletion of sodium and potassium from the muscles is involved with the problem, the primary cause of cramps is muscle fatigue. Children are particularly susceptible to heat cramps, but the condition can also occur in adults, even those who are fit. The best treatment for heat cramps is a combination of gentle stretching, replacement of fluid and electrolytes, and rest.

**Heat Exhaustion** Symptoms of **heat exhaustion** include the following:

- Rapid, weak pulse
- Low blood pressure
- Headache
- Faintness, weakness, dizziness
- Profuse sweating
- Pale face
- Psychological disorientation (in some cases)
- Normal or slightly elevated core body temperature

Heat exhaustion occurs when an insufficient amount of blood returns to the heart because so much of the body's blood volume is being directed to working muscles (for exercise) and to the skin (for cooling). Treatment for heat exhaustion includes resting in a cool area, removing excess clothing, applying cool or damp towels to the body, and drinking fluids. An affected individual should rest for the remainder of the day and drink plenty of fluids for the next 24 hours.

**Heatstroke** **Heatstroke** is a major medical emergency involving the failure of the brain's temperature regulatory center. The body does not sweat enough, and body temperature rises dramatically to extremely dangerous levels. In addition to high body temperature, symptoms can include the following:

- Hot, flushed skin (dry or sweaty), red face
- Chills, shivering
- Very high or very low blood pressure
- Confusion, erratic behavior
- Convulsions, loss of consciousness

A heatstroke victim should be cooled as rapidly as possible and immediately transported to a hospital. To lower body temperature, get out of the heat, remove excess clothing, drink cold fluids, and apply cool or damp towels to the body or immerse the body in cold water. People experiencing heatstroke during exercise may still be sweating.

## Cold Weather

In extremely cold conditions, problems can occur if a person's body temperature drops or if particular parts of the body are exposed. If the body's ability to warm itself through shivering or exercise can't keep pace with heat loss, the core body temperature begins to drop. This condition, known as **hypothermia**, depresses the central nervous system, resulting in sleepiness and a lower metabolic rate. As metabolic rate drops, body temperature declines even further, and coma and death can result. The risk of hypothermia is particularly great in cold water.

**Frostbite**—the freezing of body tissues—is another potential danger of exercise in extremely cold conditions. Frostbite most commonly occurs in exposed body parts like earlobes, fingers, and the nose, and it can cause permanent circulatory damage. Hypothermia and frostbite both require immediate medical treatment.

To exercise safely in cold conditions, don't stay out in very cold temperatures for too long. Take both the temperature and the wind into account when planning your exercise session. Frostbite is possible within 30 minutes in calm conditions when the temperature is colder than −5°F, or in windy conditions (30 mph) if the temperature is below 10°F. **Wind chill** values that reflect both the temperature and the wind speed are available as part of a local weather forecast and from the National Weather Service (http://www.weather.gov).

Appropriate clothing provides insulation and helps trap warm air next to the skin. Dress in layers so you can remove them as you warm up and can put them back on if you get cold. A substantial amount of heat loss comes from the head and neck, so keep these areas covered. In subfreezing temperatures, protect the areas of your body most susceptible to frostbite—fingers, toes, ears, nose, and cheeks—with warm socks, mittens or gloves, and a cap, hood, or ski mask. Wear clothing that breathes and will wick moisture away from your skin to avoid being cooled or overheated by trapped perspiration. Many types of comfortable, lightweight clothing that provide good insulation are available. It's also important to warm up thoroughly and to drink plenty of fluids.

| Table 3.7 | Care of Common Exercise Injuries and Discomforts | |
|---|---|---|

| INJURY | SYMPTOMS | TREATMENT |
|---|---|---|
| Blister | Accumulation of fluid in one spot under the skin | Don't pop or drain it unless it interferes too much with your daily activities. If it does pop, clean the area with antiseptic and cover with a bandage. Do not remove the skin covering the blister. |
| Bruise (contusion) | Pain, swelling, and discoloration | R-I-C-E: rest, ice, compression, elevation. |
| Fracture and/or dislocation | Pain, swelling, tenderness, loss of function, and deformity | Seek medical attention, immobilize the affected area, and apply cold. |
| Joint sprain | Pain, tenderness, swelling, discoloration, and loss of function | R-I-C-E; apply heat when swelling has disappeared. Stretch and strengthen affected area. |
| Muscle cramp | Painful, spasmodic muscle contractions | Gently stretch for 15–30 seconds at a time and/or massage the cramped area. Drink fluids and increase dietary salt intake if exercising in hot weather. |
| Muscle soreness or stiffness | Pain and tenderness in the affected muscle | Stretch the affected muscle gently; exercise at a low intensity; apply heat. Nonsteroidal anti-inflammatory drugs, such as ibuprofen, help some people. |
| Muscle strain | Pain, tenderness, swelling, and loss of strength in the affected muscle | R-I-C-E; apply heat when swelling has disappeared. Stretch and strengthen the affected area. |
| Plantar fasciitis | Pain and tenderness in the connective tissue on the bottom of the foot | Apply ice, take nonsteroidal anti-inflammatory drugs, and stretch. Wear night splints when sleeping. |
| Shin splint | Pain and tenderness on the front of the lower leg; sometimes also pain in the calf muscle | Rest; apply ice to the affected area several times a day and before exercise; wrap with tape for support. Stretch and strengthen muscles in the lower legs. Purchase good-quality footwear and run on soft surfaces. |
| Side stitch | Pain on the side of the abdomen | Stretch the arm on the affected side as high as possible; if that doesn't help, try bending forward while tightening the abdominal muscles. |
| Tendinitis | Pain, swelling, and tenderness of the affected area | R-I-C-E; apply heat when swelling has disappeared. Stretch and strengthen the affected area. |

## Poor Air Quality

Air pollution can decrease exercise performance and negatively affect health, particularly if you smoke or have respiratory problems such as asthma, bronchitis, or emphysema. The effects of smog are worse during exercise than at rest because air enters the lungs faster. Polluted air may also contain carbon monoxide, which displaces oxygen in the blood and reduces the amount of oxygen available to working muscles. In a 2007 study, scientists from the ACSM found that exercise in polluted air could decrease lung function to the same extent as heavy smoking. Symptoms of poor air quality include eye and throat irritations, difficulty breathing, and possibly headache and malaise.

Do not exercise outdoors during a smog alert or if air quality is very poor. If you have any type of cardiorespiratory difficulty, you should also avoid exertion outdoors when air quality is poor. You can avoid some smog and air pollution by exercising in indoor facilities, in parks, near water (riverbanks, lakeshores, and ocean beaches), or in residential areas with less traffic (areas with stop-and-go traffic will have lower air quality than areas where traffic moves quickly). Air quality is also usually better in the early morning and late evening, before and after the commute hours.

## Exercise Injuries

Most injuries are annoying rather than serious or permanent. However, an injury that isn't cared for properly can escalate into a chronic problem, sometimes serious enough to permanently curtail the activity. It's important to learn how to deal with injuries so they don't derail your fitness program. Strategies for the care of common exercise injuries and discomforts appear in Table 3.7; some general guidelines are given in the following sections.

**When to Call a Physician** Some injuries require medical attention. Consult a physician for the following:

- Head and eye injuries
- Possible ligament injuries
- Broken bones
- Internal disorders: chest pain, fainting, elevated body temperature, intolerance to hot weather

Also seek medical attention for ostensibly minor injuries that do not get better within a reasonable amount of time. You may need to modify your exercise program for a few weeks to allow an injury to heal.

## Wellness Tip

It may be easy to nurse some injuries yourself, but if you aren't sure what to do, call your doctor.

# Rehabilitation Following a Minor Athletic Injury

- Reduce the initial inflammation using the R-I-C-E principle (see text).

- After 36–48 hours, apply heat *if the swelling has disappeared completely.* Immerse the affected area in warm water or apply warm compresses, a hot water bottle, or a heating pad. As soon as it's comfortable, begin moving the affected joints slowly. If you feel pain, or if the injured area begins to swell again, reduce the amount of movement. Continue gently stretching and moving the affected area until you have regained normal range of motion.

- Gradually begin exercising the injured area to build strength and endurance. Depending on the type of injury, weight training, walking, and resistance training can all be effective.

- Gradually reintroduce the stress of an activity until you can return to full intensity. Don't progress too rapidly or you'll re-injure yourself. Before returning to full exercise participation, you should have a full range of motion in your joints, normal strength and balance among your muscles, normal coordinated patterns of movement (with no injury compensation movements, such as limping), and little or no pain.

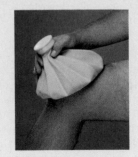

**Managing Minor Exercise Injuries** For minor cuts and scrapes, stop the bleeding and clean the wound. Treat injuries to soft tissue (muscles and joints) with the R-I-C-E principle: rest, ice, compression, and elevation.

- *Rest:* Stop using the injured area as soon as you experience pain. Avoid any activity that causes pain.

- *Ice:* Apply ice to the injured area to reduce swelling and alleviate pain. Apply ice immediately for 10–20 minutes, and repeat every few hours until the swelling disappears. Let the injured part return to normal temperature between icings, and do not apply ice to one area for more than 20 minutes. An easy method for applying ice is to freeze water in a paper cup, peel some of the paper away, and rub the exposed ice on the injured area. If the injured area is large, you can surround it with several bags of crushed ice or ice cubes, or bags of frozen vegetables. Place a thin towel between the bag and your skin. If you use a cold gel pack, limit application time to 10 minutes. Apply ice regularly for 36–48 hours or until the swelling is gone; it may be necessary to apply ice for a week or more if swelling persists.

- *Compression:* Wrap the injured area firmly with an elastic or compression bandage between icings. If the area starts throbbing or begins to change color, the bandage may be wrapped too tightly. Do not sleep with the wrap on.

- *Elevation:* Raise the injured area above heart level to decrease the blood supply and reduce swelling. Use pillows, books, or a low chair or stool to raise the injured area.

The day after the injury, some experts recommend also taking an over-the-counter medication, such as aspirin, ibuprofen, or naproxen, to decrease inflammation. To rehabilitate your body, follow the steps listed in the box "Rehabilitation Following a Minor Athletic Injury."

**Preventing Injuries** The best method for dealing with exercise injuries is to prevent them. If you choose activities for your program carefully and follow the training guidelines described here and in Chapter 2, you should be able to avoid most types of injuries. Important guidelines for preventing athletic injuries include the following:

- Train regularly and stay in condition.

- Gradually increase the intensity, duration, or frequency of your workouts.

- Avoid or minimize high-impact activities; alternate them with low-impact activities.

- Get proper rest between exercise sessions.

- Drink plenty of fluids.

- Warm up thoroughly before you exercise and cool down afterward.

- Achieve and maintain a normal range of motion in your joints.

- Use proper body mechanics when lifting objects or executing sports skills.

- Don't exercise when you are ill or overtrained.

- Use proper equipment, particularly shoes, and choose an appropriate exercise surface. If you exercise on a grass field, soft track, or wooden floor, you are less likely to be injured than on concrete or a hard track. (For information on athletic shoes, see the box "Choosing Exercise Footwear.")

- Don't return to your normal exercise program until any athletic injuries have healed. Restart your program at a lower intensity and gradually increase the amount of overload.

CRITICAL CONSUMER

## Choosing Exercise Footwear

Footwear is perhaps the most important item of equipment for almost any activity. Shoes protect and support your feet and improve your traction. When you jump or run, you place as much as six times more force on your feet than when you stand still. Shoes can help cushion against the stress that this additional force places on your lower legs, thereby preventing injuries. Some athletic shoes are also designed to help prevent ankle rollover, another common source of injury.

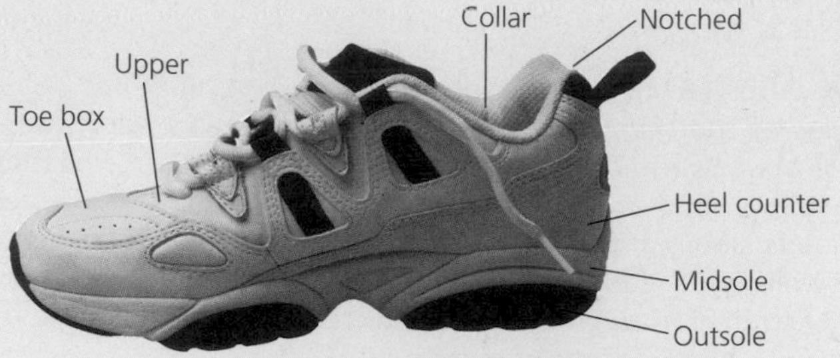

Collar
Notched
Upper
Toe box
Heel counter
Midsole
Outsole


### General Guidelines

When choosing athletic shoes, first consider the activity you've chosen for your exercise program. Shoes appropriate for different activities have very different characteristics.

Foot type is another important consideration. If your feet tend to roll inward excessively, you may need shoes with additional stability features on the inner side of the shoe to counteract this movement. If your feet tend to roll outward excessively, you may need highly flexible and cushioned shoes that promote foot motion. Most women will get a better fit if they choose shoes specifically designed for women's feet rather than downsized versions of men's shoes.

**Successful Shopping** For successful shoe shopping, keep the following strategies in mind:

- Shop late in the day or, ideally, following a workout. Your foot size increases over the course of the day and after exercise.
- Wear socks like those you plan to wear during exercise.
- Try on both shoes and wear them around for 10 or more minutes. Try walking on a noncarpeted surface. Approximate the movements of your activity: walk, jog, run, jump, and so on.
- Check the fit and style carefully:
  - Is the toe box roomy enough? Your toes will spread out when your foot hits the ground or you push off. There should be at least one thumb's width of space from the longest toe to the end of the toe box.
  - Do the shoes have enough cushioning? Do your feet feel supported when you bounce up and down? Try bouncing on your toes and on your heels.
  - Do your heels fit snugly into the shoe? Do they stay put when you walk, or do they slide up?
  - Are the arches of your feet right on top of the shoes' arch supports?
  - Do the shoes feel stable when you twist and turn on the balls of your feet? Try twisting from side to side while standing on one foot.
  - Do you feel any pressure points?
- If you exercise at dawn or dusk, choose shoes with reflective sections for added visibility and safety.
- Replace athletic shoes about every 3 months or 300–500 miles of jogging or walking.

## Ask Yourself

**QUESTIONS FOR CRITICAL THINKING AND REFLECTION**

Have you ever suffered an injury while exercising? If so, how did you treat the injury? Compare your treatment with the guidelines given in this chapter. Did you do the right things? What can you do to avoid such injuries in the future?

## TIPS FOR TODAY AND THE FUTURE

Regular, moderate exercise, even in short bouts spread through the day, can improve cardiorespiratory fitness.

**RIGHT NOW YOU CAN**

- Assess your cardiorespiratory fitness by using one of the methods discussed in this chapter and in Lab 3.1.
- Do a short bout of endurance exercise, such as 10–15 minutes of walking, jogging, or cycling.
- If you have physical activity planned for later in the day, drink some fluids now to make sure you are fully hydrated for your workout.
- Consider the exercise equipment, including shoes, you currently have on hand. If you need new equipment, start researching your options to get the best equipment you can afford.

**IN THE FUTURE YOU CAN**

- Graduate to a different, more challenging fitness assessment as your cardiorespiratory fitness improves.
- Incorporate different types of exercises into your cardiorespiratory endurance training to keep yourself challenged and motivated.

**Q** Do I need a special diet for my endurance exercise program?

**A** No. For most people, a nutritionally balanced diet contains all the energy and nutrients needed to sustain an exercise program. Don't waste your money on unnecessary supplements. (Chapter 8 provides detailed information about putting together a healthy diet.)

**Q** How can I measure how far I walk or run?

**A** The simplest and cheapest way to measure distance is with a pedometer, which counts your steps. Although stride length varies among individuals, 2000 steps typically equals about 1 mile, and 10,000 steps equals about 5 miles. To track your distance and your progress using a pedometer, follow the guidelines in Lab 2.3.

**Q** How can I avoid being so sore when I start an exercise program?

**A** Postexercise muscle soreness is caused by muscle injury followed by muscle inflammation. Muscles get stronger and larger in response to muscle tension and injury. However, excessive injury can delay progress. The best approach is to begin conservatively with low-volume, low-intensity workouts, and gradually increase the severity of the exercise sessions. If you are currently sedentary, begin with 5 to 10 minutes of exercise and gradually increase the distance and speed you walk, run, cycle, or swim.

**Q** Is it OK to do cardiorespiratory endurance exercise while menstruating?

**A** Yes. There is no evidence that exercise during menstruation is unhealthy or that it has negative effects on performance. If you have headaches, backaches, and abdominal pain during menstruation, you may not feel like exercising. For some women, exercise helps relieve these symptoms. Listen to your body and exercise at whatever intensity is comfortable for you.

**Q** Will high altitude affect my ability to exercise?

**A** At high altitudes (above 1500 meters, or about 4900 feet), there is less oxygen available in the air than at lower altitudes. High altitude doesn't affect anaerobic exercise, such as stretching and weight lifting, but it does affect aerobic activities—that is, any type of cardiovascular endurance exercise—because the heart and lungs have to work harder, even when the body is at rest, to deliver enough oxygen to body cells. The increased cardiovascular strain of exercise reduces endurance. To play it safe when at high altitudes, avoid heavy exercise—at least for the first few days—and drink plenty of water. And don't expect to reach your normal lower-altitude exercise capacity.

*For more Common Questions Answered about endurance training, visit the Online Learning Center at www.mhhe.com/fahey.*

## SUMMARY

• The cardiorespiratory system consists of the heart, blood vessels, and respiratory system; it picks up and transports oxygen, nutrients, and waste products.

• The body takes chemical energy from food and uses it to produce ATP and fuel cellular activities. ATP is stored in the body's cells as the basic form of energy.

• During exercise, the body supplies ATP and fuels cellular activities by combining three energy systems: immediate, for short periods of activity; nonoxidative (anaerobic), for intense activity; and oxidative (aerobic), for prolonged activity. Which energy system predominates depends on the duration and intensity of the activity.

• Cardiorespiratory endurance exercise improves cardiorespiratory functioning and cellular metabolism; it reduces the risk of chronic diseases such as heart disease, cancer, type 2 diabetes, obesity, and osteoporosis; and it improves immune function and psychological and emotional well-being.

• Cardiorespiratory fitness is measured by determining how well the cardiorespiratory system transports and uses oxygen. The upper limit of this measure, called maximal oxygen consumption, or $\dot{V}O_{2max}$, can be measured precisely in a laboratory, or it can be estimated reasonably well through self-assessment tests.

• To create a successful exercise program, set realistic goals, choose suitable activities, begin slowly, and always warm up and cool down. As fitness improves, exercise more often, longer, and/or harder.

• Intensity of training can be measured through target heart rate zone, METs, ratings of perceived exertion, or the talk test.

• With careful attention to fluid intake, clothing, duration of exercise, and exercise intensity, endurance training can be safe in hot and cold weather conditions.

- Serious injuries require medical attention. Application of the R-I-C-E principle (rest, ice, compression, elevation) is appropriate for treating many types of muscle or joint injuries.

## FOR FURTHER EXPLORATION

### BOOKS

American College of Sports Medicine. 2003. *ACSM Fitness Book.* 3rd ed. Champaign, Ill.: Human Kinetics. *Includes fitness assessment tests and advice on creating a complete fitness program.*

Centers for Disease Control and Prevention. 2010. *Promoting Physical Activity: A Guide for Community Action*, 2nd ed. Champaign, Ill.: Human Kinetics. *Presents a guide for community action that offers the tools and information you need to help people become more active.*

Coffman, S. 2007. *Successful Programs for Fitness and Health Clubs.* Champaign, Ill.: Human Kinetics. *Presents more than 100 ready-to-use programs for fitness centers, group exercise studios, pools, gyms, and classrooms.*

Edwards, S., and S. Reed. 2006. *Heart Zones Cycling: The Avid Cyclist's Guide to Riding Faster and Farther.* Boulder, Colo: VeloPress. *An excellent guide to using heart rate in endurance training written by a top athlete and scientist.*

Fenton, M. 2008. *The Complete Guide to Walking, New and Revised: For Health, Weight Loss, and Fitness.* Guilford, Conn.: Lyons Press. *Discusses walking as a fitness method and a way to avoid diseases such as diabetes.*

Gotlin, R. 2007. *Sports Injuries Guidebook.* Champaign, Ill.: Human Kinetics. *Provides information and care instructions on many types of sports-related injuries.*

Howley, E. T., and B. D. Franks. 2007. *Fitness Professional's Handbook*, 5th ed. Champaign, Ill.: Human Kinetics. *A comprehensive manual on physical training for professionals and people interested in exercise and sports.*

Maffetone, P. 2010. *The Big Book of Endurance Training and Racing.* New York: Skyhorse Publishing. *An excellent book for people of all levels interested in running, swimming, cycling, and triathlon.*

Marcus, B. H., and L. A. Forsyth. 2009. *Motivating People to be Physically Active*, 2nd ed. Champaign, Ill.: Human Kinetics. *Describes methods for helping people increase their level of physical activity.*

Nieman, D. C. 2010. *Exercise Testing and Prescription: A Health-Related Approach*, 7th ed. New York: McGraw-Hill. *A comprehensive discussion of the effect of exercise and exercise testing and prescription.*

Richmond, M. 2011. *The Physiology Storybook: An Owner's Manual for the Human Body.* Monterey, Calif.: Healthy Learning. *A discussion of human physiology and wellness written for the average person.*

Rothman, J., and T. LaFontaine. 2011. *The Exercise Professional's Guide to Optimizing Health: Strategies for Preventing and Reducing Chronic Disease.* Baltimore: Lippincott Williams & Wilkins. *Written for professionals in association with the American College of Sports Medicine, the book describes how exercise can help prevent and treat chronic disease.*

## ORGANIZATIONS AND WEB SITES

*American Academy of Orthopaedic Surgeons: Sports and Exercise.* Provides fact sheets on many fitness and sports topics, including how to begin a program, how to choose equipment, and how to prevent and treat many types of injuries.

http://orthoinfo.aaos.org/menus/sports.cfm

*American Cancer Society: Staying Active.* Provides tools for managing an exercise program and discusses the links between cancer and lifestyle, including the importance of physical activity in preventing some cancers.

http://www.cancer.org/docroot/PED/ped_6.asp?sitearea-PED

*American Heart Association: Exercise and Fitness.* Provides information on cardiovascular health and disease, including the role of exercise in maintaining heart health and exercise tips for people of all ages.

http://www.americanheart.org/presenter.jhtml?identifier_1200013

*Centers for Disease Control and Prevention: Physical Activity for Everyone.* Explains the latest government recommendations on exercise and physical activity and provides strategies for getting the appropriate type and amount of exercise.

http://www.cdc.gov/physicalactivity/everyone/guidelines/adults.html

*Dr. Pribut's Running Injuries Page.* Provides information about running and many types of running injuries.

http://www.drpribut.com/sports/spsport.html

*The Human Heart.* An online museum exhibit with information on the structure and function of the heart, blood vessels, and respiratory system.

http://www.fi.edu/learn/heart/index.html

*President's Challenge Adult Fitness Test: Aerobics.* Provides step-by-step instructions for taking and interpreting standard tests of aerobic fitness.

http://www.adultfitnesstest.org/testInstructions/aerobicFitness/default.aspx

*Runner's World Online.* Contains a wide variety of information about running, including tips for beginning runners, advice about training, and a shoe buyer's guide.

http://www.runnersworld.com

*Weight Control Information Network: Walking.* An online fact sheet that explains the benefits of walking for exercise, tips for starting a walking program, and techniques for getting the most from walking workouts.

http://win.niddk.nih.gov/publications/walking.htm

*Women's Sports Foundation.* Provides information and links about training and about many specific sports activities.

http://www.womenssportsfoundation.org

## SELECTED BIBLIOGRAPHY

Adler, P. A., and B. L. Roberts. 2009. The use of Tai Chi to improve health in older adults. *Orthopedic Nursing* 25(2): 122–126.

American College of Sports Medicine. 2009. *ACSM's Resource Manual for Guidelines for Exercise Testing and Prescription*, 6th ed. Philadelphia: Lippincott Williams and Wilkins.

American College of Sports Medicine. 2009. *ACSM's Guidelines for Exercise Testing and Prescription,* 8th ed. Philadelphia: Lippincott Williams and Wilkins.

American Heart Association. 2010. *Heart Disease and Stroke Statistics—2010 Update.* Dallas: American Heart Association.

Brooks, G. A., et al. 2005. *Exercise Physiology: Human Bioenergetics and Its Applications,* 4th ed. New York: McGraw-Hill.

Budde H., et al. 2008. Acute coordinative exercise improves attentional performance in adolescents. *Neuroscience Letters* 441(2): 219–223.

Cadore, E. L., et al. 2011. Effects of strength, endurance, and concurrent training on aerobic power and dynamic neuromuscular economy in elderly men. *J Strength Conditioning Research* 25(3): 758–766.

Courneya, K. S., and C. M. Friedenreich. 2011. Physical activity and cancer: an introduction. *Recent Results Cancer Research.* 186: 1–10.

Denadai, B. S., et al. 2006. Interval training at 95% and 100% of the velocity at $\dot{V}O_{2max}$: Effects on aerobic physiological indexes and running performance. *Applied Physiology, Nutrition, and Metabolism* 31(6): 737–743.

Erickson, K. I., et al. 2011. Exercise training increases size of hippocampus and improves memory. *Proceedings of the National Academy of Sciences.* 108(7): 3017–3022.

Garber, C. E., et al. 2011. Quantity and quality of exercise for developing and maintaining cardiorespiratory, musculoskeletal, and neuromotor fitness in apparently healthy adults: Guidance for prescribing exercise. *Medicine and Science in Sport and Exercise* 43(7):1334–1359.

Haskell, W. L., et al. 2007. Physical activity and public health: Updated recommendation for adults from the American College of Sports Medicine and the American Heart Association. *Medicine and Science in Sport and Exercise* 39(8): 1423–1434.

Hautala, A. J., et al. 2009. Individual responses to aerobic exercise: The role of the autonomic nervous system. *Neuroscience and Biobehavioral Reviews* 33(2): 107–115.

Keller, P., et al. 2011. A transcriptional map of the impact of endurance exercise training on skeletal muscle phenotype. *Journal of Applied Physiology* 110(1): 46–59.

Moien-Afshari, F., et al. 2009. Exercise restores endothelial function independently of weight loss or hyperglycaemic status in db/db mice. *Diabetologia* 51(7): 1327–1337.

Morikawa, M., et al. 2011. Physical fitness and indices of lifestyle-related diseases before and after interval walking training in middle-aged and older males and females. *British Journal Sports Medicine* 45(3): 216–224.

Murphy, M. H., et al. 2009. Accumulated versus continuous exercise for health benefit: A review of empirical studies. *Sports Medicine* 39(1): 29–43.

Netz, Y. T., et al. 2011. Aerobic fitness and multi-domain cognitive function in advanced age. *International Psychogeriatrics.* 23(1): 114–124.

Okura, T., et al. 2006. Effect of regular exercise on homocysteine concentrations: The HERITAGE Family Study. *European Journal of Applied Physiology* 98(4): 394–401.

Physical Activity Guidelines Advisory Committee. 2008. *Physical Activity Guidelines Advisory Committee Report, 2008.* Washington, D.C.: U.S. Department of Health and Human Services.

Ploughman, M. 2008. Exercise is brain food: The effects of physical activity on cognitive function. *Developmental Neurorehabilitation* 11(3): 236–240.

Reigle, B. S., and K. Wonders. 2009. Breast cancer and the role of exercise in women. *Methods in Molecular Biology* 472(1): 169–189.

Ruiz, J. R., et al. 2011. Strenuous endurance exercise improves life expectancy: It's in our genes. *British Journal of Sports Medicine* 45(3): 159–161.

Sui, X., et al. 2008. A prospective study of cardiorespiratory fitness and risk of type 2 diabetes in women. *Diabetes Care* 31(3): 550–555.

Suominen, H. 2006. Muscle training for bone strength. *Aging Clinical and Experimental Research* 18(2): 85–93.

U.S. Department of Health and Human Services. 2008. *Physical Activity Guidelines for Americans.* Washington, D.C.: U.S. Department of Health and Human Services.

Waterhouse, J., et al. 2010. Effects of music tempo upon submaximal cycling performance. *Scandinavian Journal of Medicine and Science in Sports* 20(4): 662–669.

Yeo, W. K., et al. 2011. Fat adaptation in well-trained athletes: effects on cell metabolism. *Applied Physiology Nutrition Metabolism* 36(1): 12–22.

Yung, L. M., et al. 2009. Exercise, vascular wall and cardiovascular diseases: An update (part 2). *Sports Medicine* 39(1): 45–63.

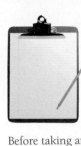

## LAB 3.1 Assessing Your Current Level of Cardiorespiratory Endurance

Before taking any of the cardiorespiratory endurance assessment tests, refer to the fitness prerequisites and cautions given in Table 3.2. Choose one of the following four tests presented in this lab:

- 1-mile walk test
- 3-minute step test
- 1.5-mile run-walk test
- 12-minute swim test

For best results, don't exercise strenuously or consume caffeine the day of the test, and don't smoke or eat a heavy meal within about 3 hours of the test.

### The 1-Mile Walk Test

#### Equipment

1. A track or course that provides a measurement of 1 mile
2. A stopwatch, clock, or watch with a second hand
3. A weight scale

#### Preparation

Measure your body weight (in pounds) before taking the test.

Body weight: _____ lb

#### Instructions

1. Warm up before taking the test. Do some walking, easy jogging, or calisthenics.
2. Cover the 1-mile course as quickly as possible. Walk at a pace that is brisk but comfortable. You must raise your heart rate above 120 beats per minute (bpm).
3. As soon as you complete the distance, note your time and take your pulse for 10 seconds.

   Walking time: _____ min _____ sec

   10-second pulse count: _____ beats
4. Cool down after the test by walking slowly for several minutes.

#### Determining Maximal Oxygen Consumption

1. Convert your 10-second pulse count into a value for exercise heart rate by multiplying it by 6.

   Exercise heart rate: _____ × 6 = _____ bpm
2. Convert your walking time from minutes and seconds to a decimal figure. For example, a time of 14 minutes and 45 seconds would be 14 + (45/60), or 14.75 minutes.

   Walking time: _____ min + (_____ sec ÷ 60 sec/min) = _____ min
3. Insert values for your age, gender, weight, walking time, and exercise heart rate in the following equation, where

   W = your weight (in pounds)

   A = your age (in years)

   G = your gender (male = 1; female = 0)

   T = your time to complete the 1-mile course (in minutes)

   H = your exercise heart rate (in beats per minute)

   $\dot{V}O_{2max} = 132.853 - (0.0769 \times W) - (0.3877 \times A) + (6.315 \times G) - (3.2649 \times T) - (0.1565 \times H)$

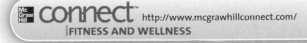

*For example, a 20-year-old, 190-pound male with a time of 14.75 minutes and an exercise heart rate of 152 bpm would calculate maximal oxygen consumption as follows:*

$$\dot{V}O_{2max} = 132.853 - (0.0769 \times 190) - (0.3877 \times 20) + (6.315 \times 1) - (3.2649 \times 14.75) - (0.1565 \times 152) = 45 \ ml/kg/min$$

$$\dot{V}O_{2max} = 132.853 - (0.0769 \times \underline{\hspace{2cm}}) - (0.3877 \times \underline{\hspace{2cm}}) + (6.315 \times \underline{\hspace{2cm}})$$
$$\underset{\text{weight (lb)}}{} \qquad \underset{\text{age (years)}}{} \qquad \underset{\text{gender}}{}$$

$$- (3.2649 \times \underline{\hspace{2cm}}) - (0.1565 \times \underline{\hspace{2cm}}) = \underline{\hspace{2cm}} ml/kg/min$$
$$\underset{\text{walking time (min)}}{} \qquad \underset{\text{exercise heart rate (bpm)}}{}$$

4. Copy this value for $\dot{V}O_{2max}$ into the appropriate place in the chart on page 92.

## The 3-Minute Step Test

### Equipment

1. A step, bench, or bleacher step that is 16.25 inches from ground level

2. A stopwatch, clock, or watch with a second hand

3. A metronome

### Preparation

Practice stepping up onto and down from the step before you begin the test. Each step has four beats: up-up-down-down. Males should perform the test with the metronome set for a rate of 96 beats per minute, or 24 steps per minute. Females should set the metronome at 88 beats per minute, or 22 steps per minute.

### Instructions

1. Warm up before taking the test. Do some walking or easy jogging.

2. Set the metronome at the proper rate. Your instructor or a partner can call out starting and stopping times; otherwise, have a clock or watch within easy viewing during the test.

3. Begin the test and continue to step at the correct pace for 3 minutes.

4. Stop after 3 minutes. Remain standing and count your pulse for the 15-second period from 5 to 20 seconds into recovery.

   15-second pulse count: _____ beats

5. Cool down after the test by walking slowly for several minutes.

### Determining Maximal Oxygen Consumption

1. Convert your 15-second pulse count to a value for recovery heart rate by multiplying by 4.

   Recovery heart rate: $\underset{\text{bpm 15-sec pulse count}}{\underline{\hspace{3cm}}} \times 4 = \underline{\hspace{3cm}}$

2. Insert your recovery heart rate in the equation below, where

   $H$ = recovery heart rate (in beats per minute)

   Males: $\dot{V}O_{2max} = 111.33 - (0.42 \times H)$

   Females: $\dot{V}O_{2max} = 65.81 - (0.1847 \times H)$

   *For example, a man with a recovery heart rate of 162 bpm would calculate maximal oxygen consumption as follows:*

   $$\dot{V}O_{2max} = 111.33 - (0.42 \times 162) = 43 \ ml/kg/min$$

   **Males:** $\dot{V}O_{2max} = 111.33 - (0.42 \times \underset{\text{recovery heart rate (bpm)}}{\underline{\hspace{3cm}}}) = \underline{\hspace{3cm}} ml/kg/min$

   **Females:** $\dot{V}O_{2max} = 65.81 - (0.1847 \times \underset{\text{recovery heart rate (bpm)}}{\underline{\hspace{3cm}}}) = \underline{\hspace{3cm}} ml/kg/min$

3. Copy this value for $\dot{V}O_{2max}$ into the appropriate place in the chart on page 92.

## The 1.5-Mile Run-Walk Test

### Equipment

1. A running track or course that is flat and provides exact measurements of up to 1.5 miles

2. A stopwatch, clock, or watch with a second hand

### Preparation

You may want to practice pacing yourself prior to taking the test to avoid going too fast at the start and becoming prematurely fatigued. Allow yourself a day or two to recover from your practice run before taking the test.

### Instructions

1. Warm up before taking the test. Do some walking or easy jogging.

2. Try to cover the distance as fast as possible without overexerting yourself. If possible, monitor your own time, or have someone call out your time at various intervals of the test to determine whether your pace is correct.

3. Record the amount of time, in minutes and seconds, it takes you to complete the 1.5-mile distance.

   Running-walking time: _____ min _____ sec

4. Cool down after the test by walking or jogging slowly for about 5 minutes.

### Determining Maximal Oxygen Consumption

1. Convert your running time from minutes and seconds to a decimal figure. For example, a time of 14 minutes and 25 seconds would be 14 + (25/60), or 14.4 minutes.

   Running-walking time: _____ min + (_____ sec ÷ 60 sec/min) = _____ min

2. Insert your running time into the equation below, where

   $T$ = running time (in minutes)

   $\dot{V}O_{2max} = (483 \div T) + 3.5$

   *For example, a person who completes 1.5 miles in 14.4 minutes would calculate maximal oxygen consumption as follows:*

   $\dot{V}O_{2max} = (483 \div 14.4) + 3.5 = 37$ *ml/kg/min*

   $\dot{V}O_{2max} = (483 \div \underline{\phantom{xxxxxxx}}_{\text{run-walk time (min)}}) + 3.5 = \underline{\phantom{xxxxxxx}}$ **ml/kg/min**

3. Copy this value for $\dot{V}O_{2max}$ into the appropriate place in the chart on page 92.

### Rating Your Cardiovascular Fitness

Record your $\dot{V}O_{2max}$ score(s) and the corresponding fitness rating from the table below.

| Women | Very Poor | Poor | Fair | Good | Excellent | Superior |
|---|---|---|---|---|---|---|
| Age: 18–29 | Below 31.6 | 31.6–35.4 | 35.5–39.4 | 39.5–43.9 | 44.0–50.1 | Above 50.1 |
| 30–39 | Below 29.9 | 29.9–33.7 | 33.8–36.7 | 36.8–40.9 | 41.0–46.8 | Above 46.8 |
| 40–49 | Below 28.0 | 28.0–31.5 | 31.6–35.0 | 35.1–38.8 | 38.9–45.1 | Above 45.1 |
| 50–59 | Below 25.5 | 25.5–28.6 | 28.7–31.3 | 31.4–35.1 | 35.2–39.8 | Above 39.8 |
| 60–69 | Below 23.7 | 23.7–26.5 | 26.6–29.0 | 29.1–32.2 | 32.3–36.8 | Above 36.8 |
| **Men** | | | | | | |
| Age: 18–29 | Below 38.1 | 38.1–42.1 | 42.2–45.6 | 45.7–51.0 | 51.1–56.1 | Above 56.1 |
| 30–39 | Below 36.7 | 36.7–40.9 | 41.0–44.3 | 44.4–48.8 | 48.9–54.2 | Above 54.2 |
| 40–49 | Below 34.6 | 34.6–38.3 | 38.4–42.3 | 42.4–46.7 | 46.8–52.8 | Above 52.8 |
| 50–59 | Below 31.1 | 31.1–35.1 | 35.2–38.2 | 38.3–43.2 | 43.3–49.6 | Above 49.6 |
| 60–69 | Below 27.4 | 27.4–31.3 | 31.4–34.9 | 35.0–39.4 | 39.5–46.0 | Above 46.0 |

**SOURCE:** Ratings based on norms from The Cooper Institute of Aerobic Research, Dallas, Texas; from *The Physical Fitness Specialist Manual*, Revised 2002. Used with permission.

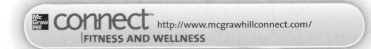

| | $\dot{V}O_{2max}$ | Cardiovascular Fitness Rating |
|---|---|---|
| 1-mile walk test | | |
| 3-minute step test | | |
| 1.5-mile run-walk test | | |

## The 12-Minute Swim Test

If you enjoy swimming and prefer to build a cardiorespiratory training program around this type of exercise, you can assess your cardiorespiratory endurance by taking the 12-minute swim test. You will receive a rating based on the distance you can swim in 12 minutes. A complete fitness program based on swimming is presented in Chapter 7.

Note, however, that this test is appropriate only for relatively strong swimmers who are confident in the water. If you are unsure about your swimming ability, this test may not be appropriate for you. If necessary, ask your school's swim coach or a qualified swimming instructor to evaluate your ability in the water before attempting this test.

### Equipment

1. A swimming pool that provides measurements in yards
2. A wall clock that is clearly visible from the pool, or someone with a watch who can time you

### Preparation

You may want to practice pacing yourself before taking the test to avoid going too fast at the start and becoming prematurely fatigued. Allow yourself a day or two to recover from your practice swim before taking the test.

### Instructions

1. Warm up before taking the test. Do some walking or light jogging before getting in the pool. Once in the water, swim a lap or two at an easy pace to make sure your muscles are warm and you are comfortable.
2. Try to cover the distance as fast as possible without overexerting yourself. If possible, monitor your own time, or have someone call out your time at various intervals of the test to determine whether your pace is correct.
3. Record the distance, in yards, that you were able to cover during the 12-minute period.
4. Cool down after the test by swimming a lap or two at an easy pace.
5. Use the following chart to gauge your level of cardiorespiratory fitness.

**DISTANCE IN YARDS**

| Women | *Needs Work* | *Better* | *Fair* | *Good* | *Excellent* |
|---|---|---|---|---|---|
| Age: 13–19 | Below 500 | 500–599 | 600–699 | 700–799 | Above 800 |
| 20–29 | Below 400 | 400–499 | 500–599 | 600–699 | Above 700 |
| 30–39 | Below 350 | 350–449 | 450–549 | 550–649 | Above 650 |
| 40–49 | Below 300 | 300–399 | 400–499 | 500–599 | Above 600 |
| 50–59 | Below 250 | 250–349 | 350–449 | 450–549 | Above 550 |
| 60 and over | Below 250 | 250–299 | 300–399 | 400–499 | Above 500 |
| **Men** | | | | | |
| Age: 13–19 | Below 400 | 400–499 | 500–599 | 600–699 | Above 700 |
| 20–29 | Below 300 | 300–399 | 400–499 | 500–599 | Above 600 |
| 30–39 | Below 250 | 250–349 | 350–449 | 450–549 | Above 550 |
| 40–49 | Below 200 | 200–299 | 300–399 | 400–499 | Above 500 |
| 50–59 | Below 150 | 150–249 | 250–349 | 350–449 | Above 450 |
| 60 and over | Below 150 | 150–199 | 200–299 | 300–399 | Above 400 |

**100 yards = 91 meters**

**SOURCE:** Cooper, K. H. 1982. *The Aerobics Program for Total Well-Being.* New York: Bantam Books.

Record your fitness rating:

| | Cardiovascular Fitness Rating |
|---|---|
| 12-minute swim test | |

## Using Your Results

*How did you score?* Are you surprised by your rating for cardiovascular fitness? Are you satisfied with your current rating?

If you're not satisfied, set a realistic goal for improvement: _____

_____

Are you satisfied with your current level of cardiovascular fitness as evidenced in your daily life—your ability to walk, run, bicycle, climb stairs, do yard work, or engage in recreational activities?

If you're not satisfied, set some realistic goals for improvement, such as completing a 5K run or 25-mile bike ride: _____

_____

*What should you do next?* Enter the results of this lab in the Preprogram Assessment column in Appendix C. If you've set goals for improvement, begin planning your cardiorespiratory endurance exercise program by completing the plan in Lab 3.2. After several weeks of your program, complete this lab again, and enter the results in the Postprogram Assessment column of Appendix C. How do the results compare? (Remember, it's best to compare $\dot{V}O_{2max}$ scores for the same test.)

**SOURCES:** Brooks, G. A., and T. D. Fahey. 1987. *Fundamentals of Human Performance.* New York: Macmillan. Kline, G. M., et al. 1987. Estimation of $\dot{V}O_{2max}$ from a one-mile track walk, gender, age, and body weight. *Medicine and Science in Sports and Exercise* 19(3): 253–259. McArdle, W. D., F. I. Katch, and V. L. Katch. 2010. *Exercise Physiology-. Energy, Nutrition, and Human Peformance.* Philadelphia: Lea and Febiger, pp. 243–246.

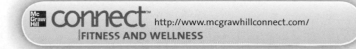

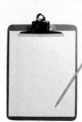

## LAB 3.2 Developing an Exercise Program for Cardiorespiratory Endurance

1. *Goals.* List goals for your cardiorespiratory endurance exercise program. Your goals can be specific or general, short or long term. In the first section, include specific, measurable goals that you can use to track the progress of your fitness program. These goals might be things like raising your cardiorespiratory fitness rating from fair to good or swimming laps for 30 minutes without resting. In the second section, include long-term and more qualitative goals, such as improving self-confidence and reducing your risk for chronic disease.

Specific Goals: Current Status                                        Final Goals

_____          _____

_____          _____

_____          _____

Other goals: _____

_____

2. *Type of Activities.* Choose one or more endurance activities for your program. These can include any activity that uses large-muscle groups, can be maintained continuously, and is rhythmic and aerobic in nature. Examples include walking, jogging, cycling, group exercise such as aerobic dance, rowing, rope skipping, stair-climbing, cross-country skiing, swimming, skating, and endurance game activities such as soccer and tennis. Choose activities that are both convenient and enjoyable. Fill in the activity names on the program plan.

3. *Frequency.* On the program plan, fill in how often you plan to participate in each activity; the ACSM recommends participating in cardiorespiratory endurance exercise 3-5 days per week.

### Program Plan

| Type of Activity | Frequency (check ✓) | | | | | | | Intensity (bpm or RPE) | Time (min) |
|---|---|---|---|---|---|---|---|---|---|
| | M | T | W | Th | F | Sa | Su | | |
| | | | | | | | | | |
| | | | | | | | | | |
| | | | | | | | | | |
| | | | | | | | | | |

4. *Intensity.* Determine your exercise intensity using one of the following methods, and enter it on the program plan. Begin your program at a lower intensity and slowly increase intensity as your fitness improves, so select a range of intensities for your program,

a. Target heart rate zone: Calculate target heart rate zone in beats per minute and then calculate the corresponding 10-second exercise count by dividing the total count by 6. For example, the 10-second exercise counts corresponding to a target heart rate zone of 122–180 bpm would be 20–30 beats.

Maximum heart rate: 220 − _____ = _____ bpm
                                         age (years)

### Maximum Heart Rate Method

65% training intensity = _____ bpm × 0.65 = _____ bpm
                                  maximum heart rate

90% training intensity = _____ bpm × 0.90 = _____ bpm
                                  maximum heart rate

**Target heart rate zone = _____ to _____ bpm      10-second count = _____ to _____**

Mc Graw Hill connect http://www.mcgrawhillconnect.com/
FITNESS AND WELLNESS

*Heart Rate Reserve Method*

Resting heart rate:_____ bpm (taken after 10 minutes of complete rest)

Heart rate reserve = _____ bpm − _____ bpm = _____ bpm
        maximum heart rate                    resting heart rate

50% training intensity = ( _____ bpm × 0.50) + _____ bpm = _____ bpm
                    heart rate reserve                       resting heart rate

85% training intensity = ( _____ bpm × 0.85) + _____ bpm = _____ bpm
                    heart rate reserve                       resting heart rate

**Target heart rate zone** = _____ to _____ **bpm**

**10-second count** = _____ to _____

b. Ratings of perceived exertion (RPE): If you prefer, determine an RPE value that corresponds to your target heart rate range (see p. 76 and Figure 3.5).

5. *Time (Duration).* A total time of 20–60 minutes is recommended; your duration of exercise will vary with intensity. For developing cardiorespiratory endurance, higher-intensity activities can be performed for a shorter duration; lower intensities require a longer duration. Enter a duration (or a range of duration) on the program plan.

6. *Monitoring Your Program.* Complete a log like the one below to monitor your program and track your progress. Note the date on top, and fill in the intensity and time (duration) for each workout. If you prefer, you can also track other variables such as distance. For example, if your cardiorespiratory endurance program includes walking and swimming, you may want to track miles walked and yards swum in addition to the duration of each exercise session.

| Activity/Date | | | | | | | | | | | | | | |
|---|---|---|---|---|---|---|---|---|---|---|---|---|---|---|
| 1 | Intentsity | | | | | | | | | | | | | |
| | Time | | | | | | | | | | | | | |
| | Distance | | | | | | | | | | | | | |
| 2 | Intentsity | | | | | | | | | | | | | |
| | Time | | | | | | | | | | | | | |
| | Distance | | | | | | | | | | | | | |
| 3 | Intentsity | | | | | | | | | | | | | |
| | Time | | | | | | | | | | | | | |
| | Distance | | | | | | | | | | | | | |
| 4 | Intentsity | | | | | | | | | | | | | |
| | Time | | | | | | | | | | | | | |
| | Distance | | | | | | | | | | | | | |

7. *Making Progress.* Follow the guidelines in the chapter and Table 3.6 to slowly increase the amount of overload in your program. Continue keeping a log, and periodically evaluate your progress.

**Progress Checkup: Week _____ of program**

Goals: Original Status                                    Current Status

_____          _____

_____          _____

_____          _____

List each activity in your program and describe how satisfied you are with the activity and with your overall progress. List any problems you've encountered or any unexpected costs or benefits of your fitness program so far.

# CHAPTER 4

# Muscular Strength and Endurance

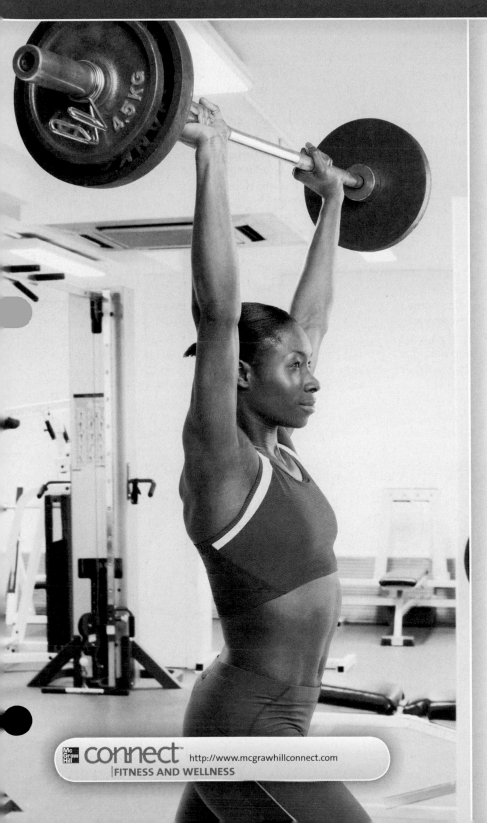

## LOOKING AHEAD...

After reading this chapter, you should be able to:

- Describe the basic physiology of muscles and explain how strength training affects muscles
- Define muscular strength and endurance, and describe how they relate to wellness
- Assess muscular strength and endurance
- Apply the FITT principle to create a safe and successful strength training program
- Describe the effects of supplements and drugs that are marketed to active people and athletes
- Explain how to safely perform common strength training exercises using free weights and weight machines

## TEST YOUR KNOWLEDGE

1. For women, weight training typically results in which of the following?
   a. bulky muscles
   b. significant increases in body weight
   c. improved body image

2. To maximize strength gains, it is a good idea to hold your breath as you lift a weight. True or false?

3. Regular strength training is associated with which of the following benefits?
   a. denser bones
   b. reduced risk of heart disease
   c. improved body composition
   d. fewer injuries
   e. improved metabolic health
   f. Increased longevity

**Answers**

1. **c.** Because the vast majority of women have low levels of testosterone, they do not develop large muscles or gain significant amounts of weight in response to a moderate-intensity weight training program. Men have higher levels of testosterone, so they can build large muscles more easily.

2. **False.** Holding one's breath while lifting weights can significantly elevate blood pressure; it also reduces blood flow to the heart and may cause faintness. You should breathe smoothly and normally while weight training. Some experts recommend that you exhale during the most difficult part of each exercise.

3. **All six.** Regular strength training has many benefits for both men and women.

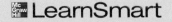

**M**uscles make up more than 40% of your body mass. You depend on them for movement, and, because of their mass, they are the site of a large portion of the energy reactions (metabolism) that take place in your body. Strong, well-developed muscles help you perform daily activities with greater ease, protect you from injury, and enhance your well-being in other ways.

As described in Chapter 2, muscular strength is the amount of force a muscle can produce with a single maximum effort; muscular endurance is the ability to hold or repeat a muscular contraction for a long time. This chapter explains the benefits of strength training (also called *resistance training* or *weight training*) and describes methods of assessing muscular strength and endurance. It then explains the basics of strength training and provides guidelines for setting up your own training program. The musculoskeletal system is depicted on pages T4-2 and T4-3 of the color transparency insert "Touring the Musculoskeletal System" in this chapter. You can refer to this illustration as you set up your program.

## BASIC MUSCLE PHYSIOLOGY AND THE EFFECTS OF STRENGTH TRAINING

Muscles move the body and enable it to exert force because they move the skeleton. When a muscle contracts (shortens), it moves a bone by pulling on the tendon that attaches the muscle to the bone, as shown in Figure 4.1. When a muscle relaxes (lengthens), the tension placed on the tendon is released and the bone moves back to—or closer to—its starting position.

## Muscle Fibers

Muscles consist of individual muscle cells, or **muscle fibers,** connected in bundles (see Figure 4.1). A single muscle is made up of many bundles of muscle fibers and is covered by layers of connective tissue that hold the fibers together. Muscle fibers, in turn, are made up of smaller protein structures called **myofibrils.** Myofibrils are made up of a series of contractile units called *sarcomeres,* which are composed largely of actin and myosin molecules. Muscle cells contract when the myosin molecules glide across the actin molecules in a ratchetlike movement.

Strength training increases the size and number of myofibrils, resulting in larger individual muscle fibers. Larger muscle fibers mean a larger and stronger muscle. The development of large muscle fibers is called **hypertrophy;** inactivity causes **atrophy,** the reversal of this process. For a depiction of the process of hypertrophy, see page T4-4 of the color transparency insert "Touring the Musculoskeletal System" in this chapter. In some species, muscles can increase in size through a separate process called **hyperplasia,** which involves an increase in the number of muscle fibers rather than the size of muscle fibers. In humans, hyperplasia is not thought to play a significant role in determining muscle size. Each muscle cell has many **nuclei** containing genes that direct the production of enzymes and structural proteins required for muscle contraction.

Muscle fibers are classified as slow-twitch or fast-twitch fibers according to their strength, speed of contraction, and energy source.

- **Slow-twitch muscle fibers** are relatively fatigue-resistant, but they don't contract as rapidly or strongly as fast-twitch fibers. The principal energy system that fuels slow-twitch fibers is aerobic (oxidative). Slow-twitch muscle fibers are typically reddish in color.

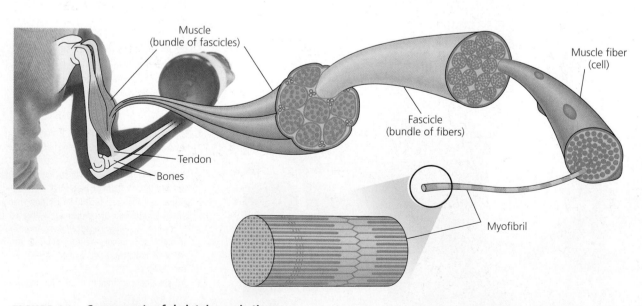

**FIGURE 4.1   Components of skeletal muscle tissue.**

### Table 4.1 — Physiological Changes and Benefits from Strength Training

| CHANGE | BENEFITS |
| --- | --- |
| Increased muscle mass* and strength | Increased muscular strength<br>Improved body composition<br>Higher rate of metabolism<br>Improved capacity to regulate fuel use with aging<br>Toned, healthy-looking muscles<br>Increased longevity<br>Improved quality of life |
| Increased utilization of motor units during muscle contractions | Increased muscular strength and power |
| Improved coordination of motor units | Increased muscular strength and power |
| Increased strength of tendons, ligaments, and bones | Lower risk of injury to these tissues |
| Increased storage of fuel in muscles | Increased resistance to muscle fatigue |
| Increased size of fast-twitch muscle fibers (from a high-resistance program) | Increased muscular strength and power |
| Increased size of slow-twitch muscle fibers (from a high-repetition program) | Increased muscular endurance |
| Increased blood supply to muscles (from a high-repetition program) and improved blood vessel health | Increased delivery of oxygen and nutrients<br>Faster elimination of wastes |
| Biochemical improvements (for example, increased sensitivity to insulin) | Enhanced metabolic health |
| Improved blood fat levels | Reduced risk of heart disease |
| Increased muscle endurance | Enhanced ability to exercise for long periods and maintain good body posture |

*Due to genetic and hormonal differences, men will build more muscle mass than women, but both genders make about the same percent gains in strength through a good program.

- **Fast-twitch muscle fibers** contract more rapidly and forcefully than slow-twitch fibers but fatigue more quickly. Although oxygen is important in the energy system that fuels fast-twitch fibers, they rely more on anaerobic (nonoxidative) metabolism than do slow-twitch fibers. (See Chapter 3 for a discussion of energy systems.) Fast-twitch muscle fibers are typically whitish in color.

Most muscles contain both slow-twitch and fast-twitch fibers. The proportion of the types of fibers varies significantly among different muscles and different individuals, and that proportion is largely fixed at birth, although fibers can contract faster or slower following a period of training or a period of inactivity. The type of fiber that acts during a particular activity depends on the type of work required. Endurance activities like jogging tend to use slow-twitch fibers, whereas strength and **power** activities like sprinting use fast-twitch fibers. Strength training can increase the size and strength of both fast-twitch and slow-twitch fibers, although fast-twitch fibers are preferentially increased.

## Motor Units

To exert force, a muscle recruits one or more motor units to contract. A **motor unit** is made up of a nerve connected to a number of muscle fibers. The number of muscle fibers in a motor unit varies from two to hundreds. Small motor units contain slow-twitch fibers, whereas large motor units contain fast-twitch fibers. When a motor unit calls on its fibers to contract, all fibers contract to their full capacity. The number of motor units recruited depends on the amount of strength required: When you pick up a small weight, you use fewer and smaller motor units than when picking up a large weight.

Strength training improves the body's ability to recruit motor units—a phenomenon called **muscle learning**—which increases strength even before muscle size increases. The physiological changes and benefits that result from strength training are summarized in Table 4.1.

**KEY TERMS**

**muscle fiber**   A single muscle cell, usually classified according to strength, speed of contraction, and energy source.

**myofibrils**   Protein structures that make up muscle fibers.

**hypertrophy**   An increase in the size of muscle fibers, usually stimulated by muscular overload, as occurs during strength training.

**atrophy**   A decrease in the size of muscle fibers.

**hyperplasia**   An increase in the number of muscle fibers.

**nucleus**   A cell structure containing DNA and genes that direct the production of proteins; plural, *nuclei*.

**slow-twitch muscle fibers**   Red muscle fibers that are fatigue resistant but have a slow contraction speed and a lower capacity for tension; usually recruited for endurance activities.

**fast-twitch muscle fibers**   White muscle fibers that contract rapidly and forcefully but fatigue quickly; usually recruited for actions requiring strength and power.

**power**   The ability to exert force rapidly.

**motor unit**   A motor nerve (one that initiates movement) connected to one or more muscle fibers.

**muscle learning**   The improvement in the body's ability to recruit motor units, brought about through strength training.

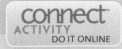

## Does Muscular Strength Reduce the Risk of Premature Death?

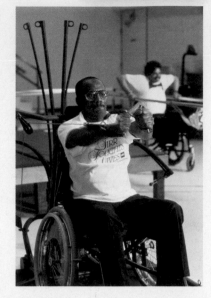

Strength training can make you stronger, but can it also help you live longer? According to a growing body of evidence, the answer is yes—especially for men.

A number of studies have associated greater muscular strength with lower rates of death from all causes, including cancer and cardiovascular disease. According to the results of a study that followed nearly 9000 men over 18 years, the stronger a man is, the lower his risk of premature death from a variety of causes. This study gauged participants' strength through exercises such as bench and leg presses; other studies have measured strength using a handgrip test, with similar outcomes. The resulting data showed significant differences in death rates among the participants, with the strongest men having the lowest death rates. This effect was particularly important for older and overweight men.

When participants in the study died, researchers analyzed causes of death and correlated the numbers of dead and surviving participants with data about their muscular fitness, the amount of time they spent exercising, and other factors (such as metabolic data, cardiovascular health, smoking status, and age). The findings revealed that, compared to men with the lowest levels of muscular strength, stronger men were

- 1.5 times less likely to die from all causes
- 1.6 times less likely to die from cardiovascular disease
- 1.25 times less likely to die from cancer

These correlations held across all age groups (ranging from age 20 to 82) and body mass indexes. They were particularly striking in older men (age 60 and older), who were more than four times more likely to die from cancer than similar-age men with greater muscular strength.

Similarly, an earlier study of more than 3000 men demonstrated an inverse relationship between muscular strength and metabolic syndrome, a cluster of symptoms that includes high blood pressure, high blood glucose levels, high triglyceride levels, low HDL cholesterol levels, and abdominal obesity. Metabolic syndrome increases risk for diabetes, heart disease, and other illnesses. The results were true regardless of participants' age, weight, or waist circumference. The findings led researchers to suggest that weight training may be a valuable way for men to avoid metabolic syndrome. Protection against metabolic syndrome is also provided by cardiorespiratory fitness, according to a 2004 study of 8570 men, in which scientists measured

each participant's level of muscular strength and cardiorespiratory fitness.

You don't have to be a power lifter or bodybuilder to enjoy the benefits of strength training. In the first study, for example, participants were advised on basic fitness techniques and healthy lifestyle behaviors. Although participants were encouraged to incorporate weight training into their fitness routine, each man chose the type and amount of weight training he felt most comfortable doing. Many researchers believe that the basic minimum recommendation of doing weight training on 2 nonconsecutive days per week may be enough to lower the average male's risk of premature death, provided he is not obese and does not already have risk factors such as diabetes, hypertension, or preexisting cancer. At the same time, as noted in Chapter 3, strength training can have negative effects on the cardiovascular system in some men, at least temporarily, if not followed by aerobic exercise. To date, only small-scale studies have been performed on women, so more research is needed to see if the same conclusions apply to women.

**SOURCES:** Physical Activity Guidelines Advisory Committee. 2008. *Physical Activity Guidelines Advisory Committee Report, 2008*. Washington, D.C.: U.S. Department of Health and Human Services; Ruiz, J. R., et al. 2008. Association between muscular strength and mortality in men: Prospective cohort study. *BMJ* 337: a439; Ruiz, J. R., et al. 2009. Muscular strength and adiposity as predictors of adulthood cancer mortality in men. *Cancer Epidemiology, Biomarkers, and Prevention* 18: 1468; Rantanen, T., et al. 2011. Midlife muscle strength and human longevity up to age 100 years: A 44-year prospective study among a decedent cohort. *Age* published online: DOI 10.1007/s11357-011-9256-y.

## BENEFITS OF MUSCULAR STRENGTH AND ENDURANCE

Enhanced muscular strength and endurance can lead to improvements in the areas of performance, injury prevention, body composition, self-image, lifetime muscle and bone health, and metabolic health. Most important, greater muscular strength and endurance reduce the risk of premature death. Stronger people—particularly men—have a lower death rate due to all causes, including cardiovascular disease and cancer (see the box "Does Muscular Strength Reduce the Risk of Premature Death?"). The link between strength and death rate is independent of age, physical activity, smoking, alcohol intake, body composition, and family history of cardiovascular disease.

## Improved Performance of Physical Activities

A person with a moderate to high level of muscular strength and endurance can perform everyday tasks—such as climbing stairs and carrying groceries—with ease. Increased strength can enhance your enjoyment of recreational sports by making it possible to achieve high levels of performance and to handle advanced techniques. Strength training also results in modest improvements in maximal oxygen consumption. People with poor muscle strength tire more easily and are less effective in both everyday and recreational activities.

## Injury Prevention

Increased muscular strength and endurance help protect you from injury in two key ways:

- By enabling you to maintain good posture
- By encouraging proper body mechanics during everyday activities such as walking and lifting

Good muscle strength and, particularly, endurance in the abdomen, hips, lower back, and legs, maintain the spine in proper alignment and help prevent low-back pain, which afflicts more than 85% of Americans at some time in their lives. (Prevention of low-back pain is discussed in Chapter 5.)

Training for muscular strength and endurance also makes the **tendons, ligaments,** and **cartilage** cells stronger and less susceptible to injury. Resistance exercise prevents injuries best when the training program is gradual and progressive and builds all the major muscle groups.

## Improved Body Composition

As Chapter 2 explained, healthy body composition means that the body has a high proportion of fat-free mass (composed primarily of muscle) and a relatively small proportion of fat. Strength training improves body composition by increasing muscle mass, thereby tipping the body composition ratio toward fat-free mass and away from fat.

Building muscle mass through strength training also helps with losing fat because metabolic rate is related to muscle mass: The greater your muscle mass, the higher your metabolic rate. A high metabolic rate means that a nutritionally sound diet coupled with regular exercise will not lead to an increase in body fat. Strength training

can boost resting metabolic rate by up to 15%, depending on how hard you train. Resistance exercise also increases muscle temperature, which in turn slightly increases the rate at which you burn calories over the hours following a weight training session.

## Enhanced Self-Image and Quality of Life

Strength training leads to an enhanced self-image in both men and women by providing stronger, firmer-looking muscles and a toned, healthy-looking body. Women tend to lose inches, increase strength, and develop greater muscle definition. Men tend to build larger, stronger muscles. The larger muscles in men combine with high levels of the hormone **testosterone** for a strong tissue-building effect; see the box "Gender Differences in Muscular Strength."

Because strength training involves measurable objectives (pounds lifted, repetitions accomplished), a person can easily recognize improved performance, leading to greater self-confidence and self-esteem. Strength training also improves quality of life by increasing energy, preventing injuries, and making daily activities easier and more enjoyable.

## Improved Muscle and Bone Health with Aging

Research has shown that good muscular strength helps people live healthier lives. A lifelong program of regular strength training prevents muscle and nerve degeneration that can compromise the quality of life and increase the risk of hip fractures and other potentially life-threatening injuries.

In the general population, people begin to lose muscle mass after age 30, a condition called *sarcopenia*. At first they may notice that they cannot play sports as well as they could in high school. After more years of inactivity and strength loss, people may have trouble performing even the simple movements of daily life, such as walking up a flight of stairs or doing yard work. By age 75, about 25% of men and 75% of women cannot lift more than 10 pounds overhead. Although aging contributes to decreased strength, inactivity causes most of the loss. Poor strength makes it much more likely that a person will be injured during everyday activities.

### Wellness Tip

Circuit training involves a series of exercises with minimal rest in between. Circuits can include almost any kind of exercises. Circuit training is an excellent way to develop strength and endurance at the same time.

---

**tendon**  A tough band of fibrous tissue that connects a muscle to a bone or other body part and transmits the force exerted by the muscle.

**ligament**  A tough band of tissue that connects the ends of bones to other bones or supports organs in place.

**cartilage**  Tough, resilient tissue that acts as a cushion between the bones in a joint.

**testosterone**  The principal male hormone, responsible for the development of secondary sex characteristics and important in increasing muscle size.

*KEY TERMS*

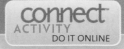

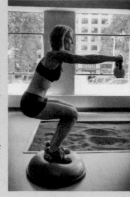

**DIMENSIONS OF DIVERSITY**

Men are generally stronger than women because they typically have larger bodies and a larger proportion of their total body mass is made up of muscle. But when strength is expressed per unit of cross-sectional area of muscle tissue, men are only 1–2% stronger than women in the upper body and about equal to women in the lower body. Men have a larger proportion of muscle tissue in the upper body, so they can more easily build upper-body strength than women can. Individual muscle fibers are larger in men, but the metabolism of cells within those fibers is the same in both sexes.

Two factors that help explain these disparities are testosterone levels and the speed of nervous control of muscle. Testosterone promotes the growth of muscle tissue in both males and females. Testosterone levels are 5–10 times higher in men than in women, so men tend to have larger muscles. Also, because the male nervous system can activate muscles faster, men tend to have more power.

Women are often concerned that they will develop large muscles from strength training. Because of hormonal differences, most women do not develop big muscles unless they train intensely over many years or take anabolic steroids. Women do gain muscle and improve body composition through strength training, but they don't develop bulky muscles or gain significant amounts of weight. A study of average women who weight trained 2–3 days per week for 8 weeks found that they gained about 1.75 pounds of muscle and lost about 3.5 pounds of fat. Losing muscle over time is a much greater health concern for women than small gains in muscle weight, especially because any gains in muscle weight are typically more than offset by loss of fat weight. Both men and women lose muscle mass and power as they age, but because men start out with more muscle and don't lose power as quickly, older women tend to have greater impairment of muscle function than older men. This may partially account for the higher incidence of life-threatening falls in older women.

The bottom line is that both men and women can increase strength through strength training. Women may not be able to lift as much weight as men, but pound for pound of muscle, they have nearly the same capacity to gain strength as men.

---

As a person ages, motor nerves can become disconnected from the portion of muscle they control. By age 70, 15% of the motor nerves in most people are no longer connected to muscle tissue. Aging and inactivity also cause muscles to become slower and therefore less able to perform quick, powerful movements. Strength training helps maintain motor nerve connections and the quickness of muscles.

Osteoporosis (bone loss) is common in people over age 55, particularly postmenopausal women. Osteoporosis leads to fractures that can be life-threatening. Hormonal changes from aging account for much of the bone loss that occurs, but lack of bone mass due to inactivity and a poor diet are contributing factors. Strength training can lessen bone loss even if it is taken up later in life, and if practiced regularly, strength training may even build bone mass in postmenopausal women and older men. Increased muscle strength can also help prevent falls, which are a major cause of injury in people with osteoporosis.

### ? Ask Yourself

QUESTIONS FOR CRITICAL THINKING AND REFLECTION

What benefits of strength training are most important to you? Are you more interested in improved physical performance? Better body composition and appearance? Long-term health benefits? How can you define your goals so they are most meaningful and motivating for you?

## Metabolic and Heart Health

Strength training helps prevent and manage both cardiovascular disease (CVD) and diabetes by:

- Improving glucose metabolism
- Increasing maximal oxygen consumption
- Reducing blood pressure
- Increasing HDL cholesterol and reducing LDL cholesterol (in some people)
- Improving blood vessel health

Stronger muscles reduce the demand on the heart during ordinary daily activities such as lifting and carrying objects. The benefits of resistance exercise to the heart are so great that the American Heart Association recommends that healthy adults and many low-risk cardiac patients do strength training 2–3 days per week. Resistance training may not be appropriate for people with some types of heart disease.

## ASSESSING MUSCULAR STRENGTH AND ENDURANCE

Muscular strength is usually assessed by measuring the maximum amount of weight a person can lift one time. This single maximum effort is called a **repetition maximum (RM).** You can assess the strength of your major muscle groups by taking the one–repetition maximum (1 RM) test

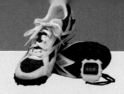

# How Strong Are You?

Tests of strength have challenged humans since the dawn of history. Strength is highly specific; one type of strength does not necessarily predict another. Strength tests help you determine your current fitness level and help you set achievable goals. You could test your capacity doing almost any exercise. Test your maximum performance on as many of the following tests as you can.

| TEST | MAXIMUM REPETITIONS OR TIME | GOAL |
|---|---|---|
| Push-ups (Modified Or Regular) | _____ | _____ |
| Pull-ups or bent-arm bar hang | _____ | _____ |
| One-arm kettlebell snatches | _____ | _____ |
| Two-arm kettlebell swings | _____ | _____ |
| Bench press for reps (at a specific weight; e.g., 135 pounds, 225 pounds) | _____ | _____ |

Write down your performance for each exercise in the second column of the list. (Note that you should wait at least a few minutes between tests.) If you aren't happy with the results, set a reasonable goal for each exercise in the third column. If you aren't sure what a reasonable goal would be, talk to your instructor or a certified personal trainer. Use these goals as a starting point for a broad-ranging strength training program.

for the bench press and by taking functional leg strength tests. You can measure 1 RM directly or estimate it by doing multiple repetitions with a submaximal (lighter) weight. It is best to train for several weeks before attempting a direct 1 RM test; once you have a baseline value, you can retest after 6–12 weeks to check your progress. See Lab 4.1 for guidelines on taking these tests. For more accurate results, avoid strenuous weight training for 48 hours beforehand.

Muscular endurance is usually assessed by counting the maximum number of **repetitions** of an exercise a person can do (such as in push-ups or kettlebell snatches) or the maximum amount of time a person can hold a muscular contraction (such as in the flexed-arm hang). You can test the muscular endurance of major muscle groups in your body by taking the curl-up test, the push-up test, and the squat endurance test. See Lab 4.2 for complete instructions on taking these assessment tests.

## CREATING A SUCCESSFUL STRENGTH TRAINING PROGRAM

When the muscles are stressed by a greater load than they are used to, they adapt and improve their function. The type of adaptation that occurs depends on the type of stress applied.

### Static Versus Dynamic Strength Training Exercises

Strength training exercises are generally classified as static or dynamic. Each involves a different way of using and strengthening muscles.

**Static Exercise** Also called **isometric** exercise, **static exercise** involves a muscle contraction without a change in the length of the muscle or the angle in the joint on which the muscle acts. In isometrics, the muscle contracts, but there is no movement. To perform an isometric exercise, a

## ? Ask Yourself

**QUESTIONS FOR CRITICAL THINKING AND REFLECTION**

Considering your lifestyle and the physical activities you most commonly do, which is more important to you—muscular strength or muscular endurance? Why is this the case? Do you think your priority may change some day?

**KEY TERMS**

**repetition maximum (RM)** The maximum amount of resistance that can be moved a specified number of times.

**repetitions** The number of times an exercise is performed during one set.

**static (isometric) exercise** Exercise involving a muscle contraction without a change in the muscle's length.

person can use an immovable object like a wall to provide resistance, or simply tighten a muscle while remaining still (for example, tightening the abdominal muscles while sitting at a desk). The spine extension and the side bridge, shown on pp. 119–120, are both isometric exercises.

Static exercises are not used as widely as dynamic exercises because they don't develop strength throughout a joint's entire range of motion. During almost all movements, however, some muscles contract statically to support the skeleton so that other muscles can contract dynamically. For example, when you throw, hit a ball, or ski, the core muscles in the abdomen and back stabilize the spine. This stability allows more powerful contractions in the lower- and upper-body muscles. The core muscles contract statically during dynamic exercises, such as squats, lunges, and overhead presses.

Static exercises are useful in strengthening muscles after an injury or surgery, when movement of the affected joint could delay healing. Isometrics are also used to overcome weak points in an individual's range of motion. Statically strengthening a muscle at its weakest point will allow more weight to be lifted with that muscle during dynamic exercise. Certain types of calisthenics and Pilates exercises (described in more detail later in the chapter) also involve static contractions. For maximum strength gains, hold the isometric contraction maximally for 6 seconds; do 2–10 repetitions.

**Dynamic Exercise** Also called **isotonic** exercise, **dynamic exercise** involves a muscle contraction with a change in the length of the muscle. Dynamic exercises are the most popular type of exercises for increasing muscle strength and seem to be most valuable for developing strength that can be transferred to other forms of physical activity. They can be performed with weight machines, free weights, or a person's own body weight (as in curl-ups or push-ups).

There are two kinds of dynamic muscle contractions:

- A **concentric muscle contraction** occurs when the muscle applies enough force to overcome resistance and shortens as it contracts.

- An **eccentric muscle contraction** (also called a *pliometric contraction*) occurs when the resistance is greater than the force applied by the muscle and the muscle lengthens as it contracts.

For example, in an arm curl, the biceps muscle works concentrically as the weight is raised toward the shoulder and eccentrically as the weight is lowered.

**CONSTANT AND VARIABLE RESISTANCE** Two of the most common dynamic exercise techniques are constant resistance exercise and variable resistance exercise.

- **Constant resistance exercise** uses a constant load (weight) throughout a joint's full range of motion. Training with free weights is a form of constant resistance exercise. A problem with this technique

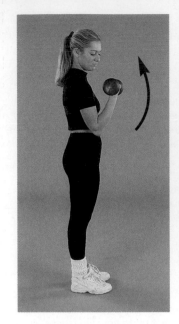
A concentric contraction.

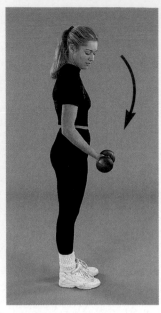
An eccentric contraction.

is that, because of differences in leverage, there are points in a joint's range of motion where the muscle controlling the movement is stronger and points where it is weaker. The amount of weight a person can lift is limited by the weakest point in the range.

- In **variable resistance exercise,** the load is changed to provide maximum load throughout the entire range of motion. This form of exercise uses machines that place more stress on muscles at the end of the range of motion, where a person has better leverage and can exert more force. Use elastic bands and chains with free weights to add variable resistance to the exercises.

Constant and variable resistance exercises are both extremely effective for building strength and endurance.

Pneumatic strength training machines use air pressure for resistance and are popular in many gyms and health clubs. They build strength in beginners but are less effective for more advanced strength trainers. The machines provide resistance only during the concentric (muscle shortening) phase of the exercise and not during the eccentric (muscle lengthening) phase. Such machines do not preload the muscles with resistance; they provide resistance only after the movement has been started.

**OTHER DYNAMIC EXERCISE TECHNIQUES** Athletes use four other kinds of isotonic techniques, primarily for training and rehabilitation.

- **Eccentric (pliometric) loading** involves placing a load on a muscle as it lengthens. The muscle contracts eccentrically in order to control the weight. Eccentric loading is practiced during most types of resistance training. For example, you are performing an eccentric movement as you lower the weight to your chest during a bench press in preparation for the active movement. You can also perform exercises designed specifically to overload muscle eccentrically, a technique called *negatives*.

• **Plyometrics** is the sudden eccentric loading and stretching of muscles followed by a forceful concentric contraction. An example would be the action of the lower-body muscles when jumping from a bench to the ground and then jumping back onto the bench. This type of exercise is used to develop explosive strength; it also helps build and maintain bone density.

• **Speed loading** involves moving a weight as rapidly as possible in an attempt to approach the speeds used in movements like throwing a softball or sprinting. In the bench press, for example, speed loading might involve doing five repetitions as fast as possible using a weight that is half the maximum load you can lift. You can gauge your progress by timing how fast you can perform the repetitions.

Training with **kettlebells** is a type of speed loading. Kettlebell training is highly ballistic, meaning that many exercises involve fast, pendulum-type motions, extreme decelerations, and high-speed eccentric muscle contractions. Kettlebell swings require dynamic concentric muscle contractions during the upward phase of the exercise followed by high-speed eccentric contractions to control the movement when returning to the starting position. Kettlebell training is very popular around the world, but more research is needed to better understand its effects on strength, power, and fitness.

• **Isokinetic** exercise involves exerting force at a constant speed against an equal force exerted by a special strength training machine. The isokinetic machine provides variable resistance at different points in the joint's range of motion, matching the effort applied by the individual while keeping the speed of the movement constant. Isokinetic exercises are excellent for building strength and endurance.

**Comparing Static and Dynamic Exercise** Static exercises require no equipment, so they can be done virtually

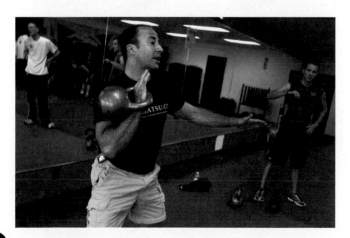

Kettlebells are growing in popularity. They provide a fast, effective workout when used properly.

# Fitness Tip

As you create a personalized weight training program, focus on specificity and eliminate training methods that do not help you achieve your goal. Follow a well-designed training program that builds strength gradually and progressively. Don't adopt the program of the week just because it's popular.

anywhere. They build strength rapidly and are useful for rehabilitating injured joints. On the other hand, they have to be performed at several different angles for each joint to improve strength throughout its entire range of motion. Dynamic exercises can be performed without equipment (calisthenics) or with equipment (weight training). They are excellent for building strength and endurance, and they tend to build strength through a joint's full range of motion. Most people develop muscular strength and endurance using dynamic exercises. Ultimately, the type of exercise a person chooses depends on individual goals, preferences, and access to equipment.

## Weight Machines Versus Free Weights

Muscles get stronger when made to work against resistance. Resistance can be provided by free weights, your own body weight, or exercise machines. Many people prefer weight machines because they are safe, convenient,

**KEY TERMS**

**dynamic (isotonic) exercise**  Exercise involving a muscle contraction with a change in the muscle's length.

**concentric muscle contraction**  A dynamic contraction in which the muscle gets shorter as it contracts.

**eccentric muscle contraction**  A dynamic contraction in which the muscle lengthens as it contracts; also called a *pliometric contraction*.

**constant resistance exercise**  A type of dynamic exercise that uses a constant load throughout a joint's full range of motion.

**variable resistance exercise**  A type of dynamic exercise that uses a changing load, providing a maximum load at the strongest point in the affected joint's range of motion.

**eccentric (pliometric) loading**  Loading the muscle while it is lengthening; sometimes called *negatives*.

**plyometrics**  Rapid stretching of a muscle group that is undergoing eccentric stress (the muscle is exerting force while it lengthens), followed by a rapid concentric contraction.

**speed loading**  Moving a load as rapidly as possible.

**kettlebell**  A large iron weight with a connected handle; used for ballistic weight training exercises such as swings and one-arm snatches.

**isokinetic**  The application of force at a constant speed against an equal force.

and easy to use. You just set the resistance, sit down at the machine, and start working. Machines make it easy to isolate and work specific muscles. You don't need a **spotter**—someone who stands by to assist when free weights are used—and you don't have to worry about dropping a weight on yourself. Many machines provide support for the back.

Free weights require more care, balance, and coordination to use, but they strengthen your body in ways that are more adaptable to real life. They are also more popular with athletes for developing functional strength for sports, especially sports that require a great deal of strength. Free weights are widely available, inexpensive, and convenient for home use.

## Other Training Methods and Types of Equipment

You don't need a fitness center or expensive equipment to strength train. If you prefer to train at home or like low-cost alternatives, consider the following options.

**Resistance Bands** Resistance or exercise bands are elastic strips or tubes of rubber material that are inexpensive, lightweight, and portable. They are available in a variety of styles and levels of resistance. Some are sold with instructional guides or DVDs, and classes may be offered at fitness centers. Many free weight exercises can be adapted for resistance bands. For example, you can do biceps curls by standing on the center of the band and holding one end of the band in each hand; the band provides resistance when you stretch it to perform the curl.

**Exercise (Stability) Balls** The exercise or stability ball is an extra-large inflatable ball. It was originally developed for use in physical therapy but has become a popular piece of exercise equipment for use in the home or gym. It can be used to work the entire body, but it is particularly effective for working the core stabilizing muscles in the abdomen, chest, and back—muscles that are important for preventing back problems. The ball's instability forces the exerciser to use the stability muscles to balance the body, even when just sitting on the ball. Moves such as crunches are more effective when performed with an exercise ball.

When choosing a ball, make sure that your thighs are parallel to the ground when you sit on it; if you are a beginner or have back problems, choose a larger ball so that your thighs are at an angle, with hips higher than knees. Beginners should use caution until they feel comfortable with the movements and take care to avoid poor form due to fatigue. See Chapter 7 for more on incorporating stability balls into a fitness program.

**Pilates** Pilates (*pil LAH teez*) was developed by German gymnast and boxer Joseph Pilates early in the twentieth

Resistance bands are a popular and inexpensive alternative to training with weights or machines.

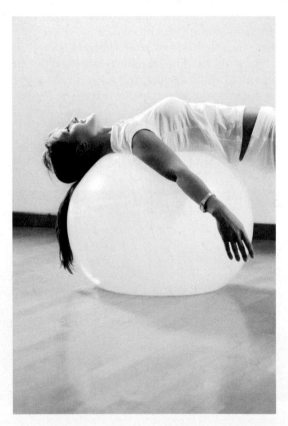

Proper fit is an important factor in choosing and using a stability ball.

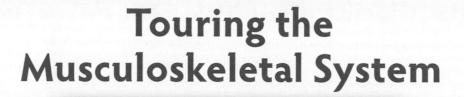

# Touring the Musculoskeletal System

**The Muscular System: Anterior View**

**The Muscular System: Posterior View**

**Muscle Hypertrophy: Gaining Muscle Through Strength Training**

**The Knee: Supporting and Maintaining Joint Stability**

## GOALS OF THE TOUR

5. **The Muscular System, Anterior View.** You will be able to use the illustration as a reference point for identifying the deep and superficial muscles of the front of the body in the context of understanding and performing strength training exercises.

6. **The Muscular System, Posterior View.** You will be able to use the illustration as a reference point for identifying the deep and superficial muscles of the back of the body in the context of understanding and performing strength training exercises.

7. **Muscle Hypertrophy.** You will be able to identify the components of skeletal muscle tissue and describe the process of muscle hypertrophy.

8. **The Knee.** You will be able to identify the muscles that support and stabilize the knee and describe the exercises that strengthen and stretch these muscles.

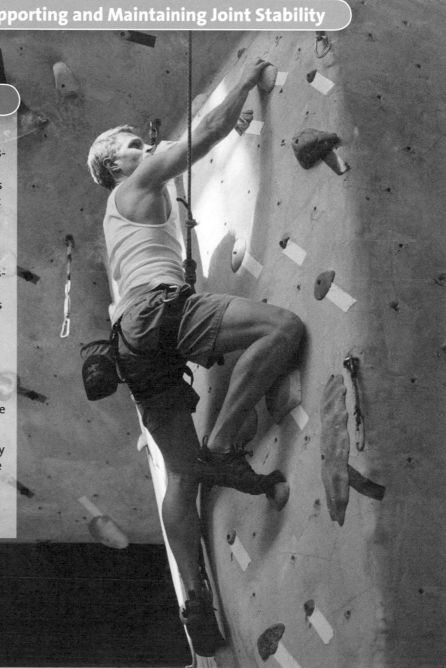

# The Musculoskeletal System: Anterior View

**5** Become familiar with and use the illustration as a reference point for identifying the deep and superficial muscles of the front of the body in the context of understanding and performing strength training exercises.

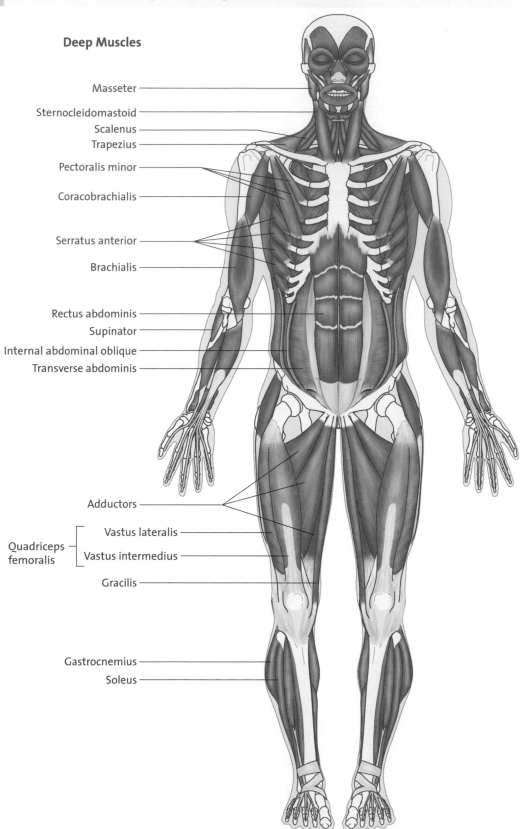

**Deep Muscles**

Masseter

Sternocleidomastoid

Scalenus

Trapezius

Pectoralis minor

Coracobrachialis

Serratus anterior

Brachialis

Rectus abdominis

Supinator

Internal abdominal oblique

Transverse abdominis

Adductors

Quadriceps femoralis — Vastus lateralis

Vastus intermedius

Gracilis

Gastrocnemius

Soleus

# The Muscular System: Posterior View

Become familiar with and use the illustration as a reference point for identifying the deep and superficial muscles of the back of the body in the context of understanding and performing strength training exercises.

**Deep Muscles**

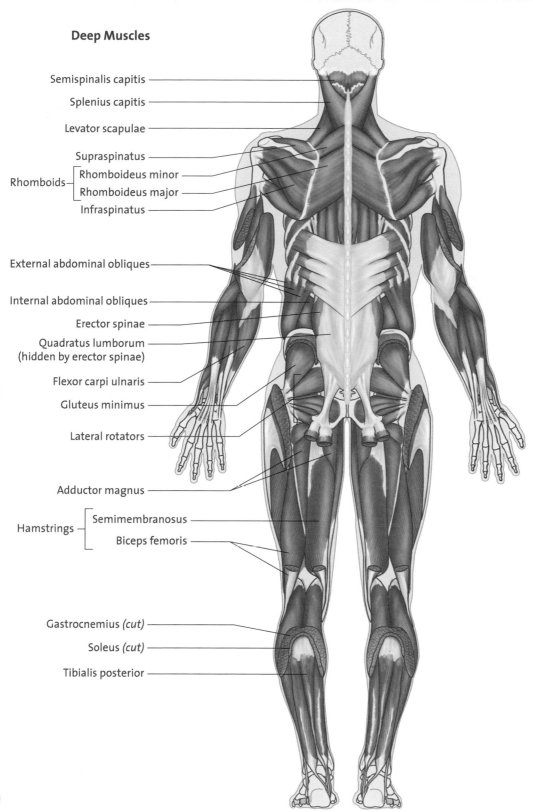

Semispinalis capitis

Splenius capitis

Levator scapulae

Supraspinatus

Rhomboids — Rhomboideus minor

Rhomboideus major

Infraspinatus

External abdominal obliques

Internal abdominal obliques

Erector spinae

Quadratus lumborum
(hidden by erector spinae)

Flexor carpi ulnaris

Gluteus minimus

Lateral rotators

Adductor magnus

Hamstrings — Semimembranosus

Biceps femoris

Gastrocnemius *(cut)*

Soleus *(cut)*

Tibialis posterior

# Muscle Hypertrophy: Gaining Muscle Through *Strength* Training

  Identify the components of skeletal muscle tissue and describe the process of muscle hypertrophy.

Skeletal muscles are found throughout the body; they are attached to bones by tendons. Contraction of skeletal muscles allows the body to maintain posture and move. The number of muscle fibers a person has is set in childhood and does not change.

Muscles consist of individual muscle cells, or muscle fibers, bundled together (*fascicles*) and covered by layers of connective tissue.

A single muscle fiber is a cylindrical cell running the length of the muscle; in some muscles, muscle fibers measure up to a foot long.

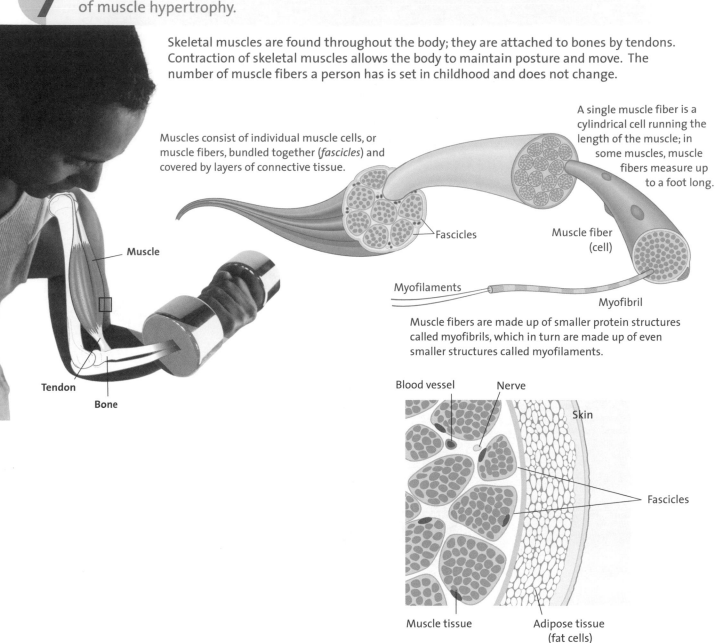

Muscle

Tendon

Bone

Fascicles

Muscle fiber (cell)

Myofilaments

Myofibril

Muscle fibers are made up of smaller protein structures called myofibrils, which in turn are made up of even smaller structures called myofilaments.

Blood vessel

Nerve

Skin

Fascicles

Muscle tissue

Adipose tissue (fat cells)

# The Knee: Supporting and Maintaining Joint Stability

Identify the muscles that support and stabilize the knee, and describe the exercises that strengthen and stretch these muscles.

The knee is important both for weight bearing and for locomotion. Because of the stresses and strains placed on this joint, it is often subject to injury. Powerful muscles help provide support for the joint. The development of strength, endurance, and flexibility in these muscles is essential for injury prevention and maintenance of stability of the joint.

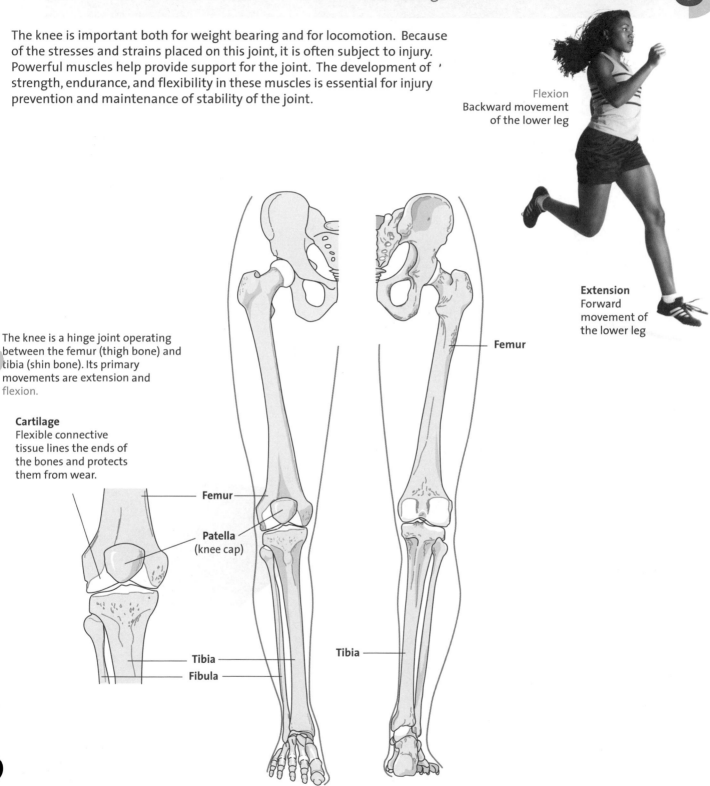

Flexion
Backward movement
of the lower leg

Extension
Forward
movement of
the lower leg

The knee is a hinge joint operating between the femur (thigh bone) and tibia (shin bone). Its primary movements are extension and flexion.

**Cartilage**
Flexible connective tissue lines the ends of the bones and protects them from wear.

**Femur**

**Femur**

**Patella**
(knee cap)

**Tibia**

**Tibia**
**Fibula**

**Anterior**     **Posterior**

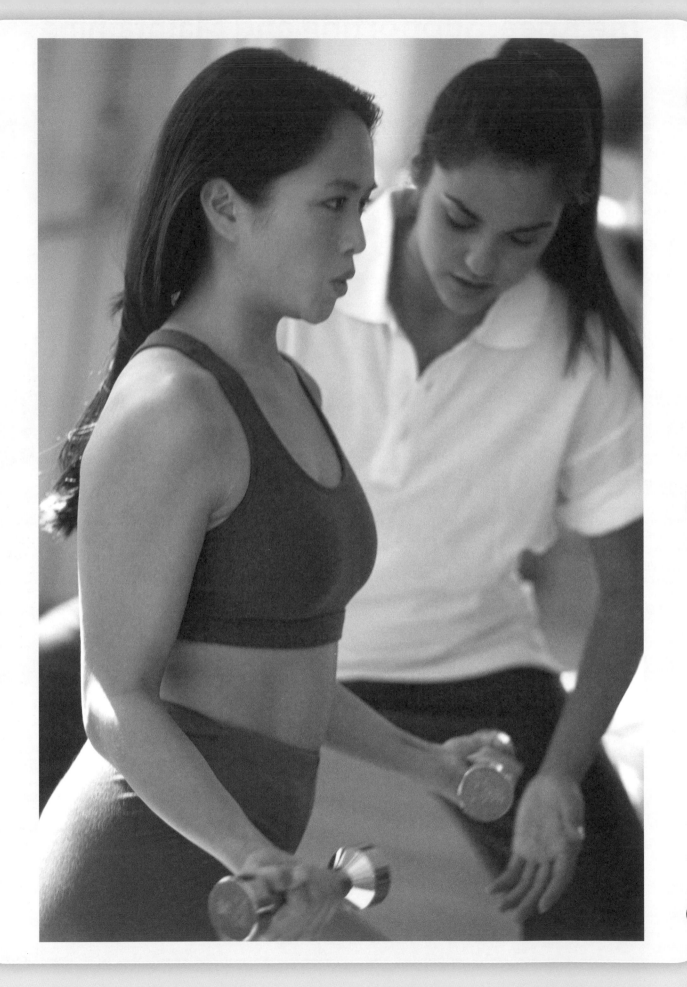

century. It often involves the use of specially designed resistance training devices, although some classes feature just mat or floor work. Pilates focuses on strengthening and stretching the core muscles in the back, abdomen, and buttocks to create a solid base of support for whole-body movement; the emphasis is on concentration, control, movement flow, and breathing. Mat exercises can be done at home, but because there are hundreds of Pilates exercises, some of them strenuous, it is best to begin with some qualified instruction. The Pilates Method Alliance (www.pilatesmethodalliance.org) offers advice on finding a qualified teacher.

### Medicine Balls, Suspension Training, Stones, and Carrying Exercises

Almost anything that provides resistance to movement will develop strength. Rubber medicine balls weigh up to 50 pounds and can be used for a variety of functional movements, such as squats and overhead throws. Suspension training uses body weight as the resistance and involves doing exercises with ropes or cords attached to a hook, bar, door jam, or sturdy tree branch. Stones can provide resistance to almost any movement, are free, and can be found in many shapes and sizes. Walking while carrying dumbbells, farmer's bars, or heavy stones is an easy and effective way to develop whole body strength.

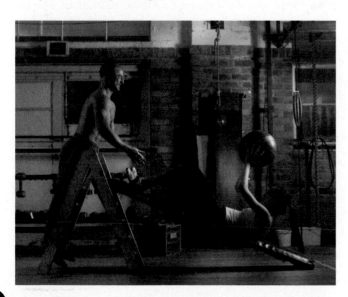

Medicine balls can be used in many ways to get an effective resistance workout.

### No-Equipment Calisthenics

You can use your own body weight as resistance for strength training. Exercises such as curl-ups, push-ups, squats, step-ups, heel raises, chair dips, and lunges can be done anywhere.

## Applying the FITT Principle: Selecting Exercises and Putting Together a Program

A complete weight training program works all the major muscle groups. It usually takes about 8–10 different exercises to get a complete full-body workout. Use the FITT principle—frequency, intensity, time, and type—to set the parameters of your program.

**Frequency of Exercise** For general fitness, the American College of Sports Medicine (ACSM) recommends a frequency of at least 2 nonconsecutive days per week for weight training. Allow your muscles at least one day of rest between workouts; if you train too often, your muscles won't be able to work with enough intensity to improve their fitness, and soreness and injury are more likely to result. If you enjoy weight training and want to train more often, try working different muscle groups on alternate days—a training plan called a *split routine*. For example, work your arms and upper body one day, work your lower body the next day, and then return to upper-body exercises on the third day.

**Intensity of Exercise: Amount of Resistance** The amount of weight (resistance) you lift in weight training exercises is equivalent to intensity in cardiorespiratory endurance training. It determines how your body will adapt to weight training and how quickly these adaptations will occur.

Choose weights based on your current level of muscular fitness and your fitness goals. Choose a weight heavy enough to fatigue your muscles but light enough for you to complete the repetitions with good form. (For tips on perfecting your form, see the box "Improving Your Technique with Video.") To build strength rapidly, you should lift weights as heavy as 80% of your maximum capacity (1 RM). If you're more interested in building endurance, choose a lighter weight (perhaps 40–60% of 1 RM), and do more repetitions.

For example, if your maximum capacity for the leg press is 160 pounds, you might lift 130 pounds to build strength and 80 pounds to build endurance. For a general fitness program to develop both strength and endurance, choose a weight in the middle of this range, perhaps 70% of 1 RM. Or you can create a program that includes

**spotter** A person who assists with a weight training exercise done with free weights.

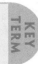

KEY TERM

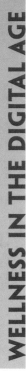

# Improving Your Technique with Video

Want to get stronger? Then you need to focus on developing your skills at least as much as you focus on lifting more weight. Improving skill is the best way to increase strength during movements such as hitting a tennis ball or baseball, performing a bench press, driving a golf ball, skiing down a slope, or carrying a bag of groceries up a flight of stairs. In the world of weight training, skill means lifting weights with proper form; the better your form, the better your results.

The brain develops precise neural pathways as you learn a skill. As you improve, the pathways conduct nervous impulses faster and more precisely until the movement almost becomes reflexive. The best way to learn a skill is through focused practice that involves identifying mistakes, correcting them, and practicing the refined movement many times. However, simply practicing the skill is not enough if you want to improve and perform more powerful movements. You must perform the movements correctly instead of practicing mistakes or poor form over and over again.

Here's where technology can help. Watch videos of people performing weight-training movements correctly. You may be able to borrow videos from your instructor, purchase low-cost training videos through magazines and sporting goods stores, or find them on the Internet. If you watch training videos online, however, make sure they were produced by an authoritative source on weight training. Otherwise, you may be learning someone else's mistakes.

Film your movements using a phone camera or inexpensive video camera. Compare your movements with those of a more skilled person performing them correctly. Make a note of poor movement patterns and try to change your technique to make it more mechanically correct. Share your videos with your instructor or a certified personal trainer, who can help you identify poor form and teach you ways to correct your form.

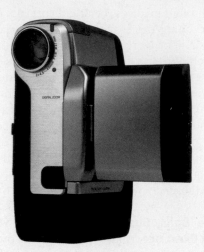

both higher-intensity exercise (80% of 1 RM for 8–10 repetitions) and lower-intensity exercise (60% of 1 RM for 15–20 repetitions); this routine will develop both fast-twitch and slow-twitch muscle fibers.

Because it can be tedious and time-consuming to continually reassess your maximum capacity for each exercise, you might find it easier to choose a weight based on the number of repetitions of an exercise you can perform with a given resistance.

**Time of Exercise: Repetitions and Sets**  To improve fitness, you must do enough repetitions of each exercise to fatigue your muscles. The number of repetitions needed to cause fatigue depends on the amount of resistance: The heavier the weight, the fewer repetitions to reach fatigue. In general, a heavy weight and a low number of repetitions (1–5) build strength and overload primarily fast-twitch fibers, whereas a light weight and a high number of repetitions (15–20) build endurance and overload primarily slow-twitch fibers.

For a general fitness program to build both strength and endurance, try to do about 8–12 repetitions of each exercise; a few exercises, such as abdominal crunches and calf raises, may require more. To avoid injury, older (approximately age 50–60 and above) and frailer people should perform more repetitions (10–15) using a lighter weight.

In weight training, a **set** refers to a group of repetitions of an exercise followed by a rest period. To develop strength and endurance for general fitness, you can make gains doing a single set of each exercise, provided you use enough resistance to fatigue your muscles. (You should just barely be able to complete the 8–12 repetitions—using good form—for each exercise.) Doing more than one set of each exercise will increase strength development, and most serious weight trainers do at least three sets of each exercise (see the section "More Advanced Strength Training Programs" for guidelines on more advanced programs).

If you perform more than one set of an exercise, you need to rest long enough between sets to allow your muscles to work with enough intensity to increase fitness. The length of the rest interval depends on the amount of resistance. In a program to develop a combination of strength and endurance for wellness, a rest period of 1–3 minutes between sets is appropriate. If you are lifting heavier loads to build strength, rest 3–5 minutes between sets. You can save time in your workouts by alternating sets of different exercises. One muscle group can rest between sets while you work on another group.

Training volume is one method of quantifying the total load lifted during weight training. Use this formula to calculate the training volume for a workout:

*repetitions* × *weight* × *sets*

For example, if you did three sets of 10 repetitions for biceps curls using 50 pounds, the training volume for the exercise would be 1500 pounds ($3 \times 10 \times 50 = 1500$). Do the same calculation for every exercise in your program and add the results together to determine the total training volume for the entire workout.

Overtraining—doing more exercise than your body can recover from—can occur in response to heavy resistance training. Possible signs of overtraining include lack of progress or decreased performance, chronic fatigue, decreased coordination, and chronic muscle soreness. The best remedy for overtraining is rest; add more days of recovery between workouts. With extra rest, chances are you'll be refreshed and ready to train again. Adding variety to your program, as discussed later in the chapter, can also help you avoid overtraining with resistance exercise.

**Type or Mode of Exercise**  For overall fitness, you need to include exercises for your neck, upper back, shoulders, arms, chest, abdomen, lower back, thighs, buttocks, and calves—about 8–10 exercises in all. If you are also training for a particular sport, include exercises to strengthen the muscles important for optimal performance *and* the muscles most likely to be injured. Weight training exercises for general fitness are presented later in this chapter, on pp. 116–124.

It is important to balance exercises between **agonist** and **antagonist** muscle groups. When a muscle contracts, it is known as the agonist; the opposing muscle, which must relax and stretch to allow contraction by the agonist, is known as the antagonist. Whenever you do an exercise that moves a joint in one direction, also select an exercise that works the joint in the opposite direction. For example, if you do knee extensions to develop the muscles on the front of your thighs, also do leg curls to develop the antagonist muscles on the back of your thighs.

The order of exercises can also be important. Do exercises for large-muscle groups or for more than one joint before you do exercises that use small-muscle groups or single joints. This allows for more effective overload of the larger, more powerful muscle groups. Small-muscle groups fatigue more easily than larger ones, and small-muscle fatigue limits your capacity to overload large-muscle groups. For example, lateral raises, which work the shoulder muscles, should be performed after bench presses, which work the chest and arms in addition to the shoulders. If you fatigue your shoulder muscles by doing lateral raises first, you won't be able to lift as much weight and effectively fatigue all the key muscle groups used during the bench press.

Also, order exercises so that you work agonist and antagonist muscle groups in sequence, one after the other. For example, follow biceps curls, which work the biceps, with triceps extensions, which exercise the triceps—the antagonist muscle to the biceps.

## The Warm-Up and Cool-Down

As with cardiorespiratory endurance exercise, you should warm up before every weight training session and cool down afterward (Figure 4.2). You should do both a general warm-up—several minutes of walking or easy jogging—and a warm-up for the weight training exercises you plan

| Warm-up 5–10 minutes | Strength training exercises for major muscle groups (8–10 exercises) | | Cool-down 5–10 minutes |
|---|---|---|---|
| | **Sample program** | | |
| | *Exercise* | *Muscle group(s) developed* | |
| | Bench press | Chest, shoulders, triceps | |
| | Pull-ups | Lats, biceps | |
| | Shoulder press | Shoulders, trapezius, triceps | |
| | Upright rowing | Deltoids, trapezius | |
| | Biceps curls | Biceps | |
| | Lateral raises | Shoulders | |
| | Squats | Gluteals, quadriceps | |
| | Heel raises | Calves | |
| | Abdominal curls | Abdominals | |
| | Spine extensions | Low- and mid-back spine extensors | |
| *Start* | Side bridges | Obliques, quadratus lumborum | *Stop* |

**Frequency:** 2–3 nonconsecutive days per week

**Intensity/Resistance:** Weights heavy enough to cause muscle fatigue when exercises are performed with good form for the selected number of repetitions

**Time: Repetitions:** 8–12 of each exercise (10–15 with a lower weight for people over age 50–60); **Sets:** 1 (doing more than 1 set per exercise may result in faster and greater strength gains); rest 1–2 minutes between exercises.

**Type of activity:** 8–10 strength training exercises that focus on major muscle groups

**FIGURE 4.2  The FITT principle for a strength training workout.**

**set**  A group of repetitions followed by a rest period.

**agonist**  A muscle in a state of contraction, opposed by the action of another muscle, its *antagonist*.

**antagonist**  A muscle that opposes the action of a contracting muscle, its *agonist*.

KEY TERMS

to perform. For example, if you plan to do one or more sets of 10 repetitions of bench presses with 125 pounds, you might do one set of 10 repetitions with 50 pounds as a warm-up. Do similar warm-up exercises for each exercise in your program.

To cool down after weight training, relax for 5–10 minutes after your workout. Although this is controversial, a few studies have suggested that including a period of postexercise stretching may help prevent muscle soreness; warmed-up muscles and joints make this a particularly good time to work on flexibility.

## Getting Started and Making Progress

The first few sessions of weight training should be devoted to learning the movements and allowing your nervous system to practice communicating with your muscles so you can develop strength effectively. To start, choose a weight that you can move easily through 8–12 repetitions, do only one set of each exercise, and rest 1–2 minutes between exercises. Gradually add weight and (if you want) sets to your program over the first few weeks until you are doing one to three sets of 8–12 repetitions of each exercise.

As you progress, add weight according to the "two-for-two" rule: When you can perform two additional repetitions with a given weight on two consecutive training sessions, increase the load. For example, if your target is to perform 8–10 repetitions per exercise, and you performed 12 repetitions in your previous two workouts, it would be appropriate to increase your load. If adding weight means you can do only 7 or 8 repetitions, stay with that weight until you can again complete 12 repetitions per set. If you can do only 4–6 repetitions after adding weight, or if you can't maintain good form, you've added too much and should take some off.

You can add more resistance in large-muscle exercises, such as squats and bench presses, than you can in small-muscle exercises, such as curls. For example, when you can complete 12 repetitions of squats with good form, you may be able to add 10–20 pounds of additional resistance; for curls, on the other hand, you might add only 3–5 pounds. As a general guideline, try increases of approximately 5%, which is half a pound of additional weight for each 10 pounds you are currently lifting.

You can expect to improve rapidly during the first 6–10 weeks of training—a 10–30% increase in the amount of weight lifted. Gains will then come more slowly. Your rate of improvement will depend on how hard you work and how your body responds to resistance training. Factors such as age, gender, motivation, and heredity also will affect your progress.

After you achieve the level of strength and muscularity you want, you can maintain your gains by training 2–3 days per week. You can monitor the progress of your program by recording the amount of resistance and the number of repetitions and sets you perform on a workout card like the one shown in Figure 4.3.

| WORKOUT CARD FOR Sara Lopez | | | | | | | | | | |
| --- | --- | --- | --- | --- | --- | --- | --- | --- | --- | --- |
| Exercise/Date | | 9/14 | 9/16 | 9/18 | 9/21 | 9/23 | 9/25 | 9/28 | 9/30 | 10/2 |
| Bench press | Wt. | 45 | 45 | 45 | 50 | 50 | 50 | 60 | 60 | 60 |
| | Sets | 1 | 1 | 1 | 1 | 1 | 1 | 1 | 1 | 1 |
| | Reps. | 10 | 12 | 12 | 10 | 12 | 12 | 10 | 9 | 12 |
| Pull-ups (assisted) | Wt. | — | — | — | — | — | — | — | — | — |
| | Sets | 1 | 1 | 1 | 1 | 1 | 1 | 1 | 1 | 1 |
| | Reps. | 5 | 5 | 5 | 6 | 6 | 6 | 7 | 7 | 7 |
| Shoulder press | Wt. | 20 | 20 | 20 | 25 | 25 | 25 | 30 | 30 | 30 |
| | Sets | 1 | 1 | 1 | 1 | 1 | 1 | 1 | 1 | 1 |
| | Reps. | 10 | 12 | 12 | 10 | 12 | 12 | 8 | 10 | 9 |
| Upright rowing | Wt. | 5 | 5 | 10 | 10 | 10 | 10 | 12 | 12 | 12 |
| | Sets | 1 | 1 | 1 | 1 | 1 | 1 | 1 | 1 | 1 |
| | Reps. | 12 | 12 | 8 | 10 | 11 | 12 | 9 | 10 | 12 |
| Biceps curls | Wt. | 15 | 15 | 15 | 20 | 20 | 20 | 25 | 25 | 25 |
| | Sets | 1 | 1 | 1 | 1 | 1 | 1 | 1 | 1 | 1 |
| | Reps. | 10 | 10 | 10 | 10 | 12 | 12 | 8 | 10 | 10 |
| Lateral raise | Wt. | 5 | 5 | 5 | 5 | 5 | 5 | 7.5 | 7.5 | 7.5 |
| | Sets | 1 | 1 | 1 | 1 | 1 | 1 | 1 | 1 | 1 |
| | Reps. | 8 | 8 | 10 | 10 | 12 | 12 | 8 | 10 | 10 |
| Squats | Wt. | — | — | — | 45 | 45 | 45 | 55 | 55 | 55 |
| | Sets | 1 | 1 | 1 | 1 | 1 | 1 | 1 | 1 | 1 |
| | Reps. | 10 | 12 | 15 | 8 | 12 | 12 | 8 | 12 | 12 |
| Heel raises | Wt. | — | — | — | 45 | 45 | 45 | 55 | 55 | 55 |
| | Sets | 1 | 1 | 1 | 1 | 1 | 1 | 1 | 1 | 1 |
| | Reps. | 15 | 15 | 15 | 8 | 12 | 12 | 10 | 12 | 12 |
| Abdominal curls | Wt. | — | — | — | — | — | — | — | — | — |
| | Sets | 1 | 1 | 1 | 1 | 1 | 1 | 1 | 1 | 1 |
| | Reps. | 20 | 20 | 20 | 20 | 20 | 20 | 25 | 25 | 25 |
| Spine extensions | Wt. | — | — | — | — | — | — | — | — | — |
| | Sets | 1 | 1 | 1 | 1 | 1 | 1 | 1 | 1 | 1 |
| | Reps. | 5 | 5 | 5 | 8 | 8 | 8 | 10 | 10 | 10 |
| Side bridge | Wt. | — | — | — | — | — | — | — | — | — |
| | Sets | 1 | 1 | 1 | 1 | 1 | 1 | 1 | 1 | 1 |
| | Seconds | 60 | 60 | 60 | 65 | 65 | 70 | 70 | 70 | 70 |

**FIGURE 4.3  A sample workout card for a general fitness strength training program.**

## More Advanced Strength Training Programs

The program just described is sufficient to develop and maintain muscular strength and endurance for general fitness. Performing more sets and fewer repetitions with a heavier load will cause greater increases in strength. Such a program might include three to five sets of 4–6 repetitions each; the load should be heavy enough to cause fatigue with the smaller number of repetitions. Rest long enough after a set (3–5 minutes) to allow your muscles to recover and work intensely during the next set.

Experienced weight trainers often practice some form of cycle training, also called *periodization,* in which the exercises, number of sets and repetitions, and intensity vary within a workout and/or between workouts. For example, you might do a particular exercise more intensely during some sets or on some days than others. You might also vary the exercises you perform for particular muscle groups. For more detailed information on these more advanced training techniques, consult a strength coach certified by the National Strength and Conditioning Association or

# Safe Weight Training

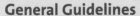

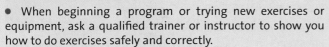
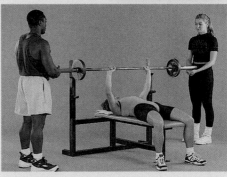

## General Guidelines

● When beginning a program or trying new exercises or equipment, ask a qualified trainer or instructor to show you how to do exercises safely and correctly.

● Lift weights from a stabilized body position; keep weights as close to your body as possible.

● Protect your back by maintaining control of your spine and avoiding dangerous positions. Don't twist your body while lifting.

● Observe proper lifting techniques and good form at all times. Don't lift beyond the limits of your strength.

● Don't hold your breath while doing weight training exercises. Doing so causes a decrease in blood returning to the heart and can make you become dizzy and faint. It can also increase blood pressure to dangerous levels. Exhale when exerting the greatest force, and inhale when moving the weight into position for the active phase of the lift. Breathe smoothly and steadily.

● Don't use defective equipment. Be aware of broken collars or bolts, frayed cables, broken chains, or loose cushions.

● Don't exercise if you're ill, injured, or overtrained. Do not try to work through the pain.

## Free Weights

● Make sure the bar is loaded evenly on both sides and that weights are secured with collars or spring clips.

● When you pick a weight up from the ground, keep your back straight and your head level. Don't bend at the waist with straight legs.

● Lift weights smoothly; don't jerk them. Control the weight through the entire range of motion.

● Do most of your lifting with your legs. Keep your hips and buttocks back. When doing standing lifts, maintain a good posture so that you protect your back. Bend at the hips, not with

the spine. Feet should be shoulder-width apart, heels and balls of the feet in contact with the floor, and knees slightly bent.

● Don't bounce weights against your body during an exercise.

## Spotting

● Use spotters for free weights exercises in which the bar crosses the face or head (e.g., the bench press), is placed on the back (e.g., squats), or is racked in front of the chest (e.g., overhead press from the rack).

● If one spotter is used, the spotter should stand behind the lifter; if two spotters are used, one spotter should stand at each end of the barbell.

● For squats with heavy resistance, use at least three spotters—one behind the lifter (hands near lifter's hips, waist, or torso) and one at each end of the bar. Squatting in a power rack will increase safety during this exercise.

● Spot dumbbell exercises at the forearms, as close to the weights as possible.

● For over-the-face and over-the-head lifts, the spotter should hold the bar with an alternate grip (one palm up and one palm down) inside the lifter's grip.

● Ensure good communication between spotter and lifter by agreeing on verbal signals before the exercise.

another reliable source. If you decide to adopt a more advanced training regimen, start off slowly to give your body a chance to adjust and to minimize the risk of injury.

### Fitness Tip

Doing three sets of resistance exercise is more anabolic than one set, meaning that doing multiple sets enhances muscle protein synthesis. If you're serious about strength training, do multiple sets of exercises to maximize muscle protein synthesis and muscle growth.

## Weight Training Safety

Injuries happen in weight training. Maximum physical effort, elaborate machinery, rapid movements, and heavy weights can combine to make the weight room a dangerous place if proper precautions aren't taken. To help ensure that your workouts are safe and productive, follow the guidelines in the box "Safe Weight Training" and the following suggestions.

**Use Proper Lifting Technique** Every exercise has a proper technique that is important for obtaining maximum benefits and preventing injury. Your instructor or weight room attendant can help explain the specific techniques for different exercises and weight machines.

## Dietary Supplements: A Consumer Dilemma

Wading through manufacturers' claims can be tricky when you are considering taking a dietary supplement. Although drugs and food products undergo stringent government testing, dietary supplements can be freely marketed without testing for safety or effectiveness. There is no guarantee that advertisements about dietary supplements are accurate or true.

What's the difference between a drug—which must be approved by the Food and Drug Administration (FDA)—and a dietary supplement? In some cases, the only real difference is in how the product is marketed. Some dietary supplements are as potentially dangerous as potent prescription drugs. But because dietary supplements have a different classification, manufacturers do not have to prove they are safe and effective before being sold; the FDA can, however, take action against any unsafe supplement product after it reaches the market.

Supplement manufacturers often make glowing claims about their products, such as "Builds lean muscle fast" or "Burns fat and gives you energy." With all the hype, how can you determine if a particular supplement might be helpful? Ask yourself the following questions:

- **Do you really need a supplement at all?** Nutritional authorities agree that most athletes and young adults can obtain all the necessary ingredients for health and top athletic performance by eating a well-balanced diet and training appropriately. No dietary supplement outperforms

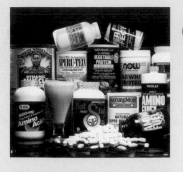

wholesome food and a good training regimen.

- **Is the product safe and effective?** The fact that a dietary supplement is available in your local store is no guarantee of safety. As described earlier, the FDA doesn't regulate supplements in the same way as drugs. The only way to determine if a supplement really works is to perform carefully controlled research on human subjects. Testimonials from individuals who claim to have benefited from the product don't count. Few dietary supplements have undergone careful human testing, so it is difficult to tell which of them may actually work.

- **Can you be sure that the product is of high quality?** There is no official agency that ensures the quality of dietary supplements. There is no guarantee that a supplement contains the desired ingredient, that dosages are appropriate, that potency is standardized, or that the product is free from contaminants. (See Chapter 8 for more information on dietary supplement labeling.)

---

Perform exercises smoothly and with good form. Lift or push the weight forcefully during the active phase of the lift and then lower it with control. Perform all lifts through the full range of motion and strive to maintain a neutral spine position during each exercise.

**Use Spotters and Collars with Free Weights** Spotters are necessary when an exercise has potential for danger; a weight that is out of control or falls can cause a serious injury. A spotter can assist you if you cannot complete a lift or if the weight tilts. A spotter can also help you move a weight into position before a lift and provide help or additional resistance during a lift. Spotting requires practice and coordination between the lifter and the spotter(s).

Collars are devices that secure weights to a barbell or dumbbell. Although people lift weights without collars, doing so is dangerous. It is easy to lose your balance or to raise one side of the weight faster than the other. Without collars, the weights can slip off and crash to the floor.

**Be Alert for Injuries** Report any obvious muscle or joint injuries to your instructor or physician, and stop exercising the affected area. Training with an injured joint or

muscle can lead to a more serious injury. Make sure you get the necessary first aid. Even minor injuries heal faster if you use the R-I-C-E principle of treating injuries described in Chapter 3.

Consult a physician if you have any unusual symptoms during exercise or if you're uncertain whether weight training is a proper activity for you. Conditions such as heart disease and high blood pressure can be aggravated during weight training. Immediately report symptoms such as headaches; dizziness; labored breathing; numbness; vision disturbances; and chest, neck, or arm pain.

## A Caution About Supplements and Drugs

Many active people use nutritional supplements and drugs in the quest for improved performance and appearance. Table 4.2 lists a selective summary of "performance aids" along with their potential side effects. Most of these substances are ineffective and expensive, and many are dangerous (see the box "Dietary Supplements: A Consumer Dilemma"). A balanced diet should be your primary nutritional strategy.

| Table 4.2 | Performance Aids Marketed to Weight Trainers |

| SUBSTANCE | SUPPOSED EFFECTS | ACTUAL EFFECTS | SELECTED POTENTIAL SIDE EFFECTS |
|---|---|---|---|
| Adrenal androgens, such as dehydroepiandros-terone (DHEA), androstenedione | Increased testosterone, muscle mass, and strength; decreased body fat | Increased testosterone, strength, and fat-free mass; decreased fat in older subjects (more studies needed in younger people) | Gonadal suppression, prostate hyper-trophy, breast development in males, masculinization in women and children; long-term effects unknown |
| Amino acids | Increased muscle mass | No effects if dietary protein intake is adequate; consuming before or after training may improve performance | Minimal side effects; unbalanced amino acid intake can cause problems with protein metabolism |
| Amphetamines | Prevention of fatigue; increased confidence and training intensity | Increased arousal, wakefulness, and confidence; feeling of enhanced decision-making ability | Depression and fatigue (after drug wears off), extreme confusion; neural and psychological effects including aggressiveness, paranoia, hallucinations, compulsive behavior, restlessness, irritability, heart arrhythmia, high blood pressure, and chest pain |
| Anabolic steroids | Increased muscle mass, strength, power, psychological aggressiveness, and endurance | Increased strength, power, fat-free mass, and aggression; no effects on endurance | Liver damage and tumors, decrease in high-density lipoprotein (good choles-terol), depressed sperm and testoster-one production, high blood pressure, depressed immune function, problems with sugar metabolism, psychological disturbances, gonadal suppression, liver disease, acne, breast development in males, masculinization in women and children, heart disease, thicker blood, and increased risk of cancer; steroids are controlled substances* |
| Beta-agonists, such as clenbuterol, salmeterol, terbutaline | Enhanced performance; prevention of muscle atrophy; increased fat-free weight; decreased body fat | Used to treat asthma, including exercise-induced asthma | Insomnia, heart arrhythmia, anxiety, an-orexia, nausea, heart enlargement, heart attack (particularly if used with steroids), and heart failure |
| Chromium picolinate | Increased muscle mass, decreased body fat; improved blood sugar control | Well-controlled studies show no significant effect on fat-free mass or body fat | Moderate doses (50–200 μg) appear safe; higher doses may cause DNA damage and other serious effects; long-term effects unknown |
| Creatine monohydrate | Increased creatine phosphate levels in muscles, muscle mass, and capacity for high-intensity exercise | Increased muscle mass and per-formance in some types of high-intensity exercise | Minimal side effects; long-term effects unknown |
| Diuretics | Promote loss of body fluid | Promote loss of body fluid to ac-centuate muscle definition; often taken with potassium supple-ments and very-low-calorie diets | Muscle cell destruction, low blood pres-sure, blood chemistry abnormalities, and heart problems |
| Energy drinks | Increased energy, strength, power | Increased training volume | Insomnia, increased blood pressure, heart palpitations |
| Ephedra | Decreased body fat; increased training intensity due to stimulant effect | Decreased appetite, particularly when taken with caffeine; some evidence for increased training intensity | Abnormal heart rhythms, nervousness, headache, gastrointestinal distress, and heatstroke; banned by the FDA |
| Erythropoietin, darbepoetin | Enhanced performance during endurance events | Stimulated growth of red blood cells; enhanced oxygen uptake and endurance | Increased blood viscosity (thickness); can cause potentially fatal blood clots |

*(Continued)*

## Table 4.2 — Performance Aids Marketed to Weight Trainers (*continued*)

| SUBSTANCE | SUPPOSED EFFECTS | ACTUAL EFFECTS | SELECTED POTENTIAL SIDE EFFECTS |
|---|---|---|---|
| Ginseng | Decreased effects of physical and emotional stress; increased oxygen consumption | Most well-controlled studies show no effect on performance | No serious side effects; high doses can cause high blood pressure, nervousness, and insomnia |
| Green tea extract | Decreased body fat | Some studies show decreases in body fat | Insomnia, headache, nausea, heart palpitations |
| Growth hormone | Increased muscle mass, strength, and power; decreased body fat | Increased muscle mass and strength; decreased fat mass; studies show no effect on muscle or exercise performance | Elevated blood sugar, high insulin levels, and carpal tunnel syndrome; enlargement of the heart and other organs; acromegaly (disease characterized by increased growth of bones in hands and face); diseases of the heart, nerves, bones, and joints; an extremely expensive controlled substance* |
| Human chorionic gonadotrophin (HCG) | Increased testosterone production; prevention of muscle atrophy during steroid withdrawal | Increased testosterone production | Interferes with normal testosterone regulation; banned in most sports |
| Beta-hydroxy beta-methylbutyrate (HMB) | Increased strength and muscle mass; decreased body fat | Some studies show increased fat-free mass and decreased fat; more research needed | No reported side effects; long-term effects unknown |
| Insulin | Increased muscle mass | Effectiveness in stimulating muscle growth unknown | Insulin shock (characterized by extremely low blood sugar), which can lead to unconsciousness and death |
| Insulin-like growth factor (IGF) | Increased muscle mass; improved cellular function | Actual effects in healthy, active people unknown | Similar to side effects of growth hormone; long-term use promotes cancer |
| "Metabolic-optimizing" meals for athletes | Increased muscle mass and energy supply; decreased body fat | No proven effects beyond those of balanced meals | No reported side effets, extremely expensive |
| Over-the-counter stimulants, such as caffeine, phenylpropanolamine (PPA) | Weight loss; improved endurance; stimulant effect | Can be used for weight control; may improve endurance; does not appear to enhance short-term maximal exercise capacity | Increased risk of heart attack and stroke in some people (in high doses); increased incidence of abnormal heart rhythm and insomnia; caffeine is addictive |
| Prescription appetite suppressants, such as diethylproprion, phentermine, sibutramine, rimonabant | Weight control, weight loss | Weight loss; typically prescribed only for short-term use | Restlessness, anxiety, dizziness, depression, tremors, increased urination, diarrhea, constipation, vomiting, high blood pressure, swelling of legs or ankles, insomnia, seizures, fast or irregular heartbeat, heart palpitations, blurred vision, rashes, and difficulty breathing; can be habit-forming |
| Protein, amino acids, polypeptide supplements | Increased muscle mass and growth hormone release; accelerated muscle development; decreased body fat | No effects if dietary protein intake is adequate; may promote protein synthesis if taken immediately before or after weight training | Can be dangerous for people with liver or kidney disease; substituting amino acid or polypeptide supplements for protein-rich food can cause nutrient deficiencies |

*Possession of a controlled substance is illegal without a prescription, and physicians are not allowed to prescribe controlled substances for the improvement of athletic performance. In addition, the use of anabolic steroids, growth hormone, or any of several other substances listed in this table is banned for athletic competition.

SOURCES: Brooks, G. A., et al. 2005. *Exercise Physiology: Human Bioenergetics and Its Applications,* 4th ed. New York: McGraw-Hill. Sports-supplement dangers. 2001. *Consumer Reports,* June. U.S. National Library of Medicine, National Institutes of Health. *MedlinePlus Medical Encyclopedia* (http://www.nlm.nih.gov/medlineplus/encyclopedia.html; retrieved).

## Wellness Tip

The FDA has issued several consumer warnings about dietary supplements—particularly the kinds that are marketed to people who want to build muscle and lose fat. A number of products have been pulled off store shelves after the FDA found they were not safe. Talk to your doctor before considering any dietary supplement.

## Ask Yourself

### QUESTIONS FOR CRITICAL THINKING AND REFLECTION

Do you think athletes should be allowed to use drugs and supplements to improve their sports performance? Would you be tempted to use a banned performance-enhancing drug if you thought you could get away with it?

## WEIGHT TRAINING EXERCISES

A general book on fitness and wellness cannot include a detailed description of all weight training exercises. The following pages present a basic program for developing muscular strength and endurance for general fitness using free weights and weight machines. Instructions for each exercise are accompanied by photographs and a listing of the muscles being trained. See pages T4-2 and T4-3 of the color transparency insert "Touring the Musculoskeletal System" in this chapter for a clear illustration of the deep and superficial muscles referenced in the exercises.

Labs 4.2 and 4.3 will help you assess your current level of muscular endurance and design your own weight training program. If you want to develop strength for a particular activity, your program should contain exercises for general fitness, exercises for the muscle groups most important for the activity, and exercises for muscle groups most often injured. Regardless of the goals of your program or the type of equipment you use, your program should be structured so that you obtain maximum results without risking injury.

## TIPS FOR TODAY AND THE FUTURE

You don't need a complicated or heavy training program to improve strength: Just one set of 8–12 repetitions of 8–10 exercises, done at least two nonconsecutive days per week, is enough for general fitness.

### RIGHT NOW YOU CAN

- Do a set of static (isometric) exercises. If you're sitting, try tightening your abdominal muscles as you press your lower back into the seat, or work your arms by placing the palms of your hands on top of your thighs and pressing down. Hold the contraction for 6 seconds and do 5–10 repetitions; don't hold your breath.
- Think of three things you've done in the past 24 hours that would have been easier or more enjoyable if you increased your level of muscular strength and endurance. Visualize improvements in your quality of life that could come from increased muscular strength and endurance.

### IN THE FUTURE YOU CAN

- Make an appointment with a trainer at your campus or neighborhood fitness facility. A trainer can help you put together an appropriate weight training program and introduce you to the equipment at the facility.
- Invest in an inexpensive set of free weights, kettlebells, a stability ball, or a resistance band. Then make a regular appointment with yourself to use your new equipment.

### EXERCISE 1

### Bench Press

**Instructions: (a)** Lying on a bench on your back with your feet on the floor, grasp the bar with palms upward and hands shoulder-width apart. If the weight is on a rack, move the bar carefully from the supports to a point over the middle of your chest or slightly above it (at the lower part of the sternum). **(b)** Lower the bar to your chest. Then press it in a straight line to the starting position. Don't arch your back or bounce the bar off your chest. You can also do this exercise with dumbbells.

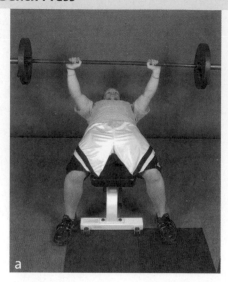
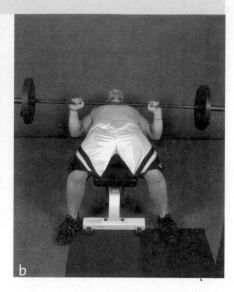

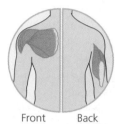

**Muscles developed:** Pectoralis major, triceps, deltoids

Front   Back

**Note:** *To allow an optimal view of exercise technique, a spotter does not appear in these demonstration photographs; however, spotters should be used for most exercises with free weights.*

### EXERCISE 2

### Pull-Up

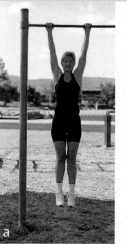
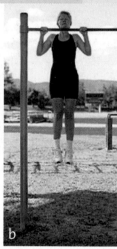
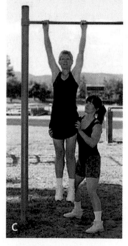

**Assisted pull-up: (c)** This is done as described for a pull-up, except that a spotter assists the person by pushing upward at the waist, hips, or legs during the exercise.

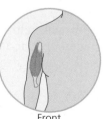

Front

Back

**Instructions: (a)** Begin by grasping the pull-up bar with both hands, palms facing forward and elbows extended fully. **(b)** Pull yourself upward until your chin goes above the bar. Then return to the starting position.

**Muscles developed:** Latissimus dorsi, biceps

## EXERCISE 3 — Shoulder Press (Overhead or Military Press)

**Instructions:** This exercise can be done standing or seated, with dumbbells or a barbell. The shoulder press begins with the weight at your chest, preferably on a rack. **(a)** Grasp the weight with your palms facing away from you. **(b)** Push the weight overhead until your arms are extended. Then return to the starting position (weight at chest). Be careful not to arch your back excessively.

If you are a more advanced weight trainer, you can "clean" the weight (lift it from the floor to your chest). The clean should be attempted only after instruction from a knowledgeable coach; otherwise, it can lead to injury.

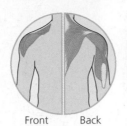

Front    Back

**Muscles developed:**
Deltoids, triceps, trapezius

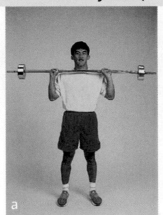

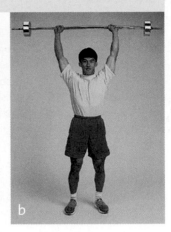

a    b

## EXERCISE 4 — Upright Rowing

**Instructions:** From a standing position with arms extended fully, grasp a barbell with a close grip (hands about 6–12 inches apart) and palms facing the body. Raise the bar to about the level of your collarbone, keeping your elbows above bar level at all times. Return to the starting position.

This exercise can be done using dumbbells, a weighted bar (shown), or a barbell.

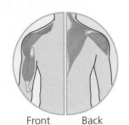

Front    Back

**Muscles developed:**
Trapezius, deltoids, biceps

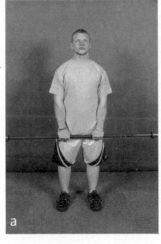

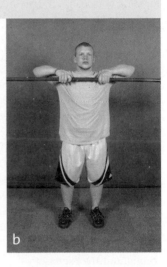

a    b

## EXERCISE 5 — Biceps Curl

**Instructions:** **(a)** From a standing position, grasp the bar with your palms facing away from you and your hands shoulder-width apart. **(b)** Keeping your upper body rigid, flex (bend) your elbows until the bar reaches a level slightly below the collarbone. Return the bar to the starting position.

This exercise can be done using dumbbells, a curl bar (shown), or a barbell; some people find that using a curl bar places less stress on the wrists.

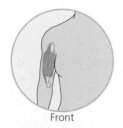

Front

**Muscles developed:**
Biceps, brachialis

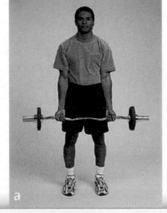

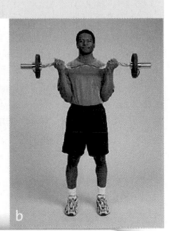

a    b

McGraw Hill connect™    http://www.mcgrawhillconnect.com/
FITNESS AND WELLNESS

## EXERCISE 6 — Lateral Raise

**Instructions:** **(a)** Stand with feet shoulder-width apart and a dumbbell in each hand. Hold the dumbbells in front of you and parallel to each other. **(b)** With elbows slightly bent, slowly lift both weights until they reach shoulder level. Keep your wrists in a neutral position, in line with your forearms. Return to the starting position.

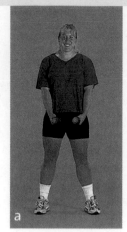

Front    Back

**Muscles developed:**
Deltoids

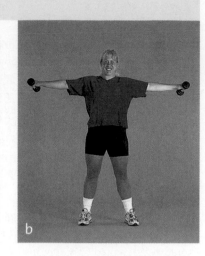

a    b

## EXERCISE 7 — Squat

**Instructions:** If the bar is racked, place the bar on the fleshy part of your upper back and grasp the bar at shoulder width. Keeping your back straight and head level, remove the bar from the rack and take a step back. Stand with feet slightly more than shoulder-width apart and toes pointed slightly outward. **(a)** Rest the bar on the back of your shoulders, holding it there with palms facing forward. **(b)** Keeping your head level and lower back straight and pelvis back, squat down until your thighs are below parallel with the floor. Let your thighs move laterally (outward) so that you "squat between your legs." This will help keep your back straight and keep your heels on the floor. Drive upward toward the starting position, hinging at the hips and keeping your back in a fixed position throughout the exercise.

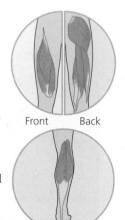

Front    Back

Back

**Muscles developed:**
Quadriceps, gluteus maximus, hamstrings, gastrocnemius

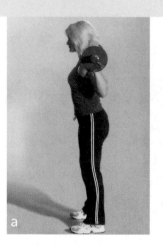

a

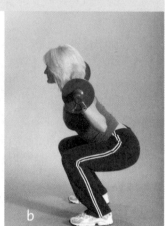

b

## EXERCISE 8 — Heel Raise

**Instructions:** Stand with feet shoulder-width apart and toes pointed straight ahead. **(a)** Rest the bar on the back of your shoulders, holding it there with palms facing forward. **(b)** Press down with your toes while lifting your heels. Return to the starting position.

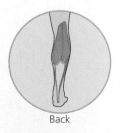

Back

**Muscles developed:**
Gastrocnemius, soleus

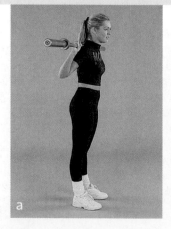

a

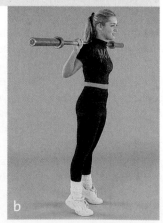

b

## EXERCISE 9 — Curl-Up or Crunch

**Instructions:** **(a)** Lie on your back on the floor with your arms folded across your chest and your feet on the floor or on a bench. **(b)** Curl your trunk up, minimizing your head and shoulder movement. Lower to the starting position. Focus on using your abdominal muscles rather than the muscles in your shoulders, chest, and neck.

This exercise can also be done using an exercise ball (see p. 106).

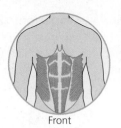

Front

**Muscles developed:**
Rectus abdominis, obliques

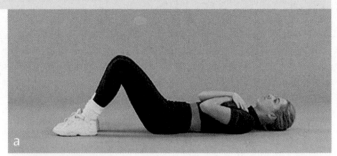

a

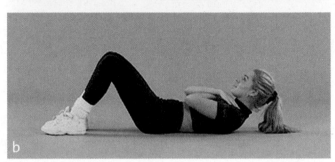

b

## EXERCISE 10 — Spine Extension ("Bird Dog") (Isometric Exercise)

**Instructions:** Begin on all fours with your knees below your hips and your hands below your shoulders.

**Unilateral spine extension:**
**(a)** Extend your right leg to the rear and reach forward with your right arm. Keep your spine neutral and your raised arm and leg in line with your torso. Don't arch your back or let your hip or shoulder sag. Hold this position for 10–30 seconds. Repeat with your left leg and left arm.

**Bilateral spine extension:**
**(b)** Extend your left leg to the rear and reach forward with your right arm. Keep your spine neutral and your raised arm and leg in line with your torso. Don't arch your back or let your hip or shoulder sag. Hold this position for 10–30 seconds. Repeat with your right leg and left arm.

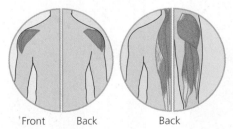

Front    Back        Back

**Muscles developed:** Erector spinae, gluteus maximus, hamstrings, deltoids

You can make this exercise more difficult by making box patterns with your arms and legs.

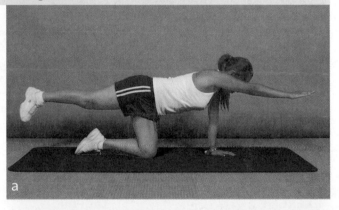

a

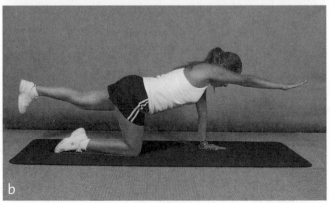

b

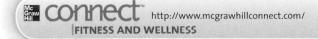

**Instructions:** Lie on the floor on your side with your knees bent and your top arm lying alongside your body. Lift and drive your hips forward so your weight is supported by your forearm and knee. Hold this position for 3–10 seconds, breathing normally. Repeat on the other side. Perform 3–10 repetitions on each side.

**Variation:** You can make the exercise more difficult by keeping your legs straight and supporting yourself with your feet and forearm (see Lab 5.3) or with your feet and hand (with elbow straight). You can also do this exercise on an exercise ball.

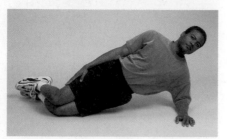

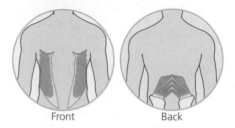

Front          Back

**Muscles developed:** Obliques, quadratus lumborum

---

## WEIGHT TRAINING EXERCISES   Weight Machines

### EXERCISE 1                          Bench Press (Chest or Vertical Press)

**Instructions:** Sit or lie on the seat or bench, depending on the type of machine and the manufacturer's instructions. Your back, hips, and buttocks should be pressed against the machine pads. Place your feet on the floor or the foot supports.

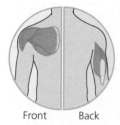

Front     Back

**Muscles developed:** Pectoralis major, anterior deltoids, triceps

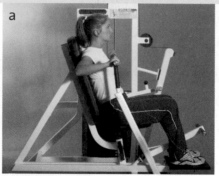

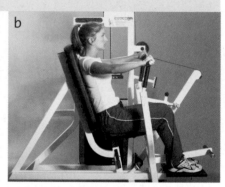

**(a)** Grasp the handles with your palms facing away from you; the handles should be aligned with your armpits.

**(b)** Push the bars until your arms are fully extended, but don't lock your elbows. Return to the starting position.

---

### EXERCISE 2                          Lat Pull

**Instructions:** Begin in a seated or kneeling position, depending on the type of lat machine and the manufacturer's instructions.

**Note:** *This exercise focuses on the same major muscles as the assisted pull-up (Exercise 3); choose an appropriate exercise for your program based on your preferences and equipment availability.*

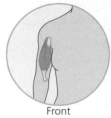
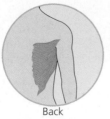

Front          Back

**Muscles developed:** Latissimus dorsi, biceps

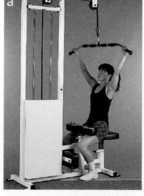
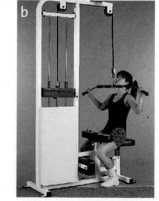

**(a)** Grasp the bar of the machine with arms fully extended.
**(b)** Slowly pull the weight down until it reaches the top of your chest. Slowly return to the starting position.

## EXERCISE 3 — Assisted Pull-Up

**Instructions:** Set the weight according to the amount of assistance you need to complete a set of pull-ups—the heavier the weight, the more assistance provided.

**(a)** Stand or kneel on the assist platform, and grasp the pull-up bar with your elbows fully extended and your palms facing away. **(b)** Pull up until your chin goes above the bar, and then return to the starting position.

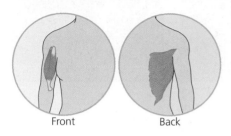

Front      Back

**Muscles developed:** Latissimus dorsi, biceps

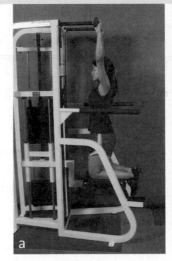

a

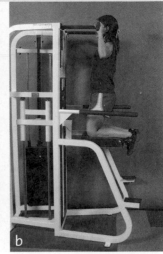

b

## EXERCISE 4 — Overhead Press (Shoulder Press)

**Instructions:** Adjust the seat so your feet are flat on the ground and the hand grips are slightly above your shoulders.

**(a)** Sit down, facing away from the machine, and grasp the hand grips with your palms facing forward. **(b)** Press the weight upward until your arms are extended. Return to the starting position.

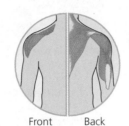

Front      Back

**Muscles developed:** Deltoids, trapezius, triceps

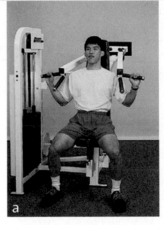

a

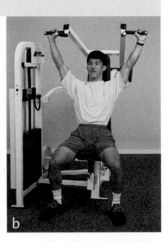

b

## EXERCISE 5 — Biceps Curl

**Instructions:** **(a)** Adjust the seat so that your back is straight and your arms rest comfortably against the top and side pads. Place your arms on the support cushions and grasp the hand grips with your palms facing up. **(b)** Keeping your upper body still, flex (bend) your elbows until the hand grips almost reach your collarbone. Return to the starting position.

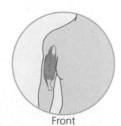

Front

**Muscles developed:** Biceps, brachialis

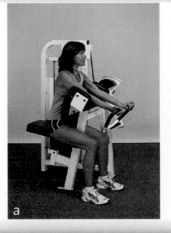

a

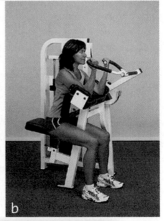

b

## EXERCISE 6　　　　Pullover

**Instructions:** Adjust the seat so your shoulders are aligned with the cams. Push down on the foot pads with your feet to bring the bar forward until you can place your elbows on the pads. Rest your hands lightly on the bar. If possible, place your feet flat on the floor. **(a)** To get into the starting position, let your arms go backward as far as possible. **(b)** Pull your elbows forward until the bar almost touches your abdomen. Return to the starting position.

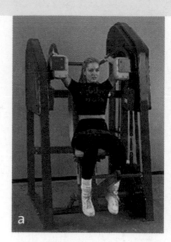

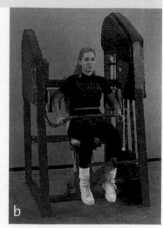

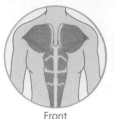

Front

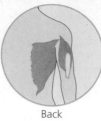

Back

**Muscles developed:**
Latissimus dorsi, pectoralis major and minor, triceps, rectus abdominis

## EXERCISE 7　　　　Lateral Raise

**Instructions: (a)** Adjust the seat so the pads rest just above your elbows when your upper arms are at your sides, your elbows are bent, and your forearms are parallel to the floor. Lightly grasp the handles. **(b)** Push outward and up with your arms until the pads are at shoulder height. Lead with your elbows rather than trying to lift the bars with your hands. Return to the starting position.

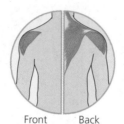

Front　　Back

**Muscles developed:**
Deltoids, trapezius

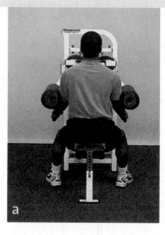

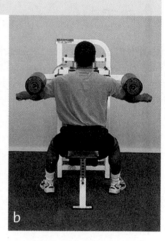

## EXERCISE 8　　　　Triceps Extension

**Note:** *This exercise focuses on some of the same muscles as the assisted dip (Exercise 9); choose an appropriate exercise for your program based on your preferences and equipment availability.*

**Instructions: (a)** Adjust the seat so your back is straight and your arms rest comfortably against the top and side pads. Place your arms on the support cushions and grasp the hand grips with palms facing inward. **(b)** Keeping your upper body still, extend your elbows as much as possible. Return to the starting position.

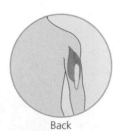

Back

**Muscles developed:**
Triceps

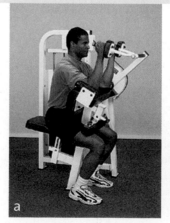

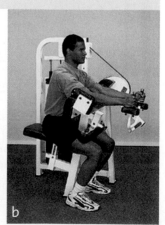

## EXERCISE 9 — Assisted Dip

**Instructions:** Set the weight according to the amount of assistance you need to complete a set of dips—the heavier the weight, the more assistance provided. **(a)** Stand or kneel on the assist platform with your body between the dip bars. With your elbows fully extended and palms facing your body, support your weight on your hands. **(b)** Lower your body until your upper arms are approximately parallel with the bars. Then push up until you reach the starting position.

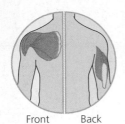

Front    Back

**Muscles developed:**
Triceps, deltoids, pectoralis major

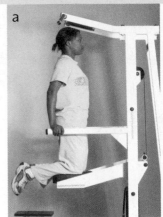

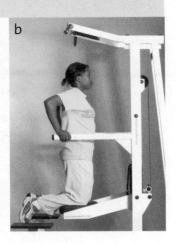

a    b

## EXERCISE 10 — Leg Press

**Instructions:** Sit or lie on the seat or bench, depending on the type of machine and the manufacturer's instructions. Your head, back, hips, and buttocks should be pressed against the machine pads. Loosely grasp the handles at the side of the machine. **(a)** Begin with your feet flat on the foot platform about shoulder-width apart. Extend your legs, but do not forcefully lock your knees. **(b)** Slowly lower the weight by bending your knees and flexing your hips until your knees are bent at about a 90-degree angle or your heels start to lift off the foot platform. Keep your lower back flat against the support pad. Then extend your knees and return to the starting position.

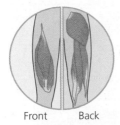

**Muscles developed:**
Gluteus maximus, quadriceps, hamstrings

Front    Back

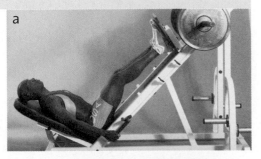
a

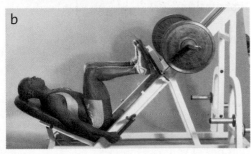
b

## EXERCISE 11 — Leg Extension (Knee Extension)

**Instructions: (a)** Adjust the seat so the pads rest comfortably on top of your lower shins. Loosely grasp the handles. **(b)** Extend your knees until they are almost straight. Return to the starting position.

Knee extensions cause kneecap pain in some people. If you have kneecap pain during this exercise, check with an orthopedic specialist before repeating it.

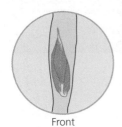

Front

**Muscles developed:**
Quadriceps

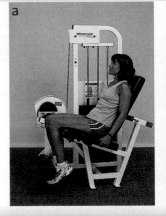

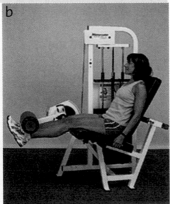

a    b

**Instructions: (a)** Sit on the seat with your back against the back pad and the leg pad below your calf muscles. **(b)** Flex your knees until your lower and upper legs form a 90-degree angle. Return to the starting position.

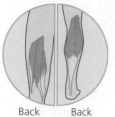

**Muscles developed:**

Hamstrings, gastrocnemius

Back          Back

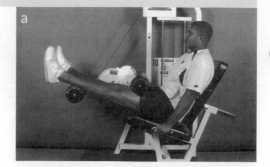
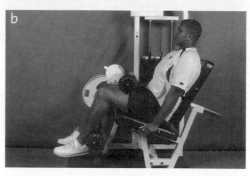

**Instructions: (a)** Stand with your head between the pads and one pad on each shoulder. The balls of your feet should be on the platform. Lightly grasp the handles. **(b)** Press down with your toes while lifting your heels. Return to the starting position. Changing the direction your feet are pointing (straight ahead, inward, and outward) will work different portions of your calf muscles.

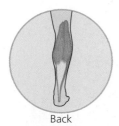

**Muscles developed:**

Gastrocnemius, soleus

Back

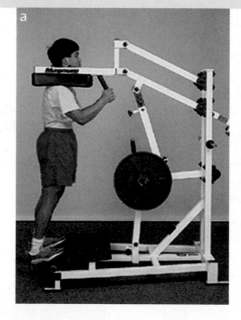
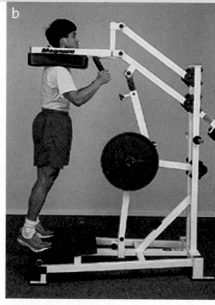

**Note:** *Abdominal machines, low-back machines, and trunk rotation machines are not recommended because of injury risk. Refer to the "Free Weights" exercise section for appropriate exercises to strengthen the abdominal and low-back muscles. For the rectus abdominus, obliques, and transvere abdominus, perform curl-ups (Exercise 9 in* the "Free Weights" section), and for the erector spinae and quadratus lumborum, perform the spine extension and the isometric side bridge (Exercises 10 and 11 in the "Free Weights" section).*

## Q Will I gain weight if I do resistance exercises?

A Your weight probably will not change significantly as a result of a general fitness program: one set of 8–12 repetitions of 8–10 exercises, performed on at least two nonconsecutive days per week. You will increase muscle mass and lose body fat, so your weight will stay about the same. You may notice a change in how your clothes fit, however, because muscle is denser than fat. Increased muscle mass will help you control body fat. Muscle increases your metabolism, which means you burn more calories every day. If you combine resistance exercises with endurance exercises, you will be on your way to developing a healthier body composition. Concentrate on fat loss rather than weight loss.

## Q Do I need more protein in my diet when I train with weights?

A No. Although there is some evidence that power athletes involved in heavy training have a higher-than-normal protein requirement, there is no reason for most people to consume extra protein. Most Americans take in more protein than they need, so even if there is an increased protein need during heavy training, it is probably supplied by the average diet. Consuming a protein-rich snack before or after training may promote muscle hypertrophy.

## Q What causes muscle soreness the day or two following a weight training workout?

A The muscle pain you feel a day or two after a heavy weight training workout is caused by injury to the muscle fibers and surrounding connective tissue. Contrary to popular belief, delayed-onset muscle soreness is not caused by lactic acid buildup. Scientists believe that injury to muscle fibers causes inflammation, which in turn causes the release of chemicals that break down part of the muscle tissue and cause pain. After a bout of intense exercise that causes muscle injury and delayed-onset muscle soreness, the muscles produce protective proteins that prevent soreness during future workouts. If you don't work out regularly, you lose these protective proteins and become susceptible to soreness again.

## Q Will strength training improve my sports performance?

A Strength developed in the weight room does not automatically increase your power in sports such as skiing, tennis, or cycling. Hitting a forehand in tennis and making a turn on skis are precise skills that require coordination between your nervous system and muscles. For skilled people, movements become reflex; you don't think about them when you do them. Increasing strength can disturb this coordination. Only by simultaneously practicing a sport and improving fitness can you expect to become more powerful in the skill. Practice helps you integrate your new strength with your skills, which makes you more powerful. Consequently, you can hit the ball harder in tennis or make more graceful turns on the ski slopes. (Refer to Chapter 2 for more on the concept of specificity in physical training.)

## Q Will I improve faster if I train every day?

A No. Your muscles need time to recover between training sessions. Doing resistance exercises every day will cause you to become overtrained, which will increase your chance of injury and impede your progress. If your strength training program reaches a plateau, try one of these strategies:

- Vary the number of sets. If you have been performing one set of each exercise, add sets.
- Train less frequently. If you are currently training the same muscle groups three or more times per week, you may not be allowing your muscles to fully recover from intense workouts.
- Change exercises. Using different exercises for the same muscle group may stimulate further strength development.
- Vary the load and number of repetitions. Try increasing or decreasing the loads you are using and changing the number of repetitions accordingly.
- If you are training alone, find a motivated training partner. A partner can encourage you and assist you with difficult lifts, forcing you to work harder.

## Q If I stop training, will my muscles turn to fat?

A No. Fat and muscle are two different kinds of tissue, and one cannot turn into the other. Muscles that aren't used become smaller (atrophy), and body fat may increase if caloric intake exceeds calories burned. Although the result of inactivity may be smaller muscles and more fat, the change is caused by two separate processes.

## Q Should I wear a weight belt when I lift?

A Until recently, most experts advised people to wear weight belts. However, several studies have shown that weight belts do not prevent back injuries and may, in fact, increase the risk of injury by encouraging people to lift more weight than they are capable of lifting with good form. Although wearing a belt may allow you to lift more weight in some lifts, you may not get the full benefit of your program because use of a weight belt reduces the effectiveness of the workout on the muscles that help support your spine.

*For more Common Questions Answered about strength training, visit the Online Learning Center at www.mhhe.com/fahey.*

- Hypertrophy (increased muscle fiber size) occurs when weight training causes the size and number of myofibrils to increase, thereby increasing total muscle size. Strength also increases through muscle learning. Most women do not develop large muscles from weight training.

- Improvements in muscular strength and endurance lead to enhanced physical performance, protection against injury, improved body composition, better self-image, improved muscle and bone health with aging, reduced risk of chronic disease, and decreased risk of premature death.

- Muscular strength can be assessed by determining the amount of weight that can be lifted in one repetition of an exercise. Muscular endurance can be assessed by determining the number of repetitions of a particular exercise that can be performed.

- Static (isometric) exercises involve contraction without movement. They are most useful when a person is recovering from an injury or surgery or needs to overcome weak points in a range of motion.

- Dynamic (isotonic) exercises involve contraction that results in movement. The two most common types are constant resistance (free weights) and variable resistance (many weight machines).

- Free weights and weight machines have pluses and minuses for developing fitness, although machines tend to be safer.

- Lifting heavy weights for only a few repetitions helps develop strength. Lifting lighter weights for more repetitions helps develop muscular endurance.

- A strength training program for general fitness includes at least one set of 8–12 repetitions (enough to cause fatigue) of 8–10 exercises, along with warm-up and cool-down periods. The program should be carried out at least 2 nonconsecutive days per week.

- Safety guidelines for strength training include using proper technique, using spotters and collars when necessary, and taking care of injuries.

- Supplements or drugs that are promoted as instant or quick "cures" usually don't work and are either dangerous, expensive, or both.

## FOR FURTHER EXPLORATION

### BOOKS

Baechle, T., and R. W. Earl. 2008. National Strength and Conditioning Association's *Essentials of Strength and Conditioning*. Champaign, Ill.: Human Kinetics. *A textbook of strength and conditioning for fitness professionals.*

Bjornlund, L. 2010. How Dangerous Are Performance-Enhancing Drugs? San Diego, Calif.: Referencepoint Press. *A discussion of the effects of performance-enhancing drugs on health, performance, and the integrity of sport. The author discusses the role of sports organizations in preventing drug use and whether they can be successful.*

Delavier, F. 2010. *Strength Training Anatomy*, 3rd ed. Champaign, Ill.: Human Kinetics. *Includes exercises for all major muscle groups as well as full anatomical pictures of the muscular system.* Women's Strength Training Anatomy, *a matching volume for women, was published in 2003.*

Fahey, T. D. 2011. *Basic Weight Training for Men and Women*, 8th ed. New York: McGraw-Hill. *A practical guide to developing training programs, using free weights, tailored to individual needs.*

Goldenberg, L., and P. Twist. 2007. *Strength Ball Training*. Champaign, Ill.: Human Kinetics. *A guide to incorporating exercise balls and medicine balls into a complete weight training program.*

Lethi, A., et al. 2007. *Free-Weight Training*. Berkeley, Calif.: Thunder Bay Press. *A complete guide to training with free weights, with special instructions for using weights with an exercise ball.*

Tsatsouline, P. 2010. *Enter the Kettlebell*. Minneapolis, Minn.: Dragon Door Publications. *A guide to basic strength training using kettlebells.*

## ORGANIZATIONS AND WEB SITES

*American College of Sports Medicine Position Stand: Progression Models in Resistance Training for Healthy Adults.* Provides an in-depth look at strategies for setting up a strength training program and making progress based on individual program goals.
http://journals.lww.com/acsm-msse/Fulltext/2009/03000/Progression_Models_in_Resistance_Training_for.26.aspx

*Dan John.* An excellent Web site for people serious about improving strength and fitness, written by a world-class athlete and coach in track and field and Highland games.
http://danjohn.net

*Georgia State University: Strength Training.* Provides information about the benefits of strength training and ways to develop a safe and effective program; also includes illustrations of a variety of exercises.
http://www2.gsu.edu/~wwwfit/strength.html

*Human Anatomy On-line.* Provides text, illustrations, and animation about the muscular system, nerve-muscle connections, muscular contraction, and other topics.
http://www.innerbody.com/htm/body.html

*Mayo Clinic: Weight Training: Improve Your Muscular Fitness.* Provides a basic overview of weight training essentials along with links to many other articles on specific weight training-related topics.
http://www.mayoclinic.com/health/weight-training/HQ01627

*National Strength and Conditioning Association.* A professional organization that focuses on strength development for fitness and athletic performance.
http://www.nsca-lift.org

*Pilates Method Alliance.* Provides information about Pilates and about instructor certification; includes a directory of instructors.
http://www.pilatesmethodalliance.org

*University of California, San Diego: Muscle Physiology Home Page.* Provides an introduction to muscle physiology, including information about types of muscle fibers and energy cycles.
http://muscle.ucsd.edu/index.shtml

*University of Michigan: Muscles in Action.* Interactive descriptions of muscle movements.
http://www.med.umich.edu/lrc/Hypermuscle/Hyper.html
See also the listings in Chapter 2.

## SELECTED BIBLIOGRAPHY

Ahtiainen, J. P., et al. 2011. Recovery after heavy resistance exercise and skeletal muscle androgen receptor and insulin-like growth factor-i isoform expression in strength trained men. *Journal of Strength and Conditioning Research* 25(3): 767–777.

American College of Sports Medicine. 2009. *ACSM's Guidelines for Exercise Testing and Prescription,* 8th ed. Philadelphia: Lippincott Williams and Wilkins.

American College of Sports Medicine. 2009. *ACSM's Resource Manual for Guidelines for Exercise Testing and Prescription,* 6th ed. Philadelphia: Lippincott Williams and Wilkins.

American College of Sports Medicine. 2009. American College of Sports Medicine position stand: Progression models in resistance training for healthy adults. *Medicine and Science in Sports and Exercise* 41(3): 687–708.

Arikawa, A. Y., et al. 2011. Adherence to a strength training intervention in adult women. *Journal of Physical Activity and Health* 8(1): 111–118.

Bellar, D. M., et al. 2011. The Effects of Combined Elastic- and Free-Weight Tension vs. Free-Weight Tension on One-Repetition Maximum Strength in the Bench Press. *Journal of Strength and Conditioning Research* 25(2): 459–463.

Blazevich, A. J., et al. 2007. Lack of human muscle architectural adaptation after short-term strength training. *Muscle and Nerve* 35(1): 78–86.

Bouchard, D. R., et al. 2011. Association between muscle mass, leg strength, and fat mass with physical function in older adults: Influence of age and sex. *Journal of Aging and Health* 23(2): 313–328.

Brentano, M. A., et al. 2011. A review on strength exercise-induced muscle damage: applications, adaptation mechanisms and limitations. *Journal of Sports Medicine and Physical Fitness* 51(1): 1–10.

Brooks, G. A., et al. 2005. *Exercise Physiology: Human Bioenergetics and Its Applications,* 4th ed. New York: McGraw-Hill.

Brooks, N., et al. 2006. Strength training improves muscle quality and insulin sensitivity in Hispanic older adults with type 2 diabetes. *International Journal of Medical Sciences* 4(1): 19–27.

Burt, J., et al. 2007. A comparison of once versus twice per week training on leg press strength in women. *Journal of Sports Medicine and Physical Fitness* 47(1): 13–17.

Cadore, E. L., et al. 2011. Effects of strength, endurance, and concurrent training on aerobic power and dynamic neuromuscular economy in elderly men. *Journal of Strength and Conditioning Research* 25(3): 758–766.

Carlsohn, A., et al. 2011. How much is too much? A case report of nutritional supplement use of a high-performance athlete. *British Journal Nutrition* 1–5.

Caserotti, P., et al. 2008. Explosive heavy-resistance training in old and very old adults: Changes in rapid muscle force, strength and power. *Scandinavian Journal of Medicine and Science in Sports* 18(6): 773–782.

Davis, W. J., et al. 2008. Concurrent training enhances athletes' strength, muscle endurance, and other measures. *Journal of Strength and Conditioning Research* 22(5): 1487–1502.

Dengel, D. R., et al. 2011. Gender differences in vascular function and insulin sensitivity in young adults. *Clinical Sciences* 120(4): 153–160.

Farrar, R. E., et al. 2010. Oxygen cost of kettlebell swings. *Journal of Strength and Conditioning Research* 24(4): 1034–1036.

Gee, T. I., et al. 2011. Strength and conditioning practices in rowing. *Journal of Strength and Conditioning Research* 25(3): 668–682.

Graham, M. R., et al. 2008. Anabolic steroid use: Patterns of use and detection of doping. *Sports Medicine* 38(6): 505–525.

Haskell, W. L., et al. 2007. Physical activity and public health: updated recommendation for adults from the American College of Sports Medicine and the American Heart Association. *Circulation* 116(9): 1081–1093.

Headley, S. A., et al. 2011. Effects of lifting tempo on one repetition maximum and hormonal responses to a bench press protocol. *Journal of Strength and Conditioning Research* 25(2): 406–413.

Heikkinen, A., et al. 2011. Use of dietary supplements in Olympic athletes is decreasing: A follow-up study between 2002 and 2009. *Journal of the International Society of Sports Nutrition* 8(1): 1.

Hoffman, J. R., et al. 2008. Nutritional supplementation and anabolic steroid use in adolescents. *Medicine and Science in Sports and Exercise* 40(1): 15–24.

Ikeda, E. R., et al. 2009. The valsalva maneuver revisited: The influence of voluntary breathing on isometric muscle strength. *Journal of Strength and Conditioning Research* 23(1): 127–132.

Jay, K., et al. 2010. Kettlebell training for musculoskeletal and cardiovascular health: A randomized controlled trial. *Scandinavian Journal of Work and Environmental Health.* Published online December 2010.

Kell, R. T. 2011. The influence of periodized resistance training on strength changes in men and women. *Journal of Strength and Conditioning Research* 25(3): 735–744.

Kirk, E. P., et al. 2007. Six months of supervised high-intensity low-volume resistance training improves strength independent of changes in muscle mass in young overweight men. *Journal of Strength and Conditioning Research* 21(1): 151–156.

Lindegaard, B., et al. 2008. The effect of strength and endurance training on insulin sensitivity and fat distribution in human immunodeficiency virus-infected patients with lipodystrophy. *Journal of Clinical Endocrinology and Metabolism* 93(10): 3860–3869.

Machado, M. V., et al. 2011. The dark side of sports: Using steroids may harm your liver. *Liver International* 31(3): 280–281.

Manore, M., et al. 2011. BJSM reviews: A-Z of nutritional supplements: dietary supplements, sports nutrition foods and ergogenic aids for health and performance—Part 16. *British Journal Sports Medicine* 45(1): /3–74.

Newsholme, P., et al. 2011. BJSM reviews: A to Z of nutritional supplements: dietary supplements, sports nutrition foods and ergogenic aids for health and performance—Part 18. *British Journal Sports Medicine* 45(3): 230–232.

Norrbrand, L., et al. 2008. Resistance training using eccentric overload induces early adaptations in skeletal muscle size. *European Journal of Applied Physiology* 102(3): 271–281.

Reitelseder, S., et al. 2011. Whey and casein labeled with L-[1-13C]leucine and muscle protein synthesis: Effect of resistance exercise and protein ingestion. *American Journal of Physiology, Endocrinology and Metabolism* 300(1): E231–242.

Ruiz, J. R., et al. 2008. Association between muscular strength and mortality in men: Prospective cohort study. *British Medical Journal* 337: a439, published online.

Saeterbakken, A. H., et al. 2011. A comparison of muscle activity and 1-RM strength of three chest-press exercises with different stability requirements. *Journal of Sports Science* 1–6.

Santos, E. J., et al. 2011. The effects of plyometric training followed by detraining and reduced training periods on explosive strength in adolescent male basketball players. *Journal of Strength and Conditioning Research* 25(2): 441–452.

Schick, E. E., et al. 2010. A comparison of muscle activation between a Smith machine and free weight bench press. *Journal of Strength and Conditioning Research* 24(3): 779–784.

Sedano, S., et al. 2011. Effects of plyometric training on explosive strength, acceleration capacity and kicking speed in young elite soccer players. *Journal of Sports Medicine and Physical Fitness* 51(1): 50–58.

Senchina, D. S., et al. 2011. BJSM reviews: A-Z of nutritional supplements: dietary supplements, sports nutrition foods and ergogenic aids for health and performance—Part 17. *British Journal Sports Medicine* 45(2): 150–151.

Wieser, M., and P. Haber. 2007. The effects of systematic resistance training in the elderly. *International Journal of Sports Medicine* 28(1): 59–65.

Winchester, J. B., et al. 2008. Eight weeks of ballistic exercise improves power independently of changes in strength and muscle fiber type expression. *Journal of Strength and Conditioning Research* 22(6): 1728–1734.

Young, W. B., et al. 2011. Enhancing foot velocity in football kicking: the role of strength training. *Journal of Strength and Conditioning Research* 25(2): 561–566.

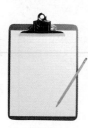

## LAB 4.1 Assessing Your Current Level of Muscular Strength

For best results, don't do any strenuous weight training within 48 hours of any test. Use great caution when completing 1-RM tests; do not take the maximum bench press test if you have any injuries to your shoulders, elbows, back, hips, or knees. In addition, do not take these tests until you have had at least one month of weight training experience.

### The Maximum Bench Press Test

#### Equipment
The free weights bench press test uses the following equipment

1. Flat bench (with or without racks)
2. Barbell
3. Assorted weight plates, with collars to hold them in place
4. One or two spotters
5. Weight scale

If a weight machine is preferred, use the following equipment:

1. Universal Gym Dynamic Variable Resistance Machine
2. Weight scale

#### Preparation
Try a few bench presses with a small amount of weight so you can practice your technique, warm up your muscles, and, if you use free weights, coordinate your movements with those of your spotters. Weigh yourself and record the results.

Body weight: _____ lb

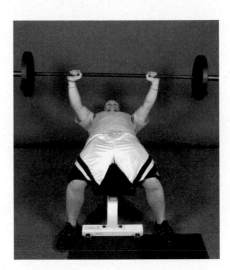

Maximum bench press test.

#### Instructions

1. Use a weight that is lower than the amount you believe you can lift. For free weights, men should begin with a weight about two-thirds of their body weight; women should begin with the weight of just the bar (45 lb).

2. Lie on the bench with your feet firmly on the floor. If you are using a weight machine, grasp the handles with palms away from you; the tops of the handles should be aligned with the tops of your armpits.

   If you are using free weights, grasp the bar slightly wider than shoulder width with your palms away from you. If you have one spotter, she or he should stand directly behind the bench; if you have two spotters, they should stand to the side, one at each end of the barbell. Signal to the spotter when you are ready to begin the test by saying "1, 2, 3." On "3," the spotter should help you lift the weight to a point over your midchest (nipple line).

3. Push the handles or barbell until your arms are fully extended. Exhale as you lift. If you are using free weights, the weight moves from a low point at the chest straight up. Keep your feet firmly on the floor, don't arch your back, and push the weight evenly with your right and left arms. Don't bounce the weight on your chest.

4. Rest for several minutes, then repeat the lift with a heavier weight. It will probably take several attempts to determine the maximum amount of weight you can lift (1 RM).

   1 RM: _____ lb     Check one: _____ Free weights _____ Universal _____ Other

5. If you used free weights, convert your free weights bench press score to an estimated value for 1 RM on the Universal bench press using the appropriate formula:

   Males: Estimated Universal 1 RM = (1.016 × free weights 1 RM _____ lb) + 18.41 = _____ lb

   Females: Estimated Universal 1 RM = (0.848 × free weights 1 RM _____ lb) + 21.37 = _____ lb

Mc Graw Hill connect™  http://www.mcgrawhillconnect.com/
FITNESS AND WELLNESS

## Rating Your Bench Press Result

1. Divide your Universal 1-RM value by your body weight.

   1 RM _____ lb ÷ body weight _____ lb = _____

2. Find this ratio in the table to determine your bench press strength rating. Record the rating here and in the chart at the end of this lab.

   Bench press strength rating: _____

## Strength Ratings for the Maximum Bench Press Test

| | Pounds Lifted/Body Weight (lb) | | | | | |
|---|---|---|---|---|---|---|
| Men | *Very Poor* | *Poor* | *Fair* | *Good* | *Excellent* | *Superior* |
| *Age:* Under 20 | Below 0.89 | 0.89–1.05 | 1.06–1.18 | 1.19–1.33 | 1.34–1.75 | Above 1.75 |
| 20–29 | Below 0.88 | 0.88–0.98 | 0.99–1.13 | 1.14–1.31 | 1.32–1.62 | Above 1.62 |
| 30–39 | Below 0.78 | 0.78–0.87 | 0.88–0.97 | 0.98–1.11 | 1.12–1.34 | Above 1.34 |
| 40–49 | Below 0.72 | 0.72–0.79 | 0.80–0.87 | 0.88–0.99 | 1.00–1.19 | Above 1.19 |
| 50–59 | Below 0.63 | 0.63–0.70 | 0.71–0.78 | 0.79–0.89 | 0.90–1.04 | Above 1.04 |
| 60 and over | Below 0.57 | 0.57–0.65 | 0.66–0.71 | 0.72–0.81 | 0.82–0.93 | Above 0.93 |
| Women | | | | | | |
| *Age:* Under 20 | Below 0.53 | 0.53–0.57 | 0.58–0.64 | 0.65–0.76 | 0.77–0.87 | Above 0.87 |
| 20–29 | Below 0.51 | 0.51–0.58 | 0.59–0.69 | 0.70–0.79 | 0.80–1.00 | Above 1.00 |
| 30–39 | Below 0.47 | 0.47–0.52 | 0.53–0.59 | 0.60–0.69 | 0.70–0.81 | Above 0.81 |
| 40–49 | Below 0.43 | 0.43–0.49 | 0.50–0.53 | 0.54–0.61 | 0.62–0.76 | Above 0.76 |
| 50–59 | Below 0.39 | 0.39–0.43 | 0.44–0.47 | 0.48–0.54 | 0.55–0.67 | Above 0.67 |
| 60 and over | Below 0.38 | 0.38–0.42 | 0.43–0.46 | 0.47–0.53 | 0.54–0.71 | Above 0.71 |

SOURCE: Based on norms from The Cooper Institute of Aerobic Research, Dallas, Texas; from *The Physical Fitness Specialist Manual,* revised 2002. Used with permission.

## Predicting 1 RM from Multiple-Repetition Lifts Using Free Weights

Instead of doing the 1-RM maximum strength bench press test, you can predict your 1 RM from multiple-repetition lifts.

## Instructions

1. Choose a weight you think you can bench press five times.

2. Follow the instructions for lifting the weight given in the maximum bench press test.

3. Do as many repetitions of the bench press as you can. A repetition counts only if done correctly

4. Refer to the chart on p. 131, or calculate predicted 1 RM using the Brzycki equation:

   1 RM = *weight* ÷ (1.0278 − [0.0278 × *number of repetitions*])

   1 RM = _____ lb ÷ (1.0278 − [0.0278 × _____ repetitions]) = _____

5. Divide your predicted 1-RM value by your body weight.

   1 RM _____ lb ÷ body weight _____ lb = _____

6. Find this ratio in the table above to determine your bench press strength rating. Record the rating here and in the chart at the end of the lab.

   Bench press strength rating: _____

| Weight Lifted (lb) | Repetitions | | | | | | | | | | | |
|---|---|---|---|---|---|---|---|---|---|---|---|---|
| | *1* | *2* | *3* | *4* | *5* | *6* | *7* | *8* | *9* | *10* | *11* | *12* |
| 66 | 66 | 68 | 70 | 72 | 74 | 77 | 79 | 82 | 85 | 88 | 91 | 95 |
| 77 | 77 | 79 | 82 | 84 | 87 | 89 | 92 | 96 | 99 | 103 | 107 | 111 |
| 88 | 88 | 91 | 93 | 96 | 99 | 102 | 106 | 109 | 113 | 117 | 122 | 127 |
| 99 | 99 | 102 | 105 | 108 | 111 | 115 | 119 | 123 | 127 | 132 | 137 | 143 |
| 110 | 110 | 113 | 116 | 120 | 124 | 128 | 132 | 137 | 141 | 147 | 152 | 158 |
| 121 | 121 | 124 | 128 | 132 | 136 | 141 | 145 | 150 | 156 | 161 | 168 | 174 |
| 132 | 132 | 136 | 140 | 144 | 149 | 153 | 158 | 164 | 170 | 176 | 183 | 190 |
| 143 | 143 | 147 | 151 | 156 | 161 | 166 | 172 | 178 | 184 | 191 | 198 | 206 |
| 154 | 154 | 158 | 163 | 168 | 173 | 179 | 185 | 191 | 198 | 205 | 213 | 222 |
| 165 | 165 | 170 | 175 | 180 | 186 | 192 | 198 | 205 | 212 | 220 | 229 | 238 |
| 176 | 176 | 181 | 186 | 192 | 198 | 204 | 211 | 219 | 226 | 235 | 244 | 254 |
| 187 | 187 | 192 | 198 | 204 | 210 | 217 | 224 | 232 | 240 | 249 | 259 | 269 |
| 198 | 198 | 204 | 210 | 216 | 223 | 230 | 238 | 246 | 255 | 264 | 274 | 285 |
| 209 | 209 | 215 | 221 | 228 | 235 | 243 | 251 | 259 | 269 | 279 | 289 | 301 |
| 220 | 220 | 226 | 233 | 240 | 248 | 256 | 264 | 273 | 283 | 293 | 305 | 317 |
| 231 | 231 | 238 | 245 | 252 | 260 | 268 | 277 | 287 | 297 | 308 | 320 | 333 |
| 242 | 242 | 249 | 256 | 264 | 272 | 281 | 290 | 300 | 311 | 323 | 335 | 349 |
| 253 | 253 | 260 | 268 | 276 | 285 | 294 | 304 | 314 | 325 | 337 | 350 | 364 |
| 264 | 264 | 272 | 280 | 288 | 297 | 307 | 317 | 328 | 340 | 352 | 366 | 380 |
| 275 | 275 | 283 | 291 | 300 | 309 | 319 | 330 | 341 | 354 | 367 | 381 | 396 |
| 286 | 286 | 294 | 303 | 312 | 322 | 332 | 343 | 355 | 368 | 381 | 396 | 412 |
| 297 | 297 | 305 | 314 | 324 | 334 | 345 | 356 | 369 | 382 | 396 | 411 | 428 |
| 308 | 308 | 317 | 326 | 336 | 347 | 358 | 370 | 382 | 396 | 411 | 427 | 444 |

**SOURCE:** Brzycki, M. 1993. Strength testing—predicting a one-rep max from reps to fatigue. *The Journal of Physical Education, Recreation and Dance* 64: 88–90. January 1993, a publication of the American Alliance for Health, Physical Education, Recreation and Dance, www.aahperd.org. Reprinted with permission.

## Functional Leg Strength Tests

The following tests assess functional leg strength using squats. Most people do squats improperly increasing their risk of knee and back pain. Before you add weight-bearing squats to your weight training program, you should determine your functional leg strength, check your ability to squat properly, and give yourself a chance to master squatting movements. The following leg strength tests will help you in each of these areas.

These tests are progressively more difficult, so do not move to the next test until you have scored at least a 3 on the current test. On each test, give yourself a rating of 0, 1, 3, or 5, as described in the instructions that follow the last test.

## 1. Chair Squat

### Instructions

1. Sit up straight in a chair with your back resting against the backrest and your arms at your sides. Your feet should be placed more than shoulder-width apart so that you can get them under the body.

2. Begin the motion of rising out of the chair by flexing (bending) at the hips—not the back. Then squat up using a hip hinge movement (no spine movement). Stand without rocking forward, bending your back, or using external support, and keep your head in a neutral position.

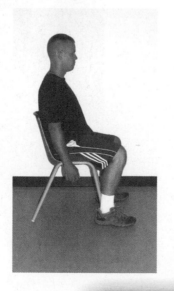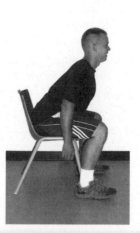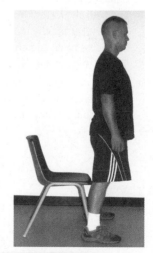

connect http://www.mcgrawhillconnect.com/ **FITNESS AND WELLNESS**

3. Return to the sitting position while maintaining a straight back and keeping your weight centered over your feet. Your thighs should abduct (spread) as you sit back in the chair. Use your rear hip and thigh muscles as much as possible as you sit.

Do five repetitions.

Your rating: _____

(See rating instructions that follow.)

## 2. Single-Leg Step-Up

### Instructions

1. Stand facing a bench, with your right foot placed on the middle of the bench, right knee bent at 90 degrees, and arms at your sides.
2. Step up on the bench until your right leg is straight, maximizing the use of the hip muscles.
3. Return to the starting position. Keep your hips stable, back straight, chest up, shoulders back, and head neutral during the entire movement.

Do five repetitions for each leg.

Your rating: _____

(See rating instructions that follow.)

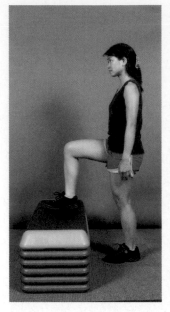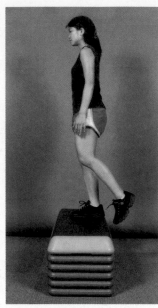

## 3. Unweighted Squat

### Instructions

1. Stand with your feet placed slightly more than shoulder-width apart, toes pointed out slightly, hands on hips or across your chest, head neutral, and back straight. Center your weight over your arches or slightly behind.
2. Squat down, keeping your weight centered over your arches and actively flexing (bending) your hips until your legs break parallel. During the movement, keep your back straight, shoulders back, and chest out, and let your thighs part to the side so that you are "squatting between your legs."
3. Push back up to the starting position, hinging at the hips and not with the spine, maximizing the use of the rear hip and thigh muscles, and maintaining a straight back and neutral head position.

Do five repetitions.

Your rating: _____

(See rating instructions that follow.)

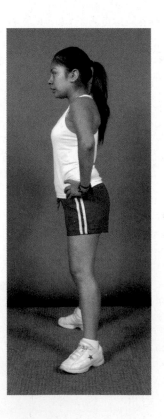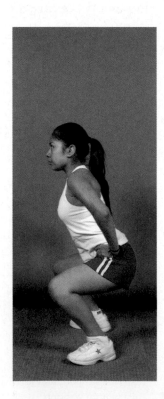

### 4. Single-Leg Lunge-Squat with Rear-Foot Support

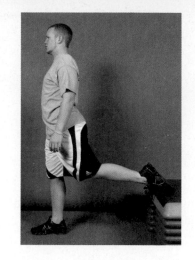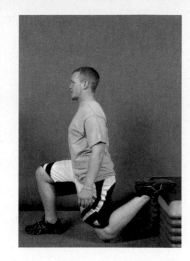

**Instructions**

1. Stand about 3 feet in front of a bench (with your back to the bench).

2. Place the instep of your left foot on the bench, and put most of your weight on your right leg (your left leg should be bent), with your hands at your sides.

3. Squat on your right leg until your thigh is parallel with the floor. Keep your back straight, chest up, shoulders back, and head neutral.

4. Return to the starting position.

Do three repetitions for each leg.

Your rating: _____

(See rating instructions that follow.)

## Rating Your Functional Leg Strength Test Results

*5 points:* Performed the exercise properly with good back and thigh position, weight centered over the middle or rear of the foot, chest out, and shoulders back; good use of hip muscles on the way down and on the way up, with head in a neutral position throughout the movement; maintained good form during all repetitions; abducted (spread) the thighs on the way down during chair squats and double-leg squats; for single-leg exercises, showed good strength on both sides; for single-leg lunge-squat with rear-foot support, maintained straight back, and knees stayed behind toes.

*3 points:* Weight was forward on the toes, with some rounding of the back; used thigh muscles excessively, with little use of hip muscles; head and chest were too far forward; showed little abduction of the thighs during double-leg squats; when going down for single-leg exercises, one side was stronger than the other; form deteriorated with repetitions; for single-leg lunge-squat with rear-foot support, could not reach parallel (thigh parallel with floor).

*1 point:* Had difficulty performing the movement, rocking forward and rounding back badly; used thigh muscles excessively, with little use of hip muscles on the way up or on the way down; chest and head were forward; on unweighted squats, had difficulty reaching parallel and showed little abduction of the thighs; on single-leg exercises, one leg was markedly stronger than the other; could not perform multiple repetitions.

*0 points:* Could not perform the exercise.

### Summary of Results

Maximum bench press test from either the 1-RM test or the multiple-repetition test: Weight pressed: _____ lb Rating: _____

Functional leg strength tests (0–5): Chair squat: _____ Single-leg step-up: _____ Unweighted squat: _____

Single-leg lunge-squat with rear-foot support: _____

Remember that muscular strength is specific: Your ratings may vary considerably for different parts of your body.

## Using Your Results

*How did you score?* Are you surprised by your ratings for muscular strength? Are you satisfied with your current ratings?

If you're not satisfied, set realistic goals for improvement:

Are you satisfied with your current level of muscular strength as evidenced in your daily life—for example, your ability to lift objects, climb stairs, and engage in sports and recreational activities?

If you're not satisfied, set realistic goals for improvement:

*What should you do next?* Enter the results of this lab in the Preprogram Assessment column in Appendix C. If you've set goals for improvement, begin planning your strength training program by completing the plan in Lab 4.3. After several weeks of your program, complete this lab again and enter the results in the Postprogram Assessment column of Appendix C. How do the results compare?

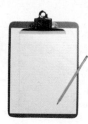

# LAB 4.2  Assessing Your Current Level of Muscular Endurance

For best results, don't do any strenuous weight training within 48 hours of any test. To assess endurance of the abdominal muscles, perform the curl-up test. To assess endurance of muscles in the upper body, perform the push-up test. To assess endurance of the muscles in the lower body, perform the squat endurance test.

## The Curl-Up Test

### Equipment

1. Four 6-inch strips of self-stick Velcro or heavy tape
2. Ruler
3. Partner
4. Mat (optional)

### Preparation

Affix the strips of Velcro or long strips of tape on the mat or testing surface. Place the strips 3 inches apart.

### Instructions

1. Start by lying on your back on the floor or mat, arms straight and by your sides, shoulders relaxed, palms down and on the floor, and fingers straight. Adjust your position so that the longest fingertip of each hand touches the end of the near strip of Velcro or tape. Your knees should be bent about 90 degrees, with your feet about 12–18 inches from your buttocks.

2. To perform a curl-up, flex your spine while sliding your fingers across the floor until the fingertips of each hand reach the second strip of Velcro or tape. Then return to the starting position; the shoulders must be returned to touch the mat between curl-ups, but the head need not touch. Shoulders must remain relaxed throughout the curl-up, and feet and buttocks must stay on the floor. Breathe easily exhaling during the lift phase of the curl-up; do not hold your breath.

3. Once your partner says "go," perform as many curl-ups as you can at a steady pace with correct form. Your partner counts the curl-ups you perform and calls a stop to the test if she or he notices any incorrect form or drop in your pace.

   Number of curl-ups: _____

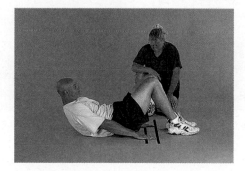 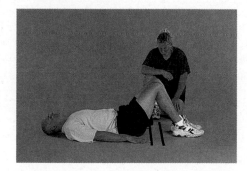

### Rating Your Curl-Up Test Result

Your score is the number of completed curl-ups. Refer to the appropriate portion of the table for a rating of your abdominal muscular endurance. Record your rating below and in the summary at the end of this lab.

Rating: _____

connect http://www.mcgrawhillconnect.com/
FITNESS AND WELLNESS

LABORATORY ACTIVITIES

| | Number of Curl-Ups | | | | | |
|---|---|---|---|---|---|---|
| **Men** | *Very Poor* | *Poor* | *Average* | *Good* | *Excellent* | *Superior* |
| Age: 16–19 | Below 48 | 48–57 | 58–64 | 65–74 | 75–93 | Above 93 |
| 20–29 | Below 46 | 46–54 | 55–63 | 64–74 | 75–93 | Above 93 |
| 30–39 | Below 40 | 40–47 | 48–55 | 56–64 | 65–81 | Above 81 |
| 40–49 | Below 38 | 38–45 | 46–53 | 54–62 | 63–79 | Above 79 |
| 50–59 | Below 36 | 36–43 | 44–51 | 52–60 | 61–77 | Above 77 |
| 60–69 | Below 33 | 33–40 | 41–48 | 49–57 | 58–74 | Above 74 |
| **Women** | | | | | | |
| Age: 16–19 | Below 42 | 42–50 | 51–58 | 59–67 | 68–84 | Above 84 |
| 20–29 | Below 41 | 41–51 | 52–57 | 58–66 | 67–83 | Above 83 |
| 30–39 | Below 38 | 38–47 | 48–56 | 57–66 | 67–85 | Above 85 |
| 40–49 | Below 36 | 36–45 | 46–54 | 55–64 | 65–83 | Above 83 |
| 50–59 | Below 34 | 34–43 | 44–52 | 53–62 | 63–81 | Above 81 |
| 60–69 | Below 31 | 31–40 | 41–49 | 50–59 | 60–78 | Above 78 |

SOURCE: Ratings based on norms calculated from data collected by Robert Lualhati on 4545 college students, 16–80 years of age, at Skyline College, San Bruno, California. Used with permission.

## The Push-Up Test

*Equipment:* Mat or towel (optional)

### Preparation

In this test, you will perform either standard push-ups or modified push-ups, in which you support yourself with your knees. The Cooper Institute developed the ratings for this test with men performing push-ups and women performing modified push-ups. Biologically, males tend to be stronger than females; the modified technique reduces the need for upper-body strength in a test of muscular endurance. Therefore, for an accurate assessment of upper-body endurance, men should perform standard push-ups and women should perform modified push-ups. However, in using push-ups as part of a strength training program, individuals should choose the technique most appropriate for increasing their level of strength and endurance—regardless of gender.

### Instructions

1. *For push-ups:* Start in the push-up position with your body supported by your hands and feet. *For-modified push-ups:* Start in the modified push-up position with your body supported by your hands and knees. *For both positions*, keep your arms and your back straight and your fingers pointed forward.

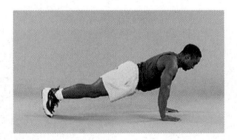 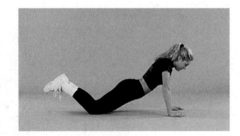

2. Lower your chest to the floor with your back straight, and then return to the starting position.

3. Perform as many push-ups or modified push-ups as you can without stopping.

   Number of push-ups: _____ or number of modified push-ups: _____

### Rating Your Push-Up Test Result

Your score is the number of completed push-ups or modified push-ups. Refer to the appropriate portion of the table for a rating of your upper-body endurance. Record your rating below and in the summary at the end of this lab.

Rating: _____

## Ratings for the Push-Up and Modified Push-Up Tests

| Men | Very Poor | Poor | Fair | Good | Excellent | Superior |
|-----|-----------|------|------|------|-----------|----------|
| | | | **Number of Push-Ups** | | | |
| Age: 18–29 | Below 22 | 22–28 | 29–36 | 37–46 | 47–61 | Above 61 |
| 30–39 | Below 17 | 17–23 | 24–29 | 30–38 | 39–51 | Above 51 |
| 40–49 | Below 11 | 11–17 | 18–23 | 24–29 | 30–39 | Above 39 |
| 50–59 | Below 9 | 9–12 | 13–18 | 19–24 | 25–38 | Above 38 |
| 60 and over | Below 6 | 6–9 | 10–17 | 18–22 | 23–27 | Above 27 |

| Women | Very Poor | Poor | Fair | Good | Excellent | Superior |
|-------|-----------|------|------|------|-----------|----------|
| | | | **Number of Modified Push-Ups** | | | |
| Age: 18–29 | Below 17 | 17–22 | 23–29 | 30–35 | 36–44 | Above 44 |
| 30–39 | Below 11 | 11–18 | 19–23 | 24–30 | 31–38 | Above 38 |
| 40–49 | Below 6 | 6–12 | 13–17 | 18–23 | 24–32 | Above 32 |
| 50–59 | Below 6 | 6–11 | 12–16 | 17–20 | 21–27 | Above 27 |
| 60 and over | Below 2 | 2–4 | 5–11 | 12–14 | 15–19 | Above 19 |

**SOURCE:** Based on norms from The Cooper Institute of Aerobic Research, Dallas, Texas; from *The Physical Fitness Specialist Manual*, revised 2002. Used with permission.

## The Squat Endurance Test

### Instructions

1. Stand with your feet placed slightly more than shoulder width apart, toes pointed out slightly hands on hips or across your chest, head neutral, and back straight. Center your weight over your arches or slightly behind.

2. Squat down, keeping your weight centered over your arches, until your thighs are parallel with the floor. Push back up to the starting position, maintaining a straight back and neutral head position.

3. Perform as many squats as you can without stopping.

   Number of squats: _____

### Rating Your Squat Endurance Test Result

Your score is the number of completed squats. Refer to the appropriate portion of the table for a rating of your leg muscular endurance. Record your rating below and in the summary at the end of this lab.
Rating: _____

### Ratings for the Squat Endurance Test

| Men | Very Poor | Poor | Below Average | Average | Above Average | Good | Excellent |
|-----|-----------|------|---------------|---------|---------------|------|-----------|
| | | | | **Number of Squats Performed** | | | |
| Age: 18–25 | <25 | 25–30 | 31–34 | 35–38 | 39–43 | 44–49 | >49 |
| 26–35 | <22 | 22–28 | 29–30 | 31–34 | 35–39 | 40–45 | >45 |
| 36–45 | <17 | 17–22 | 23–26 | 27–29 | 30–34 | 35–41 | >41 |
| 46–55 | <9 | 13–17 | 18–21 | 22–24 | 25–38 | 29–35 | >35 |
| 56–65 | <9 | 9–12 | 13–16 | 17–20 | 21–24 | 25–31 | >31 |
| 65 + | <7 | 7–10 | 11–14 | 15–18 | 19–21 | 22–28 | >28 |

| Women | Very Poor | Poor | Below Average | Average | Above Average | Good | Excellent |
|-------|-----------|------|---------------|---------|---------------|------|-----------|
| Age: 18–25 | <18 | 18–24 | 25–28 | 29–32 | 33–36 | 37–43 | >43 |
| 26–35 | <20 | 13–20 | 21–24 | 25–28 | 29–32 | 33–39 | >39 |
| 36–45 | <7 | 7–14 | 15–18 | 19–22 | 23–26 | 27–33 | >33 |
| 46–55 | <5 | 5–9 | 10–13 | 14–17 | 18–21 | 22–27 | >27 |
| 56–65 | <3 | 3–6 | 7–9 | 10–12 | 13–17 | 18–24 | >24 |
| 65+ | <2 | 2–4 | 5–10 | 11–13 | 14–16 | 17–23 | >23 |

**SOURCE:** www.topendsports.com/testing/tests/home-squat.htm

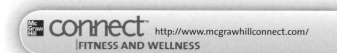

*Summary of Results*

Curl-up test: Number of curl-ups: _____ Rating: _____

Push-up test: Number of push-ups: _____ Rating: _____

Squat endurance test: Number of squats: _____ Rating: _____

Remember that muscular endurance is specific: Your ratings may vary considerably for different parts of your body.

## Using Your Results

*How did you score?* Are you surprised by your ratings for muscular endurance? Are you satisfied with your current ratings?

If you're not satisfied, set realistic goals for improvement:

Are you satisfied with your current level of muscular endurance as evidenced in your daily life—for example, your ability to carry groceries or your books, hike, and do yard work?

If you're not satisfied, set realistic goals for improvement:

*What should you do next?* Enter the results of this lab in the Preprogram Assessment column in Appendix C. If you've set goals for improvement, begin planning your strength training program by completing the plan in Lab 4.3. After several weeks of your program, complete this lab again and enter the results in the Postprogram Assessment column of Appendix C. How do the results compare?

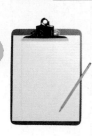

## LAB 4.3 Designing and Monitoring a Strength Training Program

1. *Set goals.* List goals for your strength training program. Your goals can be specific or general, short or long term. In the first section, include specific, measurable goals that you can use to track the progress of your fitness program—for example, raising your upper-body muscular strength rating from fair to good or being able to complete 10 repetitions of a lat pull with 125 pounds of resistance. In the second section, include long-term and more qualitative goals, such as improving self-confidence and reducing your risk for back pain.

Specific Goals: Current Status                                    Final Goals

_____                    _____

_____                    _____

_____                    _____

Other goals: _____

_____

2. *Choose exercises.* Based on your goals, choose 8–10 exercises to perform during each weight training session. If your goal is general training for wellness, use the sample program in Figure 4.2 on p. 109. List your exercises and the muscles they develop in your program plan.

3. *Frequency: Choose the number of training sessions per week.* Work out at least 2 nonconsecutive days per week. Indicate the days you will train in your program plan; be sure to include days of rest to allow your body to recover.

4. *Intensity: Choose starting weights.* Experiment with different amounts of weight until you settle on a good starting weight, one that you can lift easily for 10–12 repetitions. As you progress in your program, add more weight. Fill in the starting weight for each exercise in your program plan.

5. *Time: Choose a starting number of sets and repetitions.* Include at least 1 set of 8–12 repetitions of each exercise. (When you add weight, you may have to decrease the number of repetitions slightly until your muscles adapt to the heavier load.) If your program is focusing on strength alone, your sets can contain fewer repetitions using a heavier load. If you are over approximately age 50–60, your sets should contain more repetitions (10–15) using a lighter load. Fill in the starting number of sets and repetitions of each exercise in your program plan.

6. *Monitor your progress.* Use the workout card on the next page to monitor your progress and keep track of exercises, weights, sets, and repetitions.

### Program Plan for Weight Training

| Exercise | Muscle(s) Developed | Frequency (check ✓) | | | | | | | Intensity: Weight (lb) | Time | |
| | | M | T | W | Th | F | Sa | Su | | Repetitions | Sets |
|---|---|---|---|---|---|---|---|---|---|---|---|
| | | | | | | | | | | | |
| | | | | | | | | | | | |
| | | | | | | | | | | | |
| | | | | | | | | | | | |
| | | | | | | | | | | | |
| | | | | | | | | | | | |
| | | | | | | | | | | | |
| | | | | | | | | | | | |
| | | | | | | | | | | | |
| | | | | | | | | | | | |

connect ™  http://www.mcgrawhillconnect.com/
|FITNESS AND WELLNESS

## WORKOUT CARD FOR _____

| Exercise/Date | Wt | Sets | Reps | Wt | Sets | Reps | Wt | Sets | Reps | Wt | Sets | Reps | Wt | Sets | Reps | Wt | Sets | Reps | Wt | Sets | Reps | Wt | Sets | Reps | Wt | Sets | Reps | Wt | Sets | Reps | Wt | Sets | Reps | Wt | Sets | Reps |
|---|---|---|---|---|---|---|---|---|---|---|---|---|---|---|---|---|---|---|---|---|---|---|---|---|---|---|---|---|---|---|---|---|---|---|---|---|
| | | | | | | | | | | | | | | | | | | | | | | | | | | | | | | | | | | | | |

# CHAPTER 5

# Flexibility and Low-Back Health

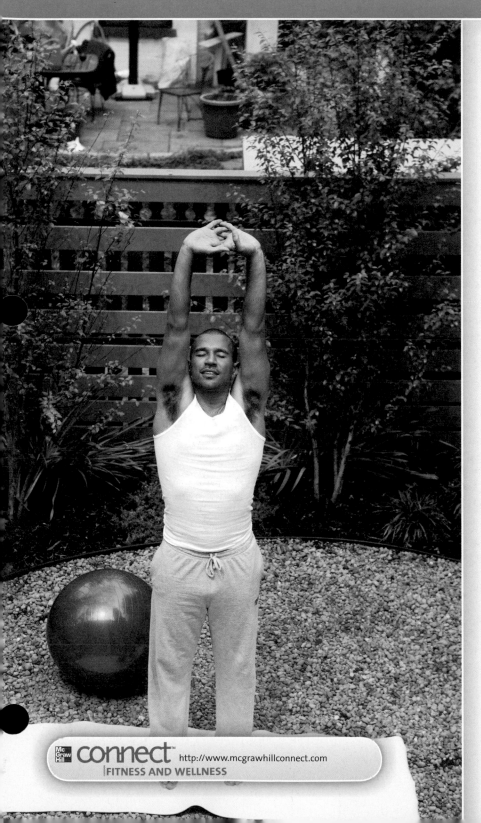

## LOOKING AHEAD...

After reading this chapter, you should be able to:

- Identify the potential benefits of flexibility and stretching exercises
- List the factors that affect a joint's flexibility
- Describe the different types of stretching exercises and how they affect muscles
- Describe the intensity, duration, and frequency of stretching exercises that will develop the most flexibility with the lowest risk of injury
- List safe stretching exercises for major joints
- Explain how low-back pain can be prevented and managed

## TEST YOUR KNOWLEDGE

1. Stretching exercises should be performed
   a. at the start of a warm-up.
   b. first thing in the morning.
   c. after endurance exercise or strength training.

2. If you injure your back, it's usually best to rest in bed until the pain is completely gone. True or false?

3. It is better to hold a stretch for a short time than to "bounce" while stretching. True or false?

**Answers**

1. **c.** It's best to do stretching exercises when your muscles are warm. Intensely stretching muscles before exercise may temporarily reduce their explosive strength and interfere with neuromuscular control.

2. **False.** Prolonged bed rest may actually worsen back pain. Limit bed rest to a day or less, treat pain and inflammation with cold and then heat, and begin moderate physical activity as soon as possible.

3. **True.** "Bouncing" during stretching can damage your muscles. This type of stretching, called ballistic stretching, should be used only by well-conditioned athletes for specific purposes. A person of average fitness should stretch slowly, holding each stretch for 10–30 seconds.

McGraw Hill **connect** http://www.mcgrawhillconnect.com
|FITNESS AND WELLNESS

McGraw Hill **LearnSmart**
GET A BETTER GRADE. TRY LEARNSMART.

flexibility—the ability of a joint to move through its normal, full **range of motion**—is important for general fitness and wellness. Flexibility is a highly adaptable physical fitness component. It increases in response to a regular program of stretching exercises and decreases with inactivity. Flexibility is also specific: Good flexibility in one joint doesn't necessarily mean good flexibility in another. You can increase your flexibility by doing regular stretching exercises for all your major joints.

This chapter describes the factors that affect flexibility and the benefits of maintaining good flexibility. It provides guidelines for assessing your current level of flexibility and putting together a successful stretching program. It also examines the common problem of low-back pain.

## TYPES OF FLEXIBILITY

There are two types of flexibility:

- *Static flexibility* is the ability to hold an extended position at one end or point in a joint's range of motion. For example, static flexibility determines how far you can extend your arm across the front of your body or out to the side. Static flexibility depends on your ability to tolerate stretched muscles; the structure of your joints; and the tightness of muscles, tendons, and ligaments.

- *Dynamic flexibility* is the ability to move a joint through its range of motion with little resistance. For example, dynamic flexibility affects your ability to pitch a ball or swing a golf club. Dynamic flexibility depends on static flexibility, but it also involves strength, coordination, and resistance to movement.

Dynamic flexibility is important for daily activities and sports. Because static flexibility is easier to measure and better researched, however, most assessment tests and stretching programs target that type of flexibility.

## WHAT DETERMINES FLEXIBILITY?

The flexibility of a joint is affected by its structure, by muscle elasticity and length, and by nervous system regulation. Some factors, such as joint structure, can't be changed. Other factors, such as the length of resting muscle fibers, can be changed through exercise; these factors should be the focus of a program to develop flexibility.

### Joint Structure

The amount of flexibility in a joint is determined in part by the nature and structure of the joint (Figure 5.1). Hinge joints such as those in your fingers and knees allow only limited forward and backward movement; they lock

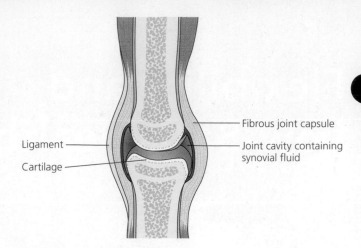

Ligament
Cartilage
Fibrous joint capsule
Joint cavity containing synovial fluid

**FIGURE 5.1   Basic joint structure.**

when fully extended. Ball-and-socket joints like the hip enable movement in many different directions and provide for a greater range of motion. Major joints are surrounded by **joint capsules**, semielastic structures that give joints strength and stability but limit movement. The bone surfaces within the joint are lined with cartilage and separated by a joint cavity containing *synovial fluid,* which cushions the bones and reduces friction as the joint moves. Ligaments, both inside and outside the joint capsule, strengthen and reinforce the joint. For an illustration of the knee joint and more about its function, see page T4-5 of the color transparency insert "Touring the Musculoskeletal System," in Chapter 4.

Heredity plays a part in joint structure and flexibility. For example, although everyone has a broad range of motion in the hip joint, not everyone can do a split. Gender may also play a role. Some studies have found that women have greater flexibility in certain joints.

### Muscle Elasticity and Length

**Soft tissues**—including skin, muscles, tendons, and ligaments—also limit the flexibility of a joint. Muscle tissue is the key to developing flexibility because it can be lengthened if it is stretched regularly. The most important component of muscle tissue related to flexibility is the connective tissue that surrounds and envelops every part of muscle tissue, from individual muscle fibers to entire muscles. Connective tissue provides structure, elasticity, and bulk and makes up about 30% of muscle mass. Two principal types of connective tissue are **collagen**—white fibers that provide structure and support—and **elastin**—yellow fibers that are elastic and flexible. Muscles contain both collagen and elastin, closely intertwined, so muscle tissue exhibits the properties of both types of fibers. A recently discovered structural protein in muscles called *titin* also has elastic properties and contributes to flexibility.

When a muscle is stretched, the wavelike elastin fibers straighten; when the stretch is relieved, they rapidly snap back to their resting position. This temporary lengthening

## Ask Yourself

is called **elastic elongation.** If stretched gently and regularly, connective tissues may lengthen and flexibility may improve. This long-term lengthening is called **plastic elongation.** Without regular stretching, the process reverses: These tissues shorten, resulting in decreased flexibility. Regular stretching may contribute to flexibility by lengthening muscle fibers through the addition of contractile units called *sarcomeres.*

The amount of stretch a muscle will tolerate is limited, and as the limits of its flexibility are reached, connective tissue becomes more brittle and may rupture if overstretched. A safe and effective program stretches muscles enough to slightly elongate the tissues but not so much that they are damaged. Research has shown that flexibility is improved best by stretching when muscles are warm (following exercise or the application of heat) and the stretch is applied gradually and conservatively. Sudden, high-stress stretching is less effective and can lead to muscle damage.

## Nervous System Regulation

**Proprioceptors** are nerves that send information about the muscular and skeletal systems to the nervous system. When these nerves detect any change in the position or force of muscles, tendons, and joints, they send signals to the spine and brain, which send signals back to coordinate muscle action in ways that protect muscles and tendons from injury. They help control the speed, strength, and coordination of muscle contractions.

When a muscle is stretched (lengthened), proprioceptors detect the amount and rate of the change in muscle length. The nerves send a signal to the spinal cord, which then sends a signal back to the muscle, triggering a muscle contraction that resists the change in muscle length. Another signal is sent to the antagonist muscle, causing it to relax and facilitate contraction of the stretched muscle. These reflexes occur frequently in active muscles and allow for fine control of muscle length and movement.

Small movements that only slightly stimulate these nerves cause small reflex actions. Rapid, powerful, and sudden changes in muscle length strongly stimulate the receptors and can cause large and powerful reflex muscle contractions. Thus, stretches that involve rapid, bouncy movements can be dangerous and cause injury because each bounce causes a reflex contraction, and so a muscle might be stretching at the same time it is contracting. Performing a gradual stretch and then holding it allows the proprioceptors to adjust to the new muscle length and to reduce the signals sent to the spine, thereby allowing muscles to lengthen and, over time, improving flexibility.

The stretching technique called *proprioceptive neuromuscular facilitation (PNF),* described later, takes advantage of nerve activity to improve flexibility. For example, contracting a muscle prior to stretching it can help allow the muscle to stretch farther. The advanced strength training technique called plyometrics (Chapter 4) also takes advantage of the nervous system action in stretching and contracting muscles.

Modifying nervous control through movement and specific exercises is the best way to improve the functional range of motion. Regular stretching trains the proprioceptors to allow greater lengthening of the muscles. Proprioceptors adapt quickly to stretching (or lack of stretching), so frequent training is beneficial for developing flexibility. Stretching before exercising, however, can disturb proprioceptors and interfere with motor control during exercise. This is another good reason to stretch after exercising.

## BENEFITS OF FLEXIBILITY

Good flexibility provides benefits for the entire musculoskeletal system. It may also prevent injuries and soreness and improve performance in all physical activities.

**KEY TERMS**

**range of motion**   The full motion possible in a joint.

**joint capsules**   Semielastic structures, composed primarily of connective tissue, that surround major joints.

**soft tissues**   Tissues of the human body that include skin, fat, linings of internal organs and blood vessels, connective tissues, tendons, ligaments, muscles, and nerves.

**collagen**   White fibers that provide structure and support in connective tissue.

**elastin**   Yellow fibers that make connective tissue flexible.

**elastic elongation**   Temporary change in the length of muscles, tendons, and supporting connective tissues.

**plastic elongation**   Long-term change in the length of muscles, tendons, and supporting connective tissues.

**proprioceptor**   A nerve that sends information about the muscular and skeletal systems to the nervous system.

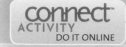

## Does Physical Activity Increase or Decrease the Risk of Bone and Joint Disease?

Most college students don't worry much about developing fall-related fractures or chronic bone-related illnesses such as osteoporosis—loss of bone mass—or osteoarthritis—degeneration of the cartilage lining the bones inside joints. Even so, bone health should be a concern throughout life. This is because girls amass 85% of their adult bone mass by age 18, and boys build the same amount by age 20, but most people begin losing bone mass around age 30. For many, bone loss is accelerated by poor diet and lack of exercise. According to the National Osteoporosis Foundation, 10 million Americans have osteoporosis. Meantime, 34 million Americans are at risk of disease because of low bone mass. Overall, osteoporosis is a health threat for about 55% of Americans aged 50 and older.

In addition to getting enough nutrients that are important for bone health (see Chapter 8), there is mounting evidence that exercise can preserve or improve bone health. For example, several studies have shown an inverse relationship between physical activity and the risk for bone fractures. That is, the more you exercise, the less likely you are to suffer fractures, especially of the upper leg and hip. Research has not determined conclusively how much exercise is required to reduce fracture risk, but reduced risk seems to become apparent when people walk at least 4 hours per week and devote at least 1 hour per week to other forms of physical activity. These findings seem to be consistent for women and men, but some studies disagree on this point, meaning that further research is needed on the sex-related response to exercise as it relates to bone fractures.

Both men and women can prevent fractures and osteoporosis by maintaining or increasing their bone mineral density throughout life, and physical activity plays a significant role in this. One way exercise helps is by increasing the mineral density of bones, or at least by decreasing the loss of mineral density over time. Several one-year-long studies found that exercise can increase bone mineral density by 1–2% per year, which is significant—especially considering that the same amount of bone mineral density can be lost every 1–4 years in older persons. Currently, the American College of Sports Medicine recommends that adults perform weight-bearing physical activities (such as walking) 3–5 days per week and strength training exercises 2–3 days per week to increase bone mass or avoid loss of mineral density. Exercise is particularly important in lactating (breastfeeding) women for preventing bone loss.

When it comes to exercise and osteoarthritis, the evidence is less conclusive but still fairly positive. All experts agree that regular, moderate-intensity exercise is necessary for joint health. However, they also warn that vigorous or too-frequent exercise may contribute to joint damage and encourage the onset of osteoarthritis. For this reason, experts try to strike a balance in their exercise recommendations, especially for persons with a family history of osteoarthritis. Research seems to support this cautious approach. Some studies

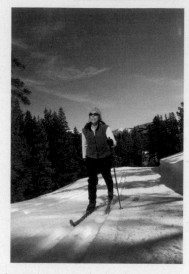

have found that regular physical activity (as recommended for general health) does not increase osteoarthritis risk. Other studies show that moderate activity may provide some protection against the disease, but this evidence is limited.

A few studies also reveal that the type of exercise you do may increase your risk. For example, competitive or strenuous sports such as ballet, orienteering, football, basketball, soccer, and tennis have been associated with the disease, whereas sports such as cross-country skiing, running, swimming, biking, and walking have not.

The bottom line is that the earlier in life you become physically active, the greater your protection against bone loss and bone-related diseases. However, if you have a family history of osteoporosis or osteoarthritis, or if you have already developed symptoms of one of these ailments, be sure to talk to your physician before beginning an exercise program.

**SOURCES:** Kemmler, W., and S. Stengel. 2011. Exercise and osteoporosis-related fractures: Perspectives and recommendations of the sports and exercise scientist. *Physician Sportsmedicine* 39(1): 142–157; Lovelady, et al. 2009. Effect of Exercise Training on Loss of Bone Mineral Density during Lactation. *Medicine and Science in Sports and Exercise* 41 (10): 1902–1907; American College of Sports Medicine. 2004. ACSM position stand: Physical activity and bone health. *Medicine and Science in Sports and Exercise* 36 (11): 1985–1996; National Osteoporosis Foundation. 2011. *Bone Basics: Fast Facts* (http://www.nof.org/node/40; retrieved March 23, 2011); Physical Activity Guidelines Advisory Committee. 2008. *Physical Activity Guidelines Advisory Committee Report, 2008.* Washington, D.C.: U.S. Department of Health and Human Services.

## Joint Health

Good flexibility is essential to good joint health. When the muscles and other tissues that support a joint are tight, the joint is subject to abnormal stresses that can cause joint deterioration. For example, tight thigh muscles cause excessive pressure on the kneecap, leading to pain in the knee joint. Poor joint flexibility can also cause abnormalities in joint lubrication, leading to deterioration of the sensitive cartilage cells lining the joint; pain and further joint injury can result.

Improved flexibility can greatly improve your quality of life, particularly as you get older. People tend to exercise less as they age, leading to loss of joint mobility and increased incidence of joint pain. Aging also decreases the natural elasticity of muscles, tendons, and joints, resulting in stiffness. The problem is often compounded by arthritis (see the box "Does Physical Activity Increase or Decrease the Risk of Bone and Joint Disease?"). Good joint flexibility may prevent arthritis, and stretching may lessen pain in people who have the condition. Another benefit of good flexibility for older adults is that it increases balance and stability.

## Prevention of Low-Back Pain and Injuries

Low-back pain can be related to poor spinal stability, which puts pressure on the nerves leading out from the spinal column. Strength and flexibility in the back, pelvis, and thighs may help prevent this type of back pain but may or may not improve back health or reduce the risk of injury. Good hip and knee flexibility protects the spine from excessive motion during the tasks of daily living.

Although scientific evidence is limited, people with either high or low flexibility seem to have an increased risk of injury. Extreme flexibility reduces joint stability, and poor flexibility limits a joint's range of motion. Persons of average fitness should try to attain normal flexibility in joints throughout the body, meaning each joint can move through its normal range of motion with no difficulty. Stretching programs are particularly important for older adults, people involved in high-power sports involving rapid changes in direction (such as football and tennis), workers involved in brief bouts of intense exertion (such as police officers and firefighters), and people who sit for prolonged periods (such as office workers and students).

However, stretching before a high-intensity activity (such as sprinting or basketball) may increase the risk of injury by interfering with neuromuscular control and reducing muscles' natural ability to stretch and contract. When injuries occur, flexibility exercises can be used in treatment: They reduce symptoms and help restore normal range of motion in affected joints.

## Additional Potential Benefits

- **Relief of aches and pains.** Studying or working in one place for a long time can make your muscles tense. Stretching helps relieve tension and joint stiffness, so you can go back to work refreshed and effective. Stretching reduces the symptoms of exercise-induced muscle damage, and flexible muscles are less susceptible to the damage.
- **Relief of muscle cramps.** Recent research suggests that exercise-related muscle cramps are caused by increased electrical activity within the affected muscle. The best treatment for muscle cramps is gentle stretching, which reduces the electrical activity and allows the muscle to relax.
- **Improved body position and strength for sports (and life).** Good flexibility lets you assume more efficient body positions and exert force through a greater range of motion. For example, swimmers with more flexible shoulders have stronger strokes because they can pull their arms through the water in the optimal position. Some studies also suggest that flexibility training enhances strength development.

- **Maintenance of good posture and balance.** Good flexibility also contributes to body symmetry and good posture. Bad posture can gradually change your body structures. Sitting in a slumped position, for example, can lead to tightness in the muscles in the front of your chest and overstretching and looseness in the upper spine, causing a rounding of the upper back. This condition, called *kyphosis*, is common in older people. It may be prevented by stretching regularly.
- **Relaxation.** Flexibility exercises, particularly when practiced in combination with yoga or tai chi, reduce mental tension, slow your breathing rate, and reduce blood pressure.
- **Improving impaired mobility.** Stretching often decreases pain and improves functional capacity in people with arthritis, stroke, or muscle and nerve diseases and in people who are recovering from surgery or injury.

## ASSESSING FLEXIBILITY

Because flexibility is specific to each joint, there are no tests of general flexibility. The most commonly used flexibility test is the sit-and-reach test, which rates the flexibility of the muscles in the lower back and hamstrings. To assess your flexibility and identify inflexible joints, complete Lab 5.1.

## CREATING A SUCCESSFUL PROGRAM TO DEVELOP FLEXIBILITY

A successful program for developing flexibility includes safe exercises executed with the most effective techniques. Your goal should be to attain normal flexibility

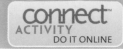

## Safe Stretching

- Do stretching exercises statically. Stretch to the point of mild discomfort, hold the position for 10–30 seconds, rest for 30–60 seconds, and then repeat, trying to stretch a bit farther.

- Do not stretch to the point of pain. Any soreness after a stretching workout should be mild and last no more than 24 hours. If you are sore for a longer period, you stretched too intensely.

- Relax and breathe easily as you stretch. Inhale through the nose and exhale through pursed lips during the stretch. Try to relax the muscles being stretched.

- Perform all exercises on both sides of your body.

- Wear loose-fitting clothing that won't inhibit movement when you're stretching.

- To prevent falls, wear athletic shoes when stretching, or stretch on a no-slip surface.

- Increase intensity and duration gradually over time. Improved flexibility takes many months to develop.

- Stretch when your muscles are warm. Do gentle warm-up exercises such as easy jogging or calisthenics before doing a stretching routine.

- There are large individual differences in joint flexibility. Don't feel you have to compete with others during stretching workouts.

- Engage in a variety of physical activities to help you develop well-rounded functional physical fitness and allow you to perform all types of training more safely and effectively.

in the major joints. Balanced flexibility (not too much or too little) provides joint stability and facilitates smooth, economical movement patterns. You can achieve balanced flexibility by performing stretching exercises regularly and by using a variety of stretches and stretching techniques.

## Applying the FITT Principle

As with other programs, the acronym FITT can be used to remember key components of a stretching program: Frequency, Intensity, Time, and Type of exercise.

**Frequency** The ACSM recommends that stretching exercises be performed at least 2–3 days per week, but more often is even better. It's best to stretch when your muscles are warm, so try incorporating stretching into your cool-down after cardiorespiratory endurance exercise or weight training.

Never stretch when your muscles are cold; doing so can increase your risk of injury as well as limit the amount of flexibility you can develop. Although stretching before exercise is a time-honored ritual practiced by athletes in many sports, many studies have found that preexercise stretching decreases muscle strength and performance and disturbs neuromuscular control. If your workout involves participation in a sport or high-performance activity, you may be better off stretching after your workout. For moderate-intensity activities like walking or cycling, stretching before your workout is unlikely to impair your performance.

**Intensity and Time (Duration)** For each exercise, slowly stretch your muscles to the point of slight tension or mild discomfort—but not to the point of pain. Hold the stretch for 10–30 seconds. As you hold the stretch, the feeling of slight tension should slowly subside; at that point, try to stretch a bit farther. Throughout the stretch, try to relax and breathe easily. Rest for about 30–60

seconds between each stretch, and do 2–4 repetitions of each stretch. A complete flexibility workout usually takes about 10–30 minutes (Figure 5.2).

**Types of Stretching Techniques** Stretching techniques vary from simply stretching the muscles during the course of normal activities to sophisticated methods based on patterns

| Warm-up 5–10 minutes or following an endurance or strength training workout | Stretching exercises for major joints | |
|---|---|---|
| | **Sample program** | |
| | *Exercise* | *Areas stretched* |
| | Head turns and tilts | Neck |
| | Towel stretch | Triceps, shoulders, chest |
| | Across-the-body and overhead stretches | Shoulders, upper back, back of arm |
| | Upper-back stretch | Upper back |
| | Lateral stretch | Trunk muscles |
| | Step stretch | Hip, front of thigh |
| | Side lunge | Inner thigh, hip, calf |
| | Inner-thigh stretch | Inner thigh, hip |
| | Hip and trunk stretch | Trunk, outer thigh, hip, buttocks, lower back |
| | Modified hurdler stretch | Back of thigh, lower back |
| | Alternate leg stretcher | Back of thigh, hip, knee, ankle, buttocks |
| | Lower-leg stretch | Calf, soleus, Achilles tendon |

**Frequency:** 2–3 days per week (minimum); 5–7 days per week (ideal)

**Intensity:** Stretch to the point of mild discomfort, not pain

**Time (duration):** All stretches should be held for 15–30 seconds and performed 2–4 times

**Type of activity:** Stretching exercises that focus on major joints

**FIGURE 5.2   The FITT principle for a flexibility program.**

of muscle reflexes. Improper stretching can do more harm than good, so it's important to understand the different types of stretching exercises and how they affect the muscles (see the box "Safe Stretching"). Four common techniques are static stretches, ballistic stretches, dynamic stretches, and PNF. These techniques can be performed passively or actively.

**STATIC STRETCHING**    In **static stretching**, each muscle is gradually stretched, and the stretch is held for 10–30 seconds. A slow stretch prompts less reaction from proprioceptors, and the muscles can safely stretch farther than usual. Static stretching is the type most often recommended by fitness experts because it is safe and effective.

The key to this technique is to stretch the muscles and joints to the point where a pull is felt, but not to the point of pain. (One note of caution: Excess static stretching can decrease joint stability and increase the risk of injury. This may be a particular concern for women, who naturally have joints that are less stable and more flexible than men.) The sample stretching program presented later in this chapter features static stretching exercises.

**BALLISTIC STRETCHING**    In **ballistic stretching**, the muscles are stretched suddenly in a forceful bouncing movement. For example, touching the toes repeatedly in rapid succession is a ballistic stretch for the hamstrings. A problem with this technique is that the heightened activity of proprioceptors caused by the rapid stretches can continue for some time, possibly causing injuries during any physical activities that follow. Another concern is that triggering strong responses from the nerves can cause a reflex muscle contraction that makes it harder to stretch. For these reasons, ballistic stretching is usually not recommended, especially for people of average fitness.

Ballistic stretching trains the muscle dynamically, so it can be an appropriate stretching technique for some well-trained athletes. For example, tennis players stretch their hamstrings and quadriceps ballistically when they lunge for a ball during a tennis match. Because this movement is part of their sport, they might benefit from ballistic training of these muscle groups.

**DYNAMIC (FUNCTIONAL) STRETCHING**    The emphasis in **dynamic stretching** is on functional movements. Dynamic stretching is similar to ballistic stretching in that it includes movement, but it differs in that it does not involve rapid bouncing. Instead, dynamic stretching involves moving the joints through the range of motion used in a specific exercise or sport in an exaggerated but controlled manner; movements are fluid rather than jerky. An example of a dynamic stretch is the lunge walk, in which a person takes slow steps with an exaggerated stride length and reaches a lunge stretch position with each step.

Slow dynamic stretches can lengthen the muscles in many directions without developing high tension in the tissues. These stretches elongate the tissues and train the neuromuscular system. Because dynamic stretches are based on sports movements or movements used in daily life, they develop functional flexibility that translates well into activities.

Dynamic stretches are more challenging than static stretches because they require balance and coordination and may carry a greater risk of muscle soreness and injury. People just beginning a flexibility program might want to start off with static stretches and try dynamic stretches only after they are comfortable with static stretching techniques and have improved their flexibility. It is also a good idea to seek expert advice on dynamic stretching technique and program development.

Serious athletes may use dynamic stretches as part of their warm-up before a competitive event or a high-intensity training session in order to move their joints through the range of motion required for the activity. Functional flexibility training can also be combined with functional strength training. For example, lunge curls, which combine dynamic lunges with free weights biceps curls, stretch the hip, thigh, and calf muscles; stabilize the core muscles in the trunk; and build strength in the arm muscles. Many activities build functional flexibility and strength at the same time, including yoga, Pilates, taijiquan, Olympic weight lifting, plyometrics, stability training (including Swiss and Bosu ball exercises), medicine ball exercises, and functional training machines (for example, Life Fitness and Cybex).

**PROPRIOCEPTIVE NEUROMUSCULAR FACILITATION (PNF)**    PNF techniques use reflexes initiated by both muscle and joint nerves to cause greater training effects. The most popular PNF stretching technique is the contract-relax stretching method, in which a muscle is contracted before it is stretched. The contraction activates proprioceptors, causing relaxation in the muscle about to be stretched. For example, in a seated stretch of calf muscles, the first step in PNF is to contract the calf muscles. The individual or a partner can provide resistance for an isometric

## Wellness Tip

You don't have to be at the gym to stretch. There are lots of simple, small-movement stretches you can do anywhere—even at your desk. For some examples, visit a good health Web site such as MayoClinic.com and search for "stretching exercises."

contraction. Following a brief period of relaxation, the next step is to stretch the calf muscles by pulling the tops of the feet toward the body. A duration of six seconds for the contraction and 10–30 seconds for the stretch is recommended. PNF appears to be most effective if the individual pushes hard during the isometric contraction.

Another example of a PNF stretch is the contract-relax-contract pattern. In this technique, begin by contracting the muscle to be stretched and then relaxing it. Next, contract the opposing muscle (the antagonist). Finally, stretch the first muscle. For example, using this technique to stretch the hamstrings (the muscles in the back of the thigh) would require the following steps: Contract the hamstrings, relax the hamstrings, contract the quadriceps (the muscles in the front of the thigh), then stretch the hamstrings.

PNF appears to allow more effective stretching and greater increases in flexibility than static stretching, but it tends to cause more muscle stiffness and soreness. It also usually requires a partner and takes more time.

PASSIVE VERSUS ACTIVE STRETCHING    Stretches can be done either passively or actively. In **passive stretching**, an outside force or resistance provided by yourself, a partner, gravity, or a weight helps your joints move through their range of motion. For example, a seated stretch of the hamstring and back muscles can be done by reaching the hands toward the feet until a pull is felt in those muscles. You can achieve a greater range of motion (a more intense stretch) using passive stretching. However, because the stretch is not controlled by the muscles themselves, there is a greater risk of injury. Communication between partners in passive stretching is important to ensure that joints aren't forced outside their normal functional range of motion.

In **active stretching**, a muscle is stretched by a contraction of the opposing muscle (the muscle on the opposite side of the limb). For example, an active seated stretch of the calf muscles occurs when a person actively contracts the muscles on the top of the shin. The contraction of this opposing muscle produces a reflex that relaxes the muscles to be stretched. The muscle can be stretched farther with a low risk of injury.

The only disadvantage of active stretching is that a person may not be able to produce enough stress (enough stretch) to increase flexibility using only the contraction of opposing muscle groups. The safest and most convenient technique is active static stretching, with an occasional passive assist. For example, you might stretch your calves both by contracting the muscles on the top of your shin and by pulling your feet toward you. This way you combine the advantages of active stretching—safety and

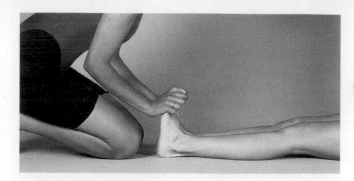

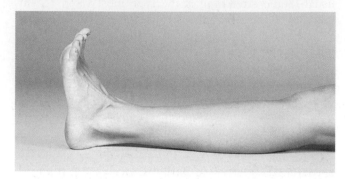

In passive stretching (top), an outside force—such as pressure exerted by another person—helps move the joint and stretch the muscles. In active stretching (bottom), the force to move the joint and stretch the muscles is provided by a contraction of the opposing muscles.

the relaxation reflex—with those of passive stretching—greater range of motion. People who are just beginning flexibility training may be better off doing active rather than passive stretches. For PNF techniques, it is particularly important to have a knowledgeable partner.

## Making Progress

As with any type of training, you will make progress and improve your flexibility if you stick with your program. Judge your progress by noting your body position while stretching. For example, note how far you can lean forward during a modified hurdler stretch. Repeat the assessment tests that appear in Lab 5.1 periodically and be sure to take the test at the same time of day each time. You will likely notice some improvement after only 2–3 weeks of stretching, but you may need at least 2 months to attain significant improvements. By then, you can expect flexibility increases of about 10–20% in many joints.

## Exercises to Improve Flexibility: A Sample Program

There are hundreds of exercises that can improve flexibility. Your program should include exercises that work all the major joints of the body by stretching their associated muscle groups (refer back to Figure 5.2). The exercises illustrated here are simple to do and pose a minimum risk of injury. Use these exercises to create a well-rounded program for developing flexibility. Be sure to perform each stretch using the proper technique. Hold each position

### EXERCISE 1 — Head Turns and Tilts

**Instructions:**

*Head turns:* Turn your head to the right and hold the stretch. Repeat to the left.

*Head tilts:* Tilt your head to the right and hold the stretch. Repeat to the left.

**Areas stretched:** Neck

**Variation:** Place your right palm on your right cheek; try to turn your head to the right as you resist with your hand. Repeat on the left side.

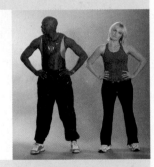

### EXERCISE 2 — Towel Stretch

**Instructions:** Roll up a towel and grasp it with both hands, palms down. With your arms straight, slowly lift the towel back over your head as far as possible. The closer together your hands are, the greater the stretch.

**Areas stretched:** Triceps, shoulders, chest

**Variation:** Repeat the stretch with your arms down and the towel behind your back. Grasp the towel with your palms forward and thumbs pointing out. Gently raise your arms behind your back. This exercise can also be done without a towel.

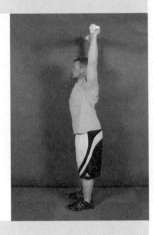

### EXERCISE 3 — Across-the-Body and Overhead Stretches

**Instructions: (a)** Keeping your back straight, cross your right arm in front of your body and grasp it with your left hand. Stretch your arm, shoulders, and back by gently pulling your arm as close to your body as possible. Hold.
**(b)** Bend your right arm over your head, placing your right elbow as close to your right ear as possible. Grasp your right elbow with your left hand over your head. Stretch the back of your arm by gently pulling your right elbow back and toward your head. Hold. Repeat both stretches on your left side.

**Areas stretched:**
Shoulders, upper back, back of the arm (triceps)

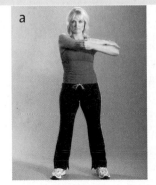

a

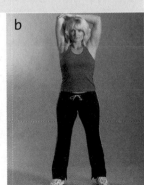

b

### EXERCISE 4 — Upper-Back Stretch

**Instructions:** Stand with your feet shoulder-width apart, knees slightly bent, and pelvis tucked under. Lace your fingers in front of your body and press your palms forward.

**Areas stretched:** Upper back

**Variation:** In the same position, wrap your arms around your body as if you were giving yourself a hug.

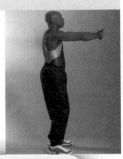

McGraw Hill **connect** http://www.mcgrawhillconnect.com/
**|FITNESS AND WELLNESS**

## EXERCISE 5     Lateral Stretch

**Instructions:** Stand with your feet shoulder-width apart, knees slightly bent, and pelvis tucked under. Raise one arm over your head and bend sideways from the waist. Support your trunk by placing the hand or forearm of your other arm on your thigh or hip for support. Be sure you bend directly sideways and don't move your body below the waist. Repeat on the other side.

**Areas stretched:** Trunk muscles

**Variation:** Perform the same exercise in a seated position.

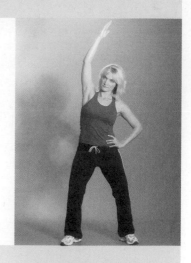

## EXERCISE 6     Step Stretch

**Instructions:** Step forward and bend your forward knee, keeping it directly above your ankle. Stretch your other leg back so that your shin is parallel to the floor. Press your hips forward and down to stretch. Your arms can be at your sides, on top of your knee, or on the ground for balance. Repeat on the other side.

**Areas stretched:** Hip, front of thigh (quadriceps)

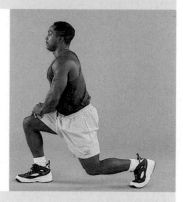

## EXERCISE 7     Side Lunge

**Instructions:** Stand in a wide straddle with your legs turned out from your hip joints and your hands on your thighs. Lunge to one side by bending one knee and keeping the other leg straight. Keep your bent knee directly over your ankle; do not bend it more than 90 degrees. Repeat on the other side.

**Areas stretched:** Inner thigh, hip, calf

**Variation:** In the same position, lift the heel of the bent knee to provide additional stretch. The exercise may also be performed with your hands on the floor for balance.

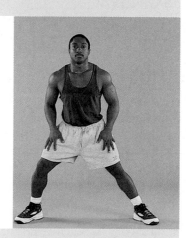

## EXERCISE 8     Inner Thigh Stretch

**Instructions:** Sit with the soles of your feet together. Push your knees toward the floor using your hands or forearms.

**Areas stretched:** Inner thigh, hip

**Variation:** When you first begin to push your knees toward the floor, use your legs to resist the movement. Then relax and press your knees down as far as they will go.

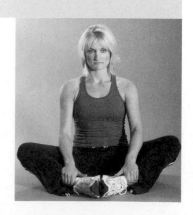

## EXERCISE 9 — Hip and Trunk Stretch

**Instructions:** Sit with your left leg straight, right leg bent and crossed over the left knee, and right hand on the floor next to your right hip. Turn your trunk as far as possible to the right by pushing against your right leg with your left fore-arm or elbow. Keep your right foot on the floor. Repeat on the other side.

**Areas stretched:** Trunk, outer thigh and hip, buttocks, lower back

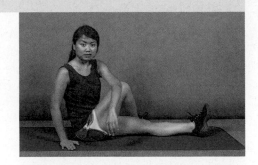

## EXERCISE 10 — Modified Hurdler Stretch (Seated Single-Leg Hamstring)

**Instructions:** Sit with your left leg straight and your right leg tucked close to your body. Reach toward your left ankle as far as possible. Repeat for the other leg.

**Areas stretched:** Back of the thigh (hamstring), lower back

**Variation:** As you stretch forward, alternately flex and point the foot of your extended leg.

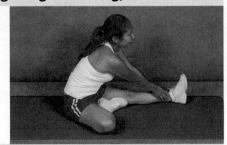

## EXERCISE 11 — Alternate Leg Stretcher

**Instructions:** Lie flat on your back with both legs straight. (**a**) Grasp your left leg behind the thigh, and pull it in to your chest. (**b**) Hold this position, and then extend your left leg toward the ceiling. (**c**) Hold this position, and then bring your left knee back to your chest and pull your toes toward your shin with your left hand. Stretch the back of the leg by attempting to straighten your knee. Repeat for the other leg.

**Areas stretched:** Back of the thigh (hamstring), hip, knee, ankle, buttocks

**Variation:** Perform the stretch on both legs at the same time.

a
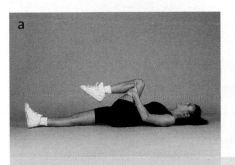

b
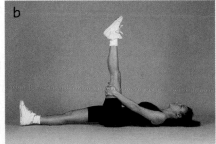

c
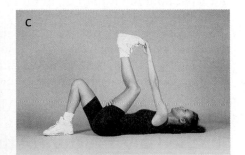

## EXERCISE 12 — Lower-Leg Stretch

**Instructions:** Stand with one foot about 1–2 feet in front of the other, with both feet pointing forward. (**a**) Keeping your back leg straight, lunge forward by bending your front knee and pushing your rear heel backward. Hold. (**b**) Then pull your back foot in slightly, and bend your back knee. Shift your weight to your back leg. Hold. Repeat on the other side.

**Areas stretched:** Back of the lower leg (calf, soleus, Achilles tendon)

**Variation:** Place your hands on a wall and extend one foot back, pressing your heel down to stretch, or stand with the balls of your feet on a step or bench and allow your heels to drop below the level of your toes.

a
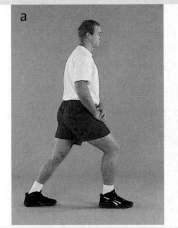

b
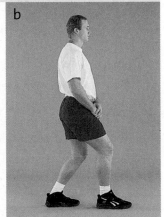

Mc Graw Hill **connect™** http://www.mcgrawhillconnect.com/
|FITNESS AND WELLNESS

## Ask Yourself

QUESTIONS FOR CRITICAL THINKING
AND REFLECTION

Why do you think improper stretching can do more harm than good? How can stretching cause injury? Of all the types of stretches described, which ones do you think would be safest for you? Which ones appeal to you most?

for 10–30 seconds and perform 2–4 repetitions of each exercise. Avoid exercises that put excessive pressure on your joints (see the box "Stretches to Avoid"). Complete Lab 5.2 when you're ready to start your program.

## PREVENTING AND MANAGING LOW-BACK PAIN

More than 85% of Americans experience back pain by age 50. Low-back pain is the second most common ailment in the United States—headache tops the list—and the second most common reason for absences from work and visits to a physician. Low-back pain is estimated to cost as much as $50 billion a year in lost productivity, medical and legal fees, and disability insurance and compensation.

Back pain can result from sudden traumatic injuries, but it is more often the long-term result of weak and inflexible muscles, poor posture, or poor body mechanics during activities like lifting and carrying. Any abnormal strain on the back can result in pain. Most cases of low-back pain clear up within a few weeks or months, but some people have recurrences or suffer from chronic pain.

### Function and Structure of the Spine

The spinal column performs many important functions in the body.

- It provides structural support for the body, especially the thorax (upper-body cavity).
- It surrounds and protects the spinal cord.
- It supports much of the body's weight and transmits it to the lower body.
- It serves as an attachment site for a large number of muscles, tendons, and ligaments.
- It allows movement of the neck and back in all directions.

The spinal column is made up of bones called **vertebrae** (Figure 5.3). The spine consists of 7 cervical vertebrae in the neck, 12 thoracic vertebrae in the upper

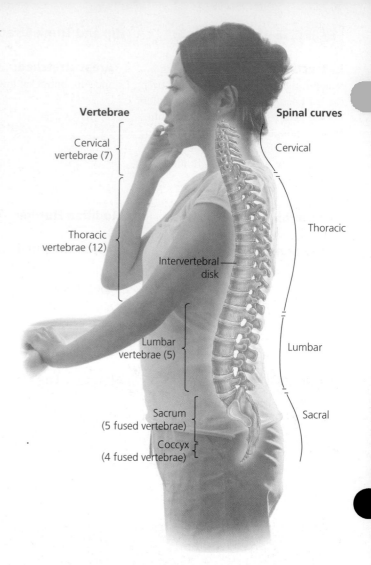

**FIGURE 5.3   The spinal column.**
The spine is made up of five separate regions and has four distinct curves. An intervertebral disk is located between adjoining vertebrae.

back, and 5 lumbar vertebrae in the lower back. The 9 vertebrae at the base of the spine are fused into two sections and form the sacrum and the coccyx (tailbone). The spine has four curves: the cervical, thoracic, lumbar, and sacral curves. These curves help bring the body weight supported by the spine in line with the axis of the body.

Although the structure of vertebrae depends on their location on the spine, the different types of vertebrae share common characteristics. Each consists of a body, an arch, and several bony processes (Figure 5.4). The vertebral body is cylindrical, with flattened surfaces where **intervertebral disks** are attached. The vertebral body is designed to carry the stress of body weight and physical activity. The vertebral arch surrounds and protects the spinal cord. The bony processes serve as joints for adjacent vertebrae and attachment sites for muscles and ligaments. **Nerve roots** from the spinal cord pass through notches in the vertebral arch.

Intervertebral disks, which absorb and disperse the stresses placed on the spine, separate vertebrae from each

## Stretches to Avoid

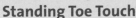

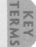

The safe alternatives listed under each stretch are described and illustrated on pp. 149–151 as part of a complete program of safe flexibility exercises.

### Standing Toe Touch

*Problem:* Puts excessive strain on the spine.

*Alternatives:* Modified hurdler stretch (Exercise 10), alternate leg stretcher (Exercise 11), and lower-leg stretch (Exercise 12).

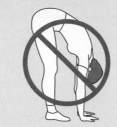

### Standing Ankle-to-Buttocks Quadriceps Stretch

*Problem:* Puts excessive strain on the ligaments of the knee.

*Alternative:* Step stretch (Exercise 6).

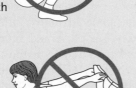

### Full Squat with Bent Back

*Problem:* Puts excessive strain on the ankles, knees, and spine.

*Alternatives:* Alternate leg stretcher (Exercise 11) and lower-leg stretch (Exercise 12).

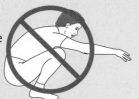

### Prone Arch

*Problem:* Puts excessive strain on the spine, knees, and shoulders.

*Alternatives:* Towel stretch (Exercise 2) and step stretch (Exercise 6).

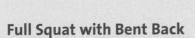

### Standing Hamstring Stretch

*Problem:* Puts excessive strain on the knee and lower back.

*Alternatives:* Modified hurdler stretch (Exercise 10) and alternate leg stretcher (Exercise 11).

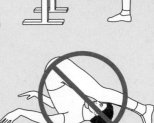

### Yoga Plow

*Problem:* Puts excessive strain on the neck, shoulders, and back.

*Alternatives:* Head turns and tilts (Exercise 1), across-the-body and overhead stretches (Exercise 3), and upper-back stretch (Exercise 4).

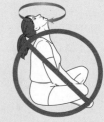

### Hurdler Stretch

*Problem:* Turning out the bent leg can put excessive strain on the ligaments of the knee.

*Alternative:* Modified hurdler stretch (Exercise 10).

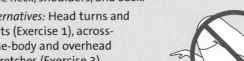

### Neck Circles

*Problem:* Puts excessive strain on the neck and cervical disks.

*Alternatives:* Head turns and tilts (Exercise 1).

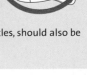

**NOTE:** Prone leg extensions, in which a person lifts both the chest and the legs while lying on the stomach but without grabbing the ankles, should also be avoided; spine extensions (p. 160) are a safe alternative.

---

other. Disks are made up of a gel- and water-filled nucleus surrounded by a series of fibrous rings. The liquid nucleus can change shape when it is compressed, allowing the disk to absorb shock. The intervertebral disks also help maintain the spaces between vertebrae where the spinal nerve roots are located.

## Core Muscle Fitness

The **core muscles** include those in the abdomen, pelvic floor, sides of the trunk, back, buttocks, hip, and

**vertebrae** Bony segments composing the spinal column that provide structural support for the body and protect the spinal cord.

**intervertebral disk** An elastic disk located between adjoining vertebrae, consisting of a gel- and water-filled nucleus surrounded by fibrous rings; serves as a shock absorber for the spinal column.

**nerve root** The base of each of the 31 pairs of spinal nerves that branch off the spinal cord through spaces between vertebrae.

**core muscles** The trunk muscles extending from the hips to the upper back.

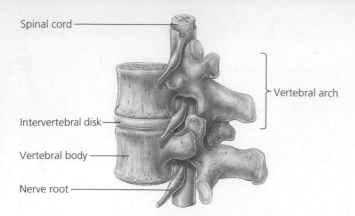

Spinal cord

Intervertebral disk

Vertebral body

Nerve root

Vertebral arch

**FIGURE 5.4** **Vertebrae and an intervertebral disk.**

**Front**

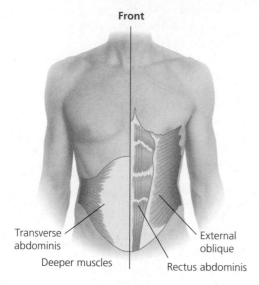

Transverse abdominis

Deeper muscles

External oblique

Rectus abdominis

**Back**

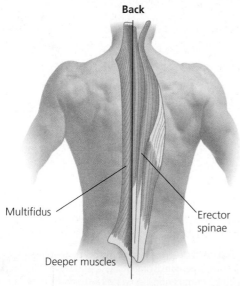

Multifidus

Deeper muscles

Erector spinae

**FIGURE 5.5** **Major core muscles.**

pelvis (Figure 5.5). There are 29 of these muscles, attaching to the ribs, hips, spinal column, and other bones in the trunk of the body. As described in Chapter 4, the core muscles stabilize the spine and help transfer force

between the upper body and lower body. They stabilize the midsection when you sit, stand, reach, walk, jump, twist, squat, throw, or bend. The muscles on the front, back, and sides of your trunk support your spine when you sit in a chair and fix your midsection as you use your legs to stand up. When hitting a forehand in tennis or batting a softball, most of the force is transferred from the legs and hips, across the core muscles, to the arms. Strong core muscles make movements more forceful and help prevent back pain.

During any dynamic movement, the core muscles work together. Some shorten to cause movement, while others contract and hold to provide stability, lengthen to brake the movement, or send signals to the brain about the movements and positions of the muscles and bones (proprioception). When specific core muscles are weak or tired, the nervous system steps in and uses other muscles. This substitution causes abnormal stresses on the joints, decreases power, and increases the risk of injury.

The best exercises for low-back health are whole-body exercises that force the core muscles to stabilize the spine in many different directions. The low-back exercises presented later in this chapter include several exercises that focus on the core muscles, including the step stretch (lunge), side bridges, and spine extensions. These exercises are generally safe for beginning exercisers and, with physician approval, people with some back pain. More challenging core exercises utilize stability balls or free weights. Stability ball exercises require the core muscles to stabilize the ball (and the body) while performing nearly any type of exercise. Many traditional exercises with free weights can strengthen the core muscles if you do them in a standing position. Weight machines train muscles in isolation, while exercises with free weights done while standing help train the body for real-world movements—an essential principle of core training.

## Causes of Back Pain

Back pain can occur at any point along your spine. The lumbar area, because it bears the majority of your weight, is the most common site. Any movement that causes excessive stress on the spinal column can cause injury and pain. The spine is well equipped to bear body weight and the force or stress of body movements along its long axis. However, it is less capable of bearing loads at an angle to its long axis or when the trunk is flexed (bent). You do not have to carry a heavy load or participate in a vigorous contact sport to injure your back. Picking a pencil up from the floor while using poor body mechanics—reaching too far out in front of you or bending over with your knees straight, for example—can also result in back pain.

Risk factors associated with low-back pain include age greater than 34 years, degenerative diseases such as arthritis or osteoporosis, a family or personal history of back pain or trauma, a sedentary lifestyle, low job satisfaction, and low socioeconomic status. Smoking increases risk because smoking appears to hasten degenerative changes in the spine. Excess body weight also increases strain on the back, and psychological stress or depression can cause muscle tension and back pain. Occupations and activities associated with low-back pain are those involving physically hard work, such as frequent lifting, twisting, bending, standing up, or straining in forced positions; those requiring high concentration demands (such as computer programming); and those involving vibrations affecting the entire body (such as truck driving).

Underlying causes of back pain include poor muscle endurance and strength in the core muscles; excess body weight; poor posture or body position when standing, sitting, or sleeping; and poor body mechanics when performing actions like lifting and carrying, or sports movements. Strained muscles, tendons, or ligaments can cause pain and can, over time, lead to injuries to vertebrae, intervertebral disks, and surrounding muscles and ligaments.

Stress can cause disks to break down and lose some of their ability to absorb shock. A damaged disk may bulge out between vertebrae and put pressure on a nerve root, a condition commonly referred to as a *slipped disk*. Painful pressure on nerves can also occur if damage to a disk narrows the space between two vertebrae. With age, you lose fluid from the disks, making them more likely to bulge and put pressure on nerve roots. Depending on the amount of pressure on a nerve, symptoms may include numbness in the back, hip, leg, or foot; radiating pain; loss of muscle function; depressed reflexes; and muscle spasm. If the pressure is severe enough, loss of function can be permanent.

## Preventing Low-Back Pain

Incorrect posture is responsible for many back injuries. Strategies for maintaining good posture are presented in the box "Good Posture and Low-Back Health." Follow the same guidelines when you engage in sports or recreational activities. Control your movements, and warm up thoroughly before you exercise. Take special care when lifting weights.

The role of exercise in preventing and treating back pain is still being investigated. However, many experts recommend exercise, especially for people who have already experienced an episode of low-back pain.

Regular exercise aimed at increasing muscle endurance and strength in the back and abdomen is often recommended to prevent back pain, as is lifestyle physical activity such as walking. Movement helps lubricate your spinal joints and increases muscle fitness in your trunk and legs. Other lifestyle recommendations for preventing back pain include the following:

- Maintain a healthy weight. Excess fat contributes to poor posture, which can place harmful stresses on the spine.
- Stop smoking, and reduce stress.
- Avoid sitting, standing, or working in the same position for too long. Stand up every hour or half-hour and move around.
- Use a supportive seat and a medium-firm mattress.
- Use lumbar support when driving, particularly for long distances, to prevent muscle fatigue and pain.
- Warm up thoroughly before exercising.
- Progress gradually when attempting to improve strength or fitness.

## Managing Acute Back Pain

Sudden (acute) back pain usually involves tissue injury. Symptoms may include pain, muscle spasms, stiffness, and inflammation. Many cases of acute back pain go away by themselves within a few days or weeks. You may be able to reduce pain and inflammation by applying cold and then heat (see Chapter 3). Apply ice several times a day; once inflammation and spasms subside, you can apply heat using a heating pad or a warm bath. If the pain is bothersome, an over-the-counter, nonsteroidal anti-inflammatory medication such as ibuprofen or naproxen may be helpful. Stronger pain medications and muscle relaxants are available by prescription.

Bed rest immediately following the onset of back pain may make you feel better, but it should be of very short duration. Prolonged bed rest—5 days or more—was once thought to be an effective treatment for back pain, but most physicians now advise against it because it may weaken muscles and actually worsen pain. Limit bed rest to one day and begin moderate physical activity as soon as possible. Exercise can increase muscular endurance and flexibility and protect disks from loss of fluid. Three of the back exercises discussed later in the chapter may be particularly helpful following an episode of acute back pain: curl-ups, side bridges, and spine extensions ("bird dogs").

See your physician if acute back pain doesn't resolve within a short time. Other warning signals of a more severe problem that requires a professional evaluation include severe pain, numbness, pain that radiates down one or both legs, problems with bladder or bowel control, fever, and rapid weight loss.

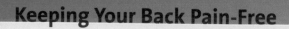
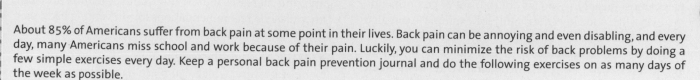
About 85% of Americans suffer from back pain at some point in their lives. Back pain can be annoying and even disabling, and every day, many Americans miss school and work because of their pain. Luckily, you can minimize the risk of back problems by doing a few simple exercises every day. Keep a personal back pain prevention journal and do the following exercises on as many days of the week as possible.

| EXERCISE | MON. | TUES. | WEDS. | THUR. | FRI. | SAT. | SUN. |
|---|---|---|---|---|---|---|---|
| Curl-ups: one set of 10 reps | ✓ | | ✓ | | ✓ | | ✓ |
| Side bridge: five sets, 3-second hold, each side | ✓ | | ✓ | | ✓ | | ✓ |
| Bird dog: five sets, 3-second hold, each side | ✓ | | ✓ | | ✓ | | ✓ |
| Walking: 15-60 minutes | | ✓ | ✓ | | ✓ | | ✓ |
| Kettlebell swings: one set 20 repetitions | ✓ | | | | ✓ | ✓ | ✓ |

Make a chart like the one shown above, and place a new copy in your training log each week. Enter a check mark every time you do the exercise. Try to enter a check mark for each exercise as often as you can during the week. In this one-week example, the person didn't do all the exercises every day, but she tried to do something on as many days a week as she could. Regularity is the key; if you miss a day, try not to miss the next one.

## Managing Chronic Back Pain

Low-back pain is considered chronic if it persists for more than 3 months. Symptoms vary—some people experience stabbing or shooting pain, and others a steady ache accompanied by stiffness. Sometimes pain is localized; in other cases, it radiates to another part of the body. Underlying causes of chronic back pain include injuries, infection, muscle or ligament strains, and disk herniations.

Because symptoms and causes are so varied, different people benefit from different treatment strategies, and researchers have found that many treatments have only limited benefits. Potential treatments include over-the-counter or prescription medications; exercise; physical therapy, massage, yoga, or chiropractic care; acupuncture; percutaneous electrical nerve stimulation (PENS), in which acupuncture-like needles are used to deliver an electrical current; education and advice about posture, exercise, and body mechanics; and surgery (see the box "Yoga for Relaxation and Pain Relief").

Psychological therapy may also be beneficial in some cases. Reducing emotional stress that causes muscle tension can provide direct benefits, and other therapies can help people deal better with chronic pain and its effects on their daily lives. Support groups and expressive writing are beneficial for people with chronic pain and other conditions.

## Exercises for the Prevention and Management of Low-Back Pain

The tests in Lab 5.3 can help you assess low-back muscular endurance. The exercises that follow are designed to help you maintain a healthy back by stretching and strengthening the major muscle groups that affect the back—the abdominal muscles, the muscles along your spine and sides, and the muscles of your hips and thighs. If you have back problems, check with your physician before beginning any exercise program. Perform the exercises slowly and progress very gradually. Stop and consult your physician if any exercise causes back pain. General guidelines for back exercise programs include the following:

- Do low-back exercises at least 3 days per week. Most experts recommend daily back exercises.

- Emphasize muscular endurance rather than muscular strength—endurance is more protective.

- Don't do spine exercises involving a full range of motion early in the morning. Your disks have a high fluid content early in the day and injuries may result.

- Engage in regular endurance exercise such as cycling or walking in addition to performing exercises that specifically build muscular endurance and flexibility. Brisk walking with a vigorous arm swing may help relieve back pain. Start with fast walking if your core muscles are weak or you have back pain.

- Be patient and stick with your program. Increased back fitness and pain relief may require as long as 3 months of regular exercise.

- The adage "no pain, no gain" does not apply to back exercises. Always use good form and stop if you feel pain.

# Good Posture and Low-Back Health

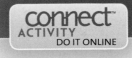
Changes in everyday posture and behavior can help prevent and alleviate low-back pain.

- **Lying down.** When resting or sleeping, lie on your side with your knees and hips bent. If you lie on your back, place a pillow under your knees. However, do not elevate your knees so much that the curve in your lower spine is flattened. Don't lie on your stomach. Use a medium-firm mattress.

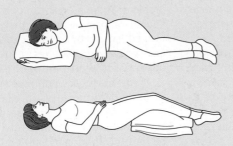

- **Sitting at a computer.** Sit in a slightly reclined position of 100–110 degrees, not an upright 90-degree position. Adjust your chair so your knees are slightly lower than your hips. If your back flattens as you sit, try using a lumbar roll to maintain your back's natural curvature. Place your feet flat on the floor or on a footrest. Place the monitor directly in front of you and adjust it so your eyes are level with the top of the screen; you should be looking slightly downward at the middle of the screen. Adjust the keyboard and mouse so your forearms and wrists are in a neutral position, parallel with the floor.

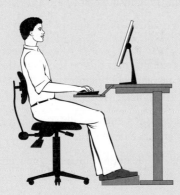

- **Lifting.** If you need to lower yourself to grasp an object, bend at the knees and hips rather than at the waist. Your feet should be about shoulder-width apart. Lift gradually, keeping your arms straight, by standing up or by pushing with your leg muscles. Keep the object close to your body. Don't twist; if you have to turn with the object, change the position of your feet.

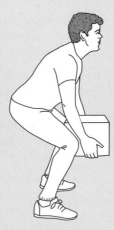

- **Standing.** When you are standing, a straight line should run from the top of your ear through the center of your shoulder, the center of your hip, the back of your kneecap, and the front of your ankle bone. Support your weight mainly on your heels, with one or both knees slightly bent. Don't let your pelvis tip forward or your back arch. Shift your weight back and forth from foot to foot. Avoid prolonged standing.

  To check your posture, stand normally with your back to a wall. Your upper back and buttocks should touch the wall; your heels may be a few inches away. Slide one hand into the space between your lower back and the wall. It should slide in easily but should almost touch both your back and the wall. Adjust your posture as needed, and try to hold this position as you walk away from the wall.

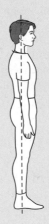

- **Walking.** Walk with your toes pointed straight ahead. Keep your back flat, head up and centered over your body, and chin in. Swing your arms freely. Don't wear tight or high-heeled shoes. Walking briskly is better for back health than walking slowly.

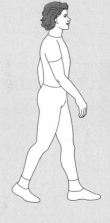

TAKE CHARGE

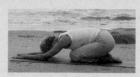

# Yoga for Relaxation and Pain Relief

Certain types of exercise can provide relief from back pain, depending on the pain's underlying cause. Effective exercises stretch the muscles and connective tissue in the hips, stabilize the spine, and strengthen and build endurance in the core muscles of the back and abdomen.

Yoga may be an option for many back pain sufferers because it offers a variety of exercises that target the spine and the core muscles. Yoga is an ancient practice involving slow, gentle movements performed with controlled breathing and focused attention. Yoga practitioners slowly move into a specific posture (called an *asana*) and hold the posture for up to 60 seconds. There are hundreds of asanas, many of which are easy to do and provide good stretches.

Yoga also involves simple breathing exercises that gently stretch the muscles of the upper back while helping the practitioner focus. Yoga experts say that breathing exercises not only encourage relaxation but also clear the mind and can help relieve mild to moderate pain. Yoga enthusiasts end their workouts energized and refreshed but calm and relaxed.

Many medical professionals now recommend yoga for patients with back pain, particularly postures that involve arching and gently stretching the back, such as the cat pose (similar to the cat stretch shown on p. 159) and the child pose (shown here). These are basic asanas that most people can perform repeatedly and hold for a relatively long time.

Because asanas must be performed correctly to be beneficial, qualified instruction is recommended. For those with back pain, physicians advise choosing an instructor who is not only accomplished in yoga but also knowledgeable about back pain and its causes. Such instructors can steer students away from exercises that do more harm than good. It is especially important to choose postures that will benefit the back without worsening the underlying problem. Some asanas can aggravate an injured or painful back if they are performed incorrectly or too aggressively. In fact, a few yoga postures should not be done at all by people with back pain.

If you have back pain, see your physician to determine its cause before beginning any type of exercise program. Even gentle exercise or stretching can be bad for an already injured back, especially if the spinal disks or nerves are involved. For some back conditions, rest or therapy may be better options than exercise, at least in the short term.

## Ask Yourself

### QUESTIONS FOR CRITICAL THINKING AND REFLECTION

Do you know anyone who suffers from chronic back pain? If so, how has it affected that person's life? Have you ever had back pain? Do you have any of the risk factors listed in the text? If so, what can you do to lower your risk and avoid developing chronic back problems?

## TIPS FOR TODAY AND THE FUTURE

To improve and maintain your flexibility, perform stretches that work the major joints at least twice a week.

### RIGHT NOW YOU CAN

- Stand up and stretch—do either the upper-back stretch or the across-the-body stretch shown in the chapter.
- Practice the recommended sitting and standing postures described in the chapter. If needed, adjust your chair or find something to use as a footrest.

### IN THE FUTURE YOU CAN

- Build up your flexibility by incorporating more sophisticated stretching exercises into your routine.
- Increase the frequency of your flexibility workouts to 5 or more days per week.
- Increase the efficiency of your workouts by adding stretching exercises to the cool-down period of your endurance or strength workouts.

## SUMMARY

- Flexibility, the ability of joints to move through their full range of motion, is highly adaptable and specific to each joint.

- Range of motion can be limited by joint structure, muscle inelasticity, and proprioceptor activity.

- Developing flexibility depends on stretching the elastic tissues within muscles regularly and gently until they lengthen. Overstretching can make connective tissue brittle and lead to rupture.

- Signals sent between muscle and tendon nerves and the spinal cord can enhance flexibility.

- The benefits of flexibility include preventing abnormal stresses that lead to joint deterioration and possibly reducing the risk of injuries.

- Stretches should be held for 10–30 seconds; perform 2–4 repetitions. Flexibility training should be done a minimum of 2–3 days per week, preferably following activity, when muscles are warm.

- Static stretching is done slowly and held to the point of mild tension; ballistic stretching consists of bouncing stretches and can lead to injury. Dynamic stretching involves moving joints slowly and fluidly through their range of motion. Proprioceptive neuromuscular facilitation uses muscle receptors in contracting and relaxing a muscle.

- Passive stretching, using an outside force in moving muscles and joints, achieves a greater range of motion (and has a higher injury risk) than active stretching, which uses opposing muscles to initiate a stretch.

### EXERCISE 1      Cat Stretch

**Instructions:** Begin on all fours with your knees below your hips and your hands below your shoulders. Slowly and deliberately move through a cycle of extension and flexion of your spine. **(a)** Begin by slowly pushing your back up and dropping your head slightly until your spine is extended (rounded). **(b)** Then slowly lower your back and lift your chin slightly until your spine is flexed (relaxed and slightly arched). *Do not press at the ends of the range of motion.* Stop if you feel pain. Do 10 slow, continuous cycles of the movement.

**Target:** Improved flexibility, relaxation, and reduced stiffness in the spine

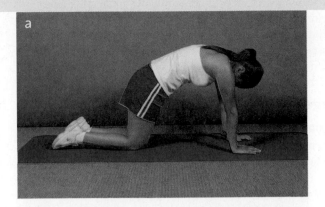

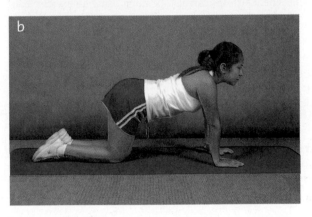

### EXERCISE 2      Step Stretch *(See Exercise 6 in the flexibility program, p. 150)*

**Instructions:** Hold each stretch for 10–30 seconds and do 2–4 repetitions on each side.

**Target:** Improved flexibility, strength, and endurance in the muscles of the hip and the front of the thigh

### EXERCISE 3      Alternate Leg Stretcher *(See Exercise 11 in the flexibility program, p. 151)*

**Instructions:** Hold each stretch for 10–30 seconds and do 2–4 repetitions on each side.

**Target:** Improved flexibility in the back of the thigh, hip, knee, and buttocks

### EXERCISE 4      Trunk Twist

**Instructions:** Lie on your side with top knee bent, lower leg straight, lower arm extended in front of you on the floor, and upper arm at your side. Push down with your upper knee while you twist your trunk backward. Try to get your shoulders and upper body flat on the floor, turning your head as well. Return to the starting position, and then repeat on the other side. Hold the stretch for 10–30 seconds and do 2–4 repetitions on each side.

**Target:** Improved flexibility in the lower back and sides

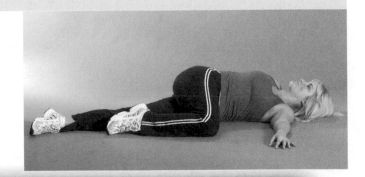

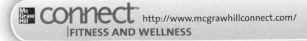
http://www.mcgrawhillconnect.com/
FITNESS AND WELLNESS

## EXERCISE 5       Curl-Up

**Instructions:** Lie on your back with one or both knees bent and arms crossed on your chest or hands under your lower back. Maintain a neutral spine. Tuck your chin in and slowly curl up, one vertebra at a time, as you use your abdominal muscles to lift your head first and then your shoulders. Stop when you can see your knees and hold for 5–10 seconds before returning to the starting position. Do 10 or more repetitions.

**Target:** Improved strength and endurance in the abdomen

**Variation:** Add a twist to develop other abdominal muscles. When you have curled up so that your shoulder blades are off the floor, twist your upper body so that one shoulder is higher than the other; reach past your knee with your upper arm. Hold and then return to the starting position. Repeat on the opposite side. Curl-ups can also be done using an exercise ball.

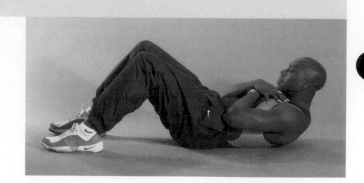

## EXERCISE 6       Isometric Side Bridge *(See Exercise 11 in the free weights program in Chapter 4, p. 120)*

**Instructions:** Hold the bridge position for 10 seconds, breathing normally. Work up to a 60-second hold. Perform one or more repetitions on each side.

**Target:** Increased strength and endurance in the muscles along the sides of the abdomen

**Variation:** You can make the exercise more difficult by keeping your legs straight and supporting yourself with your feet and forearm (see Lab 5.3) or with your feet and hand (with elbow straight).

## EXERCISE 7       Spine Extensions *("Bird dogs"; see Exercise 10 in the free weights program in Chapter 4, p. 119)*

**Instructions:** Hold each position for 10–30 seconds. Begin with one repetition on each side, and work up to several repetitions.

**Target:** Increased strength and endurance in the back, buttocks, and back of the thighs

**Variation:** If you have experienced back pain in the past or if this exercise is difficult for you, do the exercise with both hands on the ground rather than with one arm lifted. You can make this exercise more difficult by doing it balancing on an exercise ball. Find a balance point on your chest while lying face down on the ball with one arm and the opposite leg on the ground. Tense your abdominal muscles while reaching and extending with one arm and reaching and extending with the opposite leg. Repeat this exercise using the other arm and leg.

## EXERCISE 8      Wall Squat (Phantom Chair)

**Instructions:** Lean against a wall and bend your knees as though you are sitting in a chair. Support your weight with your legs. Begin by holding the position for 5–10 seconds. Squeeze your gluteal muscles together as you do the exercise. Build up to 1 minute or more. Perform one or more repetitions.

**Target:** Increased strength and endurance in the lower back, thighs, and abdomen

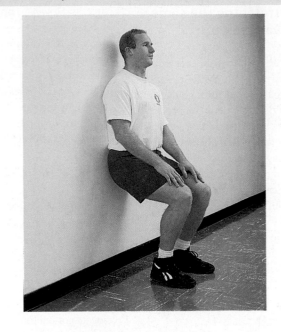

## EXERCISE 9      Pelvic Tilt

**Instructions:** Lie on your back with knees bent and arms extended to the side. Tilt your pelvis under and try to flatten your lower back against the floor. Tighten your buttock and abdominal muscles while you hold this position for 5–10 seconds. Don't hold your breath. Work up to 10 repetitions of the exercise. Pelvic tilts can also be done standing or leaning against a wall.

**Note:** *Although this is a popular exercise with many therapists, some experts question the safety of pelvic tilts. Stop if you feel pain in your back at any time during the exercise.*

**Target:** Increased strength and endurance in the abdomen and buttocks

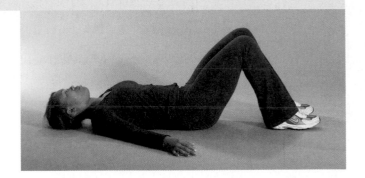

## EXERCISE 10      Back Bridge

**Instructions:** Lie on your back with knees bent and arms extended to the side. Tuck your pelvis under, contract your gluteal muscles, and then lift your tailbone, buttocks, and lower back from the floor. Hold this position for 5–10 seconds with your weight resting on your feet, arms, and shoulders, and then return to the starting position. Work up to 10 repetitions of the exercise.

**Target:** Increased strength and endurance in the hips and buttocks

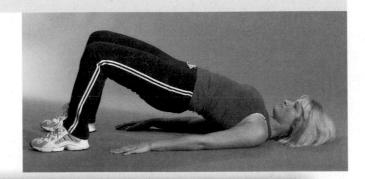

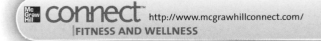

Mc Graw Hill **connect** http://www.mcgrawhillconnect.com/
|FITNESS AND WELLNESS

## Q Is stretching the same as warming up?

A No. They are two distinct activities. A warm-up is light exercise that involves moving the joints through the same motions used during a more intense activity; it increases body temperature so your metabolism works better when you're exercising at high intensity. Stretching increases the movement capability of your joints, so you can move more easily with less risk of injury. It is best to stretch at the end of your aerobic or weight training workout, when your muscles are warm. Warmed muscles stretch better than cold ones and are less prone to injury.

## Q How much flexibility do I need?

A This question is not always easy to answer. If you're involved in a sport such as gymnastics, figure skating, or ballet, you are often required to reach extreme joint motions to achieve success. However, nonathletes do not need to reach these extreme joint positions. In fact, too much flexibility may, in some cases, create joint instability and increase your risk of injury. As with other types of fitness, moderation is the key. You should regularly stretch your major joints and muscle groups but not aspire to reach extreme flexibility.

## Q Can I stretch too far?

A Yes. As muscle tissue is progressively stretched, it reaches a point where it becomes damaged and may rupture. The greatest danger occurs during passive stretching when a partner is doing the stretching for you. It is critical that your stretching partner not force your joint outside its normal functional range of motion.

## Q Can physical training limit flexibility?

A Weight training, jogging, or any physical activity will decrease flexibility if the exercises are not performed through a full range of motion. When done properly, weight training increases flexibility. However, because of the limited range of motion used during the running stride, jogging tends to compromise flexibility. It is important for runners to do flexibility exercises for the hamstrings and quadriceps regularly.

## Q Does stretching affect muscular strength?

A Flexibility training increases muscle strength over time, but preexercise stretching can cause short-term decreases in strength and power. Several recent studies have found that stretching decreases strength, power, and motor control following the stretch. This is one reason some experts suggest that people not stretch as part of their exercise warm-up. It is important to warm up before any workout by engaging in 5–10 minutes of light exercise such as walking or slow jogging.

*For more Common Questions Answered about flexibility and low-back health, visit the Online Learning Center at www.mhhe.com/fahey.*

---

• The spinal column consists of vertebrae separated by intervertebral disks. It provides structure and support for the body and protects the spinal cord. The core muscles stabilize the spine and transfer force between the upper and lower body.

• Acute back pain can be treated as a soft tissue injury, with cold treatment followed by application of heat (once swelling subsides); prolonged bed rest is not recommended. A variety of treatments have been suggested for chronic back pain, including regular exercise, physical therapy, acupuncture, education, and psychological therapy.

• In addition to good posture, proper body mechanics, and regular physical activity, a program for preventing low-back pain includes exercises that develop flexibility, strength, and endurance in the muscle groups that affect the lower back.

## FOR FURTHER EXPLORATION

### BOOKS

Anderson, B., and J. Anderson. 2010. *Stretching*, 30th anniv. ed. Bolinas, Calif.: Shelter Publications. *A best-selling exercise book, updated with more than 200 stretches for 60 sports and activities.*

Armiger, P., and M. A. Martyn. 2010. *Stretching for Functional Flexibility*. Philadelphia: Lippincott Williams & Wilkins. *Presents stretching methods for fitness, athletics, and rehabilitation.*

Blahnik, J. 2011. *Full-Body Flexibility,* 2nd ed. Champaign, Ill.: Human Kinetics. *Presents a blend of stretching techniques derived from sports training, martial arts, yoga, and Pilates.*

McGill, S. 2007. *Low Back Disorders: Evidence-Based Prevention and Rehabilitation,* 2nd ed. Champaign, Ill.: Human Kinetics. *A comprehensive guide to the prevention, diagnosis, and treatment of back pain.*

McGill, S. 2009. *Ultimate Back Fitness and Performance,* 4th ed. Waterloo, Canada: Backfit Pro. *Written by one of the premier researchers in the world on back biomechanics and back pain; describes mechanisms of back pain and exercises and movement patterns for preventing it.*

McGill, S. 2010. *Ultimate Back: Enhancing Performance* (DVD). Waterloo, Canada: Backfit Pro. *A video by the authors of* Ultimate Back Fitness and Performance.

Nelson, A. G., et al. 2006. *Stretching Anatomy*. Champaign, Ill.: Human Kinetics. *A guide to stretching that features highly detailed illustrations of the muscles that are affected by each exercise.*

### ORGANIZATIONS AND WEB SITES

*American Academy of Orthopaedic Surgeons.* Provides information about a variety of joint problems.
http://orthoinfo.aaos.org

*Back Fit Pro.* A Web site maintained by Dr. Stuart McGill, a professor of spine biomechanics at the University of Waterloo, which provides evidence-based information on preventing and treating back pain.

http://www.backfitpro.com

*CUErgo: Cornell University Ergonomics Web Site.* Provides information about how to arrange a computer workstation to prevent back pain and repetitive strain injuries, as well as other topics related to ergonomics.

http://ergo.human.cornell.edu

*Georgia State University: Flexibility.* Provides information about the benefits of stretching and ways to develop a safe and effective program; includes illustrations of stretches.

http://www2.gsu.edu/~wwwfit/flexibility.html

*Mayo Clinic: Focus on Flexibility.* Presents an easy-to-use program of basic stretching exercises for beginners, with a focus on the benefits of greater flexibility.

http://www.mayoclinic.com/health/stretching/HQ01447

*NIH Back Pain Fact Sheet.* Provides basic information on the prevention and treatment of back pain.

http://www.ninds.nih.gov/disorders/backpain/backpain.htm

*Southern California Orthopedic Institute.* Provides information on a variety of orthopedic problems, including back injuries; also has illustrations of spinal anatomy.

http://www.scoi.com

*Stretching and Flexibility.* Provides information on the physiology of stretching and different types of stretching exercises.

http://www.ifafitness.com/stretch/index.html

See also the listings for Chapters 2 and 4.

## SELECTED BIBLIOGRAPHY

American College of Sports Medicine. 2009. *ACSM's Guidelines for Exercise Testing and Prescription,* 8th ed. Philadelphia: Lippincott Williams and Wilkins.

American College of Sports Medicine. 2009. *ACSM's Resource Manual for Guidelines for Exercise Testing and Prescription,* 6th ed. Philadelphia: Lippincott Williams and Wilkins.

Aquino, C. F., et al. 2010. Stretching versus strength training in lengthened position in subjects with tight hamstring muscles: a randomized controlled trial. *Manual Therapy* 15(1): 26–31.

Ayala, F., et al. 2010. Effect of active stretch on hip flexion range of motion in female professional futbal players. *The Journal of Sports Medicine and Physical Fitness* 50(4): 428–435.

Bacurau, R. F., et al. 2009. Acute effect of a ballistic and a static stretching exercise bout on flexibility and maximal strength. *Journal of Strength and Conditioning Research* 23(1): 304–308.

Bazett-Jones, D. M., et al. 2008. Sprint and vertical jump performances are not affected by six weeks of static hamstring stretching. *Journal of Strength and Conditioning Research* 22(1): 25–31.

Bogduk, N. 2010. A cure for back pain? *Pain* 149(1): 7–8.

Carpes, F. P., et al. 2008. Effects of a program for trunk strength and stability on pain, low back and pelvis kinematics, and body balance: A pilot study. *Journal of Bodywork and Movement Therapies* 12(1): 22–30.

Chen, C. H., et al. 2011. Effects of flexibility training on eccentric exercise-induced muscle damage. *Medicine and Science in Sports and Exercise* 43(3): 491–500.

Chen, K. M., et al. 2008. Physical fitness of older adults in senior activity centers after 24-week silver yoga exercises. *Journal of Clinical Nursing* 17(19): 2634–2646.

Christiansen, C. L. 2008. The effects of hip and ankle stretching on gait function of older people. *Archive of Physical Medicine and Rehabilitation* 89(8): 1421–1428.

Costa, P. B., et al. 2009. The acute effects of different durations of static stretching on dynamic balance performance. *Journal of Strength and Conditioning Research* 23(1): 141–147.

Davis, D. S., et al. 2008. Concurrent validity of four clinical tests used to measure hamstring flexibility. *Journal of Strength and Conditioning Research* 22(2): 583–588.

Deleget, A. 2010. Overview of thigh injuries in dance. *Journal of Dance Medicine and Science* 14(3): 97–102.

Duehring, M. D., et al. 2009. Strength and conditioning practices of United States high school strength and conditioning coaches. *Journal of Strength and Conditioning Research* 23(8): 2188–2203.

Duque, I., et al. 2011. Maximal aerobic power in patients with chronic low back pain: A comparison with healthy subjects. *European Spine Journal* 20(1): 87–93.

Fasen, J. M., et al. 2009. A randomized controlled trial of hamstring stretching: comparison of four techniques. *Journal of Strength and Conditioning Research.* 23(2): 660–667.

Favero, J. P., et al. 2009. Effects of an acute bout of static stretching on 40 m sprint performance: Influence of baseline flexibility. *Research in Sports Medicine* 17(1): 50–60.

Feland, J. B., et al. 2010. Whole body vibration as an adjunct to static stretching. *International Journal of Sports Medicine* 31(8): 584–589.

Fenwick, C. M., et al. 2009. Comparison of different rowing exercises: Trunk muscle activation and lumbar spine motion, load, and stiffness. *Journal of Strength and Conditioning Research* 23(5): 1408–1417.

Field, T. 2011. Yoga clinical research review. *Complementary Therapies in Clinical Practice* 17(1): 1–8.

Garber, C. E., et al. 2011. Quantity and quality of exercise for developing and maintaining cardiorespiratory, musculoskeletal, and neuromotor fitness in apparently healthy adults: guidance for prescribing exercise. *Medicine and Science in Sports and Exercise* 43(7): 1334–1359.

Gergley, J. C. 2010. Latent effect of passive static stretching on driver club-head speed, distance, accuracy, and consistent ball contact in young male competitive golfers. *Journal of Strength and Conditioning Research* 24(12): 3326–3333.

Guidetti, L., et al. 2009. Precompetition warm-up in elite and subelite rhythmic gymnastics. *Journal of Strength and Conditioning Research.* 23(6): 1877–1882.

Guillot, A., et al. 2010. Does motor imagery enhance stretching and flexibility? *Journal of Sports Sciences* 28(3): 291–298.

Gurjao, A. L., et al. 2009. Acute effect of static stretching on rate of force development and maximal voluntary contraction in older women. *Journal of Strength and Conditioning Research* 23(7): 2149–2154.

Henchoz, Y., and A. Kai-Lik So. 2008. Exercise and nonspecific low back pain: A literature review. *Joint Bone Spine* 75(5): 533–539.

Herman, S. L., et al. 2008. Four-week dynamic stretching warm-up intervention elicits longer-term performance benefits. *Journal of Strength and Conditioning Research* 22(4): 1286–1297.

Heuser, M., et al. 2010. The effects of stretching on knee flexor fatigue and perceived exertion. *Journal of Sports Sciences* 28(2): 219–226.

Higgs, F., et al. 2009. The effect of a four-week proprioceptive neuromuscular facilitation stretching program on isokinetic torque production. *Journal of Strength and Conditioning Research* 23(5): 1442–1447.

Jaggers, J. R., et al. 2008. The acute effects of dynamic and ballistic stretching on vertical jump height, force, and power. *Journal of Strength and Conditioning Research* 22(6): 1844–1849.

Jenkins, J., et al. 2010. Flexibility for runners. *Clinics in Sports Medicine* 29(3): 365–377.

Judge, L. W., et al. 2009. An examination of the stretching practices of Division I and Division III college football programs in the midwestern United States. *Journal of Strength and Conditioning Research* 23(4): 1091–1096.

Keller, A., et al. 2008. Predictors of change in trunk muscle strength for patients with chronic low back pain randomized to lumbar fusion or cognitive intervention and exercises. *Pain Medicine* 9(6): 680–687.

Kiecolt-Glaser, J. K., et al. 2010. Stress, inflammation, and yoga practice. *Psychosomatic Medicine* 72(2): 113–121.

Lariviere, C., et al. 2010. Poor back muscle endurance is related to pain catastrophizing in patients with chronic low back pain. *Spine* 35(22): E1178–1186.

LaRoche, D. P., et al. 2008. Chronic stretching and voluntary muscle force. *Journal of Strength and Conditioning Research* 22(2): 589–596.

McGill, S. M., et al. 2009. Comparison of different strongman events: trunk muscle activation and lumbar spine motion, load, and stiffness. *Journal of Strength and Conditioning Research* 23(4): 1148–1161.

McHugh, M. P., and M. Nesse. 2008. Effect of stretching on strength loss and pain after eccentric exercise. *Medicine and Science in Sports and Exercise* 40(3): 566–573.

Meroni, R., et al. 2010. Comparison of active stretching technique and static stretching technique on-hamstring flexibility. *Clinical Journal of Sport Medicine* 20(1): 8–14.

Molacek, Z. D., et al. 2010. Effects of low- and high-volume stretching on bench press performance in collegiate football players. *Journal of Strength and Conditioning Research* 24(3): 711–716.

Monteiro, W. D., et al. 2008. Influence of strength training on adult women's flexibility. *Journal of Strength and Conditioning Research* 22(3): 672–677.

Morse, C. I., et al. 2008. The acute effect of stretching on the passive stiffness of the human gastrocnemius muscle tendon unit. *Journal of Physiology* 586(1): 97–106.

Nieman, D. C. 2011. *Exercise Testing and Prescription: A Health-Related Approach*, 7th ed. New York: McGraw-Hill.

Purcell, L. 2009. Causes and prevention of low back pain in young athletes. *Paediatrics and Child Health* 14(8): 533–538.

Rancour, J., et al. 2009. The effects of intermittent stretching following a 4-week static stretching protocol: A randomized trial. *Journal of Strength and Conditioning Research* 23(8): 2217–2222.

Rasmussen-Barr, E., et al. 2009. Graded exercise for recurrent low-back pain: A randomized, controlled trial with 6-, 12-, and 36-month follow-ups. *Spine* 34(3): 221–228.

Ryan, E. D., et al. 2008. Do practical durations of stretching alter muscle strength? A dose-response study. *Medicine and Science in Sports and Exercise* 40(8): 1529–1537.

Saeed, S. A., et al. 2010. Exercise, yoga, and meditation for depressive and anxiety disorders. *American Family Physician* 81(8): 981–986.

Samuel, M. N., et al. 2008. Acute effects of static and ballistic stretching on measures of strength and power. *Journal of Strength and Conditioning Research* 22(5): 1422–1428.

Scannell, J. P., et al. 2009. Disc prolapse: Evidence of reversal with repeated extension. *Spine* 34(4): 344–350.

Small, K., et al. 2008. A systematic review into the efficacy of static stretching as part of a warm-up for the prevention of exercise-related injury. *Research in Sports Medicine* 16(3): 213–231.

Tekur, P., et al. 2008. Effect of short-term intensive yoga program on pain, functional disability and spinal flexibility in chronic low back pain: A randomized control study. *Journal of Alternative and Complementary Medicine* 14(6): 637–644.

Torres, E. M., et al. 2008. Effects of stretching on upper-body muscular performance. *Journal of Strength and Conditioning Research* 22(4): 1279–1285.

Verbunt, J. A., et al. 2010. Cause or effect? Deconditioning and chronic low back pain. *Pain* 149(3): 428–430.

Weil, R. 2008. Exercising the aging body. Part 2: Flexibility, balance, and diabetes control. *Diabetes Self-Management* 25(1): 42–52.

Werner, G. 2010. Strength and conditioning techniques in the rehabilitation of sports injury. *Clinics in Sports Medicine* 29(1): 177–191.

Winchester, J. B., et al. 2008. Static stretching impairs sprint performance in collegiate track and field athletes. *Journal of Strength and Conditioning Research* 22(1): 13–19.

Winke, M. R., et al. 2010. Moderate static stretching and torque production of the knee flexors. *Journal of Strength and Conditioning Research* 24(3): 706–710.

Ylinen, J., et al. 2009. Effect of stretching on hamstring muscle compliance. *Journal of Rehabilitation Medicine* 41(1): 80–84.

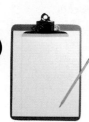

## LAB 5.1  Assessing Your Current Level of Flexibility

### Part I Sit-and-Reach Test

### Equipment

Use a modified Wells and Dillon flexometer or construct your own measuring device using a firm box or two pieces of wood about 30 centimeters (12 inches) high attached at right angles to each other. Attach a metric ruler to measure the extent of reach. With the low numbers of the ruler toward the person being tested, set the 26-centimeter mark of the ruler at the footline of the box. Individuals who cannot reach as far as the footline will have scores below 26 centimeters; those who can reach past their feet will have scores above 26 centimeters. Most studies show no relationship between performance on the sit-and-reach test and the incidence of back pain.

### Preparation

Warm up your muscles with a low-intensity activity such as walking or easy jogging. Then perform slow stretching movements.

### Instructions

1. Remove your shoes and sit facing the flexibility measuring device with your knees fully extended and your feet flat against the device about 10 centimeters (4 inches) apart.

2. Reach as far forward as you can, with palms down, arms evenly stretched, and knees fully extended; hold the position of maximum reach for about 2 seconds.

3. Perform the stretch 2 times, recording the distance of maximum reach to the nearest 0.5 centimeters: _____ cm

### Rating Your Flexibility

Find the score in the table below to determine your flexibility rating. Record it here and on the final page of this lab.
Rating: _____

### Ratings for Sit-and-Reach Test

| Men | Rating/Score (cm)* | | | | |
|---|---|---|---|---|---|
| | Needs Improvement | Fair | Good | Very Good | Excellent |
| Age: 15–19 | Below 24 | 24–28 | 29–33 | 34–38 | Above 38 |
| 20–29 | Below 25 | 25–29 | 30–33 | 34–39 | Above 39 |
| 30–39 | Below 23 | 23–27 | 28–32 | 33–37 | Above 37 |
| 40–49 | Below 18 | 18–23 | 24–28 | 29–34 | Above 34 |
| 50–59 | Below 16 | 16–23 | 24–27 | 28–34 | Above 34 |
| 60–69 | Below 15 | 15–19 | 20–24 | 25–32 | Above 32 |
| **Women** | | | | | |
| Age: 15–19 | Below 29 | 29–33 | 34–37 | 38–42 | Above 42 |
| 20–29 | Below 28 | 28–32 | 33–36 | 37–40 | Above 40 |
| 30–39 | Below 27 | 27–31 | 32–35 | 36–40 | Above 40 |
| 40–49 | Below 25 | 25–29 | 30–33 | 34–37 | Above 37 |
| 50–59 | Below 25 | 25–29 | 30–32 | 33–38 | Above 38 |
| 60–69 | Below 23 | 23–26 | 27–30 | 31–34 | Above 34 |

*Footline is set at 26 cm.

SOURCE: *The Canadian Physical Activity, Fitness & Lifestyle Approach: CSEP-Health & Fitness Program's Health-Related Appraisal and Counselling Strategy,* 3rd edition, 2003. Adapted with permission from the Canadian Society for Exercise Physiology.

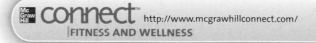

## Part II  Range-of-Motion Assessment

This portion of the lab can be completed by doing visual comparisons or by measuring joint range of motion with a goniometer or other instrument.

### Equipment

1. A partner to do visual comparisons or to measure the range of motion of your joints. (You can also use a mirror to perform your own visual comparisons.)
2. For the measurement method, you need a goniometer, flexometer, or other instrument to measure range of motion.

### Preparation

Warm up your muscles with some low-intensity activity such as walking or easy jogging.

### Instructions

On the following pages, the average range of motion is illustrated and listed quantitatively for some of the major joints. Visually assess the range of motion in your joints, and compare it to that shown in the illustrations. For each joint, note (with a check mark) whether your range of motion is above average, average, or below average and in need of improvement. Average values for range of motion are given in degrees for each joint in the assessment. You can also complete the assessment by measuring your range of motion with a goniometer, flexometer, or other instrument. If you are using this measurement method, identify your rating (above average, average, or below average) and record your range of motion in degrees next to the appropriate category. Although the measurement method is more time-consuming, it allows you to track the progress of your stretching program more precisely and to note changes within the broader ratings categories (below average, above average).

Record your ratings on the following pages and on the chart on the final page of this lab. (Ratings were derived from several published sources.)

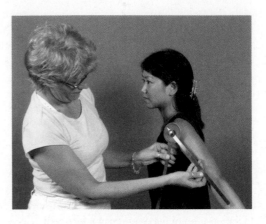

Assessment of range of motion using a goniometer

### 1. Shoulder Abduction and Adduction

For each position and arm, check one of the following; fill in degrees if using the measurement method.

***Shoulder abduction***—raise arm up to the side.

| Right | Left | |
|-------|------|---|
| _____ | _____ | Below average/needs improvement |
| _____ | _____ | Average (92–95°) |
| _____ | _____ | Above average |

***Shoulder abduction***—move arm down and in front of body.

| Right | Left | |
|-------|------|---|
| _____ | _____ | Below average/needs improvement |
| _____ | _____ | Average (124–127°) |
| _____ | _____ | Above average. |

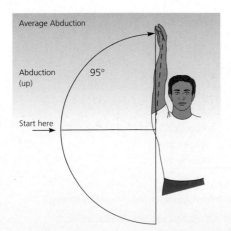

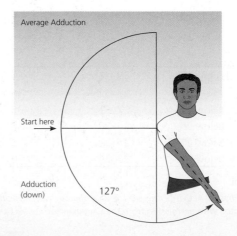

## 2. Shoulder Flexion and Extension

For each position and arm, check one of the following; fill in degrees if using the measurement method.

*Shoulder flexion*—raise arm up in front of the body.

Right     Left

_____   _____   Below average/needs improvement

_____   _____   Average (92–95°)

_____   _____   Above average

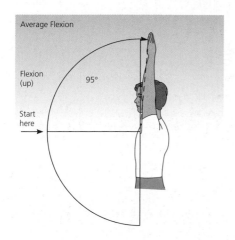

*Shoulder extension*—move arm down and behind the body.

Right     Left

_____   _____   Below average/needs improvement

_____   _____   Average (145–150°)

_____   _____   Above average

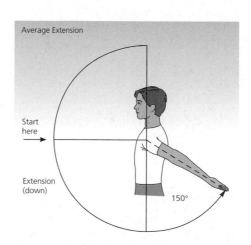

## 3. Trunk/Low-Back Lateral Flexion

Bend directly sideways at your waist. To prevent injury, keep your knees slightly bent, and support your trunk by placing your hand or forearm on your thigh. Check one of the following for each side; fill in degrees if using the measurement method.

Right     Left

_____   _____   Below average/needs improvement

_____   _____   Average (36–40°)

_____   _____   Above average

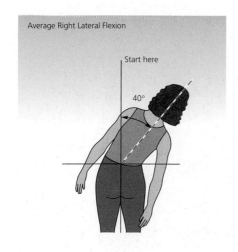

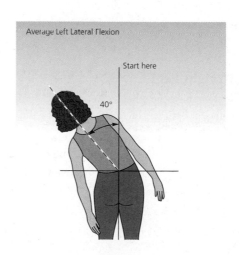

McGraw Hill **connect** http://www.mcgrawhillconnect.com/
|FITNESS AND WELLNESS

### 4. Hip Abduction

Raise your leg to the side at the hip. Check one of the following for each leg; fill in degrees if using the measurement method.

*Right*      *Left*

_____    _____    Below average/needs improvement

_____    _____    Average (40–45°)

_____    _____    Above average

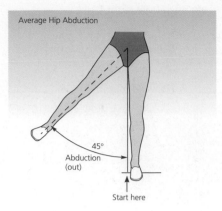

### 5. Hip Flexion (Bent Knee)

With one leg flat on the floor, bend the other knee and lift the leg up at the hip. Check one of the following for each leg; fill in degrees if using the measurement method.

*Right*      *Left*

_____    _____    Below average/needs improvement

_____    _____    Average (121–125°)

_____    _____    Above average

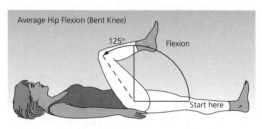

### 6. Hip Flexion (Straight Leg)

With one leg flat on the floor, raise the other leg at the hip, keeping both legs straight. Take care not to put excess strain on your back. Check one of the following for each leg; fill in degrees if using the measurement method.

*Right*      *Left*

_____    _____    Below average/needs improvement

_____    _____    Average (79–81°)

_____    _____    Above average

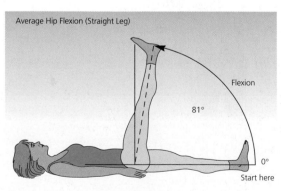

## 7. Ankle Dorsiflexion and Plantar Flexion

For each position and foot, check one of the following; fill in degrees if using the measurement method.

*Ankle dorsiflexion*—pull your toes toward your shin.

*Right*        *Left*

_____    _____    Below average/needs improvement

_____    _____    Average (9–13°)

_____    _____    Above average

*Plantar flexion*—point your toes.

*Right*        *Left*

_____    _____    Below average/needs improvement

_____    _____    Average (50–55°)

_____    _____    Above average

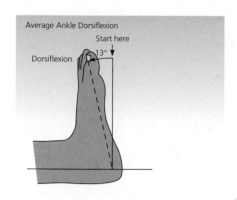

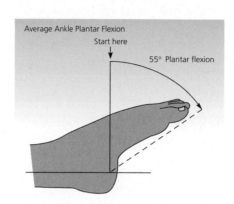

## Rating Your Flexibility

Sit-and-reach test:   Score: _____ cm   Rating: _____

## Range-of-Motion Assessment

Identify your rating for each joint on each side of the body. If you used the comparison method, put check marks in the appropriate categories; if you measured range of motion, enter the degrees for each joint in the appropriate category.

| Joint/Assessment | | Right | | | Left | | |
|---|---|---|---|---|---|---|---|
| | | Below Average | Average | Above Average | Below Average | Average | Above Average |
| 1. Shoulder abduction and adduction | Abduction | | | | | | |
| | Adduction | | | | | | |
| 2. Shoulder flexion and extension | Flexion | | | | | | |
| | Extension | | | | | | |
| 3. Trunk/low-back lateral flexion | Flexion | | | | | | |
| 4. Hip abduction | Abduction | | | | | | |
| 5. Hip flexion (bent knee) | Flexion | | | | | | |
| 6. Hip flexion (straight leg) | Flexion | | | | | | |
| 7. Ankle dorsiflexion and plantar flexion | Dorsiflexion | | | | | | |
| | Plantar flexion | | | | | | |

## Using Your Results

*How did you score?* Are you surprised by your ratings for flexibility? Are you satisfied with your current ratings?

If you're not satisfied, set a realistic goal for improvement.

Are you satisfied with your current level of flexibility as expressed in your daily life—for example, your ability to maintain good posture and move easily and without pain?

If you're not satisfied, set some realistic goals for improvement:

*What should you do next?* Enter the results of this lab in the Preprogram Assessment column in Appendix C. If you've set goals for improvement, begin planning your flexibility program by completing the plan in Lab 5.2. After several weeks of your program, complete this lab again and enter the results in the Postprogram Assessment column of Appendix C. How do the results compare?

Name _____  Section _____  Date _____

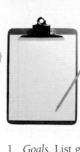

## LAB 5.2 Creating a Personalized Program for Developing Flexibility

1. *Goals.* List goals for your flexibility program. On the left, include specific, measurable goals that you can use to track the progress of your fitness program. These goals might be things like raising your sit-and-reach score from fair to good or your bent-leg hip flexion rating from below average to average. On the right, include long-term and more qualitative goals, such as reducing your risk for back pain.

Specific Goals: Current Status                          Final Goals

_____          _____

_____          _____

_____          _____

Other Goals: _____

_____

2. *Exercises.* The exercises in the program plan below are from the general stretching program presented in Chapter 5. You can add or delete exercises depending on your needs, goals, and preferences. For any exercises you add, fill in the areas of the body affected.

3. *Frequency.* A minimum frequency of 2–3 days per week is recommended; 5–7 days per week is ideal. You may want to do your stretching exercises the same days you plan to do cardiorespiratory endurance exercise or weight training, because muscles stretch better following exercise, when they are warm.

4. *Intensity.* All stretches should be done to the point of mild discomfort, not pain.

5. *Time/duration.* All stretches should be held for 15–30 seconds. (PNF techniques should include a 6-second contraction followed by a 10–30-second assisted stretch.) All stretches should be performed 2–4 times.

### Program Plan for Flexibility

| Exercise | Areas Stretched | Frequency (check ✓) | | | | | | |
|---|---|---|---|---|---|---|---|---|
| | | M | T | W | Th | F | Sa | Su |
| Head turns and tilts | Neck | | | | | | | |
| Towel stretch | Triceps, shoulders, chest | | | | | | | |
| Across-the-body and overhead stretches | Shoulders, upper back, back of the arm | | | | | | | |
| Upper-back stretch | Upper back | | | | | | | |
| Lateral stretch | Trunk muscles | | | | | | | |
| Step stretch | Hip, front of thigh | | | | | | | |
| Side lunge | Inner thigh, hip, calf | | | | | | | |
| Inner-thigh stretch | Inner thigh, hip | | | | | | | |
| Trunk rotation | Trunk, outer thigh and hip, lower back | | | | | | | |
| Modified hurdler stretch | Back of the thigh, lower back | | | | | | | |
| Alternate leg stretcher | Back of the thigh, hip, knee, ankle, buttocks | | | | | | | |
| Lower-leg stretch | Back of the lower leg | | | | | | | |
| | | | | | | | | |

You can monitor your program using a chart like the one on the next page.

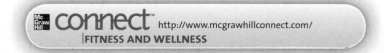

# Flexibility Program Chart

Fill in the dates you perform each stretch, the number of seconds you hold each stretch (should be 15–30), and the number of repetitions of each (should be 2–4). For an easy check on the duration of your stretches, count "one thousand one, one thousand two," and so on. You will probably find that over time you'll be able to hold each stretch longer (in addition to being able to stretch farther).

| Exercise/Date | | | | | | | | | | | | | | | | | | | | | | |
|---|---|---|---|---|---|---|---|---|---|---|---|---|---|---|---|---|---|---|---|---|---|---|
| | Duration | | | | | | | | | | | | | | | | | | | | | |
| | Reps | | | | | | | | | | | | | | | | | | | | | |
| | Duration | | | | | | | | | | | | | | | | | | | | | |
| | Reps | | | | | | | | | | | | | | | | | | | | | |
| | Duration | | | | | | | | | | | | | | | | | | | | | |
| | Reps | | | | | | | | | | | | | | | | | | | | | |
| | Duration | | | | | | | | | | | | | | | | | | | | | |
| | Reps | | | | | | | | | | | | | | | | | | | | | |
| | Duration | | | | | | | | | | | | | | | | | | | | | |
| | Reps | | | | | | | | | | | | | | | | | | | | | |
| | Duration | | | | | | | | | | | | | | | | | | | | | |
| | Reps | | | | | | | | | | | | | | | | | | | | | |
| | Duration | | | | | | | | | | | | | | | | | | | | | |
| | Reps | | | | | | | | | | | | | | | | | | | | | |
| | Duration | | | | | | | | | | | | | | | | | | | | | |
| | Reps | | | | | | | | | | | | | | | | | | | | | |
| | Duration | | | | | | | | | | | | | | | | | | | | | |
| | Reps | | | | | | | | | | | | | | | | | | | | | |
| | Duration | | | | | | | | | | | | | | | | | | | | | |
| | Reps | | | | | | | | | | | | | | | | | | | | | |
| | Duration | | | | | | | | | | | | | | | | | | | | | |
| | Reps | | | | | | | | | | | | | | | | | | | | | |
| | Duration | | | | | | | | | | | | | | | | | | | | | |
| | Reps | | | | | | | | | | | | | | | | | | | | | |
| | Duration | | | | | | | | | | | | | | | | | | | | | |
| | Reps | | | | | | | | | | | | | | | | | | | | | |
| | Duration | | | | | | | | | | | | | | | | | | | | | |
| | Reps | | | | | | | | | | | | | | | | | | | | | |
| | Duration | | | | | | | | | | | | | | | | | | | | | |
| | Reps | | | | | | | | | | | | | | | | | | | | | |
| | Duration | | | | | | | | | | | | | | | | | | | | | |
| | Reps | | | | | | | | | | | | | | | | | | | | | |
| | Duration | | | | | | | | | | | | | | | | | | | | | |
| | Reps | | | | | | | | | | | | | | | | | | | | | |
| | Duration | | | | | | | | | | | | | | | | | | | | | |
| | Reps | | | | | | | | | | | | | | | | | | | | | |

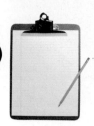

## LAB 5.3  Assessing Muscular Endurance for Low-Back Health

The three tests in this lab evaluate the muscular endurance of major spine-stabilizing muscles.

### Side Bridge Endurance Test

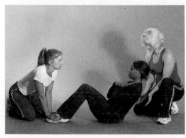

#### Equipment

1. Stopwatch or clock with a second hand
2. Exercise mat
3. Partner

#### Preparation

Warm up your muscles with some low-intensity activity such as walking or easy jogging. Practice assuming the side bridge position described below.

#### Instructions

1. Lie on the mat on your side with your legs extended. Place your top foot in front of your lower foot for support. Lift your hips off the mat so that you are supporting yourself on one elbow and your feet (see photo). Your body should maintain a straight line. Breathe normally; don't hold your breath.

2. Hold the position as long as possible. Your partner should keep track of the time and make sure that you maintain the correct position. Your final score is the total time you are able to hold the side bridge with correct form—from the time you lift your hips until your hips return to the mat.

3. Rest for 5 minutes and then repeat the test on the other side. Record your times here and on the chart at the end of the lab. Right side bridge time: _____ sec     Left side bridge time: _____ sec

### Trunk Flexors Endurance Test

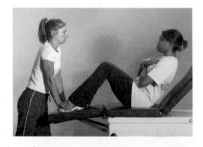

#### Equipment

1. Stopwatch or clock with a second hand
2. Exercise mat or padded exercise table
3. Two helpers
4. Jig angled at 60 degrees from the floor or padded bench (optional)

#### Preparation

Warm up with some low-intensity activity such as walking or easy jogging.

#### Instructions

1  To start, assume a sit-up posture with your back supported at an angle of 60 degrees from the floor; support can be provided by a jig, a padded bench, or a spotter (see photos). Your knees and hips should both be flexed at 90 degrees, and your arms should be folded across your chest with your hands placed on the opposite shoulders. Your toes should be secured under a toe strap or held by a partner.

2  Your goal is to hold the starting position (isometric contraction) as long as possible after the support is pulled away. To begin the test, a helper should pull the jig or other support back about 10 centimeters (4 inches). The helper should keep track of the time; if a spotter is acting as your support, she or he should be ready to support your weight as soon as your torso begins to move back. Your final score is the total time you are able to hold the contraction—from the time the support is removed until any part of your back touches the support. Remember to breathe normally throughout the test.

3  Record your time here and on the chart at the end of the lab. Trunk flexors endurance time: _____ sec

McGraw Hill **connect**™  http://www.mcgrawhillconnect.com/
|FITNESS AND WELLNESS

## Back Extensors Endurance Test

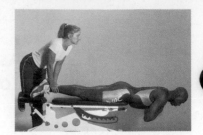

### Equipment

1. Stopwatch or clock with a second hand
2. Extension bench with padded ankle support or any padded bench
3. Partner

### Preparation

Warm up with some low-intensity activity such as walking or easy jogging.

### Instructions

1. Lie face down on the test bench with your upper body extending out over the end of the bench and your pelvis, hips, and knees flat on the bench. Your arms should be folded across your chest with your hands placed on the opposite shoulders. Your feet should be secured under a padded strap or held by a partner.

2. Your goal is to hold your upper body in a straight horizontal line with your lower body as long as possible. Keep your neck straight and neutral; don't raise your head and don't arch your back. Breathe normally. Your partner should keep track of the time and watch your form. Your final score is the total time you are able to hold the horizontal position—from the time you assume the position until your upper body drops from the horizontal position.

3. Record your time here and on the chart below. Back extensors endurance time: _____ sec

### Rating Your Test Results for Muscular Endurance for Low-Back Health

The table below shows mean endurance test times for healthy young college students with a mean age of 21 years. Compare your scores with the times shown in the table. (If you are older or have suffered from low-back pain in the past, these ratings are less accurate; however, your time scores can be used as a point of comparison.)

| | Mean Endurance Times (sec) | | | |
|---|---|---|---|---|
| | Right side bridge | Left side bridge | Trunk flexors | Back extensors |
| Men | 95 | 99 | 136 | 161 |
| Women | 75 | 78 | 134 | 185 |

**SOURCE:** Adapted with permission from S. M. McGill, 2007, *Low Back Disorders: Evidence-Based Prevention and Rehabilitation,* 2nd ed., p. 211. Champaign, IL: Human Kinetics.

Right side bridge: _____ sec          Rating (above mean, at mean, below mean): _____

Left side bridge: _____ sec          Rating (above mean, at mean, below mean): _____

Trunk flexors: _____ sec          Rating (above mean, at mean, below mean): _____

Back extensors: _____ sec          Rating (above mean, at mean, below mean): _____

## Using Your Results

*How did you score?* Are you surprised by your scores for the low-back tests? Are you satisfied with your current ratings?

If you're not satisfied, set a realistic goal for improvement. The norms in this lab are based on healthy young adults, so a score above the mean may or may not be realistic for you. Instead, you may want to set a specific goal based on time rather than rating; for example, set a goal of improving your time by 10%. Imbalances in muscular endurance have been linked with back problems, so if your rating is significantly lower for one of the three tests, you should focus particular attention on that area of your body.
Goal:

*What should you do next?* Enter the results of this lab in the Preprogram Assessment column in Appendix C. If you've set a goal for improvement, begin a program of low-back exercises such as that suggested in this chapter. After several weeks of your program, complete this lab again and enter the results in the Postprogram Assessment column of Appendix C. How do the results compare?

# CHAPTER 6

# Body Composition

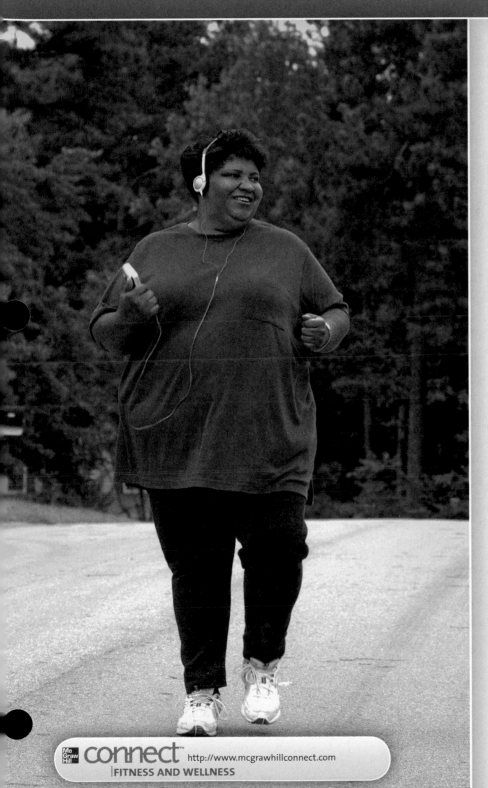

## LOOKING AHEAD...

After reading this chapter, you should be able to:

- Define fat-free mass and body fat, and describe their functions in the body
- Explain how body composition affects overall health and wellness
- Describe how body mass index, body composition, and body fat distribution are measured and assessed
- Explain how to determine recommended body weight and body fat distribution

## TEST YOUR KNOWLEDGE

1. Exercise helps reduce the risks associated with overweight and obesity even if it doesn't result in improvements in body composition. True or false?

2. Which of the following is the most significant risk factor for the most common type of diabetes (type 2 diabetes)?
   a. smoking
   b. low-fiber diet
   c. overweight or obesity
   d. inactivity

3. In women, excessive exercise and low energy (calorie) intake can cause which of the following?
   a. unhealthy reduction in body fat levels
   b. amenorrhea (absent menstruation)
   c. bone density loss and osteoporosis
   d. muscle wasting and fatigue

### Answers

1. **True.** Regular physical activity provides protection against the health risks of overweight and obesity. It lowers the risk of death for people who are overweight or obese as well as for those at a normal weight.

2. **c.** All four are risk factors for diabetes, but overweight/obesity is the most significant. It's estimated that 90% of cases of type 2 diabetes could be prevented if people adopted healthy lifestyle behaviors.

3. **All four.** Very low levels of body fat, and the behaviors used to achieve them, have serious health consequences for both men and women.

**B**ody composition, the body's relative amounts of fat and fat-free mass, is an important component of fitness for health and wellness. People with an optimal body composition tend to be healthier, to move more efficiently, and to feel better about themselves. They also have a lower risk of many chronic diseases.

Many people, however, don't succeed in their efforts to obtain a fit and healthy body because they set unrealistic goals and emphasize short-term weight loss rather than permanent lifestyle changes that lead to fat loss and a healthy body composition. Successful management of body composition requires the long-term, consistent coordination of many aspects of a wellness program. Even in the absence of changes in body composition, an active lifestyle improves wellness and decreases the risk of disease and premature death (see the box "Why Is Physical Activity Important Even if Body Composition Doesn't Change?").

This chapter focuses on defining and measuring body composition. The aspects of lifestyle that affect body composition are discussed in detail in other chapters: physical activity and exercise in Chapters 2–5 and 7, nutrition in Chapter 8, weight management in Chapter 9, and stress management in Chapter 10.

## WHAT IS BODY COMPOSITION, AND WHY IS IT IMPORTANT?

The human body can be divided into fat-free mass and body fat. As defined in Chapter 2, fat-free mass is composed of all the body's nonfat tissues: bone, water, muscle, connective tissue, organ tissues, and teeth.

A certain amount of body fat is necessary for the body to function. Fat is incorporated into the nerves, brain, heart, lungs, liver, mammary glands, and other body organs and tissues. It is the main source of stored energy in the body; it also cushions body organs and helps regulate body temperature. This **essential fat** makes up about 3–5% of total body weight in men and about 8–12% in women (Figure 6.1). The percentage is higher in women due to fat deposits in the breasts, uterus, and other sex-specific sites.

Most of the fat in the body is stored in fat cells, or **adipose tissue,** located under the skin (**subcutaneous fat**) and around major organs (**visceral** or **intra-abdominal fat**). People have a genetically determined number of fat cells, but these cells can become larger or smaller depending on how much fat is being stored. The amount of stored fat depends on several factors, including age, sex, metabolism, diet, and activity level. The primary source of excess body fat is excess calories consumed in the diet—that is, calories consumed in excess of calories expended in metabolism, physical activity, and exercise. A pound of body fat is equal to 3500 calories, so an intake of just 100 calories a day in excess of calories expended will result

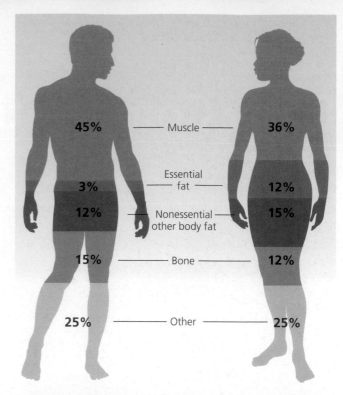

**FIGURE 6.1** **Body composition of a typical man and woman, 20–24 years old.**
**SOURCE:** Adapted from Brooks, G. A., et al. 2005. *Exercise Physiology: Human Bioenergetics and Its Applications,* 4th ed. New York: McGraw-Hill.

in a 10-pound weight gain over the course of a year. Excess stored body fat is associated with increased risk of chronic diseases like diabetes and cardiovascular disease, as described later in this chapter.

## Overweight and Obesity Defined

Some of the most commonly used methods of assessing and classifying body composition are described later in this chapter. Some methods are based on body fat and others on total body weight. Methods based on total body weight are less accurate than those based on body fat, but they are commonly used because body weight is easier to measure than body fat.

In the past, many people relied on height/weight tables (which were based on insurance company mortality statistics) to determine whether they were at a healthy weight. Such tables, however, can be highly inaccurate for some people. Because muscle tissue is denser and heavier than fat, a fit person can easily weigh more than the recommended weight on a height/weight table. For the same reason, an unfit person may weigh less than the table's recommended weight.

When looking at body composition, the most important consideration is the proportion of the body's total weight that is fat—the **percent body fat.** For example, two women may both be 5 feet, 5 inches tall and weigh 130 pounds. But one woman may have only 15%

# Why Is Physical Activity Important Even if Body Composition Doesn't Change?

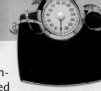

Physical activity is important for health even if it produces no changes in body composition—that is, even if a person remains overweight or obese. Physical activity confers benefits no matter how much you weigh; conversely, physical inactivity operates as a risk factor for health problems independently of body composition.

Regular physical activity and exercise block many of the destructive effects of obesity. For example, physical activity improves blood pressure, blood glucose levels, cholesterol levels, and body fat distribution. It also lowers the risk of cardiovascular disease, diabetes, and premature death. Although physical activity and exercise produce these improvements quickly in some people and slowly in others, due to genetic differences, the improvements do occur. Physical activity is particularly important for the many people who have metabolic syndrome or pre-diabetes, both of which are characterized by insulin resistance. Exercise encourages the body's cells to take up and use insulin efficiently for converting nutrients into usable energy. Being physically inactive for just one day decreases the capacity of the cells to take up and use blood sugar.

Although being physically active and not being sedentary may sound identical, experts describe them as different dimensions of the same health issue. Data suggest that it is important not only to be physically active but also to avoid prolonged sitting. In one study, people who watched TV or used a computer 4 or more hours a day had twice the risk of having metabolic syndrome as those who spent less than 1 hour a day in these activities; other studies reported similar results. Thus, in addition to increasing physical activity, avoiding or reducing sedentary behavior is an important—and challenging—health goal.

Although physical activity is important even if it doesn't change body composition, at a certain level, physical activity and exercise do improve body composition (meaning less fat and more lean muscle mass). Evidence supports a *dose-response* relation between exercise and fat loss: The more you exercise, the more fat you will lose. This includes both total body fat and abdominal fat. Additionally, the more body fat a person has, the greater is the loss of abdominal fat with exercise. Studies show that, even without calorie reduction, walking 150 minutes per week at a pace of 4 miles per hour, or jogging 75 minutes a week at 6 miles per hour, produces a decrease in total fat and abdominal fat that is associated with improved metabolic health.

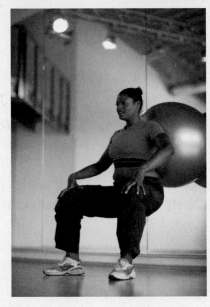

Studies also show, however, that combining exercise with an appropriate reduction in calories is an even better way to reduce levels of body fat and increase lean muscle mass. The results of combining exercise and calorie reduction may not show up as expected on the scale, because the weight of body fat lost is partially offset by the weight of muscle mass gained. Still, your body composition, physical fitness, and overall health have improved.

The question is sometimes asked, Which is more important in combating the adverse health effects of obesity—physical activity or physical fitness? Many studies suggest that both are important; the more active and fit you are, the lower your risk of having health problems and dying prematurely. Of the two, however, physical activity appears to be more important for health than physical fitness.

**SOURCES**: Baer, H. J., et al. 2011. Risk factors for mortality in the nurses' health study: A competing risks analysis. *American Journal of Epidemiology* 173(3): 319–329; Farrell, S. W. 2010. Cardiorespiratory fitness, adiposity, and all-cause mortality in women. *Medicine and Science in Sports and Exercise* 42(11): 2006–2012; Physical Activity Guidelines Advisory Committee. 2008. *Physical Activity Guidelines Advisory Committee Report, 2008*. Washington, D.C.: U.S. Department of Health and Human Services; Stephens, B. R., et al. 2011. Effects of 1 day of inactivity on insulin action in healthy men and women: interaction with energy intake. *Metabolism Clinical and Experimental*. 60: 941–949.

## Wellness Tip

Sleep problems increase the risk of obesity, especially in children and young adults. Sleep loss increases production of the hormone ghrelin, which boosts appetite and slows metabolic rate. Fatigue can also make it hard to live a healthy lifestyle and maintain a healthy weight.

**essential fat**   Fat incorporated in various tissues of the body; critical for normal body functioning.

**adipose tissue**   Tissue in which fat is stored; fat cells.

**subcutaneous fat**   Fat located under the skin.

**visceral fat**   Fat located around major organs; also called *intra-abdominal fat*.

**percent body fat**   The percentage of total body weight that is composed of fat.

of her body weight as fat, whereas the other woman could have 34% body fat. Although neither woman is overweight by most standards, the second woman is overfat. Too much body fat (not just total weight) has a negative effect on health and well-being. Just as the amount of body fat is important, so is its location on your body. Visceral fat is more harmful to health than subcutaneous fat.

**Overweight** is usually defined as total body weight above the recommended range for good health as determined by large-scale population surveys. **Obesity** is defined as a more serious degree of overweight that carries multiple major health risks. The cutoff point for obesity may be set in terms of percent body fat or in terms of some measure of total body weight.

## Prevalence of Overweight and Obesity Among Americans

By any measure, Americans are getting fatter. Since 1960, the average American man's weight has increased from 166 to 191 pounds, and the average American woman's weight has increased from 140 to 164 pounds. The prevalence of obesity has increased from about 13% in 1960 to about 34% today, and about 67% of adult Americans are now overweight (Figures 6.2 and 6.3). In June 2010, the National Center for Health Statistics reported that for the first time ever, more Americans are obese than overweight. According to these statistics, about 33% of adult men and 35% of adult women are obese. Experts predict that, by 2015, 75% of adults will be overweight and 41% will be obese.

Possible explanations for this increase include more time spent in sedentary work and leisure activities, fewer short trips on foot and more by automobile, fewer daily gym classes for students, more meals eaten outside the home, greater consumption of fast food, increased portion sizes, and increased consumption of soft drinks and convenience foods. According to the USDA, average calorie intake among Americans increased by more than 500 calories per day between 1970 and 2010. Further, the CDC says that nearly 40% of adult Americans are physically inactive and get no exercise at all.

## Excess Body Fat and Wellness

As rates of overweight and obesity increase, so do the problems associated with them. Obesity doubles mortality rates and can reduce life expectancy by 10–20 years. In fact, if the current trends in overweight and obesity (and their related health problems) continue, scientists believe the average American's life expectancy will soon decline by 5 years.

### Metabolic Syndrome, Diabetes, and Premature Death
Many overweight and obese people—especially those who are sedentary and eat a poor diet—suffer from a group of

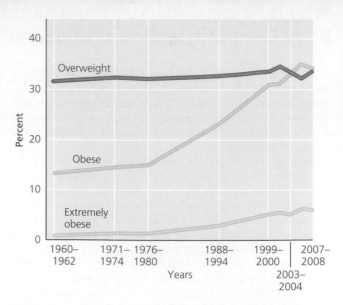

**FIGURE 6.2  Trends in overweight, obesity, and extreme obesity in adults aged 20–74 in the United States, 1960–2008.**
SOURCE: National Center for Health Statistics. 2010. *2007-2008 National Health and Nutrition Examination Survey (NHANES)*. Hyattsville, Md.: National Center for Health Statistics.

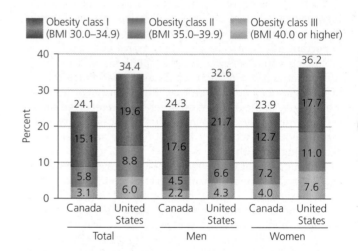

**FIGURE 6.3  Prevalence of obesity in people aged 20–79, by sex, in the U.S. and Canada, 2007–2009.**
SOURCE: National Center for Health Statistics. March 2011.

symptoms called **metabolic syndrome** (or *insulin resistance syndrome*). Symptoms include a resistance to the effects of insulin, high blood pressure, high blood glucose levels, abnormal blood fat levels (high triglycerides and low HDLs, or "good" cholesterol), **chronic inflammation**, and fat deposits in the abdominal region. Metabolic syndrome increases the risk of heart disease, more so in men than in women. According to the American Heart Association, about 34% of adult Americans have metabolic syndrome.

Even mild to moderate overweight is associated with a substantial increase in the risk of type 2 diabetes. Obese people are more than three times as likely as nonobese people to develop type 2 diabetes, and the incidence of this disease among Americans has increased dramatically as the

As obesity rates have increased, so have rates of infertility. Obese men and women are both at greater risk of infertility because obesity interferes with normal hormone levels and functions.

How do you view your own body composition? Where do you think you've gotten your ideas about how your body should look and perform? In light of what you've learned in this chapter, do the ideals and images promoted in our culture seem reasonable? Do they seem healthy?

rate of obesity has climbed (see the box "Diabetes" and the depiction of diabetes on page T3-5 of the color transparency insert "Touring the Cardiorespiratory System" in Chapter 3).

Obesity is also associated with increased risk of death from many types of cancer. Other health problems associated with obesity include hypertension, impaired immune function, gallbladder and kidney diseases, skin problems, sleep and breathing disorders, erectile dysfunction, pregnancy complications, back pain, arthritis, and other bone and joint disorders.

**Body Fat Distribution and Health** The distribution of body fat (the locations of fat on the body) is also an important indicator of health. Men and postmenopausal women tend to store fat in the upper regions of their bodies, particularly in the abdominal area (the "apple shape"). Premenopausal women usually store fat in the hips, buttocks, and thighs (the "pear shape"). Excess fat in the abdominal area increases risk of high blood pressure, diabetes, early-onset heart disease, stroke, certain cancers, and mortality. The reason for this increase in risk is not entirely clear, but it appears that abdominal fat is more easily mobilized and sent into the bloodstream, increasing disease-related blood fat levels.

The risks from body fat distribution are usually assessed by measuring waist circumference. A total waist measurement of more than 40 inches (102 cm) for men and more than 35 inches (88 cm) for women is associated with a significantly increased risk of disease. In the United States, waist circumference increased by about 1 inch in men and women between 1999 and 2008. Waist circumference tends to be higher in taller people, so waist-to-height ratio is a more accurate measure than waist circumference alone. Your waist measurement should be less than half your height. Using this index, a person who is 5 feet 8 inches (68 inches) tall should have a waist circumference of less than 34 inches. A person who is 6 feet 4 inches (76 inches) tall should have a waist circumference of less than 38 inches.

**Performance of Physical Activities** Too much body fat makes physical activity difficult because moving the body through everyday activities means working harder and using more energy. In general, overfat people are less fit than others and don't have the muscular strength, endurance, and flexibility that make normal activity easy. Because exercise is more difficult, they do less of it, depriving themselves of an effective way to improve body composition.

**Emotional Wellness and Self-Image** Obesity can affect psychological as well as physical wellness. Being perceived as fat can be a source of judgment, ostracism, and sometimes discrimination by others; it can contribute to psychological problems such as depression, anxiety, and low self-esteem.

The popular image of the "ideal" body has changed greatly in the past 50 years, evolving from slightly plump to unhealthily thin. The ideal body—as presented by the media—is an unrealistic goal for most Americans. This is because one's ability to change body composition depends on heredity as well as diet and exercise. Body image, problems with body image, and unhealthy ways of dealing with a negative body image are all discussed in Chapter 9.

## Problems Associated with Very Low Levels of Body Fat

Though not as prevalent a problem as overweight or obesity, having too little body fat is also dangerous. Essential fat is necessary for the functioning of the body, and health experts generally view too little body fat—less than 8–12% for women and 3–5% for men—as a threat to health. Extreme leanness is linked with reproductive, respiratory, circulatory, and immune system disorders and with premature death. Extremely lean people may experience muscle wasting and fatigue. They are also more likely to have eating disorders, which are described in more detail

**overweight** Body weight above the recommended range for good health; sometimes defined as a body mass index between 25 and 29.9.

**obesity** Severely overweight, characterized by an excessive accumulation of body fat; may also be defined in terms of some measure of total body weight or a body mass index of 30 or more.

**metabolic syndrome** A cluster of symptoms present in many overweight and obese people that greatly increases their risk of heart disease, diabetes, and other chronic illnesses; symptoms include insulin resistance, abnormal blood fats, abdominal fat deposition, type 2 diabetes, high blood pressure, and chronic inflammation.

**chronic inflammation** A response of blood vessels to harmful substances, such as germs, damaged cells, or irritants that can lead to heart disease, cancer, allergies, and muscle degeneration.

KEY TERMS

# Diabetes

*Diabetes mellitus* is a disease that causes a disruption of normal metabolism. The pancreas normally secretes the hormone insulin, which stimulates cells to take up glucose (blood sugar) to produce energy. Diabetes disrupts this process, causing a buildup of glucose in the bloodstream. Diabetes is associated with kidney failure, nerve damage, circulation problems, retinal damage and blindness, and increased rates of heart attack, stroke, and hypertension. The incidence of diabetes among Americans has increased dramatically as the rate of obesity has climbed. Diabetes is currently the seventh leading cause of death in the United States.

## Types of Diabetes

About 25.8 million Americans (8.3% of the population) have one of two major forms of diabetes. About 5–10% of people with diabetes have the more serious form, known as *type 1 diabetes*. In this type of diabetes, the pancreas produces little or no insulin, so daily doses of insulin are required, and people with type 1 diabetes may require other medications to control their blood sugar levels and other complications of the disease. (Without insulin, a person with type 1 diabetes can lapse into a coma.) Type 1 diabetes usually strikes before age 30.

The remaining 90–95% of Americans with diabetes have *type 2 diabetes*. This condition can develop slowly, and about 25% of affected individuals are unaware of their condition. In type 2 diabetes, the pancreas doesn't produce enough insulin, cells are resistant to insulin, or both. This condition is usually diagnosed in people over age 40, although there has been a tenfold increase in type 2 diabetes in children in the past two decades. About one-third of people with type 2 diabetes must take insulin; others may take medications that increase insulin production or stimulate cells to take up glucose.

A third type of diabetes occurs in 2–10% of women during pregnancy. *Gestational diabetes* usually disappears after pregnancy, but 5–10% of women with gestational diabetes go on to have type 2 diabetes immediately after pregnancy. Women who had gestational diabetes during pregnancy have up to a 60% chance of developing diabetes in the next 10–20 years.

The term *pre-diabetes* describes blood glucose levels that are higher than normal but not high enough for a diagnosis of full-blown diabetes. According to 2010 estimates from the American Diabetes Association, about 79 million Americans have pre-diabetes; experts warn that most people with the condition will develop type 2 diabetes unless they adopt preventive lifestyle measures.

The major factors involved in the development of diabetes are age, obesity, physical inactivity, a family history of diabetes, and lifestyle. Excess body fat reduces cell sensitivity to insulin, and insulin resistance is usually a precursor of type 2 diabetes. Ethnicity also plays a role. According to the CDC, the rate of diagnosed diabetes cases is highest among Native Americans and Alaska Natives, followed by blacks, Hispanics, Asian Americans, and white Americans. Across all races, about 27% of Americans age 60 and older have diabetes, either diagnosed or undiagnosed.

## Treatment

There is no cure for diabetes, but it can be managed successfully by keeping blood sugar levels within safe limits through diet, exercise, and, if necessary, medication. Blood sugar levels can be monitored using a home test, and close control of glucose levels can significantly reduce the rate of serious complications.

Nearly 90% of people with type 2 diabetes are overweight when diagnosed, including 55% who are obese. An important step in treatment is to lose weight. Even a small amount of exercise and weight loss can be beneficial. Regular exercise and a healthy diet are often sufficient to control type 2 diabetes.

## Prevention

It is estimated that 90% of cases of type 2 diabetes could be prevented if people adopted healthy lifestyle behaviors, including regular physical activity, a moderate diet, and modest weight loss. For people with pre-diabetes, lifestyle measures are more effective than medication for delaying or preventing the development of diabetes. Studies of people with pre-diabetes show that a 5–7% weight loss can lower diabetes onset by nearly 60%.

Exercise (endurance and/or strength training) makes cells more sensitive to insulin and helps stabilize blood glucose levels; it also helps keep body fat at healthy levels.

A moderate diet to control body fat is perhaps the most important dietary recommendation for the prevention of diabetes. However, the composition of the diet may also be important. Studies have linked diets low in fiber and high in sugar, refined carbohydrates, saturated fat, red meat, and high-fat dairy products to increased risk of diabetes; diets rich in whole grains, fruits, vegetables, legumes, fish, and poultry may be protective. Specific foods linked to higher diabetes risk include soft drinks, white bread, white rice, french fries, processed meats, and sugary desserts.

## Warning Signs and Testing

Be alert for the warning signs of diabetes:

- Frequent urination
- Extreme hunger or thirst
- Unexplained weight loss
- Extreme fatigue
- Blurred vision
- Frequent infections
- Cuts and bruises that are slow to heal
- Tingling or numbness in the hands or feet
- Generalized itching with no rash

The best way to avoid complications is to recognize these symptoms and get early diagnosis and treatment. Type 2 diabetes is often asymptomatic in the early stages, however, and major health organizations now recommend routine screening for people over age 45 and anyone younger who is at high risk, including anyone who is obese.

Screening involves a blood test to check glucose levels after either a period of fasting or the administration of a set dose of glucose. A fasting glucose level of 126 mg/dl or higher indicates diabetes; a level of 100–125 mg/dl indicates pre-diabetes. If you are concerned about your risk for diabetes, talk with your physician about being tested.

**DIMENSIONS OF DIVERSITY**

While obesity is at epidemic levels in the United States, many girls and women strive for unrealistic thinness in response to pressure from peers and a society obsessed with appearance. This quest for thinness has led to an increasingly common, underreported condition called the **female athlete triad.**

The triad consists of three interrelated disorders: abnormal eating patterns (and excessive exercising), followed by lack of menstrual periods (amenorrhea), followed by decreased bone density (premature osteoporosis). Left untreated, the triad can lead to decreased physical performance, increased incidence of bone fractures, disturbances of heart rhythm and metabolism, and even death.

Abnormal eating is the event from which the other two components of the triad flow. Abnormal eating ranges from moderately restricting food intake, to binge eating and purging (bulimia), to severely restricting food intake (anorexia nervosa). Whether serious or relatively mild, eating disorders prevent women from getting enough calories to meet their bodies' needs.

Disordered eating, combined with intense exercise and emotional stress, can suppress the hormones that control the menstrual cycle. If the menstrual cycle stops for three consecutive months, the condition is called amenorrhea. Prolonged amenorrhea can lead to

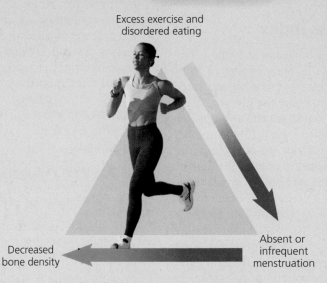

Excess exercise and disordered eating

Decreased bone density

Absent or infrequent menstruation

osteoporosis. Bone density may erode to the point that a woman in her twenties has the bone density of a woman in her sixties. Women with osteoporosis have fragile, easily fractured bones. Some researchers have found that even a few missed menstrual periods can decrease bone density.

All physically active women and girls have the potential to develop one or more components of the female athlete triad. For example, it is estimated that 5–20% of women who exercise regularly and vigorously may develop amenorrhea. But the triad is most prevalent among athletes who participate in certain sports: those in which appearance is highly important, those that emphasize a prepubertal body shape, those that require contour-revealing clothing for competition, those

that require endurance, and those that use weight categories for participation. Such sports include gymnastics, figure skating, swimming, distance running, cycling, cross-country skiing, track, volleyball, rowing, horse racing, and cheerleading.

The female athlete triad can be life-threatening. Typical signs of the eating disorders that trigger the condition are extreme weight loss, dry skin, loss of hair, brittle fingernails, cold hands and feet, low blood pressure and heart rate, swelling around the ankles and hands, and weakening of the bones. Female athletes who have repeated stress fractures may be suffering from the condition.

Early intervention is the key to stopping this series of interrelated conditions. Unfortunately, once the condition has progressed, long-term consequences, especially bone loss, are unavoidable. Teenagers may need only to learn about good eating habits; college-age women with a long-standing problem may require psychological counseling.

**SOURCES:** Ackerman, K. E., et al. 2011. Bone health and the female athlete triad in adolescent athletes. *Physician Sportsmedicine* 39(1): 131–141; Nattiv, A., et al. 2007. American College of Sports Medicine position stand: The female athlete triad. *Medicine and Science in Sports and Exercise* 39(10): 1867–1882; Witkop, C. T., et al. 2010. Understanding the spectrum of the female athlete triad. *Obstetrics and Gynecology* 116(6): 1444–1448.

in Chapter 9. For women, an extremely low percentage of body fat is associated with **amenorrhea** and loss of bone mass (see the box "The Female Athlete Triad").

## ASSESSING BODY MASS INDEX, BODY COMPOSITION, AND BODY FAT DISTRIBUTION

Although a scale can tell your total weight, it can't reveal whether a fluctuation in weight is due to a change in muscle, body water, or fat. Most important, a scale can't differentiate between overweight and overfat.

There are a number of simple, inexpensive ways to estimate healthy body weight and healthy body composition. These assessments can provide you with information about the health risks associated with your current body weight and body composition. They can also help you establish

**amenorrhea** Absent or infrequent menstruation, sometimes related to low levels of body fat and excessive quantity or intensity of exercise.

**female athlete triad** A condition consisting of three interrelated disorders: abnormal eating patterns (and excessive exercising) followed by lack of menstrual periods (amenorrhea) and decreased bone density (premature osteoporosis).

KEY TERMS

reasonable goals and set a starting point for current and future decisions about weight loss and weight gain.

## Calculating Body Mass Index

**Body mass index (BMI)** is a measure of body weight that is useful for classifying the health risks of body weight if you don't have access to more sophisticated methods. Though more accurate than height-weight tables, body mass index is also based on the concept that weight should be proportional to height. BMI is a fairly accurate measure of the health risks of body weight for average (nonathletic) people, and it is easy to calculate and rate. Researchers frequently use BMI in conjunction with waist circumference in studies that examine the health risks associated with body weight (Table 6.1).

Because BMI doesn't distinguish between fat weight and fat-free weight, however, it is inaccurate for some groups. For example, athletes who weight train have more muscle mass—and thus weigh more—than average people and may be classified as overweight by the BMI scale. Because their "excess" weight is in the form of muscle, however, it is healthy. Further, BMI is not particularly useful for tracking changes in body composition—gains in muscle mass and losses of fat. Women are likely to have more body fat for a given BMI

than men. BMI measurements have also over- and underestimated the prevalence of obesity in several ethnic groups. If you are an athlete, a serious weight trainer, or a person of short stature, do not use BMI as your primary means of assessing whether your current weight is healthy. Instead, try one of the methods described in the next section for estimating percent body fat.

BMI is calculated by dividing your body weight (expressed in kilograms) by the square of your height (expressed in meters). The following example is for a person who is 5 feet, 3 inches tall (63 inches) and weighs 130 pounds:

1. Divide body weight in pounds by 2.2 to convert weight to kilograms:
   $130 \div 2.2 = 59.1$

2. Multiply height in inches by 0.0254 to convert height to meters:
   $63 \times 0.0254 = 1.6$

3. Multiply the result of step 2 by itself to get the square of the height measurement:
   $1.6 \times 1.6 = 2.56$

4. Divide the result of step 1 by the result of step 3 to determine BMI:
   $59.1 \div 2.56 = 23$

An alternative equation, based on pounds and inches, is

$$BMI = [weight/(height \times height)] \times 703$$

Space for your own calculations can be found in Lab 6.1, and a complete BMI chart appears in Lab 6.2.

Under separate standards from the National Institutes of Health (NIH) and the World Health Organization (WHO), a BMI between 18.5 and 24.9 is considered healthy. A person with a BMI of 25 or above is classified as overweight, and someone with a BMI of 30 or above is classified as obese (Table 6.1). A person with a BMI below 18.5 is classified as underweight, although low BMI values may be healthy in some cases if they are not the result of smoking, an eating disorder, or an underlying disease. A BMI of 17.5 or less is sometimes used as a diagnostic criterion for the eating disorder anorexia nervosa (Chapter 9).

In classifying the health risks associated with overweight and obesity, the NIH and WHO guidelines consider body fat distribution and other disease risk factors in addition to BMI. As described earlier, excess fat in the abdomen is of greater concern than excess fat in other areas. Methods of assessing body fat distribution are discussed later in the chapter; the NIH and WHO guidelines use measurement of waist circumference (see Table 6.1). At a given level of overweight, people with a large waist circumference and/or additional disease risk factors are at greater risk for health problems. For example, a man with a BMI of 27, a waist circumference of more than 40 inches, and high blood pressure is at greater risk for health problems than another man who

| Table 6.1 | Classifications from the World Health Organization |
|---|---|

### Body Mass Index (BMI) Classifications

| WEIGHT STATUS CLASSIFICATION | BODY MASS INDEX |
|---|---|
| Underweight | <18.5 |
| Severe thinness | <16.0 |
| Moderate thinness | 16.0–16.9 |
| Mild thinness | 17.0–18.4 |
| Normal | 18.5–24.9 |
| Overweight | 25.0–29.9 |
| Obese, Class I | 30.0–34.9 |
| Obese, Class II | 35.0–39.9 |
| Obese, Class III | ≥40.0 |

### Waist Circumference Classifications

| CLASSIFICATION | WAIST CIRCUMFERENCE IN INCHES (CENTIMETERS) WOMEN | MEN |
|---|---|---|
| Normal | <32 in. (80 cm) | <37 in. (94 cm) |
| Increased | ≥32 in. (80 cm) | ≥37 in. (94 cm) |
| Substantially increased | ≥35 in. (88 cm) | ≥40 in. (102 cm) |

**SOURCE:** Wormser, D., et al. 2011. Separate and combined associations of body-mass index and abdominal adiposity with cardiovascular disease: Collaborative analysis of 58 prospective studies. *Lancet.* 377(9771): 1085–1095; table adapted from World Health Organization. 2000. *Obesity: Preventing and Managing the Global Epidemic. Report of a WHO Consultation.* Geneva: World Health Organization Technical Report Series 894: i–xii, 1.

has a BMI of 27 but has a smaller waist circumference and no other risk factors.

Thus, optimal BMI for good health depends on many factors; if your BMI is 25 or above, consult a physician for help in determining a healthy BMI for you. While BMI and waist circumference are important measures of health, they must be considered with other factors such as high blood pressure, diabetes, blood fats, and insulin resistance.

## Estimating Percent Body Fat

Assessing body composition involves estimating percent body fat. The only method for directly measuring the percentage of body weight that is fat is an autopsy—the dissection and chemical analysis of the body. However, there are indirect techniques that can provide an estimate of percent body fat. One of the most accurate is underwater weighing. Other techniques include skinfold measurements, the Bod Pod, bioelectrical impedance analysis, and dual-energy X-ray absorptiometry.

All of these methods have a margin of error, so it is important not to focus too much on precise values. For example, underwater weighing has a margin of error of about ±3%, meaning that if a person's percent body fat is actually 17%, the test result may be between 14% and 20%. The results of different methods may also vary, so if you plan to track changes in body composition over time, be sure to perform the assessment using the same method each time. See Table 6.2 for body composition ratings based on percent body fat. As with BMI, the percent body fat ratings indicate cutoff points for health risks associated with underweight and obesity.

**Underwater Weighing** In hydrostatic (underwater) weighing, an individual is submerged and weighed under water. The percentages of fat and fat-free weight are calculated from body density. Muscle has a higher density and fat a lower density than water (1.1 grams per cubic centimeter for fat-free mass, 0.91 gram per cubic centimeter for fat, and 1 gram per cubic centimeter for water). Therefore, people with more body fat tend to float and weigh less

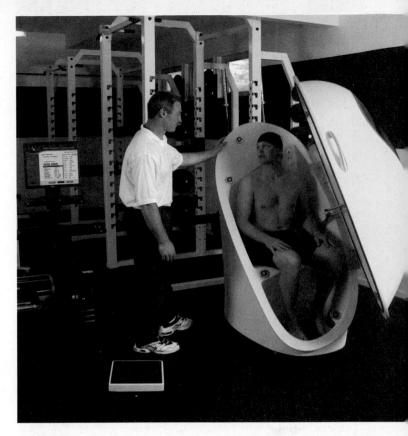

The Bod Pod.

under water, and lean people tend to sink and weigh more under water. Most university exercise physiology departments or sports medicine laboratories have an underwater weighing facility. For an accurate assessment of your body composition, find a place that does underwater weighing or has a BodPod (described in the next section).

**The Bod Pod** The Bod Pod, a small chamber containing computerized sensors, measures body composition by air displacement. The technique's technical name is *plethysmography*. It determines the percentage of fat by calculating body density from how much air is displaced by the person sitting inside the chamber. The Bod Pod has an error rate of about ± 2–4% in determining percent body fat.

**Skinfold Measurements** Skinfold measurement is a simple, inexpensive, and practical way to assess body composition. Skinfold measurements can be used to assess body composition because equations can link the thickness of skinfolds at various sites to percent body fat calculations from more precise laboratory techniques.

Skinfold assessment typically involves measuring the thickness of skinfolds at several different sites on the body.

| Table 6.2 | Percentage of Body Fat as the Criterion for Obesity | |
|---|---|---|
| | PERCENT BODY FAT | |
| CATEGORY | MALES | FEMALES |
| Normal | 12–20% | 20–30% |
| Borderline | 21–25% | 31–33% |
| Obese | > 25% | > 33% |

**SOURCE:** Bray, G. A. 2003. *Contemporary Diagnosis and Management of Obesity and the Metabolic Syndrome*, 3rd ed. Newton, Pa.: Handbooks in Health Care.

**body mass index (BMI)** A measure of relative body weight correlating highly with more direct measures of body fat, calculated by dividing total body weight (in kilograms) by the square of body height (in meters).

KEY TERM

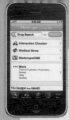

## Using BIA at Home

Scientists can use several techniques to accurately measure body composition. As described in the chapter, these techniques include underwater weighing, air displacement, and Dual-energy X-ray absorptiometry (DEXA). These methods, however, are costly and require technical expertise.

You can estimate your body fat and fat-free weight simply and accurately, at home, without the help of a technician. All you need is a digital home scale with a built-in bioelectrical impedance analyzer (BIA). BIA works by measuring the resistance in the body to a small electric current. Electricity flows more slowly through fat tissue than through muscle, so the more fat you have, the more slowly such a current will flow through your body. Conversely, a current will pass through your body more quickly if you have more fat-free (muscle) weight.

To use a BIA scale, just stand on the scale with bare feet. As it checks your weight, the scale sends a low-voltage electrical current through your body and analyzes the speed at which the current travels. Checking your weight and body composition takes no longer than checking your weight alone. Most BIA scales can remember your last weight and body composition measurement, making it easy to compare the measurements from day to day or week to week. Some scales can remember measurements for multiple people, as well.

A study of 22 weight-trained men showed that BIA compared favorably to underwater weighing for measuring body composition. Measurements of fat and lean mass are most valuable for measuring changes in body composition during diet and exercise programs.

Popular BIA scales are manufactured by Taylor, Whynter, Omron, RemedyT, and Tanita. These scales are available in most department stores and online, and cost between $50 and $200 depending on features.

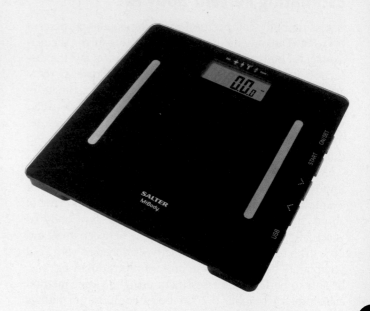

You can sum the skinfold values as an indirect measure of body fatness. For example, if you plan to create a fitness (and dietary change) program to improve body composition, you can compare the sum of skinfold values over time as an indicator of your program's progress and of improvements in body composition. You can also plug your skinfold values into equations like those in Lab 6.1 that predict percent body fat. When using these equations, however, remember that they have a fairly substantial margin of error ($\pm 4\%$ if performed by a skilled technician), so don't focus too much on specific values. The sum represents only a relative measure of body fatness.

Skinfolds are measured with a device called a **caliper**, which is a pair of spring-loaded, calibrated jaws. High-quality calipers are made of metal and have parallel jaw surfaces and constant spring tension. Inexpensive plastic calipers are also available; to ensure accuracy, plastic calipers should be spring-loaded and have metal jaws. Refer to Lab 6.1 for instructions on how to take skinfold measurements.

Taking accurate measurements with calipers requires patience, experience, and considerable practice. It's best to take several measurements at each site (or have several different people take each measurement) to help ensure accuracy. Be sure to take the measurements in the exact

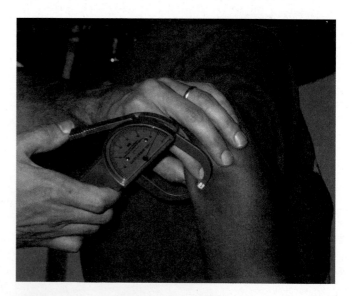

Taking skinfold measurements with calipers.

**caliper**  A pressure-sensitive measuring instrument with two jaws that can be adjusted to determine thickness.

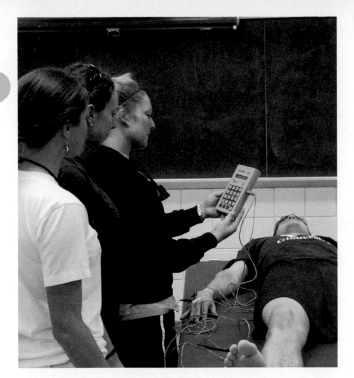

Using bioelectrical impedance analysis to estimate percent body fat.

location called for in the procedure. Because the amount of water in your body changes during the day, skinfold measurements taken in the morning and evening often differ. If you repeat the measurements in the future to track changes in your body composition, measure skinfolds at approximately the same time of day.

**Bioelectrical Impedance Analysis (BIA)** The BIA technique works by sending a small electrical current through the body and measuring the body's resistance to it. Fat-free tissues, where most body water is located, are good conductors of electrical current, whereas fat is not (see the box "Using BIA at Home"). Thus, the amount of resistance to electrical current is related to the amount of fat-free tissue in the body (the lower the resistance, the greater the fat-free mass) and can be used to estimate percent body fat.

Bioelectrical impedance analysis has an error rate of about ± 4–5%. To reduce error, follow the manufacturer's instructions carefully and avoid overhydration or underhydration (more or less body water than normal). Because measurement varies with the type of BIA analyzer, use the same instrument to compare measurements over time.

**Advanced Techniques: DEXA and TOBEC** Dual-energy X-ray absorptiometry (DEXA) works by measuring the tissue absorption of high- and low-energy X-ray beams. The procedure has an error rate of about ± 2%. Total body electrical conductivity (TOBEC) estimates lean body mass by passing a body through a magnetic field. Some fitness centers and sports medicine research facilities offer these body composition assessment techniques.

## Assessing Body Fat Distribution

Researchers have studied many different methods for measuring body fat distribution. Two of the simplest to perform are waist circumference measurement and waist-to-hip ratio calculation. In the first method, you measure your waist circumference; in the second, you divide your waist circumference by your hip circumference. Waist circumference has been found to be a better indicator of abdominal fat than waist-to-hip ratio. More research is needed to determine the precise degree of risk associated with specific values for these two assessments of body fat distribution. However, as noted earlier, a total waist measurement of more than 40 inches (102 cm) for men and 35 inches (88 cm) for women and a waist-to-hip ratio above 0.94 for young men and 0.82 for young women are associated with a significantly increased risk of heart disease and diabetes. Lab 6.1 shows you how to measure your body fat distribution.

## SETTING BODY COMPOSITION GOALS

If assessment tests indicate that fat loss would be beneficial for your health, your first step is to establish a goal. You can use the ratings in Table 6.1 or Table 6.2 to choose a target value for BMI or percent body fat (depending on which assessment you completed).

Make sure your goal is realistic and will ensure good health. Heredity limits your capacity to change your body composition, and few people can expect to develop the body of a fashion model or competitive bodybuilder. However, you can improve your body composition through a

### Fitness Tip

For most people, walking and running are better activities for weight loss than swimming. But this might not be true for older women. Recent research revealed that older women who swam lost more weight and controlled their blood sugar better than similar-aged women who walked.

Some studies have found that recording body weight every day helps keep you accountable to your weight-loss program and helps you make faster progress. An easy way to track your weight daily is to write it down in a table like the following:

| | | |
|---|---|---|
| 1. _____ | 11. _____ | 21. _____ |
| 2. _____ | 12. _____ | 22. _____ |
| 3. _____ | 13. _____ | 23. _____ |
| 4. _____ | 14. _____ | 24. _____ |
| 5. _____ | 15. _____ | 25. _____ |
| 6. _____ | 16. _____ | 26. _____ |
| 7. _____ | 17. _____ | 27. _____ |
| 8. _____ | 18. _____ | 28. _____ |
| 9. _____ | 19. _____ | 29. _____ |
| 10. _____ | 20. _____ | 30. _____ |

To make things more interesting, track your weight like this for a few weeks, and then convert the information into a line chart. A chart can help you visualize the data and make it easier for you to gauge your progress. You can easily track daily weights and convert them into charts in a spreadsheet program.

program of regular exercise and a healthy diet. If your body composition is in or close to the recommended range, you may want to set a lifestyle goal rather than a specific percent body fat or BMI goal. For example, you might set a goal of increasing your daily physical activity from 20 to 60 minutes or beginning a program of weight training, and then let any improvements in body composition occur as a secondary result of your primary target (physical activity). Remember, a lifestyle that includes regular exercise may be more important for health than trying to reach any ideal weight.

If you are significantly overfat or if you have known risk factors for disease (such as high blood pressure or high cholesterol), consult your physician to determine a body composition goal for your individual risk profile. For people who are obese, small losses of body weight (5–15%) over a 6–12 month period can result in significant health improvements.

Once you've established a body composition goal, you can then set a target range for body weight. Although body weight is not an accurate method of assessing body composition, it's a useful method for tracking progress in a program to change body composition. If you're losing a small or moderate amount of weight and exercising, you're probably losing fat while building muscle mass. Lab 6.2 will help you determine a range for recommended body weight.

Using percent body fat or BMI will generate a fairly accurate target body weight for most people. However, it's best not to stick rigidly to a recommended body weight calculated from any formula; individual genetic, cultural, and lifestyle factors are also important. Decide whether the body weight

that the formulas generate for you is realistic, meets all your goals, is healthy, *and* is reasonable for you to maintain.

## MAKING CHANGES IN BODY COMPOSITION

Chapter 9 includes specific strategies for losing or gaining weight and improving body composition. In general, lifestyle should be your focus—regular physical activity, endurance exercise, strength training, and a moderate energy intake. Making significant cuts in food intake in order to lose weight and body fat is a difficult strategy to maintain; focusing on increased physical activity is a better approach for many people. In studies of people who have lost weight and maintained the loss, physical activity was the key to long-term success.

You can track your progress toward your target body composition by checking your body weight regularly. Also, focus on how much energy you have and how your clothes fit.

To get a more accurate idea of your progress, you should directly reassess your body composition occasionally during your program: Body composition changes as weight changes. Losing a lot of weight usually includes losing some muscle mass no matter how hard a person exercises, partly because carrying less weight requires the muscular system to bear a smaller burden. Conversely, a large gain in weight without exercise still causes some gain in muscle mass because muscles are working harder to carry the extra weight.

## TIPS FOR TODAY AND THE FUTURE

A wellness lifestyle can lead naturally to a body composition that is healthy and appropriate for you.

### RIGHT NOW YOU CAN

- Find out what types of body composition assessment techniques are available at facilities on your campus or in your community.
- Do 30 minutes of physical activity—walk, jog, bike, swim, or climb stairs.
- Drink a glass of water instead of a soda, and include a high-fiber food such as whole-grain bread or cereal, popcorn, apples, berries, or beans in your next snack or meal.

### IN THE FUTURE YOU CAN

- Think about your image of the ideal body type for your sex. Consider where your idea comes from, whether you use this image to judge your own body, and whether it is a realistic goal for you.
- Be aware of media messages (especially visual images) that make you feel embarrassed or insecure about your body. Remind yourself that these messages are usually designed to sell a product; they should not form the basis of your body image.

## SUMMARY

- The human body is composed of fat-free mass (which includes bone, muscle, organ tissues, and connective tissues) and body fat.

- Having too much body fat has negative health consequences, especially in terms of cardiovascular disease and diabetes. Distribution of fat is also a significant factor in health.

- A fit and healthy-looking body, with the right body composition for a particular person, develops from habits of proper nutrition and exercise.

- Measuring body weight is not an accurate way to assess body composition because it does not differentiate between muscle weight and fat weight.

- Body mass index (calculated from weight and height measurements) and waist circumference can help classify the health risks associated with overweight. BMI is sometimes inaccurate, however, particularly in muscular people.

- Techniques for estimating percent body fat include underwater weighing, skinfold measurements, the Bod Pod, bioelectrical impedance analysis, DEXA, and TOBEC.

- Body fat distribution can be assessed through waist measurement or the waist-to-hip ratio.

- Recommended body composition and weight can be determined by choosing a target BMI or target body fat percentage. Keep heredity in mind when setting a goal, and focus on positive changes in lifestyle.

## FOR FURTHER EXPLORATION

### BOOKS

Acevedo, E., and M. Starks. 2011. *Exercise Testing and Prescription Lab Manual,* 2nd ed. Champaign, Ill.: Human Kinetics. *A book on physical fitness measurement techniques for students in kinesiology and physical education.*

American College of Sports Medicine. 2009. *ACSM's Health Related Physical Fitness Assessment Manual.* Philadelphia: Lippincott Williams and Wilkins. *A book written for professionals on assessing physical fitness in healthy adults.*

Bagchi, D., and H. G. Preuss. 2007. *Obesity: Epidemiology, Pathophysiology, and Prevention.* London: CRC Press. *A comprehensive guide for health professionals on the incidence, health risks, and prevention of obesity.*

Heyward, V. H. 2006. *Advanced Fitness Assessment and Exercise Prescription,* 5th ed. Champaign, Ill.: Human Kinetics. *Detailed coverage of assessing body composition, fitness, flexibility, and other aspects of fitness.*

Korbonit, M. 2008. *Obesity and Metabolism.* Basel, Switzerland: S Karger Pub. *Describes the physiology of weight control and metabolism.*

Lean, M., et al. 2007. *ABC of Obesity.* Boston: Blackwell Publishing Limited. *Examines the impact of obesity on the average person's life and discusses some of the most current options for preventing and treating obesity.*

### ORGANIZATIONS AND WEB SITES

*American Diabetes Association.* Provides information, a free newsletter, and referrals to local support groups; the Web site includes an online diabetes risk assessment.
   http://www.diabetes.org

*American Heart Association: Body Composition Tests.* Offers detailed information about body composition, testing and analysis, and the impact of body composition on heart health.
   http://www.heart.org/HEARTORG/GettingHealthy
      /NutritionCenter/Body-Composition-Tests_UCM_305883
      _Article.jsp

*Methods of Body Composition Analysis Tutorials.* Provides information about body composition assessment techniques, including underwater weighing, BIA, and DEXA.
   http://nutrition.uvm.edu/bodycomp

*National Heart, Lung, and Blood Institute: Obesity Education Initiative.* Provides information on the latest federal obesity standards and a BMI calculator.
   http://www.nhlbi.nih.gov/about/oei/index.htm

*National Institute of Diabetes and Digestive and Kidney Diseases Weight-Control Information Network.* Provides information about adult obesity: how it is defined and assessed, the risk factors associated with it, and its causes.
   http://win.niddk.nih.gov

*National Health and Nutrition Examination Survey (NHANES).* Ongoing survey and assessment of health status and practices in the United States.
   http://www.cdc.gov/nchs/nhanes/new_nhanes.htm

*Robert Wood Johnson Foundation.* Promotes the health and health care of Americans through research and distribution of information on healthy lifestyles.
   http://www.rwjf.org

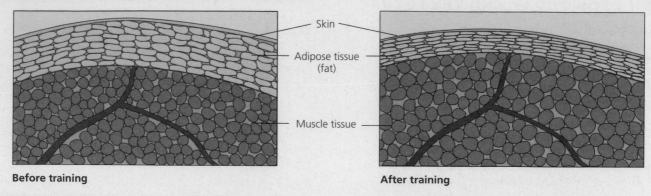

Before training · After training

**EFFECTS OF EXERCISE ON BODY COMPOSITION.** Endurance exercise and strength training both reduce body fat and increase muscle mass.

## Q Is spot reducing effective?

A *Spot reducing* refers to attempts to lose body fat in specific parts of the body by doing exercises for those parts. Danish researchers have shown that fat use increases in adipose tissue surrounding active muscle, but it is not known if short-term fat use helps reduce fat in specific sites. Most studies show that spot-reducing exercises contribute to fat loss only to the extent that they burn calories. The best way to reduce fat in any specific area is to create an overall negative energy balance: Take in less energy (food) than you use through exercise and metabolism.

## Q How does exercise affect body composition?

A Cardiorespiratory endurance exercise burns calories, thereby helping create a negative energy balance. Weight training does not use many calories and therefore is of little use in creating a negative energy balance. However, weight training increases muscle mass, which maintains a higher metabolic rate (the body's rate of energy use) and helps improve body composition. To minimize body fat and increase muscle mass,

thereby improving body composition, combine cardiorespiratory endurance exercise and weight training (see figure).

## Q Are people who have a desirable body composition physically fit?

A Having a healthy body composition is not necessarily associated with overall fitness. For example, many bodybuilders have very little body fat but have poor cardiorespiratory capacity and flexibility. Some athletes, such as NFL linemen, weigh 300 pounds or more; they have to lose the weight when they retire if they don't want to jeopardize their health. To be fit, you must rate high on all the components of fitness.

## Q What is liposuction, and will it help me lose body fat?

A Suction lipectomy, popularly known as *liposuction*, has become the most popular type of elective surgery in the world. The procedure involves removing limited amounts of fat from specific areas. Typically, no more than 2.5 kilograms (5.5 pounds) of adipose tissue are removed at a time. The procedure

is usually successful if the amount of excess fat is limited and skin elasticity is good. The procedure is most effective if integrated into a program of dietary restriction and exercise. Side effects include infection, dimpling, and wavy skin contours. Liposuction has a death rate of 1 in 5000 patients, primarily from pulmonary thromboembolism (a blood clot in the lungs) or fat embolism (circulatory blockage caused by a dislodged piece of fat). Other serious complications include shock, bleeding, and impaired blood flow to vital organs.

## Q What is cellulite, and how do I get rid of it?

A *Cellulite* is the name commonly given to ripply, wavy fat deposits that collect just under the skin. The "cottage cheese" appearance stems from the breakdown of tissues supporting the fat. These rippling fat deposits are really the same as fat deposited anywhere else in the body. The only way to control them is to create a negative energy balance— that is, burn more calories than you take in. There are no creams or lotions that will rub away surface (subcutaneous) fat deposits, and spot reducing is also ineffective. The solution is sensible eating habits and exercise.

*For more Common Questions Answered about body composition, visit the Online Learning Center at www.mhhe.com/fahey.*

*USDA Food and Nutrition Information Center: Weight and Obesity.*
Provides links to recent reports and studies on the issue of obesity among Americans.

> http://fnic.nal.usda.gov/nal_display/index.php?info_center=
> 4&tax_level=1&tax_subject=271

See also the listings for Chapters 2, 8, and 9.

## SELECTED BIBLIOGRAPHY

Ackerman, K. E., et al. 2011. Bone health and the female athlete triad in adolescent athletes. *Physician Sportsmedicine* 39(1): 131–141.

Alexander, S. C., et al. 2011. Do the five As work when physicians counsel about weight loss? *Family Medicine* 43(3): 179–184.

Allen, T. W., et al. 2010. Body size, body composition, and cardiovascular disease risk factors in NFL players. *Physician Sportsmedicine* 38(1): 21–27.

American College of Sports Medicine. 2009. *ACSM's Resource Manual for Guidelines for Exercise Testing and Prescription*, 6th ed. Philadelphia: Lippincott Williams and Wilkins.

American Heart Association. 2011. *Heart Disease and Stroke Statistics—2011 Update*. Dallas, Tx.: American Heart Association.

Baer, H. J., et al. 2011. Risk factors for mortality in the Nurses' Health Study: A competing risks analysis. *American Journal of Epidemiology* 173(3): 319–329.

Beeson, W. L., et al. 2010. Comparison of body composition by bioelectrical impedance analysis and dual-energy X-ray absorptiometry in Hispanic diabetics. *International Journal of Body Composition Research* 8(2): 45–50.

Blair, S. N. 2009. Physical inactivity: The biggest public health problem of the 21st century. *British Journal of Sports Medicine* 43(1): 1–2.

Borrud, L. G., et al. 2010. Body composition data for individuals 8 years of age and older: U.S. population, 1999–2004. *Vital Health Statistics* 11(250): 1–87.

Bouchla, A., et al. 2011. The addition of strength training to aerobic interval training: Effects on muscle strength and body composition in CHF patients. *Journal of Cardiopulmonary Rehabilitation and Prevention* 31(1): 47–51.

Caldwell, K., et al. 2010. Developing mindfulness in college students through movement-based courses: Effects on self-regulatory self-efficacy, mood, stress, and sleep quality. *Journal of American College of Health* 58(5): 433–442.

Centers for Disease Control and Prevention. 2011. *National diabetes fact sheet: National estimates and general information on diabetes and pre-diabetes in the United States, 2011*. Atlanta: Centers for Disease Control and Prevention.

Farrell, S. W., et al. 2010. Cardiorespiratory fitness, adiposity, and all-cause mortality in women. *Medicine and Science in Sports and Exercise* 42(11): 2006–2012.

Flegal, K. M., et al. 2007. Cause-specific excess deaths associated with underweight, overweight, and obesity. *Journal of the American Medical Association* 298 (17): 2028–2037.

Ford, E. S., et al. 2011. Trends in obesity and abdominal obesity among adults in the United States from 1999–2008. *International Journal of Obesity* 35: 736–743.

Gallagher, K. M., et al. 2011. When 'fit' leads to fit, and when 'fit' leads to fat: How message framing and intrinsic vs. extrinsic exercise outcomes interact in promoting physical activity. *Psychological Health* 1–16.

Hainer, V., et al. 2009. Fat or fit: What is more important? *Diabetes Care* 32 (Suppl 2): S392–S397.

Harvey, S. B., et al. 2010. Physical activity and common mental disorders. *British Journal of Psychiatry*. 197: 357–364.

Hjgaard, B., et al. 2008. Waist circumference and body mass index as predictors of health care costs. *PLoS ONE* 3(7): e2619.

Hurvitz, M., et al. 2009. The young female athlete. *Pediatrics Endocrinology Reviews* 7(2): 123–129.

Lee, D. C., et al. 2009. Does physical activity ameliorate the health hazards of obesity? *British Journal of Sports Medicine* 43(1): 49–51.

Malina, R. M. 2007. Body composition in athletes: Assessment and estimated fatness. *Clinics in Sports Medicine* 26(1): 37–68.

Mattsson, S., and B. J. Thomas. 2006. Development of methods for body composition studies. *Physics in Medicine and Biology* 51(13): R203–R228.

Moon, J. R. 2008. Percent body fat estimations in college men using field and laboratory methods: A three-compartment model approach. *Dynamic Medicine* 7:7.

Murphy, M. H., et. al. 2009. Accumulated versus continuous exercise for health benefit: A review of empirical studies. *Sports Medicine* 39(1): 29–43.

Ode, J. J., et al. 2007. Body mass index as a predictor of percent fat in college athletes and nonathletes. *Medicine and Science in Sports and Exercise* 39(3): 403–409.

Pauli, S. A., et al. 2010. Athletic amenorrhea: Energy deficit or psychogenic challenge? *Annals of the New York Academy of Sciences* 1205: 33–38.

Puterman, E., et al. 2010. The power of exercise: Buffering the effect of chronic stress on telomere length. *PLoS One* 5(5): e10837.

Romero-Corral, A., et al. 2008. Accuracy of body mass index in diagnosing obesity in the adult general population. *International Journal of Obesity* 32(6): 959–966.

Stephens, B. R., et al. 2011. Effects of 1 day of inactivity on insulin action in healthy men and women: Interaction with energy intake. *Metabolism Clinical and Experimental* 60: 941–949.

Varady, K., et al. 2007. Validation of hand-held bioelectrical impedance analysis with magnetic resonance imaging for the assessment of body composition in overweight women. *American Journal of Human Biology* 19(3): 429–433.

Wada, R., et al. 2010. Body composition and wages. *Economics and Human Biology* 8(2): 242–254.

Wang, X., et al. 2008. Weight regain is related to decreases in physical activity during weight loss. *Medicine and Science in Sports and Exercise* 40(10): 1781–1788.

Wormser, D., et al. 2011. Separate and combined associations of body-mass index and abdominal adiposity with cardiovascular disease: Collaborative analysis of 58 prospective studies. *Lancet* 377(9771): 1085–1095.

Zanovec, M., et al. 2009. Self-reported physical activity improves prediction of body fatness in young adults. *Medicine and Science in Sports and Exercise* 41(2): 328–335.

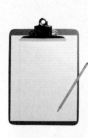

**LAB 6.1  Assessing Body Mass Index and Body Composition**

## Body Mass Index

### Equipment
1. Weight scale
2. Tape measure or other means of measuring height

### Instructions
Measure your height and weight, and record the results. Be sure to record the unit of measurement.

Height: _____   Weight: _____

### Calculating BMI (see also the shortcut chart of BMI values in Lab 6.2)
1. Convert your body weight to kilograms by dividing your weight in pounds by 2.2.

   Body weight _____ lb ÷ 2.2 lb/kg = body weight _____ kg
2. Convert your height measurement to meters by multiplying your height in inches by 0.0254.

   Height _____ in. × 0.0254 m/in. = height _____ m
3. Square your height measurement.

   Height _____ m × height _____ m = height _____ m²
4. BMI equals body weight in kilograms divided by height in meters squared (kg/m²).

   Body weight _____ kg ÷ height _____ m² = BMI _____ kg/m²
   (from step 1)                              (from step 3)

### Rating Your BMI
Refer to the table for a rating of your BMI. Record the results below and on the final page of this lab.

| Classification | BMI (kg/m²) |
|---|---|
| Underweight | <18.5 |
| Normal | 18.5−24.9 |
| Overweight | 25.0−29.9 |
| Obesity (I) | 30.0−34.9 |
| Obesity (II) | 35.0−39.9 |
| Extreme obesity (III) | ≥40.0 |

BMI _____ kg/m²

Classification _____

## Skinfold Measurements

### Equipment
1. Skinfold calipers
2. Partner to take measurements
3. Marking pen (optional)

Mc Graw Hill **connect**  http://www.mcgrawhillconnect.com/
|FITNESS AND WELLNESS

## Instructions

1. *Select and locate the correct sites for measurement*. All measurements should be taken on the right side of the body with the subject standing. Skinfolds are normally measured on the natural fold line of the skin, either vertically or at a slight angle. The skinfold measurement sites for males are chest, abdomen, and thigh; for females, triceps, suprailium, and thigh. If the person taking skinfold measurements is inexperienced, it may be helpful to mark the correct sites with a marking pen.

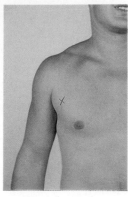 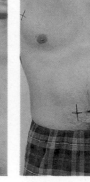 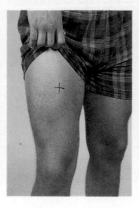 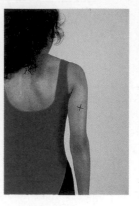 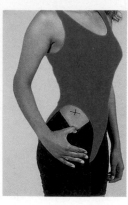

(a) Chest        (b) Abdomen        (c) Thigh        (d) Triceps        (e) Suprailium

*(a) Chest*. Pinch a diagonal fold halfway between the nipple and the shoulder crease. *(b) Abdomen*. Pinch a vertical fold about 1 inch to the right of the umbilicus (navel). *(c) Thigh*. Pinch a vertical fold midway between the top of the hipbone and the kneecap. *(d) Triceps*. Pinch a vertical skinfold on the back of the right arm midway between the shoulder and elbow. The arm should be straight and should hang naturally. *(e) Suprailium*. Pinch a fold at the top front of the right hipbone. The skinfold here is taken slightly diagonally according to the natural fold tendency of the skin.

2. *Measure the appropriate skinfolds*. Pinch a fold of skin between your thumb and forefinger. Pull the fold up so that no muscular tissue is included; don't pinch the skinfold too hard. Hold the calipers perpendicular to the fold and measure the skinfold about 0.25 inch away from your fingers. Allow the tips of the calipers to close on the skinfold and let the reading settle before marking it down. Take readings to the nearest half-millimeter. Continue to repeat the measurements until two consecutive measurements match, releasing and repinching the skinfold between each measurement. Make a note of the final measurement for each site.

Time of day of measurements: _____

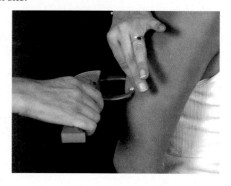

| Men | | Women | |
|---|---|---|---|
| Chest: _____ mm | | Triceps: _____ mm | |
| Abdomen: _____ mm | | Suprailium: _____ mm | |
| Thigh: _____ mm | | Thigh: _____ mm | |

## Determining Percent Body Fat

Add the measurements of your three skinfolds. Use this sum as a point of comparison for future assessments and/or to find the percent body fat that corresponds to your total in the appropriate table. For example, a 20-year-old female with measurements of 17 mm, 21 mm, and 22 mm would have a skinfold sum of 60 mm; according to the following table her percent body fat is 23.5.

Sum of three skinfolds: _____ mm        Percent body fat: _____ %

*Prediction of Fat Percentage in Females from the Sum of Three Skinfolds*

| Sum of Skinfolds (mm) | Age (Years) 20 | 25 | 30 | 35 | 40 | 45 | 50 | 55 | 60 and over |
|---|---|---|---|---|---|---|---|---|---|
| 20 | 9.3 | 9.6 | 9.9 | 10.2 | 10.5 | 10.8 | 11.1 | 11.4 | 11.7 |
| 25 | 11.2 | 11.5 | 11.8 | 12.1 | 12.4 | 12.7 | 13.0 | 13.3 | 13.6 |
| 30 | 13.1 | 13.4 | 13.7 | 14.0 | 14.3 | 14.6 | 14.9 | 15.2 | 15.5 |
| 35 | 14.9 | 15.2 | 15.5 | 15.8 | 16.1 | 16.4 | 16.7 | 17.0 | 17.3 |
| 40 | 16.7 | 17.0 | 17.3 | 17.6 | 17.9 | 18.2 | 18.5 | 18.8 | 19.1 |
| 45 | 18.4 | 18.8 | 19.1 | 19.4 | 19.7 | 20.0 | 20.3 | 20.6 | 20.9 |
| 50 | 20.2 | 20.5 | 20.8 | 21.1 | 21.4 | 21.7 | 22.0 | 22.4 | 22.7 |
| 55 | 21.9 | 22.2 | 22.5 | 22.8 | 23.1 | 23.4 | 23.7 | 24.1 | 24.4 |
| 60 | 23.5 | 23.8 | 24.1 | 24.4 | 24.8 | 25.1 | 25.4 | 25.7 | 26.0 |
| 65 | 25.1 | 25.4 | 25.7 | 26.1 | 26.4 | 26.7 | 27.0 | 27.3 | 27.7 |
| 70 | 26.7 | 27.0 | 27.3 | 27.6 | 27.9 | 28.3 | 28.6 | 28.9 | 29.2 |
| 75 | 28.2 | 28.5 | 28.8 | 29.1 | 29.5 | 29.8 | 30.1 | 30.4 | 30.8 |
| 80 | 29.7 | 30.0 | 30.3 | 30.6 | 31.0 | 31.3 | 31.6 | 31.9 | 32.3 |
| 85 | 31.1 | 31.4 | 31.7 | 32.1 | 32.4 | 32.7 | 33.0 | 33.4 | 33.7 |
| 90 | 32.5 | 32.8 | 33.1 | 33.5 | 33.8 | 34.1 | 34.4 | 34.8 | 35.1 |
| 95 | 33.8 | 34.1 | 34.5 | 34.8 | 35.1 | 35.5 | 35.8 | 36.1 | 36.5 |
| 100 | 35.1 | 35.4 | 35.8 | 36.1 | 36.4 | 36.8 | 37.1 | 37.4 | 37.8 |
| 105 | 36.3 | 36.7 | 37.0 | 37.3 | 37.7 | 38.0 | 38.3 | 38.7 | 39.0 |
| 110 | 37.5 | 37.9 | 38.2 | 38.5 | 38.9 | 39.2 | 39.5 | 39.9 | 40.2 |
| 115 | 38.7 | 39.0 | 39.3 | 39.7 | 40.0 | 40.4 | 40.7 | 41.0 | 41.4 |
| 120 | 39.8 | 40.1 | 40.4 | 40.8 | 41.1 | 41.5 | 41.8 | 42.1 | 42.5 |
| 125 | 40.8 | 41.2 | 41.5 | 41.8 | 42.2 | 42.5 | 42.9 | 43.2 | 43.5 |
| 130 | 41.8 | 42.1 | 42.5 | 42.8 | 43.2 | 43.5 | 43.9 | 44.2 | 44.5 |
| 135 | 42.7 | 43.1 | 43.4 | 43.8 | 44.1 | 44.5 | 44.8 | 45.1 | 45.5 |

**SOURCES:** Table generated from equations in Jackson, A. S., and M. L. Pollock. 1978. Generalized equations for predicting body density in men, *British Journal of Nutrition* 40: 497–504; Jackson, A. S., M. L. Pollock, and A. Ward. 1980. Gerneralized equations for predicting body density in women, *Medicine and Science in Sports and Exercise* 12: 175–182; Seri, W. E. 1956. Gross composition of the body. In J. H. Lawrence and C. A. Tobias. (eds.), *Advances in Biological and Medical Physics*, IV. New York: Academic Press.

connect http://www.mcgrawhillconnect.com/
|FITNESS AND WELLNESS

*Prediction of Fat Percentage in Males from the Sum of Three Skinfolds*

| Sum of Skinfolds (mm) | Age (Years) | | | | | | | | |
|---|---|---|---|---|---|---|---|---|---|
| | 20 | 25 | 30 | 35 | 40 | 45 | 50 | 55 | 60 and over |
| 10 | 1.6 | 2.1 | 2.7 | 3.2 | 3.7 | 4.3 | 4.8 | 5.3 | 5.9 |
| 15 | 3.2 | 3.8 | 4.3 | 4.8 | 5.4 | 5.9 | 6.4 | 7.0 | 7.5 |
| 20 | 4.8 | 5.4 | 5.9 | 6.4 | 7.0 | 7.5 | 8.1 | 8.6 | 9.2 |
| 25 | 6.4 | 6.9 | 7.5 | 8.0 | 8.6 | 9.1 | 9.7 | 10.2 | 10.8 |
| 30 | 8.0 | 8.5 | 9.1 | 9.6 | 10.2 | 10.7 | 11.3 | 11.8 | 12.4 |
| 35 | 9.5 | 10.0 | 10.6 | 11.2 | 11.7 | 12.3 | 12.8 | 13.4 | 13.9 |
| 40 | 11.0 | 11.6 | 12.1 | 12.7 | 13.2 | 13.8 | 14.4 | 14.9 | 15.5 |
| 45 | 12.5 | 13.1 | 13.6 | 14.2 | 14.7 | 15.3 | 15.9 | 16.4 | 17.0 |
| 50 | 14.0 | 14.5 | 15.1 | 15.6 | 16.2 | 16.8 | 17.3 | 17.9 | 18.5 |
| 55 | 15.4 | 16.0 | 16.5 | 17.1 | 17.7 | 18.2 | 18.8 | 19.4 | 19.9 |
| 60 | 16.8 | 17.4 | 17.9 | 18.5 | 19.1 | 19.7 | 20.2 | 20.8 | 21.4 |
| 65 | 18.2 | 18.8 | 19.3 | 19.9 | 20.5 | 21.1 | 21.6 | 22.2 | 22.8 |
| 70 | 19.5 | 20.1 | 20.7 | 21.3 | 21.9 | 22.4 | 23.0 | 23.6 | 24.2 |
| 75 | 20.9 | 21.5 | 22.0 | 22.6 | 23.2 | 23.8 | 24.4 | 24.9 | 25.5 |
| 80 | 22.2 | 22.8 | 23.3 | 23.9 | 24.5 | 25.1 | 25.7 | 26.3 | 26.9 |
| 85 | 23.4 | 24.0 | 24.6 | 25.2 | 25.8 | 26.4 | 27.0 | 27.6 | 28.2 |
| 90 | 24.7 | 25.3 | 25.9 | 26.5 | 27.0 | 27.6 | 28.2 | 28.8 | 29.4 |
| 95 | 25.9 | 26.5 | 27.1 | 27.7 | 28.3 | 28.9 | 29.5 | 30.1 | 30.7 |
| 100 | 27.1 | 27.7 | 28.3 | 28.9 | 29.5 | 30.1 | 30.7 | 31.3 | 31.9 |
| 105 | 28.2 | 28.8 | 29.4 | 30.0 | 30.6 | 31.2 | 31.8 | 32.4 | 33.0 |
| 110 | 29.3 | 29.9 | 30.5 | 31.1 | 31.7 | 32.4 | 33.0 | 33.6 | 34.2 |
| 115 | 30.4 | 31.0 | 31.6 | 32.2 | 32.8 | 33.5 | 34.1 | 34.7 | 35.3 |
| 120 | 31.5 | 32.1 | 32.7 | 33.3 | 33.9 | 34.5 | 35.1 | 35.7 | 36.4 |
| 125 | 32.5 | 33.1 | 33.7 | 34.3 | 34.9 | 35.6 | 36.2 | 36.8 | 37.4 |

SOURCES: Table generated from equations in Jackson, A. S., and M. L. Pollock, 1978. Generalized equations for predicting body density in men, *British Journal of Nutrition* 40: 497–504; Jackson, A. S., M. L. Pollock, and A. Ward. 1980. Generalized equations for predicting body density in women, *Medicine and Science in Sports and Exercise* 12: 175–182; Seri, W. E. 1956. Gross composition of the body. In J. H. Lawrence and C. A. Tobias. (eds.), *Advances in Biological and Medical Physics*, IV. New York: Academic Press.

# Rating Your Body Composition

Refer to the chart to rate your percent body fat. Record it below and in the chart at the end of this lab.

Rating: _____

*Percent Body Fat Classification*

| | Percent Body Fat (%) | | | | Percent Body Fat (%) | | |
| --- | --- | --- | --- | --- | --- | --- | --- |
| | *20–39 Years* | *40–59 Years* | *60–79 Years* | | *20–39 Years* | *40–59 Years* | *60–79 Years* |
| **Women** | | | | **Men** | | | |
| Essential* | 8–12 | 8–12 | 8–12 | Essential* | 3–5 | 3–5 | 3–5 |
| Low/athletic** | 13–20 | 13–22 | 13–23 | Low/athletic** | 6–7 | 6–10 | 6–12 |
| Recommended | 21–32 | 23–33 | 24–35 | Recommended | 8–19 | 11–21 | 13–24 |
| Overfat† | 33–38 | 34–39 | 36–41 | Overfat† | 20–24 | 22–27 | 25–29 |
| Obese† | ≥39 | ≥40 | ≥42 | Obese† | ≥25 | ≥28 | ≥30 |

**NOTE:** The cutoffs for recommended, overfat, and obese ranges in this table are based on a study that linked body mass index classifications from the National Institutes of Health with predicted percent body fat (measured using dual-energy X-ray absorptiometry).

*Essential body fat is necessary for the basic functioning of the body.
**Percent body fat in the low/athletic range may be appropriate for some people as long as it is not the result of illness or disordered eating habits.
†Health risks increase as percent body fat exceeds the recommended range.

**SOURCES:** Gallagher, D., et al. 2009. Healthy percentage body fat ranges: An approach for developing guidelines based on body mass index. *American Journal of Clinical Nutrition* 72: 694–701. American College of Sports Medicine. 2009. *ACSM's Resource Manual for Guidelines for Exercise Testing and Prescription,* 6th ed. Philadelphia: Lippincott Williams and Wilkins.

## Other Methods of Assessing Percent Body Fat

If you use a different method, record the name of the method and the result below and in the chart at the end of this lab. Find your body composition rating on the chart above.

Method used: _____    Percent body fat: _____ %    Rating (from chart above): _____

## Waist Circumference and Waist-to-Hip Ratio

*Equipment*

1. Tape measure
2. Partner to take measurements

*Preparation*

Wear clothes that will not add significantly to your measurements.

## Instructions

Stand with your feet together and your arms at your sides. Raise your arms only high enough to allow for taking the measurements. Your partner should make sure the tape is horizontal around the entire circumference and pulled snugly against your skin. The tape shouldn't be pulled so tight that it causes indentations in your skin. Record measurements to the nearest millimeter or one-sixteenth of an inch.

*Waist.* Measure at the smallest waist circumference. If you don't have a natural waist, measure at the level of your navel.

Waist measurement: _____

*Hip.* Measure at the largest hip circumference. Hip measurement: _____

*Waist-to-Hip Ratio:* You can use any unit of measurement (for example, inches or centimeters) as long as you're consistent. Waist-to-hip ratio equals waist measurement divided by hip measurement.

Waist-to-hip ratio: _____ ÷ _____ = _____
                     (waist measurement)   (hip measurement)

connect™  http://www.mcgrawhillconnect.com/
FITNESS AND WELLNESS

### Determining Your Risk

The table below indicates values for waist circumference and waist-to-hip ratio above which the risk of health problems increases significantly. If your measurement or ratio is above either cutoff point, put a check on the appropriate line below and in the chart at the end of this lab.

Waist circumference: _____ (✓ high risk) Waist-to-hip ratio: _____ (✓ high risk)

### Body Fat Distribution

**Cutoff Points for High Risk**

|  | Waist Circumference | Waist-to-Hip Ratio |
|---|---|---|
| Men | More than 40 in. (102 cm) | More than 0.94 |
| Women | More than 35 in. (88 cm) | More than 0.82 |

**SOURCE:** National Heart, Lung, and Blood Institute. 1998. *Clinical Guidelines on the Identification, Evaluation, and Treatment of Overweight and Obesity in Adults: The Evidence Report. Bethesda*, Md.: National Institutes of Health. Heyward, V. H., and D. R. Wagner. 2004. *Applied Body Composition Assessment*, 2nd ed. Champaign, Ill.: Human Kinetics.

### Rating Your Body Composition

| Assessment | Value | Classification |
|---|---|---|
| BMI | _____ kg/m$^2$ | _____ |
| Skinfold measurements or alternative method of determining percent body fat Specify method: _____ | _____ % body fat | _____ |
| Waist circumference Waist-to-hip ratio | _____ in. or cm _____ (ratio) | _____ (✓ high risk) _____ (✓ high risk) |

## Using Your Results

*How did you score?* Are you surprised by your ratings for body composition and body fat distribution? Are your current ratings in the range for good health? Are you satisfied with your current body composition? Why or why not?

If you're not satisfied, set a realistic goal for improvement:

*What should you do next?* Enter the results of this lab in the Preprogram Assessment column in Appendix C. If you've determined that you need to improve your body composition, set a specific goal by completing Lab 6.2, and then plan your program using the labs in Chapters 8 and 9. After several weeks or months of an exercise and/or dietary change program, complete this lab again and enter the results in the Postprogram Assessment column of Appendix C. How do the results compare?

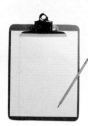

# LAB 6.2  Setting Goals for Target Body Weight

This lab is designed to help you set body weight goals based on a target BMI or percent body fat. If the results of Lab 6.1 indicate that a change in body composition would be beneficial for your health, you may want to complete this lab to help you set goals.

Remember, though, that a wellness lifestyle—including a balanced diet and regular exercise—is more important for your health than achieving any specific body weight, BMI, or percent body fat. You may want to set goals for improving your diet and increasing physical activity and let your body composition change as a result. If so, use the labs in Chapters 3, 4, 8, and 9 as your guides.

## Equipment

Calculator (or pencil and paper for calculations)

## Preparation

Determine percent body fat and/or calculate BMI as described in Lab 6.1. Keep track of height and weight as measured for these calculations.

Height: _____ Weight: _____

### Instructions: Target Body Weight from Target BMI

Use the chart below to find the target body weight that corresponds to your target BMI. Find your height in the left column, and then move across the appropriate row until you find the weight that corresponds to your target BMI. Remember, BMI is only an indirect measurement of body composition. It is possible to improve body composition without any significant change in weight. For example, a weight training program may result in increased muscle mass and decreased fat mass without any change in overall weight. For this reason, you may want to set alternative or additional goals, such as improving the fit of your clothes or decreasing your waist measurement.

| | <18.5 Underweight | | 18.5–24.9 Normal | | | | | | 25–29.9 Overweight | | | | | 30–34.9 Obesity (Class I) | | | | | 35–39.9 Obesity (Class II) | | | | | ≥40 Extreme Obesity |
|---|---|---|---|---|---|---|---|---|---|---|---|---|---|---|---|---|---|---|---|---|---|---|---|---|
| **BMI** | 17 | 18 | 19 | 20 | 21 | 22 | 23 | 24 | 25 | 26 | 27 | 28 | 29 | 30 | 31 | 32 | 33 | 34 | 35 | 36 | 37 | 38 | 39 | 40 |
| **Height** | | | | | | | | | | | Body Weight (pounds) | | | | | | | | | | | | | |
| 4' 10" | 81 | 86 | 91 | 96 | 101 | 105 | 110 | 115 | 120 | 124 | 129 | 134 | 139 | 144 | 148 | 153 | 158 | 163 | 168 | 172 | 177 | 182 | 187 | 192 |
| 4' 11" | 84 | 89 | 94 | 99 | 104 | 109 | 114 | 119 | 124 | 129 | 134 | 139 | 144 | 149 | 154 | 159 | 163 | 168 | 173 | 178 | 183 | 188 | 193 | 198 |
| 5' | 87 | 92 | 97 | 102 | 108 | 113 | 118 | 123 | 128 | 133 | 138 | 143 | 149 | 154 | 159 | 164 | 169 | 174 | 179 | 184 | 190 | 195 | 200 | 205 |
| 5' 1" | 90 | 95 | 101 | 106 | 111 | 117 | 122 | 127 | 132 | 138 | 143 | 148 | 154 | 159 | 164 | 169 | 175 | 180 | 185 | 191 | 196 | 201 | 207 | 212 |
| 5' 2" | 93 | 98 | 104 | 109 | 115 | 120 | 126 | 131 | 137 | 142 | 148 | 153 | 159 | 164 | 170 | 175 | 181 | 186 | 191 | 197 | 202 | 208 | 213 | 219 |
| 5' 3" | 96 | 102 | 107 | 113 | 119 | 124 | 130 | 136 | 141 | 147 | 153 | 158 | 164 | 169 | 175 | 181 | 186 | 192 | 198 | 203 | 209 | 215 | 220 | 226 |
| 5' 4" | 99 | 105 | 111 | 117 | 122 | 128 | 134 | 140 | 146 | 152 | 157 | 163 | 169 | 175 | 181 | 187 | 192 | 198 | 204 | 210 | 216 | 222 | 227 | 233 |
| 5' 5" | 102 | 108 | 114 | 120 | 126 | 132 | 138 | 144 | 150 | 156 | 162 | 168 | 174 | 180 | 186 | 192 | 198 | 204 | 210 | 216 | 222 | 229 | 235 | 241 |
| 5' 6" | 105 | 112 | 118 | 124 | 130 | 136 | 143 | 149 | 155 | 161 | 167 | 174 | 180 | 186 | 192 | 198 | 205 | 211 | 217 | 223 | 229 | 236 | 242 | 248 |
| 5' 7" | 109 | 115 | 121 | 128 | 134 | 141 | 147 | 153 | 160 | 166 | 173 | 179 | 185 | 192 | 198 | 204 | 211 | 217 | 224 | 230 | 236 | 243 | 249 | 256 |
| 5' 8" | 112 | 118 | 125 | 132 | 138 | 145 | 151 | 158 | 165 | 171 | 178 | 184 | 191 | 197 | 204 | 211 | 217 | 224 | 230 | 237 | 244 | 250 | 257 | 263 |
| 5' 9" | 115 | 122 | 129 | 136 | 142 | 149 | 156 | 163 | 169 | 176 | 183 | 190 | 197 | 203 | 210 | 217 | 224 | 230 | 237 | 244 | 251 | 258 | 264 | 271 |
| 5' 10" | 119 | 126 | 133 | 139 | 146 | 153 | 160 | 167 | 174 | 181 | 188 | 195 | 202 | 209 | 216 | 223 | 230 | 237 | 244 | 251 | 258 | 265 | 272 | 279 |
| 5' 11" | 122 | 129 | 136 | 143 | 151 | 158 | 165 | 172 | 179 | 187 | 194 | 201 | 208 | 215 | 222 | 230 | 237 | 244 | 251 | 258 | 265 | 273 | 280 | 287 |
| 6' | 125 | 133 | 140 | 148 | 155 | 162 | 170 | 177 | 184 | 192 | 199 | 207 | 214 | 221 | 229 | 236 | 243 | 251 | 258 | 266 | 273 | 280 | 288 | 295 |
| 6' 1" | 129 | 137 | 144 | 152 | 159 | 167 | 174 | 182 | 190 | 197 | 205 | 212 | 220 | 228 | 235 | 243 | 250 | 258 | 265 | 273 | 281 | 288 | 296 | 303 |
| 6' 2" | 132 | 140 | 148 | 156 | 164 | 171 | 179 | 187 | 195 | 203 | 210 | 218 | 226 | 234 | 242 | 249 | 257 | 265 | 273 | 281 | 288 | 296 | 304 | 312 |
| 6' 3" | 136 | 144 | 152 | 160 | 168 | 176 | 184 | 192 | 200 | 208 | 216 | 224 | 232 | 240 | 248 | 256 | 264 | 272 | 280 | 288 | 296 | 304 | 312 | 320 |
| 6' 4" | 140 | 148 | 156 | 164 | 173 | 181 | 189 | 197 | 206 | 214 | 222 | 230 | 238 | 247 | 255 | 263 | 271 | 280 | 288 | 296 | 304 | 312 | 321 | 329 |

**SOURCE:** Ratings from the National Heart, Lung, and Blood Institute. 1998. *Clinical Guidelines on the Identification, Evaluation, and Treatment of Overweight and Obesity in Adults.* Bethesda, Md.: National Institutes of Health.

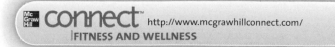

Current BMI: _____ Target BMI: _____ Target body weight (from chart): _____

Alternative/additional goals: _____

_____

*Note:* You can calculate target body weight from target BMI more precisely by using the following formula: (1) convert your height measurement to meters, (2) square your height measurement, (3) multiply this number by your target BMI to get your target weight in kilograms, and (4) convert your target weight from kilograms to pounds:

1. Height _____ in. × 0.0254 m/in. = height _____ m

2. Height _____ m × height _____ m = _____ $m^2$

3. Target BMI _____ × height _____ $m^2$ = target weight _____ kg

4. Target weight _____ kg × 2.2 lb/kg = target weight _____ lb

*Instructions: Target Body Weight from Target Body Fat Percentages*
Use the formula below to determine the target body weight that corresponds to your target percent body fat.
Current percent body fat: _____ Target percent body fat: _____

*Formula*

*Example: 180-lb male,*
*current percent body fat of 24%, goal of 21%*

1. To determine the fat weight in your body, multiply your current weight by percent body fat (determined through skinfold measurements and expressed as a decimal).

180 lb × 0.24 = 43.2 lb

2. Subtract the fat weight from your current weight to get your current fat-free weight.

180 lb − 43.2 lb = 136.8 lb

3. Subtract your target percent body fat from 1 to get target percent fat-free weight.

1 − 0.21 = 0.79

4. To get your target body weight, divide your fat-free weight by your target percent fat-free weight.

136.8 lb ÷ 0.79 = 173 lb

*Note:* Weight can be expressed in either pounds or kilograms, as long as the unit of measurement is used consistently.

1. Current body weight _____ × percent body fat _____ = fat weight _____

2. Current body weight _____ − fat weight _____ = fat-free weight _____

3. 1 − target percent body fat _____ = target percent fat-free weight _____

4. Fat-free weight _____ ÷ target percent fat-free weight _____ = target body weight_____

## Setting a Goal

Based on these calculations and other factors (including heredity, individual preference, and current health status), select a target weight or range of weights for yourself.

Target body weight: _____

# CHAPTER 7

# Putting Together a Complete Fitness Program

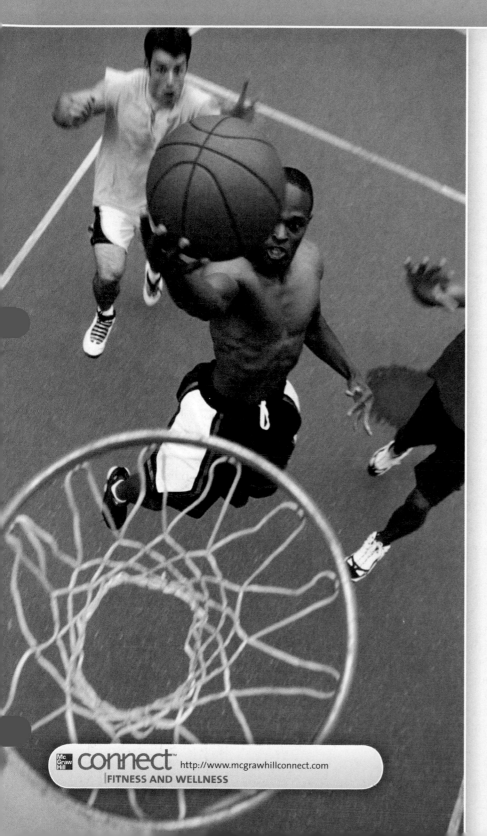

## LOOKING AHEAD...

After reading this chapter, you should be able to:

- List the steps you can follow to put together a successful personal fitness program
- Describe strategies that can help you maintain a fitness program over the long term
- Tailor a fitness program to accommodate different life stages

## TEST YOUR KNOWLEDGE

1. Which of the following physical activities is considered a high-intensity exercise?
   a. hiking uphill
   b. singles tennis
   c. jumping rope

2. Older adults should avoid exercise to protect themselves against falls and injuries. True or false?

3. Swimming is a total fitness activity that develops all the components of health-related fitness. True or false?

**Answers**

1. **All Three.** According to the U.S. Department of Health and Human Services, you can perform any of these activities for 75 minutes per week to obtain health and wellness benefits.

2. **False.** Older adults receive the same health benefits from exercise as younger adults, including improvements in strength, body composition, cardiorespiratory health, flexibility, balance, stability, and cognitive functioning. A far greater danger is posed by inactivity.

3. **False.** Swimming is excellent for developing cardiorespiratory endurance and muscular endurance, but because it is not a weight-bearing activity, it tends to reduce bone density. Swimmers are advised to include weight training in their exercise program to maintain bone mass.

Understanding the benefits of physical fitness, as explained in Chapters 1–6, is the first step toward creating a well-rounded exercise program. The next challenge is to choose activities and combine them into a program that develops all the components of fitness and helps you stay motivated. This chapter presents a step-by-step plan for creating and maintaining a well-rounded fitness program. At the end of this chapter, you'll find sample programs based on popular activities. These programs provide structure that can be helpful if you're beginning an exercise program for the first time.

## DEVELOPING A PERSONAL FITNESS PLAN

If you're ready to create a complete fitness program based on the activities you enjoy most, begin by preparing the program plan and contract in Lab 7.1. By carefully developing your plan and signing a contract, you'll increase your chances of success. The step-by-step procedure outlined here will guide you through the steps of Lab 7.1 to create an exercise program that's right for you. (See Figure 7.1 for a sample personal fitness program plan and contract.)

If you'd like additional help in setting up your program, choose one of the sample programs at the end of this chapter. Sample programs are provided for walking/jogging/running, cycling, swimming, and rowing. They include detailed instructions for starting a program and developing and maintaining fitness.

### 1. Set Goals

Ask yourself, "What do I want from my fitness program?" Develop different types of goals—general and specific, long term and short term. General or long-term goals might include lowering your risk for chronic disease, improving posture, having more energy, or improving the fit of your clothes.

It's also a good idea to develop some specific, short-term goals based on measurable factors. Specific goals might be:

- Raising cardiorespiratory capacity ($\dot{V}O_{2max}$) by 10%.
- Reducing the time it takes you to jog 2 miles from 22 minutes to 19 minutes.
- Increasing the number of push-ups you can do from 15 to 25.
- Lowering your BMI from 26 to 24.5.

Having specific goals will allow you to track your progress and enjoy the measurable changes brought about by your fitness program. Finally, break your specific goals into several smaller steps (mini-goals), such as those shown in Figure 7.1. (For detailed discussions of goals and goal setting in a behavior change or fitness program, refer back to Chapters 1 and 2.)

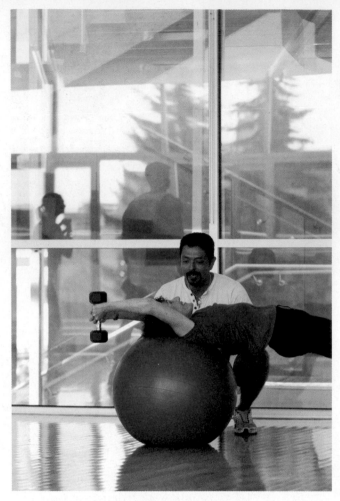

An overall fitness program includes activities to develop all the components of physical fitness.

Physical fitness assessment tests—as described in Chapters 3–6—are essential to determining your goals. They help you decide which types of exercise you should emphasize, and they help you understand the relative difficulty of attaining specific goals. If you have health problems, such as high blood pressure, heart disease, obesity, or serious joint or muscle disabilities, see your physician before taking assessment tests. Measure your progress by taking these tests about every 3 months.

### 2. Select Activities

If you have already chosen activities and created separate program plans for different fitness components in

**Fitness Tip**

Although some research indicates that pre-workout stretching can reduce muscle power and interfere with motor control, there are benefits to stretching after running. You can increase flexibility by doing stretching exercises as part of your cool-down.

A. I [Tracie Kaufman] am contracting with myself to follow a physical
(name)
fitness program to work toward the following goals:

### Specific or short-term goals

1. Improving cardiorespiratory fitness by raising my $\dot{V}O_{2max}$ from 34 to 37 ml/kg/min
2. Improving upper body muscular strength and endurance rating from fair to good
3. Improving body composition (from 28% to 25% body fat)
4. Improving my tennis game (hitting 20 playable shots in a row against the ball machine)

### General or long-term goals

1. Developing a more positive attitude about myself
2. Improving the fit of my clothes
3. Building and maintaining bone mass to reduce my risk of osteoporosis
4. Increasing my life expectancy and reducing my risk for diabetes and heart disease

B. **My program plan is as follows:**

| Activities | Components (Check X) | | | | | Time | Frequency (Check X) | | | | | | | Intensity* |
| | CRE | MS | ME | F | BC | | M | Tu | W | Th | F | S | S | |
| --- | --- | --- | --- | --- | --- | --- | --- | --- | --- | --- | --- | --- | --- | --- |
| Swimming | X | X | X | X | X | 35min | X | | X | | X | | | 140–170 bpm |
| Tennis | X | X | X | X | X | 90min | | | | | X | | | RPE = 13–16 |
| Weight training | | X | X | X | X | 30min | | X | | X | | X | | see Lab 4.3 |
| Stretching | | | | X | | 25min | X | | X | | X | X | | — |

*List your target heart rate range or an RPE value if appropriate.

C. My program will begin on [Sept.] [21] My program includes the following schedule of mini-goals. For each step in my program, I will give myself the reward listed.

| | | | |
| --- | --- | --- | --- |
| Completing 2 full weeks of program (mini-goal 1) | Oct. | 5 | movie with friends (reward) |
| $\dot{V}O_{2max}$ of 35 ml/kg/min (mini-goal 2) | Nov. | 2 | new CD (reward) |
| Completing 10 full weeks of program (mini-goal 3) | Nov. | 30 | new sweater (reward) |
| Percent body fat of 27% (mini-goal 4) | Dec. | 22 | weekend away (reward) |
| $\dot{V}O_{2max}$ of 36 ml/kg/min (mini-goal ) | Jan. | 18 | new CD (reward) |

D. My program will include the addition of physical activity to my daily routine (such as climbing stairs or walking to class):

1. Walking to and from campus job
2. Taking the stairs to dorm room instead of elevator
3. Bicycling to the library instead of driving
4. Doing one active chore a day
5.

E. I will use the following tools to monitor my program and my progress toward my goals:

I'll use a chart that lists the number of laps and minutes I swim and the charts for strength and flexibility from Labs 4.3 & 5.2.

I sign this contract as an indication of my personal commitment to reach my goal.

_Tracie Kaufman_                                        [Sep.] [10]
(your signature)

I have recruited a helper who will witness my contract and

swim with me three days per week

(list any way your helper will participate in your program)

_Russell Walker_                                        [Sep.] [10]
(witness's signature)

**FIGURE 7.1    A sample personal fitness program plan and contract.**

| Table 7.1 | Examples of Different Aerobic Activities and Their Intensities |
|---|---|

| MODERATE-INTENSITY ACTIVITIES | VIGOROUS-INTENSITY ACTIVITIES |
|---|---|
| • Walking briskly (3 miles per hour or faster, but not race-walking) | • Race-walking, jogging, or running |
| • Water aerobics | • Swimming laps |
| • Bicycling slower than 10 miles per hour | • Singles tennis |
| • Doubles tennis | • Aerobic dancing |
| • Ballroom dancing | • Bicycling 10 miles per hour or faster |
| • General gardening | • Jumping rope |
| | • Heavy gardening (continuous digging or hoeing) |
| | • Hiking uphill or with a heavy backpack |

**SOURCES:** Physical Activity Guidelines Advisory Committee. 2008. *Physical Activity Guidelines Advisory Committee Report,* 2008. Washington, D.C.: U.S. Department of Health and Human Services.

Chapters 3–5, you can put those plans together into a single program. It's usually best to include exercises to develop each of the health-related components of fitness, as follows:

- Cardiorespiratory endurance is developed by activities that involve continuous rhythmic movements of large-muscle groups, like those in the legs (see Chapter 3).
- Muscular strength and endurance are developed by training against resistance (see Chapter 4).
- Flexibility is developed by stretching the major muscle groups (see Chapter 5).
- Healthy body composition can be developed by combining a sensible diet and a program of regular exercise, including cardiorespiratory endurance exercise to burn calories and resistance training to build muscle mass (see Chapter 6).

Table 7.1 shows the intensity levels of several popular activities that promote health. Check the intensity levels of the activities you're considering to make sure the program you put together will help you achieve your goals.

If you select activities that support your commitment rather than activities that turn exercise into a chore, your program will provide plenty of incentive for continuing. Consider the following factors in making your choices:

- ***Fun and interest.*** Your fitness program is much more likely to be successful if you choose activities that you currently engage in and enjoy. Often you can modify your current activities to fit your fitness program. If you want to add a new activity to your program, it is a good idea to try it for a while before committing to it. (See the box "Can Stability Balls Be Part of a Safe and Effective Fitness Program?")

- ***Your current skill and fitness level.*** Although many activities are appropriate for beginners, some sports and activities require a certain level of skill to obtain fitness benefits. For example, if you are a beginning tennis player, you will probably not be able to sustain rallies long enough to develop cardiorespiratory endurance. A better choice might be a walking program while you improve your tennis game. To build skill for a particular activity, consider taking a class or getting some instruction from a coach or fellow participant.

- ***Time and convenience.*** You are more likely to maintain a long-term exercise program if you can easily fit exercise into your daily routine. As you consider activities, think about whether a special location or facility is required. Can you participate in the activity close to your home, school, or job? Are the necessary facilities available at convenient times (see Lab 7.2)? Can you participate in the activity year-round, or will you need to find an alternative during the summer or winter? Would a home treadmill make you more likely to exercise regularly?

- ***Cost.*** Some sports and activities require equipment, fees, or some type of membership investment. If you are on a tight budget, limit your choices to activities that are inexpensive or free. Investigate the facilities on your campus, which you may be able to use at little or no cost. Many activities require no equipment beyond an appropriate pair of shoes.

- ***Special health needs.*** If you have special exercise needs due to a particular health problem, choose activities that will conform to your needs and enhance your ability to cope. Ask your physician about how to tailor an exercise program to your needs and goals. Appendix B provides guidelines and safety tips for exercisers with common chronic conditions.

## 3. Set a Target Frequency, Intensity, and Time (Duration) for Each Activity

The next step is to apply the FITT principle and set a starting frequency, intensity, and time (duration) for each type

**? Ask Yourself**

**QUESTIONS FOR CRITICAL THINKING AND REFLECTION**

Consider the list of physical activities and sports in Table 7.1. Given your current fitness and skill level, which ones could you reasonably incorporate into your exercise program?

# Can Stability Balls Be Part of a Safe and Effective Fitness Program?

As you create a personalized exercise program, you might consider incorporating a stability ball into your workouts. Stability balls add variety and challenge to a workout and can help you target certain muscle groups more effectively than is possible with some other workout strategies. But what is the real purpose of stability balls, and what is the best way to use them?

When most people think of exercising with stability balls, they think of *core training*—exercises that target the muscles of the trunk. These core muscles, as described in Chapter 5, surround your internal organs and provide support for your spine. The core muscles enable you to stand straight, sit up, twist and bend, and perform countless types of movements, both large and small. If you play any type of competitive sport, from golf to figure skating, your core muscles are essential to your performance. In everyday living, a strong, stable core helps you maintain good posture and balance and provides some protection against injuries.

Core training can be done on a stable surface, such as a floor or bench, or on an unstable surface, such as a stability ball. A stability ball—which is actually an unstable platform—gets its name from the fact that it forces the user's body to stabilize itself to compensate for the ball's instability. Using a stability ball, therefore, is sometimes called *instability training*. Stability ball exercises activate muscle and nerve groups that might not otherwise get involved in the exercise. Depending on the specific exercises being done, instability training improves core strength and enhances the stability of supporting joints throughout the body.

There are many ways to incorporate a stability ball into a typical workout. For example, you can perform crunches or curl-ups while lying on a ball instead of on the floor. Lying face-down across a ball provides different leverage points for push-ups. A variety of resistance training exercises can be performed on a stability ball, but experts recommend using dumbbells rather than barbells when lifting weights on a ball.

Although stability balls are an excellent workout tool, they have drawbacks. For example, if you lift weights while resting on a ball instead of on a stable bench, much of your muscles' effort is devoted to keeping your body stable, reducing the muscles' ability to exert force. This effort can enhance your overall stability, but it can also slow your gains in strength. Research has shown that some exercises (such as curl-ups) can be more

stressful to certain joints and muscles when performed on a ball, at least in some people. Further, there is always a risk of falling off an unstable surface; this can cause serious injury, especially if you are holding weights in your hands.

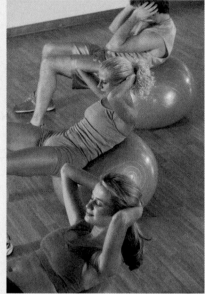

Finally, while instability training is a valuable aid in building up the core stabilizing muscles, it contributes little to the development of dynamic strength or power in the core. This strength and power are essential to total core fitness (especially in athletes) and must be developed through other types of exercise. For these reasons, many experts recommend instability training as part of an overall exercise program but do not suggest that all exercises be performed on a ball. For example, it's probably more effective to do curl-ups on the floor 2 days per week and on a ball 1 day per week, instead of using the ball every day. If you want to work with stability balls, it's a good idea to join a class where you can learn about this method from a qualified instructor and make sure instability training is appropriate for you.

SOURCES: Behm, D. G., et al. 2010. Canadian Society for Exercise Physiology position stand: The use of instability to train the core in athletic and non-athletic conditioning. *Applied Physiology Nutrition and Metabolism*. 35(1): 109–112; Marshall, P. W., et al. 2010. Electromyographic analysis of upper body, lower body, and abdominal muscles during advanced Swiss ball exercises. *Journal of Strength and Conditioning Research*. 24(6): 1537–1545; Okada, T., et al. 2011. Relationship between core stability, functional movement, and performance. *Journal of Strength and Conditioning Research*. 25(1): 252–261.

---

of activity you've chosen (see the summary in Figure 7.2 and the sample in Figure 7.1).

**Cardiorespiratory Endurance Exercise** As noted in earlier chapters, based on more than 50 years of research on exercise and health, the U.S. Department of Health and Human Services concluded that most health benefits occur with at least 150 minutes per week of moderate-intensity physical activity (such as brisk walking) or 75 minutes per week of vigorous-intensity activity (such as jogging). Additional benefits occur with more exercise. An appropriate frequency for cardiorespiratory endurance exercise is 3–5 days per week. For intensity, note your target heart rate

zone or RPE value. Your target total workout time (duration) should be about 20–60 minutes per day, depending on the intensity of the activity. You can exercise in a single session or in multiple sessions of 10 or more minutes.

**Muscular Strength and Endurance Training** A frequency of at least 2 nonconsecutive days per week for strength training is recommended. As described in Chapter 4, a general fitness strength training program includes 1 or more sets of 8–12 repetitions of 8–10 exercises that work all major muscle groups. For intensity, choose a weight that is heavy enough to fatigue your muscles but not so heavy that you cannot complete the full number of repetitions

|  | Cardiorespiratory endurance training | Strength training | Flexibility training |
|---|---|---|---|
| **F**requency | 3–5 days per week | 2–3 nonconsecutive days per week | 2–3 days per week (minimum); 5–7 days per week (ideal) |
| **I**ntensity | 55/65–90% of maximum heart rate | Sufficient resistance to fatigue muscles | Stretch to the point of tension |
| **T**ime | 20–60 minutes in sessions lasting 10 minutes or more | 8–12 repetitions of each exercise, 1 or more sets | 2–4 repetitions of each exercise, held for 1·5–30 seconds |
| **T**ype | Continuous rhythmic activities using large muscle groups | Resistance exercises for all major muscle groups | Stretching exercises for all major joints |

**FIGURE 7.2  A summary of the FITT principle for the health-related components of fitness.**

### Fitness Tip

Want to lift weights without going to a gym? Try using resistance bands. Research shows that—especially for young women—resistance bands are just as effective as weight machines or free weights for increasing muscular strength.

with proper form. Exercises that use body weight for resistance also build strength and muscle endurance.

**Flexibility Training**  Stretches should be performed when muscles are warm at least 2–3 days per week (5–7 days per week is ideal). Stretches should be performed for all major muscle groups. For each exercise, stretch to the point of slight tension or mild discomfort, and hold the stretch for 10–30 seconds; do 2–4 repetitions of each exercise.

## 4. Set Up a System of Mini-Goals and Rewards

To keep your program on track, set up a system of goals and rewards. Break your specific goals into several steps, and set a target date for each step. For example, if one of the goals of an 18-year-old male student's program is to improve upper-body strength and endurance, he could use the push-up test in Lab 4.2 to set intermediate goals. If he can currently perform 15 push-ups (for a rating of "very poor"), he might set intermediate goals of 17, 20, 25, and 30 push-ups (for a final rating of "fair"). By allowing several weeks between mini-goals and specifying rewards, he'll be able to track his progress and reward himself as he moves toward his final goal. Reaching a series of small goals is more satisfying than working toward a single, more challenging goal that may take months to achieve. For more on choosing appropriate rewards, see Chapter 1 and Activity 4 in the Behavior Change Workbook at the end of the text.

## 5. Include Lifestyle Physical Activity in Your Program

Daily physical activity is a simple but important way to improve your overall wellness. As part of your fitness program plan, specify ways to be more active during your daily routine. You may find it helpful to first use your health journal to track your activities for several days. Review the records in your journal, identify routine opportunities to be more active, and add these to your program plan in Lab 7.1.

## 6. Develop Tools for Monitoring Your Progress

A record that tracks your daily progress will help remind you of your ongoing commitment to your program and give you a sense of accomplishment. Figure 7.3 shows you how to create a general program log and record the activity type, frequency, and times (durations). Or, if you wish, complete specific activity logs like those in Labs 3.2, 4.3, and 5.2 in addition to, or instead of, a general log. Post your log in a place where you'll see it often as a reminder and as an incentive for improvement. If you have specific, measurable goals, you can also graph your weekly or monthly progress toward your goal (Figure 7.4). To monitor the overall progress of your fitness program, you may choose to reassess your fitness every 3 months or so during the improvement phase of your program. Because the results of different fitness tests vary, be sure to compare results for the same assessments over time.

## 7. Make a Commitment

Your final step in planning your program is to make a commitment by signing a contract. Find a witness for your contract—preferably someone who will be actively involved in your program. Keep your contract in a visible spot to remind you of your commitment.

Name  Tracie Kaufman

Enter time, distance, or another factor (such as heart rate or perceived exertion) to track your progress.

| Activity/Date | M | Tu | W | Th | F | S | S | Weekly Total | M | Tu | W | Th | F | S | S | Weekly Total |
|---|---|---|---|---|---|---|---|---|---|---|---|---|---|---|---|---|
| 1 Swimming | 800 yd | | 725 yd | | 800 yd | | | 2325 yd | 800 yd | | 800 yd | | 850 yd | | | 2450 yd |
| 2 Tennis | | | | | | 90 min | | 90 min | | | | | | 95 min | | 95 min |
| 3 Weight Training | | X | | X | | X | | | | X | | X | | X | | |
| 4 Stretching | X | | X | | X | X | | . | X | | X | X | X | X | | |

**FIGURE 7.3   A sample program log.**

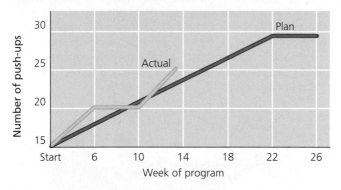

**FIGURE 7.4   A sample program progress chart.**

# PUTTING YOUR PLAN INTO ACTION

Once you've developed a detailed plan and signed your contract, you are ready to begin your fitness program. Refer to the specific training suggestions provided in Chapters 2–5 for advice on beginning and maintaining your program. Many people find it easier to plan a program than to put their plan into action and stick with it over time. For that reason, adherence to healthy lifestyle programs has become an important area of study for psychologists and health researchers. The guidelines below and in the next section reflect research into strategies that help people succeed in sticking with an exercise program.

• *Start slowly and increase fitness gradually.* Over-zealous exercising can result in discouraging discomforts and injuries. Your program is meant to last a lifetime. The important first step is to break your established pattern of inactivity. Be patient and realistic. Once your body has adjusted to your starting level of exercise, slowly increase the amount of overload. Small increases are the key—achieving a large number of small improvements will eventually result in substantial gains in fitness. It's usually best to increase duration and frequency before increasing intensity.

• *Find an exercise buddy.* The social side of exercise is an important factor for many regular exercisers. Working out with a friend will make exercise more enjoyable and increase your chances of sticking with your program.

Find an exercise partner who shares your goals and general fitness level. On days when a partner isn't available, a smartphone or MP3 player can be your workout buddy; see the box "Digital Motivation" for more information.

• *Ask for support from others.* You have a much greater chance of exercising consistently if you have the support of important people in your life, such as parents, spouse, partner, and friends. Talk with them about your program, and let them know the importance of exercise and wellness in your life. Exercise needs to be a critical component of your day (just like sleeping and eating). Good communication will help others become more supportive of and enthusiastic about the time you spend on your wellness program.

• *Vary your activities.* You can make your program more fun over the long term if you participate in a variety of activities that you enjoy. You can also add interest by varying the routes you take when walking, finding a new tennis partner, or switching to a new volleyball or basketball court. Varying your activities, a strategy known as *cross-training,* has other benefits. It can help you develop balanced, total-body fitness. For example, by alternating running with swimming, you build both upper- and lower-body strength. Cross-training can reduce the risk of injury and overtraining because the same muscles, bones, and joints are not continuously subjected to the stresses of the same activity. Cross-training can be done either by choosing different activities on different days or by alternating activities within a single workout.

• *Cycle the duration and intensity of your workouts.* Olympic athletes use a technique called periodization of training, meaning that they vary the duration and intensity of their workouts. Sometimes they exercise very intensely; other times they train lightly or rest. You can use the same technique to improve fitness more quickly and make your training program more varied and enjoyable. For example, if your program consists of walking, weight training, and stretching, pick one day a week for each activity to train a little harder or longer than you normally do. If you usually walk 2 miles at 16 minutes per mile, increase the pace to 15 minutes per mile once a week. If you lift weights twice a week, train more intensely during one of the workouts by using more resistance or performing multiple sets.

• *Adapt to changing environments and schedules.* Most people are creatures of habit and have trouble adjusting to

## Digital Motivation

If you ever have trouble getting inspired to work out, motivation may be as close as your smartphone.

Since the iPhone's advent, dozens of interactive motivational applications ("apps") have been developed for use on smart cell phones. Coaching and motivational recordings are available for use on MP3 players, as well. These apps and recordings can substitute for an exercise partner when your workout buddy isn't around and can inspire you to keep your program on track. Some smartphone apps can monitor your workouts, track your progress, and even provide on-the-spot coaching to help you keep going.

Here are just a few examples of low-cost or free smartphone apps that can help you keep exercising:

● **The "Fu" series.** Featuring titles like "CrunchFu," "Push-upFu," and others, each app in this series focuses on one type of exercise and motivates you to excel at it. Using the accelerometers built into your smartphone, these apps can count your reps and monitor your speed as you exercise. A built-in coach offers suggestions and can challenge you to improve your performance.

● **RunKeeper.** This app works with a variety of activities, including walking, running, cycling, skiing, and others. The app uses your phone's built-in GPS to tell you how far and fast you are moving and to calculate your average and overall pace. The coaching feature offers tips and advice in real time, and you can listen to your favorite music while RunKeeper functions in the background. When you're finished exercising, the program can automatically upload data about your session to the RunKeeper Web site, which offers more tools for tracking your fitness program.

● **BeatBurn Trainer.** If you like to exercise in time to music, this app can be a big help. BeatBurn features coaching and tracking capabilities like many other smartphone apps, but it also includes beat-tracking technology. The app analyzes the pace (in beats per minute) of your music, and automatically speeds or slows the music to keep it in time with your movement. Music quality is not affected by the speed shifting.

If you don't have a smartphone—or don't want to risk breaking your phone while exercising—look for motivational albums and podcasts to play on an inexpensive MP3 player. Hundreds of titles, many of them free, can be found online and already in MP3 format. Although they are not interactive, albums can provide music that inspires you to keep moving, motivational commentary, and coaching tips.

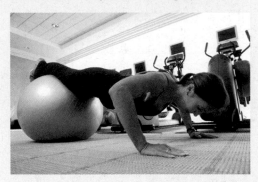

---

### Wellness Tip

Are you into intervals? Interval training can dramatically boost muscle performance and maximal oxygen consumption, but it doesn't do that much for certain measures of heart health. This is one reason it's important to vary your workouts; blend intervals with higher-volume workouts for optimal results.

### Ask Yourself

**QUESTIONS FOR CRITICAL THINKING AND REFLECTION**

How do you typically deal with setbacks? For example, if you have trouble getting motivated to study for exams, what strategies do you use to get back on track? Could those strategies work for keeping your fitness program moving forward? If so, how?

---

change. Don't use bad weather or a new job as an excuse to give up your exercise program. If you walk in the summer, put on a warm coat and walk in the winter. If you can't go out because of darkness, join a gym and walk on a treadmill.

● **Expect fluctuations and lapses.** On some days, your progress will be excellent, but on others, you'll barely be able to drag yourself through your scheduled activities. Don't let off-days or lapses discourage you or make you feel guilty (see the box "Getting Your Fitness Program Back on Track").

● **Choose other healthy lifestyle behaviors.** Exercise provides huge benefits for your health, but other behaviors are also important. Choose a nutritious diet, and avoid harmful habits like smoking and overconsumption of alcohol. Be sure to stay hydrated with water or other healthy beverages (see the box "Choosing Healthy Beverages"). Don't skimp on sleep, which has a mutually beneficial relationship with exercise. Physical activity improves sleep, and adequate sleep can improve physical performance.

## EXERCISE GUIDELINES FOR LIFE STAGES

A fitness program may need to be adjusted to accommodate the requirements of different life stages.

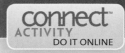

# Getting Your Fitness Program Back on Track

Lapses are a normal part of any behavior change program. The important point is to move on and avoid becoming discouraged. Try again and keep trying. Know that continued effort will lead to success. Here are some tips to help you keep going:

- Don't judge yourself too harshly. Some people make faster gains in fitness than others. Focus on the improvements you've already made from your program and how good you feel after exercise—both physically and mentally.

- Visualize what it will be like to reach your goals. Keep these images in mind as an incentive to stick with your program.

- Use your exercise journal to identify thoughts and behaviors that are causing noncompliance. Devise strategies to combat these problematic patterns. If needed, make additional changes in your environment or find more social support. For example, call a friend to walk with you, or keep exercise clothes in your car or backpack.

- Make changes in your plan and reward system to help renew your enthusiasm for and commitment to your program. Try changing fitness activities or your exercise schedule. Build in more opportunities to reward yourself.

- Plan ahead for difficult situations. Think about what circumstances might make it tough to keep up your fitness routine. Develop strategies to increase your chances of sticking with your program. For example, figure out ways to continue your program during vacation, travel, bad weather, and so on.

- If you're in a bad mood or just don't feel like exercising, remind yourself that physical activity is probably the one thing you can do that will make you feel better. Even if you can only do half your scheduled workout, you'll boost your energy, improve your mood, and help keep your program on track.

**TAKE CHARGE**

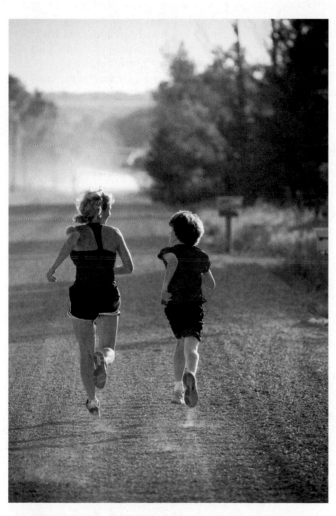

People of all ages benefit from exercise. Simply by playing actively with their children, parents can set a positive example that will lead to a lifetime of physical activity.

## Children and Adolescents

Lack of physical activity has led to alarming increases in overweight and obesity in children and adolescents. If you have children or are in a position to influence children, keep these guidelines in mind:

- Provide opportunities for children and adolescents to exercise every day. Minimize sedentary activities, such as watching television. Children and adolescents should aim for at least 60 minutes of moderate activity every day. Less fit kids should start with 30 minutes a day until their fitness improves and they can exercise longer.

- During family outings, choose dynamic activities. For example, go for a walk or park away from a mall, and then walk to the stores.

- For children younger than 12, emphasize skill development and fitness rather than excellence in competitive sports. For adolescents, combine participation and training in lifetime sports with traditional, competitive sports.

- Make sure children are developmentally capable of participating in an activity. For example, catching skills are difficult for young children because their nervous system is not developed enough to fully master the skill. Gradually increase the complexity of the skill once the child has mastered the simpler skill.

- Make sure children get plenty of water when exercising in the heat. Make sure they are dressed properly when exercising in the cold.

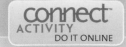

# Choosing Healthy Beverages

As discussed in other chapters, it's important to stay hydrated at all times, but especially when you are exercising. Too little water intake can leave you feeling fatigued, reduce your body's performance, and leave you vulnerable to heat-related sicknesses in hot weather. But *what* you drink is as significant as how much you drink, both when you are exercising and when you are going about your normal routine.

## The Great Water Controversy

Wherever you see people exercising, you will see bottled water in abundance. For several years, a debate has been raging about the quality and safety of commercially bottled water. Recently, new evidence has emerged showing that most bottled waters are no better for you than regular tap water, and some bottled waters may actually be bad for you. To make matters worse, bottled water costs up to 1900 times more than tap water.

In a 2011 analysis of 173 bottled water products, the Environmental Working Group, found 38 different contaminants in ten popular brands of bottled water. Contaminants included heavy metals such as arsenic, pharmaceutical residues and other pollutants commonly found in urban wastewater, and a variety of industrial chemicals. Bottled water companies are notoriously secretive about their products. Overall, 18% of bottled waters failed to list the location of their source, and 32% disclosed nothing about the treatment or purity of the water.

Many commercially bottled water products are tap water drawn from municipal water systems. Such revelations have caused some bottlers to put statements on their products' labels, identifying them as having been drawn from a standard water supply. Although these products are priced many times higher than water from a residential tap, they provide no benefit over standard tap water.

An even bigger issue is that plastic water bottles have become a huge environmental problem, with billions of bottles now filling landfills and floating in the world's oceans. Many kinds of plastic bottles will never decompose at all; at best, some types of plastic take years to biodegrade. Newer types of plastic bottles can decompose significantly faster than older bottles, but fast-degrading plastics have not yet come into widespread use in the bottled water industry.

Experts say that when you're exercising, the cheapest and safest way to stay hydrated is to drink filtered tap water. If you need to carry water with you, buy a reusable container (preferably made of stainless steel) that can be cleaned after each use. If you drink from plastic bottles, be sure they are recyclable, and dispose of them by recycling.

## Other Choices

Instead of water, many people choose to drink sodas, juice, tea, or flavored water. While these kinds of beverages have their place, it's important not to drink them too often or in large amounts, especially if they are high in sugar or caffeine. Sugary drinks add empty calories to your diet, and caffeine is a psychoactive drug with a variety of side effects.

Regular (nondiet) sodas are now the leading source of calories in the American diet; most people don't count the calories from beverages as part of their daily caloric intake, leading them to underestimate their total intake. For this reason and others, many experts believe that soda consumption is a major factor in the increasing levels of obesity, metabolic syndrome, diabetes, and other chronic diseases among Americans.

If you're concerned that the liquid portion of your diet is not as healthy as it should be, choose water, fat-free milk, or unsweetened herbal tea more often. Avoid regular soda, sweetened bottled iced tea, flavored water, and fruit beverages made with little fruit juice. To make water more appealing, try adding slices of citrus fruit with sparkling water. With some imagination, you can make sure you stay hydrated without consuming excess calories, spending money unnecessarily, or hurting the environment.

**SOURCE:** Leiba, N., et. al. 2011. The Environmental Working Group's 2011 Bottled Water Scorecard (http://www.ewg.org/bottled-water -2011-home; retrieved April 5, 2011).

# Pregnant Women

Exercise is important during pregnancy, but women should be cautious because some types of exercise can pose increased risk to the mother and the unborn child. The following guidelines are consistent with the recommendations of the American College of Obstetrics and Gynecology:

- See your physician about possible modifications needed for your particular pregnancy.

- Continue mild to moderate exercise routines at least three times a week. (For most women, this means maintaining an exercise heart rate of 100–160 beats per minute.) Avoid exercising vigorously or to exhaustion, especially in the third trimester. Monitor exercise intensity by assessing how you feel rather than by monitoring your heart rate; RPE levels of 11–13 are appropriate.

- Favor non- or low-weight-bearing exercises such as swimming or cycling over weight-bearing exercises, which can carry increased risk of injury.

- Avoid exercise in a supine position—lying on your back—after the first trimester. This position restricts blood flow to the uterus. Also avoid prolonged periods of motionless standing.

- Avoid exercise that could cause loss of balance, especially in the third trimester, and exercise that might injure the abdomen, stress the joints, or carry a risk of falling (such as contact sports, vigorous racquet sports, skiing, and in-line skating).

- Avoid activities involving extremes in barometric pressure, such as diving and mountain climbing.

- Especially during the first trimester, drink plenty of fluids and exercise in well-ventilated areas to avoid heat stress.

## Q Should I exercise every day?

**A** Some daily exercise is beneficial, but if you train intensely every day without giving yourself a rest, you will likely get injured or become over-trained. When strength training, for example, rest at least 48 hours between workouts before exercising the same muscle group. For cardiorespiratory endurance exercise, rest or exercise lightly the day after an intense or lengthy work-out. Balancing the proper amount of rest and exercise will help you feel better and improve your fitness faster.

## Q If exercise is so good for my health, why hasn't my physician ever mentioned it to me?

**A** A recent study by the ACSM suggests that most people would benefit from getting a physician's advice about exercising. According to the study, 65% of patients said they would be more interested in exercising if their physicians suggested it. About 40% of physicians said they talk to their patients about exercise.

To encourage physicians and patients to talk more often about exercise and its benefits, the ACSM and the American Medical Association have launched the Exercise Is Medicine program. The program advises physicians to give more guidance to patients about exercise and suggests that everyone try to exercise at least 5 days each week. For more information on the program, visit www.exerciseismedicine.org.

*For more Common Questions Answered about developing and maintaining a fitness program, visit the Online Learning Center at www.mhhe.com/fahey.*

---

- Do 3–5 sets of 10 Kegel exercises daily. These exercises involve tightening the muscles of the pelvic floor for 5–15 seconds per repetition. Kegel exercises are thought to help prevent incontinence (involuntary loss of urine) and speed recovery after giving birth.
- After giving birth, resume prepregnancy exercise routines gradually, based on how you feel.

## Older Adults

Older people readily adapt to endurance exercise and strength training. Exercise principles are the same as for younger people, but some specific guidelines apply:

- According to the American College of Sports Medicine (ACSM), older adults should follow the same guidelines for aerobic exercise as younger adults, but they should judge intensity on a 10-point scale of perceived exertion rather than by heart rate.
- For strength training, older adults should use a lighter weight and perform more (10–15) repetitions than young adults.
- Older adults should perform flexibility exercises at least 2 days per week for at least 10 minutes. Exercises that improve balance should also be performed 2 days per week.
- Drink plenty of water and avoid exercising in excessively hot or cold environments. Wear clothes that speed heat loss in warm environments and prevent heat loss in cold environments.

- Warm up slowly and carefully. Increase intensity and duration of exercise gradually.
- Cool down slowly, continuing very light exercise until the heart rate is below 100.
- Older adults with physical disabilities or limitations who cannot meet the recommendation of at least 150 minutes of moderate-intensity exercise should do as much exercise as they can.

### TIPS FOR TODAY AND THE FUTURE

A complete fitness program includes activities to build and maintain cardiorespiratory endurance, muscular strength and endurance, and flexibility.

#### RIGHT NOW YOU CAN

- Get a journal to track your daily physical activity and exercise routine.
- Put away your remote control devices—every bit of physical activity can benefit your health.
- Set up your next workout with your training partner.
- Plan to go to bed 15 minutes earlier than usual.

#### IN THE FUTURE YOU CAN

- Create a schedule that incorporates your workouts into your daily routine. Each week, update the schedule for the upcoming week.
- Develop strategies for dealing with setbacks in your exercise program. Having strategies in place ahead of time can prepare you to cope with lapses as they occur.

- Steps for putting together a complete fitness program include (1) setting realistic goals; (2) selecting activities to develop all the health-related components of fitness; (3) setting a target frequency, intensity, and time (duration) for each activity; (4) setting up a system of mini-goals and rewards; (5) making lifestyle physical activity a part of the daily routine; (6) developing tools for monitoring progress; and (7) making a commitment.

- In selecting activities, consider fun and interest, your current skill and fitness levels, time and convenience, cost, and any special health concerns.

- Keys to beginning and maintaining a successful program include starting slowly, increasing intensity and duration gradually, finding a buddy, varying the activities and intensity of the program, and expecting fluctuations and lapses.

- Regular exercise is appropriate and beneficial for people in particular stages of life, although program modifications may be necessary for safety.

## FOR FURTHER EXPLORATION

### BOOKS, ORGANIZATIONS, AND WEB SITES

*American Academy of Orthopaedic Surgeons.* Provides information about injuries, treatment, and rehabilitation along with exercise guidelines for people with bone, muscle, and joint pain.
  http://www.aaos.org

*American College of Obstetricians and Gynecologists.* Provides guidelines for promoting a healthy pregnancy and postpartum recovery, including exercise during pregnancy.
  http://www.acog.org

*American Diabetes Association.* Promotes diabetes education, research, and advocacy; includes guidelines for diet and exercise for people with diabetes.
  http://www.diabetes.org

*American Heart Association.* Includes information on fitness for kids as well as diet, exercise, fitness, and weight management for adults.
  http://www.americanheart.org

For additional listings, see Chapters 2–6.

## SELECTED BIBLIOGRAPHY

Almstedt, H. C., et al. 2011. Changes in bone mineral density in response to 24 weeks of resistance training in college-age men and women. *Journal of Strength and Conditioning Research* 25(4): 1098–1103.

American College of Sports Medicine. 2009. *ACSM's Guidelines for Exercise Testing and Prescription*, 8th ed. Philadelphia: Lippincott Williams and Wilkins.

American College of Sports Medicine. 2009. *ACSM's Resource Manual for Guidelines for Exercise Testing and Prescription*, 6th ed. Philadelphia: Lippincott Williams and Wilkins.

Behm, D. G., et al. 2010. Canadian Society for Exercise Physiology position stand: The use of instability to train the core in athletic and nonathletic conditioning. *Applied Physiology, Nutrition and Metabolism* 35(1): 109–112.

Behm, D. G., et al. 2010. The use of instability to train the core musculature. *Applied Physiology, Nutrition and Metabolism* 35(1): 91–108.

Boarnet, M. G., et al. 2011. Retrofitting the suburbs to increase walking: Evidence from a land-use-travel study. *Urban Studies* 48(1): 129–159.

Boone-Heinonen, J., et al. 2011. Neighborhood socioeconomic status predictors of physical activity through young to middle adulthood: The CARDIA study. *Social Science and Medicine* 72(5): 641–649.

Canadian Society for Exercise Physiology. 2011. *Public Health Agency of Canada Physical Activity Guidelines* (www.publichealth.gc.ca; retrieved April 6, 2011).

Clark, P. G., et al. 2011. Maintaining exercise and healthful eating in older adults: The SENIOR project II: Study design and methodology. *Contemporary Clinical Trials* 32(1): 129–139.

Finkelstein, E. A., et al. 2008. A randomized study of financial incentives to increase physical activity among sedentary older adults. *Preventive Medicine* 47(2): 182–187.

Hamer, M., and Y. Chida. 2008. Walking and primary prevention: A meta-analysis of prospective cohort studies. *British Journal of Sports Medicine* 42(4): 238–243.

Hurley, B. F., et al. 2011. Strength training as a countermeasure to aging muscle and chronic disease. *Sports Medicine* 41(4): 289–306.

Ingham, S. A., et al. 2008. Physiological and performance effects of low- versus mixed-intensity rowing training. *Medicine and Science in Sports and Exercise* 40(3): 579–584.

Kilpatrick, M. W., et al. 2009. Heart rate and metabolic responses to moderate-intensity aerobic exercise: A comparison of graded walking and ungraded jogging at a constant perceived exertion. *Journal of Sports Sciences* 27(5): 509–516.

Kokkinos, P. 2008. Physical activity and cardiovascular disease prevention: Current recommendations. *Angiology* 59(2 Supplement): 26S–29S.

Levine, J. A., et al. 2008. The role of free-living daily walking in human weight gain and obesity. *Diabetes* 57(3): 548–554.

Marshall, P. W., et al. 2010. Electromyographic analysis of upper body, lower body, and abdominal muscles during advanced Swiss ball exercises. *Journal of Strength and Conditioning Research* 24(6): 1537–1545.

McGinn, A. P., et al. 2008. Walking speed and risk of incident ischemic stroke among postmenopausal women. *Stroke* 39(4): 1233–1239.

Mozumdar, A., et al. 2011. Persistent increase of prevalence of metabolic syndrome among U.S. adults: NHANES III to NHANES 1999–2006. *Diabetes Care* 34(1): 216–219.

Okada, T., et al. 2011. Relationship between core stability, functional movement, and performance. *Journal of Strength and Conditioning Research* 25(1): 252–261.

Pascual, C., et al. 2009. Socioeconomic environment, availability of sports facilities, and jogging, swimming and gym use. *Health and Place* 15(2): 553–561.

Plisiene, J., et al. 2008. Moderate physical exercise: A simplified approach for ventricular rate control in older patients with atrial fibrillation. *Clinical Research in Cardiology* 97(11): 820–826.

Reis, J. P., et al. 2008. Prevalence of total daily walking among US adults, 2002–2003. *Journal of Physical Activity and Health* 5(3): 337–346.

Richardson, C. R., et al. 2008. A meta-analysis of pedometer-based walking interventions and weight loss. *Annals of Family Medicine* 6(1): 69–77.

Suminski, R. R., et al. 2008. Observing physical activity in suburbs. *Health and Place* 14(4): 894–899.

Troped, P. J., et al. 2008. Prediction of activity mode with global positioning system and accelerometer data. *Medicine and Science in Sports and Exercise* 40(5): 972–978.

U.S. Department of Health and Human Services. 2008. *Physical Activity Guidelines for Americans*. Washington, D.C.: U.S. Department of Health and Human Services.

Westhoff, T. H., et al. 2008. The cardiovascular effects of upper-limb aerobic exercise in hypertensive patients. *Journal of Hypertension* 26(7): 1336–1342.

Xu, D. Q., et al. 2008. Tai Chi exercise and muscle strength and endurance in older people. *Medicine and Sports Science* 52: 20–29.

Yabroff, K. R., et al. 2008. Walking the dog: Is pet ownership associated with physical activity in California? *Journal of Physical Activity and Health* 5(2): 216–228.

# SAMPLE PROGRAMS FOR POPULAR ACTIVITIES

The following sections present four sample programs based on different types of cardiorespiratory activities—walking/jogging/running, bicycling, swimming, and rowing. Each sample program includes regular cardiorespiratory endurance exercise, resistance training, and stretching. Read the descriptions of the programs you're considering, and decide which will work best for you based on your present routine, the potential for enjoyment, and adaptability to your lifestyle. If you choose one of these programs, complete the personal fitness program plan in Lab 7.1, just as if you had created a program from scratch.

No program will produce enormous changes in your fitness level in the first few weeks. Follow the specifics of the program for 3–4 weeks. Then, if the exercise program doesn't seem suitable, make adjustments to adapt it to your particular needs. But retain the basic elements of the program that make it effective for developing fitness.

## GENERAL GUIDELINES

The following guidelines can help make the activity programs more effective for you:

- **Frequency and time.** To improve physical fitness, exercise for 20–60 minutes at least three times a week.

- **Intensity.** To work effectively for cardiorespiratory endurance training or to improve body composition, raise your heart rate into its target zone. Monitor your pulse or use rates of perceived exertion to monitor your intensity. If you've been sedentary, begin very slowly. Give your muscles

a chance to adjust to their increased workload. It's probably best to keep your heart rate below target until your body has had time to adjust to new demands. At first you may not need to work very hard to keep your heart rate in its target zone, but as your cardiorespiratory endurance improves, you will probably need to increase intensity.

- **Interval training.** Some of the sample programs involve continuous activity. Others rely on interval training, which calls for alternating a relief interval with exercise (walking after jogging, for example, or coasting after biking uphill). Interval training is an effective method of progressive overload and improves fitness rapidly (see the box "Interval Training: Pros and Cons" in Chapter 3).

- **Resistance training and stretching guidelines.** For the resistance training and stretching parts of the program, remember the general guidelines for safe and effective exercise. See the summary of guidelines in Figure 7.2.

- **Warm-up and cool-down.** Begin each exercise session with a 10-minute warm-up. Begin your activity at a slow pace, and work up gradually to your target heart rate. Always slow down gradually at the end of your exercise session to bring your system back to its normal state. It's a good idea to do stretching exercises to increase your flexibility after cardiorespiratory exercise or strength training because your muscles will be warm and ready to stretch.

Follow the guidelines presented in Chapter 3 for exercising in hot or cold weather. Drink enough liquids to stay adequately hydrated, particularly in hot weather.

- **Record keeping.** After each exercise session, record your daily distance or time on a progress chart.

## WALKING/JOGGING/RUNNING SAMPLE PROGRAM

Walking is the perfect exercise. It increases longevity, builds fitness, expends calories, prevents weight gain, and protects against heart disease, stroke, and back pain. You don't need to join a gym, and you can walk almost anywhere. People who walk 30 minutes five times per week will lose an average of 5 pounds in 6–12 months—without dieting, watching what they eat, or exercising intensely.

Jogging takes walking to the next level. Jogging only 75 minutes per week will increase fitness, promote weight control, and provide health benefits that will prevent disease and increase longevity. Your ultimate goal for promoting wellness is to walk at a moderate intensity for 150–300 minutes per week or jog at 70% effort or more for 75–150 minutes per week.

It isn't always easy to distinguish among walking, jogging, and running. For clarity and consistency, we'll consider walking to be any on-foot exercise of less than 5 miles per hour, jogging any pace between 5 and 7.5 miles per hour, and running any pace faster than that. The faster

your pace or the longer you exercise, the more calories you burn (Table 1). The greater the number of calories burned, the higher the potential training effects of these activities. Table 2 contains a sample walking/jogging program.

### Equipment and Technique

These activities require no special skills, expensive equipment, or unusual facilities. Comfortable clothing, well-fitted walking or running shoes (see Chapter 3), and a stopwatch or ordinary watch with a second hand are all you need.

When you advance to jogging, use proper technique:

- Run with your back straight and your head up. Look straight ahead, not at your feet. Shift your pelvis forward and tuck your buttocks in.

- Hold your arms slightly away from your body. Your elbows should be bent so that your forearms are parallel to the ground. You may cup your hands, but do not clench

| Table 1 | Estimated Calories Expended by a 165-pound Adult at Different Intensities of Walking and Running for 150 and 300 minutes per week (min/wk) |
|---|---|

| | SPEED (MILES PER HOUR) | SPEED (MINUTES PER MILE) | CALORIES EXPENDED EXERCISING 150 MIN/WK | CALORIES EXPENDED EXERCISING 300 MIN/WK |
|---|---|---|---|---|
| | Rest | — | 190 | 380 |
| Walking | 2.5 | 24 | 565 | 1130 |
| | 3.0 | 20 | 620 | 1240 |
| | 4.0 | 15 | 940 | 1880 |
| | 4.3 | 14 | 1125 | 2250 |
| Jogging/Running | 5.0 | 12 | 1500 | 3000 |
| | 6.0 | 10 | 1875 | 3750 |
| | 7.0 | 8.6 | 2155 | 4310 |
| | 8.0 | 6.7 | 2530 | 5060 |
| | 10.0 | 6 | 3000 | 6000 |

**NOTE:** Heavier people will expend slightly more calories, while lighter people will expend slightly fewer.

**SOURCE:** Adapted from Physical Activity Guidelines Advisory Committee. 2008. *Physical Activity Guidelines Advisory Committee Report, 2008.* Washington, D. C.: U.S. Department of Health and Human Services.

| Table 2 | Sample Walking/Jogging Fitness Program |
|---|---|

| DAY | ACTIVITIES |
|---|---|
| Monday | • **Walking/Jogging:** Walk briskly for 30 minutes or jog for 25 minutes.<br>• **Stretching:** Stretch major muscle groups for 10 minutes after exercise. Do each exercise 2 times; hold stretch for 10–30 seconds. |
| Tuesday | • **Resistance workout:** Using body weight for resistance, perform the following exercises:<br>  • Push-ups: 2 sets, 20 reps per set<br>  • Pull-ups: 2 sets, 5 reps per set<br>  • Unloaded squats: 2 sets, 10 reps per set<br>  • Curl-ups: 2 sets, 20 reps per set<br>  • Side bridges: 3 sets, 10-second hold (left and right sides)<br>  • Spine extensions: 3 sets, 10-second hold (left and right sides) |
| Wednesday | • Repeat Monday activities. |
| Thursday | • Repeat Tuesday activities. |
| Friday | • Repeat Monday activities. |
| Saturday | • Rest. |
| Sunday | • Rest. |

your fists. Allow your arms to swing loosely and rhythmically with each stride.

• Let your heel hit the ground first in each stride. Then roll forward onto the ball of your foot and push off for the next stride. If you find this difficult, you can try a more flat-footed style, but don't land on the balls of your feet.

• Keep your steps short by allowing your foot to strike the ground in line with your knee. Keep your knees bent at all times.

• Breathe deeply through your mouth. Try to use your abdominal muscles rather than just your chest muscles to take deep breaths.

• Stay relaxed.

Find a safe, convenient place to walk or jog. Exercise on a trail, path, or sidewalk to stay clear of bicycles and cars. Make sure your clothes are brightly colored so others can see you easily.

## Beginning A Walking/Jogging Program

Start slowly if you have not been exercising, are overweight, or are recovering from an illness or surgery. At first, walk for 15 minutes at a slow pace, below your target heart rate zone. Gradually increase to 30-minute sessions. You will probably cover 1 to 2 miles. At the beginning, walk every other day.

You can gradually increase to walking 5 days per week or more if you want to expend more calories (which is helpful if you want to change body composition). Depending on your weight, you will expend ("burn") 90–135 calories during each 30-minute walking session. To increase the calories that you expend, walk for a longer time or for a longer distance instead of sharply increasing speed.

Start at the level of effort that is most comfortable for you. Maintain a normal, easy pace and stop to rest as often as you need to. Never prolong a walk past the point of comfort. When walking with a friend (a good motivator), let a comfortable conversation be your guide to pace. If you find that you cannot carry on a conversation without getting out of breath, you are walking too quickly.

Once your muscles have become adjusted to the exercise program, increase the duration of your sessions by no more than 10% each week. Keep your heart rate just below your target zone. Don't be discouraged by a lack of immediate progress, and don't try to speed things up by overdoing it. Remember that pace and heart rate can vary with the terrain, the weather, and other factors.

## Advanced Walking

Advanced walking involves walking more quickly for longer times. You should feel an increased perception of effort, but the exercise intensity should not be too stressful. Vary your pace to allow for intervals of slow, medium, and fast walking. Keep your heart rate toward the lower end of your target zone with brief periods in the upper levels. At first, walk for 30 minutes and increase your walking time gradually until eventually you reach 60 minutes at a brisk pace and can walk 2–4 miles. Try to walk at least 5 days per week. Vary your program by changing the pace and distance or by walking routes with different terrains and views. You can expect to burn 200–350 calories or more during each advanced walking session.

## Making the Transition to Jogging

Increase the intensity of exercise by gradually introducing jogging into your walking program. During a 2-mile walk, for example, periodically jog for 100 yards and then resume walking. Increase the number and distance of your jogging segments until you can jog continuously for the entire distance. More physically fit people may be capable of jogging without walking first. However, people unaccustomed to jogging should initially combine walking with short bouts of jogging.

A good strategy is to exercise on a 400-meter track at a local high school or college. Begin by jogging the straightaways and walking the turns for 800 meters (two laps). Progress to walking 200 meters (half lap) and jogging 200 meters; jogging 400 meters and walking 200 meters; jogging 800 meters, walking 800 meters; and jogging 1200

meters, walking 400 meters. Continue until you can run 2 miles without stopping.

During the transition to jogging, adjust the ratio of walking to jogging to keep within your target heart rate zone as much as possible. Most people who sustain a continuous jog/run program will find that they can stay within their target heart rate zone with a speed of 5.5–7.5 miles per hour (8–11 minutes per mile). Exercise at least every other day. Increasing frequency by doing other activities on alternate days will place less stress on the weight-bearing parts of your lower body than will a daily program of jogging/running.

## Developing Muscular Strength and Endurance and Flexibility

Walking, jogging, and running provide muscular endurance workouts for your lower body; they also develop muscular strength of the lower body to a lesser degree. If you'd like to increase your running speed and performance, you might want to focus your program on lower-body exercises. (Don't neglect upper-body strength. It is important for overall wellness.) For flexibility, pay special attention to the hamstrings and quadriceps, which are not worked through their complete range of motion during walking or jogging.

## Staying with Your Walking/Jogging Program

Health experts have found that simple motivators such as using a pedometer, walking a dog, parking farther from the office or grocery store, or training for a fun run help people stay with their programs. Use a pedometer or GPS exercise device to track your progress and help motivate you to increase distance and speed. Accurate pedometers for walking, such as those made by Omron, Yamax, and New Lifestyles, cost $20–40 and are accurate to about 5%. Sophisticated GPS-based devices made by Polar and Garmin keep track of your exercise speed and distance via satellite, monitor heart rate, and store data that can be downloaded wirelessly to your computer. Several of these units can be plugged into programs such as Google Earth, which give you a satellite view of your walking or jogging route.

A pedometer can also help you increase the number of steps you walk each day. Most sedentary people take only 2000 to 3000 steps per day. Adding 1000 steps per day and increasing gradually until you reach 10,000 steps can increase fitness and help you manage your weight. The nonprofit organization Shape Up America! has developed the 10,000 Steps program to promote walking as a fitness activity (www.shapeup.org).

## BICYCLING SAMPLE PROGRAM

Bicycling can also lead to large gains in physical fitness. For many people, cycling is a pleasant and economical alternative to driving and a convenient way to build fitness.

### Equipment and Technique

Cycling has its own special array of equipment, including helmets, lights, safety gear, and biking shoes. The bike is the most expensive item, ranging from about $100 to $1000 or more. Avoid making a large investment until you're sure you'll use your bike regularly. While investigating what the marketplace has to offer, rent or borrow a bike. Consider your intended use of the bike. Most cyclists who are interested primarily in fitness are best served by a sturdy 10-speed rather than a mountain bike or sport bike. Stationary cycles are good for rainy days and areas that have harsh winters.

Clothing for bike riding shouldn't be restrictive or binding; nor should it be so loose that it catches the wind and slows you down. Shirts made from materials that wick moisture away from your skin and padded biking shorts make for a more comfortable ride. Wear glasses or goggles to protect your eyes from dirt, small objects, and irritation from wind. Wear a pair of well-padded gloves if your hands tend to become numb while riding or if you begin to develop blisters or calluses.

To avoid saddle soreness and injury, choose a soft or padded saddle, and adjust it to a height that allows your legs to almost reach full extension while pedaling. To prevent backache and neck strain, warm up thoroughly and periodically shift the position of your hands on the handlebars and your body in the saddle. Keep your arms relaxed and don't lock your elbows. To protect your knees from strain, pedal with your feet pointed straight ahead or very slightly inward, and don't pedal in high gear for long periods.

Bike riding requires a number of precise skills that practice makes automatic. If you've never ridden before, consider taking a course. In fact, many courses are not just for beginners. They'll help you develop skills in braking, shifting, and handling emergencies, as well as teach you ways of caring for and repairing your bike. For safe cycling, follow these rules:

- Always wear a helmet.
- Keep on the correct side of the road. Bicycling against traffic is usually illegal and always dangerous.
- Obey all the same traffic signs and signals that apply to autos.
- On public roads, ride in single file, except in low-traffic areas (if the law permits). Ride in a straight line; don't swerve or weave in traffic.
- Be alert; anticipate the movements of other traffic and pedestrians. Listen for approaching traffic that is out of your line of vision.
- Slow down at street crossings. Check both ways before crossing.
- Use hand signals—the same as for automobile drivers—if you intend to stop or turn. Use audible signals to warn those in your path.
- Maintain full control. Avoid anything that interferes with your vision. Don't jeopardize your ability to steer by carrying anything (including people) on the handlebars.
- Keep your bicycle in good shape. Brakes, gears, saddle, wheels, and tires should always be in good condition.
- See and be seen. Use a headlight at night and equip your bike with rear reflectors. Use side reflectors on pedals, front and rear. Wear light-colored clothing or use reflective tape at night; wear bright colors or use fluorescent tape by day.
- Be courteous to other road users. Anticipate the worst and practice preventive cycling.
- Use a rear-view mirror.

### Developing Cardiorespiratory Endurance

Cycling is an excellent way to develop and maintain cardiorespiratory endurance and a healthy body composition.

**FIT—frequency, intensity, and time:** If you've been inactive for a long time, begin your cycling program at a heart rate that is 10–20% below your target zone. Beginning cyclists should pedal at about 80–100 revolutions per minute; adjust the gear so you can pedal at that rate easily. You can equip your bicycle with a cycling computer that displays different types of useful information, such as speed, distance traveled, heart rate, altitude, and revolutions per minute.

Once you feel at home on your bike, try cycling 1 mile at a comfortable speed, and then stop and check your heart rate. Increase your speed gradually until you can cycle at 12–15 miles per hour (4–5 minutes per mile), a speed fast enough to bring most new cyclists' heart rate into their target zone. Allow your pulse rate to be your guide: More highly fit individuals may need to ride faster to achieve their target heart rate. Cycling for at least 20 minutes 3 days per week will improve your fitness.

**At the beginning:** It may require several outings to get the muscles and joints of your legs and hips adjusted to this new activity. Begin each outing with a 10-minute warm-up. When your muscles are warm, stretch your hamstrings and your back and neck muscles. Until you become a skilled cyclist, select routes with the fewest hazards and avoid heavy automobile traffic.

**As you progress:** Interval training is also effective with bicycling. Simply increase your speed for periods of 4–8 minutes or for specific distances, such as 1–2 miles. Then coast for 2–3 minutes. Alternate the speed intervals and slow intervals for a total of 20–60 minutes, depending on your level of fitness. Biking over hilly terrain is also a form of interval training.

### Developing Muscular Strength and Endurance and Flexibility

Bicycling develops a high level of endurance and a moderate level of strength in the muscles of the lower body. If one of your goals is to increase your cycling speed and performance, be sure to include exercises for the quadriceps, hamstrings, and buttocks muscles in your strength training program. For flexibility, pay special attention to the hamstrings and quadriceps, which are not worked through their complete range of motion during bike riding, and to the muscles in your lower back, shoulders, and neck.

## SWIMMING SAMPLE PROGRAM

Swimming works every major muscle group in the body. It increases upper- and lower-body strength, promotes cardiovascular fitness, and is excellent for rehabilitating athletic injuries and preventing day-to-day aches and pains. It promotes weight control; builds powerful lungs, heart, and blood vessels; and promotes metabolic health. People weigh only 6–10 pounds in the water, so swimming places less stress on the knees, hips, and back than jogging, hiking, volleyball, or basketball.

Swimming is one of the most popular recreational and competitive sports in the world. Over 120 million Americans swim regularly. More than 165,000 of these are competitive age-group swimmers (ages 5–18), and over 30,000 competitors are over 19 years of age. You don't need a backyard pool to swim. Almost every town and city in America has a public pool. Pools are standard in many health clubs, YMCAs, and schools. Ocean and lake swimming may be options in the summer. High-tech wet suits make it possible to swim outdoors even in the middle of winter in many parts of the country.

### Training Methods

Improved fitness from swimming depends on the quantity, quality, and frequency of training. Most swimmers use interval training to increase swimming fitness, speed, and endurance. Interval training involves repeated fast swims at fixed distances followed by rest. Distance or endurance training builds stamina, mental toughness, and endurance. Interval and distance training each play important and different roles in improving fitness for swimming. Interval training improves overall swimming speed and the ability to swim fast at the beginning of a swim. Endurance training helps to maintain a faster average pace during a swim without becoming overly fatigued. Endurance training becomes more important when you want to compete in long, open-water swims or triathlons.

In swimming workouts, however, quality is better than quantity. Thirty years ago, elite swimmers from East Germany sometimes swam as much as 20,000 meters in a single workout (more than 12 miles). Recent studies found that competitive athletes who swam 4000 to 6000 meters per workout produced results similar to those who swam much farther. Likewise, recreational swimmers can improve fitness, strength, and power by swimming around 1000–2000 meters (approximately 1100–2200 yards) per workout. Swim fast to get maximum benefits, but maintain good technique to maximize efficiency and minimize the risk of injury.

**Interval training:** Interval training involves repeated fast swims at fixed distances, followed by rest. Interval training increases sprinting speed so that swimmers can accelerate faster at the beginning of a swim. It also helps the body cope with metabolic waste products so that you can maintain your speed during the workout. To increase speed, swim intervals between 25 and 200 meters (or yards) at 80–90% effort. An example of a beginning program might be to swim four sets of 50 meters using the sidestroke at 70% of maximum effort, with a 1-minute rest between sets. A more advanced program would be to swim ten sets of 100 meters using the freestyle stroke at 85–95% maximum effort with 30 seconds of rest between sets.

**Endurance training:** Include longer swims—1000 meters or more at a time—to build general stamina for swimming. Endurance training will improve aerobic capacity and help your cells use fuels and clear metabolic wastes. This will allow you to swim faster and longer. Longer swims promote metabolic health and build physical fitness.

**Cross-training:** Cross-training combines more than one type of endurance exercise, such as swimming and jogging, in your program at a time. It is a good training method for people who prefer swimming but don't have daily access to a swimming pool or open water. Including multiple exercises, such as swimming and running, stair stepping, or cycling, adds variety to the program. It also prepares you for a greater variety of physical challenges.

### Technique: The Basic Swimming Strokes for General Conditioning

The best strokes for conditioning are the freestyle and sidestroke. Competitive athletes also swim the breaststroke, butterfly, and backstroke (but not the sidestroke). Learning efficient swimming strokes helps increase enjoyment and results in better workouts. Take a class from the Red Cross, local recreation department, or private coach if you are not a strong swimmer or need help with the basic strokes.

**Freestyle:** While freestyle technically includes any unregulated stroke (such as the sidestroke), it generally refers to the front (Australian) crawl or overhand stroke. Freestyle is the fastest stroke and is best for general conditioning. Swim this stroke in a prone (face-down) position with arms stretched out in front and legs extended to the back. Move through the water by pulling first with the right arm and then with the left, while performing a kicking motion generated from the hips. During the stroke, rotate the thumb and palm 45 degrees toward the bottom of the pool. Pull in a semicircle downward toward the center of the body with the elbow higher than the hand. When the hand reaches the beginning of the ribcage, push the palm backward underneath the body as far as possible. Don't begin to stroke with the other hand until the first stroke is completed. Maximize the distance with each stroke by pulling fully and maintaining good posture.

The crawl uses a flutter kick, which involves moving the legs alternately with the force generated from the hips and a slight bend of the knees. Maintain a neutral spine during the stroke. A strong kick is important to minimize body roll during the stroke. For this reason, some of your training should include kicking without using the arms.

Breathing is almost always a problem for novice swimmers. Don't hold your breath! You will fatigue rapidly if you have poor air exchange during swimming. Breathe by turning the head to the side of a recovering stroke. Do not lift the head out of the water. Exhale continuously through the nose and mouth in between breaths. Beginners should breathe on the same side following each stroke cycle (left and right arm strokes).

**Sidestroke:** Even novices can get a good workout with minimal skill using the sidestroke. This is a good choice for beginners because you keep your head out of water and can swim great distances without fatigue. Lie in the water on your right side and stretch your right arm and hand in front of you in the direction you want to swim and place your left hand across your chest. Draw your right arm toward you, pulling at the water until your hand reaches your waist. At the same time, make a scissors kick with your legs. Repeat the stroke as your forward speed slows. Swim half the distance on your right side and the rest on your left side.

### Beginning Swim Program

Take swimming lessons from a certified teacher or coach if you are a nonswimmer or have not used swimming as your primary form of exercise. A swim teacher can help you develop good technique, make more rapid progress, and avoid injuries.

To assess your starting fitness, take the 12-minute swim test described in Lab 3.1. Use the swim test table to help you measure progress in your program. Take the test every 1 or 2 months to help establish short-term goals.

Start your program by swimming one-half lap at a time, using either freestyle or sidestroke. If you can't swim the length of a standard pool (25 meters or yards), begin by swimming the width. As soon as you can, swim one length of the pool, rest for 30 seconds, and then repeat. Build up your capacity until you can swim 20 lengths with a short rest interval between each length. If you start your program with the sidestroke, try to switch to the freestyle stroke as quickly as you can.

Increase the distance of each swim to a full lap (50 meters or yards) with 30 seconds to 1 minute of rest between laps. Build up until you can swim 20 sets of 50-meter swims with 30 seconds of rest between sets. Gradually increase the distance of each set to 100-meter swims. You are ready for the next level when you can swim 10 sets of 100 meters with 30 seconds of rest between sets.

### Swimming Program for Higher Levels of Fitness

This program includes a warm-up, specific conditioning drills for strokes and kicking, and a cool-down. It involves interval training 3 days a week and distance training 2 days per week.

Warm up before each workout by swimming 2–4 laps at an easy pace. It is also a good idea to warm up your legs and hips by holding on to the side of the pool and gently moving your legs using a flutter-kick motion. At the end of the workout, cool down by swimming 100–200 meters at a slow pace.

On Monday, Wednesday, and Friday, do interval training. Your goal is to swim intervals totaling 2000 meters per workout (20 sets of 100 meters each) at a fast pace with 30 seconds of rest between intervals. Every fifth interval, swim 25 meters using your legs alone, with your arms extended in front of you. Have someone watch you during the legs-only swims to make sure you are kicking mainly from the hips and maintaining a neutral spine. Add variety to your interval training workouts by using gloves, swim paddles, or fins.

If you are unable to do the interval workout at first, modify it by increasing rest intervals, decreasing speed, or decreasing the number of sets as you gradually increase the volume and intensity.

On Tuesday and Thursday, do distance training. Swim 1000–2000 meters continuously at a comfortable pace. Although distance days will help develop endurance, they are used mainly to help you recover from intense interval training days.

Rest on Saturday and Sunday. Rest is very important to help your muscles and metabolism recover and build fitness. Rest will also prevent overtraining and overuse injuries. Include 2 rest days per week. Rest days can be consecutive (such as Saturday and Sunday) or interspersed during the normal workout schedule.

### Integrating Swimming into a Total Fitness Program

You will develop fitness best and maintain interest in continuing your exercise program by varying the structure of your workouts. Incorporate kick boards, pull-buoys, hand paddles, and fins into some of your training sessions. Cross-training is a good option for developing well-rounded fitness. Swimming results in moderate gains in strength and large gains in endurance.

| Table 3 | Sample Swimming Program |
|---------|-------------------------|
| **DAY** | **ACTIVITIES** |
| Monday | • **Warm-up:** Swim 100–200 meters (2–4 laps of a standard pool) at an easy pace. <br> • **Intervals:** Swim 10–20 sets of 100-meter swims at 90% effort, with 30 seconds of rest between sets. After every 5 sets, swim 25 meters using your legs alone. <br> • **Cool-down:** Swim 100–200 meters at a slow pace. <br> • **Weight training:** Do at least 1 set of 10 repetitions of 8–10 exercises that work the body's major muscle groups. <br> • **Flexibility:** Do standard stretching exercises for the shoulders, chest, back, hips, and thighs. |
| Tuesday | • **Distance:** Swim 1000–2000 meters continuously at a comfortable pace. |
| Wednesday | • Repeat Monday activities. |
| Thursday | • Repeat Tuesday activities. |
| Friday | • Repeat Monday activities. |
| Saturday | • **Rest.** |
| Sunday | • Rest. |

Because swimming is not a weight-bearing activity and is not done in an upright position, it elicits a lower heart rate per minute. Therefore, swimmers need to adjust their target heart rate zone. To calculate your target heart rate for swimming, use this formula:

Maximum swimming heart rate (MSHR) = 205 − age

Target heart rate zone = 65–90% of MSHR

For example, a 19-year-old swimmer would calculate his or her target heart rate zone for swimming as follows:

MSHR: 205 − 19 = 186 bpm

65% intensity: 0.65 × 186 = 121 bpm

90% intensity: 0.90 × 186 = 167 bpm

Swimming tends to reduce bone density, so swimmers are advised to include weight training in their exercise program. Do at least one set of 10 repetitions for 8–10 exercises that use the major muscle groups in the body. To improve swimming performance, include exercises that work key muscles. For example, if you primarily swim the freestyle stroke, include exercises to increase strength in your shoulders, arms, upper back, and hips. Training the muscles you use during swimming can also help prevent injuries. In your flexibility training, pay special attention to the muscles you use during swimming, particularly the shoulders, hips, and back. Table 3 shows a basic sample swimming program that incorporates all these types of exercises.

## ROWING MACHINE SAMPLE PROGRAM

Rowing is a whole-body exercise that overloads the cardiorespiratory system and strengthens the major muscles of the body. The beauty and serenity of rowing on flat water in the morning is indescribable, but few people have access to a lake and rowing shell. Fortunately, sophisticated rowing machines simulate the rowing motion and make it possible to do this exercise at the fitness center or at a health club.

Modern rowing machines are very much like the real thing. They provide resistance with hydraulic pistons, magnets, air, or water. The best machines are solid and comfortable, provide a steady stroke, and allow you to maintain a neutral spine so you don't injure your back. Many rowing machines come with LCD displays that show heart rate, stroke rate, power output, and estimated caloric expenditure. They are also preprogrammed with workouts for interval training, cardiovascular conditioning, and moderate-intensity physical activity. Good rowing mechanics are essential because, if done incorrectly, rowing can cause severe overuse injuries that can damage the back, hips, knees, elbows, and shoulders.

### Technique: Basic Rowing Movement

Most of the power for rowing comes from the thigh and hip muscles and finishes with a pulling motion with the upper body. Maintain a neutral spine (that is, with normal curves) during the movement. Hinge at the hips and not at the back during the rowing motion.

The rowing movement includes the following phases:

• **The catch.** The catch involves sliding the seat forward on the track with arms straight as far as you can while keeping the spine neutral.

• *The drive.* The drive begins by pushing with the legs and keeping your arms straight.

• *The finish.* Finish by leaning back slightly (still maintaining a neutral spine) and pulling the handle to your abdomen.

• *The recovery.* Recover by extending your arms forward, hinging forward at the hips with a neutral spine, and sliding forward again on the seat for another "catch."

## Training Methods

Your rowing program should include both continuous training and interval training. Continuous training involves rowing for a specific amount of time—typically 20–90 minutes without stopping. Most people enjoy rowing at about 70% of maximum heart rate.

Interval training involves a series of exercise bouts followed by rest. The method manipulates distance, intensity, repetitions, and rest. An example of an interval workout would be to row for eight sets of 4-minute exercise bouts at 85% effort with 2 minutes of rest between intervals. During interval training, changing one factor affects the others. For example, if you increase the intensity of exercise, you will need more rest between intervals and won't be able to do as many repetitions. High-intensity exercise builds fitness best but also increases the risk of injury and loss of motivation. Make intervals challenging but not so difficult that you get injured or discouraged.

## Beginning Rowing Program

During the first few workouts, start conservatively by rowing for 10 minutes at a rate of about 20 strokes per minute with a moderate resistance. Exercise at about 60% effort. Do this workout three times during the first week. The movement is deceptively easy and invigorating. You are, however, using all the major muscle groups in the body and are probably not ready for a more intense exercise program.

After the first workout, do a series of 5-minute intervals during the first few weeks of training. For example, row for 5 minutes, rest 3 minutes, row 5 minutes, then rest 3 minutes. Build up until you can do 4–6 repetitions of 5-minute exercise intervals, resting only 1 minute between sets. Gradually, increase the time for each interval to 15 minutes and vary the rowing cadence from 20 to 25 strokes per minute. Your first short-term goal is to complete 30 minutes of continuous rowing without stopping.

## Rowing Program for Higher Levels of Fitness

Vary your training methods after you can row continuously for 30 minutes, gain some fitness, and get used to the technique. Alternate between interval training and distance training. Doing both will help you develop fitness rapidly and improve rowing efficiency. A good strategy is to row continuously at about 70% effort for 30-60 minutes 3 days per week and practice interval training at 80–90% effort for 2 days per week. Do resistance and flexibility training 2–3 days per week. A basic but complete rowing machine program that includes continuous and interval training as well as resistance and flexibility exercises is shown in Table 4.

| Table 4 | Sample Rowing Machine Fitness Program |
|---|---|

| DAY | ACTIVITIES |
|---|---|
| Monday | • **Warm-up:** Row at low intensity for 2 minutes.<br>• **Continuous rowing:** Row for 30 minutes at 70% effort (20–22 strokes per minute).<br>• **Weight training (1–2 sets of 10 repetitions):** Squats, leg curls, bench press, lat pulls, raises, biceps curls, triceps extensions, curl-ups, side bridge (10 seconds per side), spine extensions (10 seconds per side).<br>• **Stretching:** Do static stretching exercises for the shoulders, chest, back, hips, and thighs. Hold each stretch for 10–30 seconds. |
| Tuesday | • **Warm-up:** Row at low intensity for 2 minutes.<br>• **Continuous rowing:** Row at 60–70% of maximum effort for 5 minutes. Rest for 3 minutes.<br>• **Interval rowing:** Row 6 sets, for 5 minutes per set, at 25 strokes per minute (90% effort). Rest for 3 minutes between intervals. |
| Wednesday | • **Warm-up:** Row at low intensity for 2 minutes.<br>• **Continuous rowing:** Row for 45 minutes at 70% effort (20–22 strokes per minute).<br>• **Stretching:** Repeat Monday stretches. |
| Thursday | • **Warm-up:** Row at low intensity for 2 minutes.<br>• **Continuous rowing:** Row for 30 minutes at 70% effort (20–22 strokes per minute).<br>• **Weight training (1–2 sets of 10 repetitions):** Repeat Monday weight training exercises. |
| Friday | • **Warm-up:** Row at low intensity for 2 minutes.<br>• **Continuous rowing:** Row for 30 minutes at 70% effort (20–22 strokes per minute).<br>• **Stretching:** Repeat Monday stretches. |
| Saturday | • **Rest.** |
| Sunday | • **Rest.** |

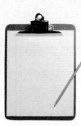

**LAB 7.1** **A Personal Fitness Program Plan and Contract**

A. I, _____, am contracting with myself to follow a physical fitness program to
   (name)

work toward the following goals:

Specific or short-term goals (include current status for each):

1. _____

2. _____

3. _____

4. _____

General or long-term goals:

1. _____

2. _____

3. _____

4. _____

B. My program plan is as follows:

| Activities | Components (Check ✓) | | | | | Frequency (Check ✓) | | | | | | | Intensity* | Time (duration) |
|---|---|---|---|---|---|---|---|---|---|---|---|---|---|---|
| | CRE | MS | ME | F | BC | M | Tu | W | Th | F | Sa | Su | | |
| | | | | | | | | | | | | | | |
| | | | | | | | | | | | | | | |
| | | | | | | | | | | | | | | |
| | | | | | | | | | | | | | | |
| | | | | | | | | | | | | | | |

*Conduct activities for achieving CRE goals in your target range for heart rate or RPE.

C. My program will begin on _____. My program includes the following schedule of mini-goals. For each step in my
   (date)

program, I will give myself the reward listed.

| _____ | _____ | _____ |
|---|---|---|
| (mini-goal 1) | (date) | (reward) |

| _____ | _____ | _____ |
|---|---|---|
| (mini-goal 2) | (date) | (reward) |

| _____ | _____ | _____ |
|---|---|---|
| (mini-goal 3) | (date) | (reward) |

| _____ | _____ | _____ |
|---|---|---|
| (mini-goal 4) | (date) | (reward) |

| _____ | _____ | _____ |
|---|---|---|
| (mini-goal 5) | (date) | (reward) |

connect
http://www.mcgrawhillconnect.com/
FITNESS AND WELLNESS

D. My program will include the addition of physical activity to my daily routine (such as climbing stairs or walking to class):

1. _____

2. _____

3. _____

4. _____

5. _____

E. I will use the following tools to monitor my program and my progress toward my goals:

_____

(list any charts, graphs, or journals you plan to use)

_____

_____

I sign this contract as an indication of my personal commitment to reach my goal.

_____   _____

(your signature)                              (date)

I have recruited a helper who will witness my contract and _____

_____

(list any way your helper will participate in your program)

_____

_____   _____

(witness's signature)                         (date)

Name _____  Section _____  Date _____

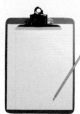

## LAB 7.2  Getting to Know Your Fitness Facility

To help create a successful training program, take time to learn more about the fitness facility you plan to use.

### Basic Information

Name and location of facility: _____

Hours of operation: _____

Times available for general use: _____

Times most convenient for your schedule: _____

Can you obtain an initial session or consultation with a trainer to help you create a program? _____ yes _____ no

If so, what does the initial planning session involve? _____

_____

Are any of the staff certified? Do any have special training? If yes, list/describe: _____

_____

What types of equipment are available for the development of cardiorespiratory endurance? Briefly list/describe: _____

_____

_____

_____

Are any group activities or classes available? If so, briefly describe: _____

_____

_____

What types of weight training equipment are available for use? _____

_____

| Yes | No | |
|-----|-----|-----|
| _____ | _____ | Is there a fee for using the facility? If so, how much? $ _____ |
| _____ | _____ | Is a student ID required for access to the facility? |
| _____ | _____ | Do you need to sign up in advance to use the facility or any of the equipment? |
| _____ | _____ | Is there typically a line or wait to use the equipment during the times you use the facility? |
| _____ | _____ | Is there a separate area with mats for stretching and/or cool-down? |
| _____ | _____ | Do you need to bring your own towel? |
| _____ | _____ | Are lockers available? If so, do you need to bring your own lock? _____ yes _____ no |
| _____ | _____ | Are showers available? If so, do you need to bring your own soap and shampoo? _____ yes _____ no |
| _____ | _____ | Is drinking water available? (If not, be sure to bring your own bottle of water.) |

What other amenities, such as vending machines or saunas, are available at the facility? Briefly list/describe: _____

_____

Mc Graw Hill **connect** http://www.mcgrawhillconnect.com/
|FITNESS AND WELLNESS

## Information About Equipment

Fill in the specific equipment and exercise(s) that you can use to develop cardiorespiratory endurance and each of the major muscle groups. For cardiorespiratory endurance, list the type(s) of equipment and a sample starting workout: frequency, intensity, time, and other pertinent information (such as a setting for resistance or speed). For muscular strength and endurance, list the equipment and exercises, and indicate the order in which you'll complete them during a workout session.

### Cardiorespiratory Endurance Equipment

| Equipment | Sample Starting Workout |
|---|---|
|  |  |
|  |  |
|  |  |

### Muscular Strength and Endurance Equipment

| Order | Muscle Groups | Equipment | Exercise(s) |
|---|---|---|---|
|  | Neck |  |  |
|  | Chest |  |  |
|  | Shoulders |  |  |
|  | Upper back |  |  |
|  | Front of arms |  |  |
|  | Back of arms |  |  |
|  | Buttocks |  |  |
|  | Abdomen |  |  |
|  | Lower back |  |  |
|  | Front of thighs |  |  |
|  | Back of thighs |  |  |
|  | Calves |  |  |
|  | *Other:* |  |  |
|  | *Other:* |  |  |

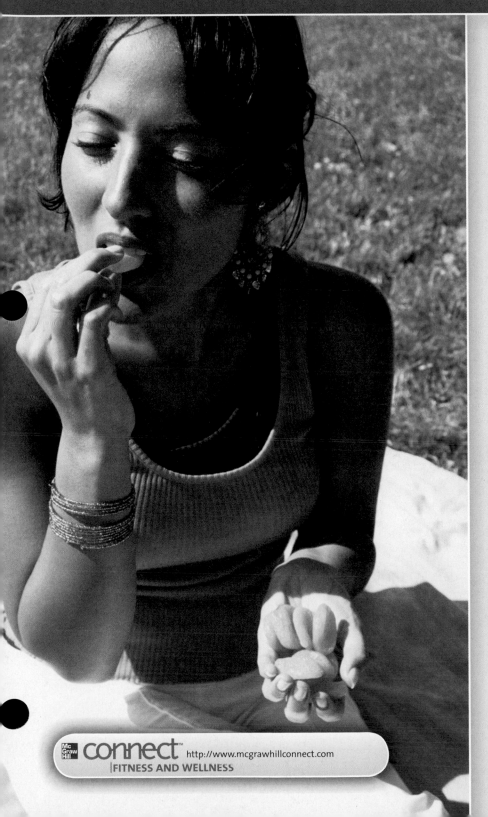

# CHAPTER 8

# Nutrition

## LOOKING AHEAD...

After reading this chapter, you should be able to:

- List the essential nutrients and describe the functions they perform in the body

- Describe the guidelines that have been developed to help people choose a healthy diet, avoid nutritional deficiencies, and reduce their risk of diet-related chronic diseases

- Describe nutritional guidelines for vegetarians and for special population groups

- Explain how to use food labels and other consumer tools to make informed choices about foods

- Put together a personal nutrition plan based on affordable foods that you enjoy and that will promote wellness, today and in the future

## TEST YOUR KNOWLEDGE

1. It is recommended that all adults consume 1–2 servings each of fruits and vegetables every day. True or false?

2. Candy is the leading source of added sugars in the American diet. True or false?

3. Which of the following is not a whole grain?
   a. brown rice
   b. wheat flour
   c. popcorn

**Answers**

1. **False.** For someone consuming 2000 calories per day, a minimum of 9 servings per day—4 of fruits and 5 of vegetables—is recommended. This is the equivalent of 4 1/2 cups per day.

2. **False.** Regular (nondiet) sodas are the leading source of added sugars. Together with energy drinks and sports drinks, they account for 36% of the added sugars in the American diet, and added sugars contribute an average of 16% of the total calories in American diets. Each 12-ounce soda supplies about 10 teaspoons of sugar, or nearly 10% of the calories in a 2000-calorie diet.

3. **b.** Unless labeled "whole wheat," wheat flour is processed to remove the bran and germ and is not a whole grain.

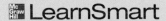

In your lifetime, you will spend about 6 years eating—about 70,000 meals and 60 tons of food. What you eat affects your energy level, well-being, and overall health. Your nutritional habits help determine your risk of major chronic diseases, including heart disease, cancer, stroke, and diabetes. Choosing foods that provide the nutrients you need while limiting the substances linked to disease should be an important part of your daily life.

Choosing a healthy diet is a two-part process. First, you have to know which nutrients you need and in what amounts. Second, you have to translate those requirements into a diet consisting of foods you like that are both available and affordable. Once you know what constitutes a healthy diet for you, you can adjust your current diet to bring it into line with your goals.

This chapter explains the basic principles of **nutrition.** It introduces the six classes of essential nutrients, explaining their role in the functioning of the body. It also provides guidelines that you can use to design a healthy eating plan. Finally, it offers practical tools and advice to help you apply the guidelines to your life.

## NUTRITIONAL REQUIREMENTS: COMPONENTS OF A HEALTHY DIET

You probably think about your diet in terms of the foods you like to eat. More important for your health, though, are the nutrients contained in those foods. Your body requires proteins, fats, carbohydrates, vitamins, minerals, and water—about 45 **essential nutrients.** In this context, the word *essential* means that you must get these substances from food because your body is unable to manufacture them, or at least not fast enough to meet your physiological needs. The six classes of nutrients, along with their functions and major sources, are listed in Table 8.1

The body needs some essential nutrients in relatively large amounts; these **macronutrients** include protein, fat, carbohydrate, and water. **Micronutrients,** such as vitamins and minerals, are required in much smaller amounts. Your body obtains nutrients through the process of **digestion,** which breaks down food into compounds that the gastrointestinal tract can absorb and the body can use (Figure 8.1, p. 226). A diet that provides enough essential nutrients is vital because they provide energy, help build and maintain body tissues, and help regulate body functions.

## Calories

The energy in foods is expressed as **kilocalories.** One kilocalorie represents the amount of heat it takes to raise the temperature of one liter of water 1°C. A person needs about 2000 kilocalories a day to meet his or her energy needs. In common usage, people refer to kilocalories as *calories,* which is a much smaller energy unit: 1 kilocalorie contains 1000 calories. This text uses the familiar word *calorie* to stand for the larger energy unit; you'll also find *calorie* used on food labels.

Of the six classes of essential nutrients, three supply energy:

- Fat = 9 calories per gram
- Protein = 4 calories per gram
- Carbohydrate = 4 calories per gram

Alcohol, though not an essential nutrient, also supplies energy, providing 7 calories per gram. (One gram equals a little less than 0.04 ounce.) The high caloric content of fat is one reason experts often advise against high fat consumption; most of us do not need the extra calories to meet energy needs. Regardless of their source, calories consumed in excess of energy needs can be converted to fat and stored in the body.

| Table 8.1 | The Six Classes of Essential Nutrients | |
|---|---|---|
| NUTRIENT | FUNCTION | MAJOR SOURCES |
| Proteins products, (4 calories/gram) | Form important parts of muscles, bone, blood, enzymes, some hormones, and cell membranes; repair tissue; regulate water and acid-base balance; help in growth; supply energy | Meat, fish, poultry, eggs, milk legumes, nuts |
| Carbohydrates (4 calories/gram) | Supply energy to cells in brain, nervous system, and blood; supply energy to muscles during exercise | Grains (breads and cereals), fruits, vegetables, milk |
| Fats (9 calories/gram) | Supply energy; insulate, support, and cushion organs; provide medium for absorption of fat-soluble vitamins | Animal foods, grains, nuts, seeds, fish, vegetables |
| Vitamins | Promote (initiate or speed up) specific chemical reactions within cells | Abundant in fruits, vegetables, and grains; also found in meat and dairy products |
| Minerals | Help regulate body functions; aid in growth and maintenance of body tissues; act as catalysts for release of energy | Found in most food groups |
| Water | Makes up 50–60% of body weight; provides medium for chemical reactions; transports chemicals; regulates temperature; removes waste products | Fruits, vegetables, liquids |

# Tracking Your Junk Food Intake

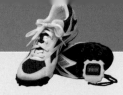

How much junk food do you eat on any given day? Let's find out. Write down all the different kinds of junk food you eat during the day today:

_____

_____

_____

_____

_____

Now, write down your reason for eating each of those items:

_____

_____

_____

_____

_____

_____

Whether you eat junk for pleasure or to help cope with stress, it pays to be mindful of your eating habits. Consider your reasons for eating junk food, and try to catch yourself the next time you're tempted to reach for some. If you're able to stop yourself, you can make healthier choices.

## Fitness Tip

A pound of body fat is equal to 3500 calories. If you eat 100 calories more than you expend every day, you will gain more than 10 pounds in a year.

Just meeting energy needs is not enough. Our bodies need enough of the essential nutrients to grow and function properly. Practically all foods contain combinations of nutrients, although foods are commonly classified according to their predominant nutrients. For example, spaghetti is considered a carbohydrate food, although it contains small amounts of other nutrients. The following sections discuss the functions and sources of each class of nutrients.

## Proteins—The Basis of Body Structure

**Proteins** form important parts of the body's main structural components: muscles and bones. Proteins also form

**nutrition**   The science of food and how the body uses it in health and disease.

**essential nutrients**   Substances the body must get from foods because it cannot manufacture them at all or fast enough to meet its needs. These nutrients include proteins, fats, carbohydrates, vitamins, minerals, and water.

**macronutrient**   An essential nutrient required by the body in relatively large amounts.

**micronutrient**   An essential nutrient required by the body in minute amounts.

**digestion**   The process of breaking down foods into compounds the gastrointestinal tract can absorb and the body can use.

**kilocalorie**   A measure of energy content in food; 1 kilocalorie represents the amount of heat needed to raise the temperature of 1 liter of water 1°C; commonly referred to as *calorie*.

**protein**   An essential nutrient that forms important parts of the body's main structures (muscles and bones) as well as blood, enzymes, hormones, and cell membranes; also provides energy.

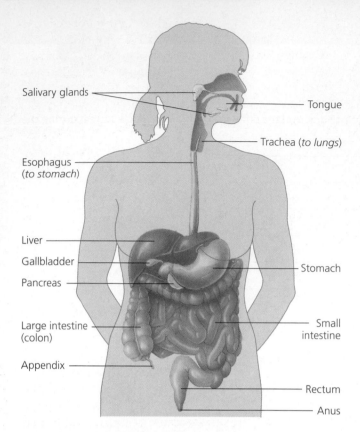

Salivary glands

Tongue

Trachea (*to lungs*)

Esophagus
(*to stomach*)

Liver

Gallbladder

Pancreas

Stomach

Large intestine
(colon)

Small
intestine

Appendix

Rectum

Anus

**FIGURE 8.1  The digestive system.**
Food is partially broken down by being chewed and mixed with saliva
in the mouth. After traveling to the stomach via the esophagus,
food is broken down further by stomach acids and other secretions.
As food moves through the digestive tract, it is mixed by muscular
contractions and broken down by chemicals. Most absorption of
nutrients occurs in the small intestine, aided by secretions from
the pancreas, gallbladder, and intestinal lining. The large intestine
reabsorbs excess water; the remaining solid wastes are collected in
the rectum and excreted through the anus.

important parts of blood, enzymes, cell membranes, and
some hormones. As mentioned earlier, proteins also provide energy (4 calories per gram) for the body.

**Amino Acids**  The building blocks of proteins are called
**amino acids**. Twenty common amino acids are found in
food. Nine of these are essential (or indispensable). The
other 11 amino acids can be produced by the body as
long as the necessary components are supplied by foods.

**Complete and Incomplete Proteins**  Individual protein sources are considered "complete" if they supply
all the essential amino acids in adequate amounts and
"incomplete" if they do not. Meat, fish, poultry, eggs, milk,
cheese, and soy provide complete proteins. Incomplete
proteins, which come from plant sources such as nuts
and **legumes** (dried beans and peas), are good sources
of most essential amino acids but are usually low in one
or two.

Certain combinations of vegetable proteins, such as
wheat and peanuts in a peanut butter sandwich, allow

| Table 8.2 | Protein Content of Common Food Items | |
|---|---|---|
| **ITEM** | | **PROTEIN (GRAMS)** |
| 3 ounces lean meat, poultry, or fish | | 20–25 |
| ⅓ cup tofu | | 20–25 |
| 1 cup dried beans | | 15–20 |
| 1 cup milk, yogurt | | 8–12 |
| 1½ ounces cheese | | 8–12 |
| 1 serving of cereals, grains, nuts, vegetables | | 2–4 |

each vegetable protein to make up for the amino acids
missing in the other protein. The combination yields a
complete protein. It was once believed that vegetarians had
to "complement" their proteins at each meal in order to
receive the benefit of a complete protein. It is now known,
however, that proteins consumed throughout the course
of the day can complement each other to form a pool of
amino acids the body can draw from to produce proteins.
Vegetarians should include a variety of vegetable protein
sources in their diets to make sure they get all the essential amino acids in adequate amounts. (Healthy vegetarian
diets are discussed later in the chapter.)

**Recommended Protein Intake**  Adequate daily intake
of protein for adults is 0.8 gram per kilogram (0.36 gram
per pound) of body weight, corresponding to 50 grams of
protein per day for someone who weighs 140 pounds and
65 grams of protein for someone who weighs 180 pounds.
Table 8.2 lists some popular food items and the amount
of protein each provides.

Most Americans meet or exceed the protein intake
needed for adequate nutrition. If you consume more
protein than your body needs, the extra protein is synthesized into fat for energy storage or burned for energy
requirements. A little extra protein is not harmful, but it
can contribute fat to the diet because protein-rich foods
are often fat-rich, as well.

A fairly broad range of protein intakes is associated
with good health, and the Food and Nutrition Board of
the Institute of Medicine recommends that the amount of
protein adults eat should fall within the range of 10–35%
of total daily calories, depending on the individual's age.
The average American diet includes about 15–16% of
total daily calories as protein.

**Wellness Tip**

Research shows that some protein-rich foods can give
you a quick mental boost, which can be helpful before
an exam.

# Fats—Essential in Small Amounts

Fats, also known as *lipids,* are the most concentrated source of energy, at 9 calories per gram. The fats stored in your body represent usable energy, help insulate your body, and support and cushion your organs. Fats in the diet help your body absorb fat-soluble vitamins, and they add flavor and texture to foods. Fats are the major fuel for the body during rest and light activity.

Two fats—linoleic acid and alpha-linolenic acid—are essential components of the diet. They are used to make compounds that are key regulators of such body functions as the maintenance of blood pressure and the progress of a healthy pregnancy.

**Types and Sources of Fats** Most of the fats in foods are fairly similar in composition, generally including a molecule of glycerol (an alcohol) with three fatty acid chains attached to it. The resulting structure is called a *triglyceride.* Animal fat, for example, is primarily made of triglycerides. Within a triglyceride, differences in the fatty acid structure result in different types of fats. Depending on this structure, a fat may be unsaturated, monounsaturated, polyunsaturated, or saturated. (The essential fatty acids—linoleic and alpha-linolenic acids—are both polyunsaturated.) The different types of fatty acids have different characteristics and different effects on your health.

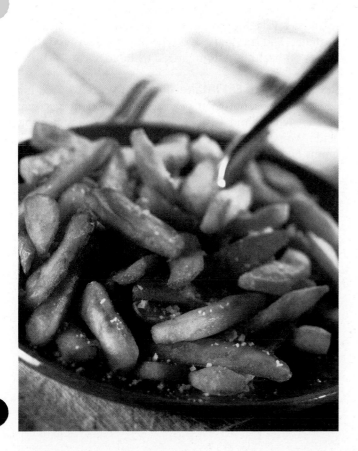

Food fats are often composed of both saturated and unsaturated fatty acids; the dominant type of fatty acid determines the fat's characteristics. Food fats containing large amounts of saturated fatty acids are usually solid at room temperature; they are generally found naturally in animal products. The leading sources of saturated fat in the American diet are red meats (hamburger, steak, roasts), whole milk, cheese, hot dogs, and lunch meats. Food fats containing large amounts of monounsaturated and polyunsaturated fatty acids usually come from plant sources and are liquid at room temperature. Olive, canola, safflower, and peanut oils contain mostly monounsaturated fatty acids. Corn, soybean, and cottonseed oils contain mostly polyunsaturated fatty acids.

**Hydrogenation** There are notable exceptions to these generalizations. When unsaturated vegetable oils undergo the process of **hydrogenation,** a mixture of saturated and unsaturated fatty acids is produced, creating a more solid fat from a liquid oil. Hydrogenation also changes some unsaturated fatty acids into **trans fatty acids (trans fats),** unsaturated fatty acids with an atypical shape that affects their behavior in the body. Food manufacturers use hydrogenation to increase the stability of an oil so it can be reused for deep frying, to improve the texture of certain foods (to make pastries and pie crusts flakier, for example), and to extend the shelf life of foods made with oil. Hydrogenation is also used to transform liquid vegetable oils into margarine or shortening.

Many baked and fried foods are prepared with hydrogenated vegetable oils, which means they can be relatively high in saturated and trans fatty acids. Leading sources of trans fats in the American diet are deep-fried fast foods such as french fries and fried chicken (typically fried in vegetable shortening rather than oil), baked and snack foods, and stick margarine.

In general, the more solid a hydrogenated oil is, the more saturated and trans fats it contains. For example, stick margarines typically contain more saturated and trans fats than do tub or squeeze margarines. Small amounts of trans fatty acids are also found naturally in meat and milk.

Hydrogenated vegetable oils are not the only plant fats that contain saturated fats. Palm and coconut oils, although derived from plants, are also highly saturated. Yet fish oils, derived from an animal source, are rich in polyunsaturated fats.

**Fats and Health** Different types of fats have very different effects on health. Many studies have examined the effects of dietary fat intake on blood **cholesterol** levels and the risk of heart disease. However, the results of a recent analysis concluded that dietary saturated fat is not associated with an increased risk of certain forms of heart disease, and that the benefits of diets low in saturated fat may come from the higher amounts of polyunsaturated fats that these diets provide.

Saturated and trans fatty acids raise blood levels of **low-density lipoprotein (LDL)**, or "bad" cholesterol, thereby increasing a person's risk of heart disease. Unsaturated fatty acids lower LDL. Monounsaturated fatty acids, such as those found in olive and canola oils, may also increase levels of **high-density lipoprotein (HDL)**, or "good" cholesterol, providing even greater benefits for heart health. In large amounts, trans fatty acids may lower HDL. Saturated fats impair the ability of HDLs to prevent inflammation of the blood vessels, a key factor in vascular disease. Saturated fats also reduce the blood vessels' ability to react normally to stress. Thus, to reduce the risk of heart disease, it is important to choose unsaturated fats instead of saturated and trans fats. (See Chapter 11 for more on cholesterol.)

Most Americans consume 4–5 times as much saturated fat as trans fat (8–10% versus 2% of total daily calories). However, health experts are particularly concerned about trans fats because of their double-negative effect on heart health—they not only raise LDL but also lower HDL—and because there is less public awareness of trans fats, although awareness is growing. Since 2006, federal law has required food labels to include trans fat content, and numerous states and cities have banned the use of trans fats in restaurant food. Consumers can also check for the presence of trans fats by examining a food's ingredient list for partially hydrogenated oil or vegetable shortening.

For heart health, it's important to limit your consumption of both saturated and trans fats. The best way to reduce saturated fat in your diet is to eat less meat and full-fat dairy products (whole milk, cream, butter, cheese, ice cream). To lower trans fats, eat fewer deep-fried foods and baked goods made with hydrogenated vegetable oils (such as many kinds of crackers and cookies), use liquid oils for cooking, and favor tub or squeeze margarines over stick margarines. Remember: The softer or more liquid a fat is, the less saturated and trans fat it is likely to contain.

Although saturated and trans fats pose health hazards, other fats can be beneficial. When used in place of saturated fats, monounsaturated fatty acids—as found in avocados, most nuts, and olive, canola, peanut, and safflower oils—improve cholesterol levels and may help protect against some cancers.

*Omega-3* fatty acids, a form of polyunsaturated fat found primarily in fish, may be even more healthful. Omega-3s and the compounds the body makes from them have a number of heart-healthy effects: They reduce the tendency of blood to clot, inhibit inflammation and abnormal heart rhythms, and reduce blood pressure and the risk of heart attack and stroke in some people. Because of these benefits, nutritionists recommend that Americans increase the proportion of omega-3s in their diet by eating fish two or more times a week. Salmon, tuna, trout, mackerel, herring, sardines, and anchovies are all good sources of omega-3s. Lesser amounts are found in plant foods, including dark green leafy vegetables; walnuts; flaxseeds; and canola, walnut, and flaxseed oils.

Most of the polyunsaturated fats currently consumed by Americans are *omega-6* fatty acids, primarily from corn oil and soybean oil. The American Heart Association (AHA) recommends consuming at least 5–10% of energy from omega-6 fatty acids as part of a low-saturated-fat and low-cholesterol diet to reduce the risk of coronary heart disease.

In addition to its effects on heart disease risk, dietary fat can affect health in other ways. Diets high in fatty red meat are associated with an increased risk of certain forms of cancer, especially colon cancer. A high-fat diet can also make weight management more difficult. Because fat is a concentrated source of calories, a high-fat diet is often a high-calorie diet that can lead to weight gain.

Although more research is needed on the precise effects of different types and amounts of fat on overall health, a great deal of evidence points to the fact that most people benefit from lowering their overall fat intake to recommended levels and choosing unsaturated fats instead of saturated and trans fats. The types of fatty acids and their effects on health are summarized in Table 8.3.

**Recommended Fat Intake** To meet the body's need for essential fats, adult men need about 17 grams per day of linoleic acid and 1.6 grams per day of alpha-linolenic acid. Women need 12 grams of linoleic acid and 1.1 grams of alpha-linolenic acid. It takes only 3–4 teaspoons (15–20 grams) of vegetable oil per day incorporated into your diet to supply the essential fats. Most Americans get enough essential fats. Limiting unhealthy fats is a much greater health concern.

Limits for total fat, saturated fat, and trans fat intake have been set by a number of government and research organizations. The Institute of Medicine's Food and Nutrition Board has released recommendations for the balance of energy sources in a healthful diet. These recommendations—called Acceptable Macronutrient Distribution Ranges (AMDRs)—are based on ensuring adequate intake of essential nutrients while reducing the risk of chronic diseases. As with protein, a range of levels of fat intake is associated with good health. The AMDR for total fat is 20–35% of total calories. Although more difficult for consumers to monitor, AMDRs have also been set for omega-6 fatty acids (5–10%) and omega-3 fatty acids (0.6–1.2%) as part of total fat intake.

## Table 8.3 — Types of Fatty Acids and Their Possible Effects on Health

| TYPE OF FATTY ACID | FOUND IN[a] | POSSIBLE EFFECTS ON HEALTH |
|---|---|---|
| **SATURATED** *(Keep Intake Low)* | • Animal fats (especially fatty meats and poultry fat and skin)<br>• Butter, cheese, and other high-fat dairy products<br>• Palm and coconut oils | • Raises total cholesterol and LDL cholesterol<br>• May increase risk of heart disease<br>• May increase risk of colon and prostate cancers |
| **TRANS** *(Keep Intake Low)* | • Deep-fried fast foods<br>• Stick margarines, shortening<br>• Packaged cookies and crackers<br>• Processed snacks and sweets | • Raises total cholesterol and LDL cholesterol<br>• Lowers HDL cholesterol<br>• May increase risk of heart disease and breast cancer |
| **MONOUNSATURATED** *(Keep Intake Low)* | • Olive, canola, and safflower oils<br>• Avocados, olives<br>• Peanut butter (without added fat)<br>• Many nuts, including almonds, cashews, pecans, and pistachios | • Lowers total cholesterol and LDL cholesterol<br>• May reduce blood pressure and lower triglycerides (a risk factor for heart disease)<br>• May reduce risk of heart disease, stroke, and some cancers |
| **POLYUNSATURATED (two groups)[b]** *(Choose Moderate Amounts)* | | |
| Omega-3 | • Fatty fish, including salmon, white albacore tuna, mackerel, anchovies, and sardines<br>• Lesser amounts in walnut, flaxseed, canola, and soybean oils; tofu, walnuts; flaxseeds; and dark green leafy vegetables | • Reduces blood clotting and inflammation and inhibits abnormal heart rhythms<br>• Lowers triglycerides<br>• May lower blood pressure in some people<br>• May reduce the risk of fatal heart attack, stroke, and some cancers |
| Omega-6 | • Corn, soybean, and cottonseed oils (often used in margarine, mayonnaise, and salad dressings) | • Lowers total cholesterol and LDL cholesterol<br>• May lower HDL cholesterol<br>• May reduce risk of heart disease<br>• May slightly increase risk of cancer if omega-6 intake is high and omega-3 is low |

[a] Food fats contain a combination of types of fatty acids in various proportions. For example, canola oil is composed mainly of monounsaturated fatty acids (62%) but also contains polyunsaturated (32%) and saturated (6%) fatty acids. Food fats are categorized here according to their predominant fatty acid.

[b] The essential fatty acids are polyunsaturated: Linoleic acid is an omega-6 fatty acid and alpha-linolenic acid is an omega-3 fatty acid.

Because any amount of saturated and trans fat increases the risk of heart disease, the Food and Nutrition Board recommends that saturated and trans fat intake be kept as low as possible; most fat in a healthy diet should be unsaturated.

For advice on setting individual intake goals, see the box "Setting Intake Goals for Protein, Fat, and Carbohydrate." To determine how close you are to meeting your personal intake goals for fat, keep a running total over the course of the day. For prepared foods, food labels list the number of grams of fat, protein, and carbohydrate. Nutrition information is also available in many grocery stores, in published nutrition guides, and online (see For Further Exploration at the end of the chapter). By checking these resources, you can keep track of the total grams of fat, protein, and carbohydrate you eat and assess your current diet.

In reducing fat intake to recommended levels, the emphasis should be on lowering saturated and trans fats (see Table 8.3). You can still eat high-fat foods, but it makes sense to limit the size of your portions and to balance your intake with low-fat foods. For example, peanut butter is high in fat, with 8 grams (72 calories) of fat in each 90-calorie tablespoon. Two tablespoons of peanut butter eaten on whole-wheat bread and served with a banana, carrot sticks, and a glass of nonfat milk make a nutritious lunch—high in protein and carbohydrate, relatively low in total and saturated fat (500 calories, 18 grams of total fat, 4 grams of saturated fat). By comparison, four tablespoons of peanut butter on high-fat crackers with potato chips, cookies, and whole milk is a less healthy combination (1000 calories, 62 grams of total fat, 15 grams of saturated fat). So although it's important to evaluate individual food items for their fat content, it is more important to look at them in the context of your overall diet.

**cholesterol**   A waxy substance found in the blood and cells and needed for synthesis of cell membranes, vitamin D, and hormones.

**low-density lipoprotein (LDL)**   Blood fat that transports cholesterol to organs and tissues; excess amounts result in the accumulation of fatty deposits on artery walls.

**high-density lipoprotein (HDL)**   Blood fat that helps transport cholesterol out of the arteries, thereby protecting against heart disease.

# Setting Intake Goals for Protein, Fat, and Carbohydrate

The Food and Nutrition Board has established goals to help ensure adequate intake of the essential amino acids, fatty acids, and carbohydrate. The daily goals for adequate intake for adults follow:

| | MEN | WOMEN |
|---|---|---|
| Protein | 56 grams | 46 grams |
| Fat: Linoleic acid | 17 grams | 12 grams |
| Alpha-linoleic acid | 1.6 grams | 1.1 grams |
| Carbohydrate | 130 grams | 130 grams |

Protein intake goals can be calculated more specifically by multiplying your body weight in kilograms by 0.8 or your body weight in pounds by 0.36. (Refer to the Nutrition Resources section at the end of the chapter for information for specific age groups and life stages.)

To meet your daily energy needs, you need to consume more than the minimally adequate amounts of the energy-providing nutrients listed above, which alone supply only about 800–900 calories.

The Food and Nutrition Board provides additional guidance in the form of Acceptable Macronutrient Distribution Ranges (AMDRs). These ranges can help you balance your intake of energy-providing nutrients in ways that ensure adequate intake and reduce the risk of chronic disease.

The AMDRs for protein, total fat, and carbohydrate are as follows:

| | |
|---|---|
| Protein | 10–35% of total daily calories |
| Total fat | 20–35% of total daily calories |
| Carbohydrate | 45–65% of total daily calories |

To set individual goals, begin by estimating your total daily energy (calorie) needs. If your weight is stable, your current energy intake is the number of calories you need to maintain your weight at your current activity level. Next, select percentage goals for protein, fat, and carbohydrate. You can allocate your total daily calories among the three classes of macronutrients to suit your preferences; just make sure that the three percentages you select total 100% and that you meet the minimum intake goals listed. Two samples reflecting different total energy intake and nutrient intake goals are shown in the table below.

To translate your percentage goals into daily intake goals expressed in calories and grams, multiply the appropriate percentages by total calorie intake, and then divide the results by the corresponding calories per gram. For example, a fat limit of 35% applied to a 2200-calorie diet would be calculated as follows: 0.35 x 2200 = 770 calories of total fat; 770 ÷ 9 calories per gram = 86 grams of total fat. (Remember that fat has 9 calories per gram and that protein and carbohydrate have 4 calories per gram.)

**Two Sample Macronutrient Distributions**

| | | SAMPLE 1 | | SAMPLE 2 | |
|---|---|---|---|---|---|
| NUTRIENT | AMDR | INDIVIDUAL GOALS | AMOUNTS FOR A 1600-CALORIE DIET | INDIVIDUAL GOALS | AMOUNTS FOR A 2800-CALORIE DIET |
| PROTEIN | 10–35% | 15% | 240 calories = 60 grams | 30% | 840 calories = 210 grams |
| FAT | 20–35% | 30% | 480 calories = 53 grams | 25% | 700 calories = 78 grams |
| CARBOHYDRATE | 45–65% | 55% | 880 calories = 220 grams | 45% | 1260 calories = 315 grams |

**SOURCE:** Food and Nutrition Board, Institute of Medicine, National Academies. 2002. *Dietary Reference Intakes: Applications in Dietary Planning.* Washington, D.C.: National Academies Press. © 2003 by the National Academy of Sciences. Reprinted with permission from the National Academies Press, Washington, D.C.

## Carbohydrates—An Ideal Source of Energy

**Carbohydrates** ("carbs") are needed in the diet primarily to supply energy to body cells. Some cells, such as those in the brain and other parts of the nervous system and in the blood, use only carbohydrates for fuel. During high-intensity exercise, muscles also get most of their energy from carbohydrates.

**Simple and Complex Carbohydrates** Carbohydrates are classified into two groups: simple and complex. *Simple carbohydrates* include sucrose (table sugar), fructose (fruit sugar, honey), maltose (malt sugar), and lactose (milk sugar). Simple carbohydrates provide much of the sweetness in foods. They are found naturally in fruits and milk and are added to soft drinks, fruit drinks, candy, and sweet desserts. There is no evidence that any type of simple carbohydrate is more nutritious than others.

*Complex carbohydrates* include starches and most types of dietary fiber. Starches are found in a variety of plants, especially grains (wheat, rye, rice, oats, barley, and millet), legumes (dried beans, peas, and lentils), and tubers (potatoes and yams). Most other vegetables contain a mix of complex and simple carbohydrates. Fiber, which is discussed later in this chapter, is found in fruits, vegetables, and grains.

During digestion, your body breaks down carbohydrates into simple sugar molecules, such as **glucose**, for absorption. Once glucose is in the bloodstream, the

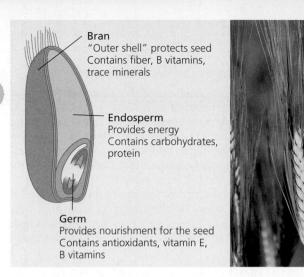

**FIGURE 8.2   The parts of a whole grain kernel.**

pancreas releases the hormone insulin, which allows cells to take up glucose and use it for energy. The liver and muscles also take up glucose and store it in the form of a starch called **glycogen.** The muscles use glucose from glycogen as fuel during endurance events or long workouts.

**Refined Carbohydrates Versus Whole Grains** Complex carbohydrates can be further divided between refined, or processed, carbohydrates and unrefined carbohydrates, or whole grains. Before they are processed, all grains are **whole grains,** consisting of an inner layer of germ, a middle layer called the endosperm, and an outer layer of bran (Figure 8.2). During processing, the germ and bran are often removed, leaving just the starchy endosperm. The refinement of whole grains transforms whole-wheat flour into white flour, brown rice into white rice, and so on.

Refined carbohydrates usually retain all the calories of their unrefined counterparts, but they tend to be much lower in fiber, vitamins, minerals, and other beneficial compounds. Refined grain products are often enriched or fortified with vitamins and minerals, but many of the nutrients lost in processing are not replaced.

Unrefined carbohydrates tend to take longer to chew and digest than refined ones; they also enter the bloodstream more slowly. This slower digestive pace tends to make people feel full sooner and for a longer period. Also, a slower rise in blood glucose levels following consumption of complex carbohydrates may help in the

management of diabetes. Whole grains are also high in dietary fiber (discussed later).

Consumption of whole grains has been linked to a reduced risk of heart disease, diabetes, high blood pressure, stroke, and certain forms of cancer. For all these reasons, whole grains are recommended over those that have been refined. This does not mean you should never eat refined carbohydrates such as white bread or white rice; it simply means that whole-wheat bread, brown rice, and other whole grains are healthier choices. See the box "Choosing More Whole-Grain Foods" for tips on increasing your intake of whole grains.

**Glycemic Index and Glycemic Response** Insulin and glucose levels rise following a meal or snack containing any type of carbohydrate. Some foods cause a quick and dramatic rise in glucose and insulin levels, while others have a slower, more moderate effect. A food that has a rapid effect on blood glucose levels is said to have a high **glycemic index.** The glycemic index of a food indicates the type of carbohydrate in that food. High-glycemic-index foods do not, as some popular diets claim, directly cause weight gain beyond the calories they contain.

Attempting to base food choices on glycemic index is a difficult task. Unrefined complex carbohydrates and high-fiber foods generally tend to have a lower glycemic index, but patterns are less clear for other types of foods. The fat content of a food also affects its glycemic index; the higher in fat a food is, the lower its effect on glucose levels. Ripeness, storage time, processing, and food preparation are other factors that can affect a food's glycemic index. The body's response to carbohydrates also depends on other factors, such as what other foods are consumed at the same time, as well as the individual's fitness status.

For people with particular health concerns, such as diabetes, glycemic index may be an important consideration in choosing foods. Still, it should not be the sole criterion for food choices. Carbohydrate choices (low versus high glycemic index) that replace dietary saturated fat may also be an important factor in determining the effects of diet on the risk of cardiovascular disease. Some unrefined grains, fruits, vegetables, and legumes are rich in nutrients, have a relatively low energy density, and have a

**carbohydrate**   An essential nutrient; sugars, starches, and dietary fiber are all carbohydrates.

**glucose**   A simple sugar that is the body's basic fuel.

**glycogen**   A starch stored in the liver and muscles.

**whole grain**   The entire edible portion of a grain (such as wheat, rice, or oats), including the germ, endosperm, and bran; processing removes parts of the grain, often leaving just the endosperm.

**glycemic index**   A measure of how a particular food affects blood glucose levels.

**KEY TERMS**

# Choosing More Whole-Grain Foods

## What Are Whole Grains?

The first step in increasing your intake of whole grains is to correctly identify them. The following are whole grains:

- whole wheat
- whole rye
- whole oats
- oatmeal

- whole-grain corn
- popcorn
- brown rice
- whole-grain barley

Other choices include bulgur (cracked wheat), millet, kasha (roasted buckwheat kernels), quinoa, wheat and rye berries, amaranth, wild rice, graham flour, whole-grain kamut, whole-grain spelt, and whole-grain triticale.

Wheat flour, unbleached flour, enriched flour, and degerminated corn meal are not whole grains. Wheat germ and wheat bran are also not whole grains, but they are the constituents of wheat typically left out when wheat is processed and so are healthier choices than regular wheat flour, which typically contains just the grain's endosperm.

## Checking Packages for Whole Grains

To find packaged foods—such as bread or pasta—that are rich in whole grains, read the list of ingredients and check for special health claims related to whole grains. The *first* item in the list of ingredients should be one of the whole grains in the preceding list. Product names and food color can be misleading. *When in doubt, always check the list of ingredients and make sure "whole" is the first word in the list.*

The U.S. Food and Drug Administration (FDA) allows manufacturers to include special health claims for foods that contain 51% or more whole-grain ingredients. Such products may contain a statement such as the following on their packaging:

- "Rich in whole grain"

- "Made with 100% whole grain"

- "Diets rich in whole-grain foods may help reduce the risk of heart disease and certain cancers."

However, many whole-grain products will not carry such claims. This is one more reason to check the ingredient list to make sure you're buying a product made from one or more whole grains.

---

low to moderate glycemic index. Your best bet, therefore, is to choose a variety of vegetables daily and limit refined grains as well as foods that are high in added sugars but low in other nutrients.

**Recommended Carbohydrate Intake** On average, Americans consume 200–300 grams of carbohydrate per day, well above the 130 grams needed to meet the body's requirement for essential carbohydrate. A range of intakes is associated with good health, and experts recommend that adults consume 45–65% of total daily calories as carbohydrate. (That's about 225–325 grams of carbohydrate for someone who consumes 2000 calories per day.) The focus should be on consuming a variety of foods rich in complex carbohydrates, especially whole grains.

Athletes in training can especially benefit from high-carbohydrate diets (60–70% of total daily calories), which enhance the amount of carbohydrates stored in their muscles as glycogen and therefore provide more carbohydrate fuel for use during endurance events or long workouts. Carbohydrates consumed during prolonged athletic events (often in the form of sports beverages) can help fuel muscles and extend the availability of the glycogen stored in muscles. Caution is in order, however, because overconsumption of carbohydrates can lead to feelings of fatigue and underconsumption of other nutrients.

Although the Food and Nutrition Board set an AMDR for added sugars of 25% or less of total daily calories,

many health experts recommend an even lower intake. (Recall that sugars are a form of carbohydrate.) World Health Organization guidelines suggest a limit of 10% of total daily calories from added sugars. Limits set by the U.S. Department of Agriculture (USDA) are even lower, with a maximum of about 8 teaspoons (32 grams) suggested for someone consuming 2000 calories per day. Foods high in added sugar are generally high in calories and low in nutrients and fiber, thus providing "empty" calories.

To reduce your intake of added sugars, limit soft drinks, candy, desserts, and sweetened fruit drinks. The simple carbohydrates in your diet shoulde come mainly from fruits, which are excellent sources of vitamins and minerals, and from low-fat or fat-free milk and other dairy products, which are high in protein and calcium.

## Fiber—A Closer Look

*Fiber* is the term given to nondigestible carbohydrates provided by plants. Instead of being digested, like starch, fiber moves through the intestinal tract and provides bulk for feces in the large intestine, which in turn facilitates elimination. In the large intestine, some types of fiber are broken down by bacteria into acids and gases, which explains why eating too much fiber-rich food can lead to intestinal gas. Even though humans don't digest fiber, it is necessary for good health.

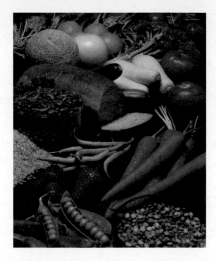

Fruits, vegetables, and whole grains are excellent sources of carbohydrates and fiber.

**Types of Dietary Fiber** The Food and Nutrition Board has defined two types of fiber:

- **Dietary fiber** is the nondigestible carbohydrates (and the noncarbohydrate substance lignin) that are present naturally in plants such as grains, legumes, and vegetables.
- **Functional fiber** is any nondigestible carbohydrate that has been either isolated from natural sources or synthesized in a lab and then added to a food product or supplement.
- **Total fiber** is the sum of dietary and functional fiber in a person's diet.

Fibers have different properties that lead to different physiological effects in the body. **Soluble (viscous) fiber** such as that found in oat bran or legumes can delay stomach emptying, slow the movement of glucose into the blood after eating, and reduce absorption of cholesterol. **Insoluble fiber**, such as that found in wheat bran or psyllium seed, increases fecal bulk and helps prevent constipation, hemorrhoids, and other digestive disorders.

A high-fiber diet can help reduce the risk of type 2 diabetes, heart disease, and pulmonary disease, as well as improve gastrointestinal health and aid in weight management. Some studies have linked high-fiber diets with a reduced risk of colon and rectal cancer. Other studies have suggested that other characteristics of diets rich in fruits, vegetables, and whole grains may be responsible for this reduction in risk.

**Sources of Fiber** All plant foods contain some dietary fiber. Fruits, legumes, oats (especially oat bran), and barley all contain the viscous types of fiber that help lower blood glucose and cholesterol levels. Wheat (especially wheat bran), cereals, grains, and vegetables are all good sources of cellulose and other fibers that help prevent

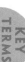

constipation. Psyllium, which is often added to cereals or used in fiber supplements and laxatives, improves intestinal health and also helps control glucose and cholesterol levels. The processing of packaged foods can remove fiber, so it's important to depend on fresh fruits and vegetables and foods made from whole grains as your main sources of fiber.

**Recommended Fiber Intake** To reduce the risk of chronic disease and maintain intestinal health, the Food and Nutrition Board recommends a daily fiber intake of 38 grams for adult men and 25 grams for adult women. Americans currently consume about half this amount. Fiber should come from foods, not supplements, which should be used only under medical supervision.

## Vitamins—Organic Micronutrients

**Vitamins** are organic (carbon-containing) substances required in small amounts to regulate various processes within living cells (Table 8.4). Humans need 13 vitamins; of these, four are fat-soluble (A, D, E, and K), and nine are water-soluble (C and the B-complex vitamins thiamin, riboflavin, niacin, vitamin B-6, folate, vitamin B-12, biotin, and pantothenic acid).

Solubility affects how a vitamin is absorbed, transported, and stored in the body. The water-soluble vitamins are absorbed directly into the bloodstream, where they travel freely. Excess water-soluble vitamins are removed by the kidneys and excreted in urine. Fat-soluble vitamins require a more complex absorptive process. They are usually carried in the blood by special proteins and are stored in the liver and in fat tissues rather than excreted.

**dietary fiber** Nondigestible carbohydrates and lignin that are intact in plants.

**functional fiber** Nondigestible carbohydrates either isolated from natural sources or synthesized; these may be added to foods and dietary supplements.

**total fiber** The total amount of dietary fiber and functional fiber in the diet.

**soluble (viscous) fiber** Fiber that dissolves in water or is broken down by bacteria in the large intestine.

**insoluble fiber** Fiber that does not dissolve in water and is not broken down by bacteria in the large intestine.

**vitamins** Carbon-containing substances needed in small amounts to help promote and regulate chemical reactions and processes in the body.

KEY TERMS

| Table 8.4 | Facts About Vitamins |

| VITAMIN | IMPORTANT DIETARY SOURCES | MAJOR FUNCTIONS | SIGNS OF PROLONGED DEFICIENCY | TOXIC EFFECTS OF MEGADOSES |
|---|---|---|---|---|
| **FAT-SOLUBLE** | | | | |
| Vitamin A | Liver, milk, butter, cheese, fortified margarine; carrots, spinach, and other orange and deep green vegetables and fruits | Maintenance of vision, skin, linings of the nose, mouth, digestive and urinary tracts, immune function | Night blindness; dry, scaling skin; increased susceptibility to infection; loss of appetite; anemia; kidney stones | Liver damage, miscarriage and birth defects, headache, vomiting and diarrhea, vertigo, double vision, bone abnormalities |
| Vitamin D | Fortified milk and margarine, fish oils, butter, egg yolks (sunlight on skin also produces vitamin D) | Development and maintenance of bones and teeth; promotion of calcium absorption | Rickets (bone deformities) in children; bone softening, loss, fractures in adults | Kidney damage, calcium deposits in soft tissues, depression, death |
| Vitamin E | Vegetable oils, whole grains, nuts and seeds, green leafy vegetables, asparagus, peaches | Protection and maintenance of cellular membranes | Red blood cell breakage and anemia, weakness, neurological problems, muscle cramps | Relatively nontoxic, but may cause excess bleeding or formation of blood clots |
| Vitamin K | Green leafy vegetables; smaller amounts widespread in other foods | Production of factors essential for blood clotting and bone metabolism | Hemorrhaging | None reported |
| **WATER-SOLUBLE** | | | | |
| Biotin | Cereals, yeast, egg yolks, soy flour, liver; widespread in foods | Synthesis of fat, glycogen, and amino acids | Rash, nausea, vomiting, weight loss, depression, fatigue, hair loss | None reported |
| Folate | Green leafy vegetables, yeast, oranges, whole grains, legumes, liver | Amino acid metabolism, synthesis of RNA and DNA, new cell synthesis | Anemia, weakness, fatigue, irritability, shortness of breath, swollen tongue | Masking of vitamin B-12 deficiency |
| Niacin | Eggs, poultry, fish, milk, whole grains, nuts, enriched breads and cereals, meats, legumes | Conversion of carbohydrates, fats, and proteins into usable forms of energy | Pellagra (symptoms include diarrhea, dermatitis, inflammation of mucous membranes, dementia) | Flushing of skin, nausea, vomiting, diarrhea, liver dysfunction, glucose intolerance |
| Pantothenic acid | Animal foods, whole grains, broccoli, potatoes; widespread in foods | Metabolism of fats, carbohydrates, and proteins | Fatigue, numbness and tingling of hands and feet, gastrointestinal disturbances | None reported |
| Riboflavin | Dairy products, enriched breads and cereals, lean meats, poultry, fish, green vegetables | Energy metabolism; maintenance of skin, mucous membranes, nervous system structures | Cracks at corners of mouth, sore throat, skin rash, hypersensitivity to light, purple tongue | None reported |
| Thiamin | Whole-grain and enriched breads and cereals, organ meats, lean pork, nuts, legumes | Conversion of carbohydrates into usable forms of energy; maintenance of appetite and nervous system function | Beriberi (symptoms include muscle wasting, mental confusion, anorexia, enlarged heart, nerve changes) | None reported |
| Vitamin B-6 | Eggs, poultry, fish, whole grains, nuts, soybeans, liver, kidney, pork | Metabolism of amino acids and glycogen | Anemia, convulsions, cracks at corners of mouth, dermatitis, nausea, confusion | Neurological abnormalities and damage |
| Vitamin B-12 | Meat, fish, poultry, fortified cereals | Synthesis of blood cells; other metabolic reactions | Anemia, fatigue, nervous system damage, sore tongue | None reported |
| Vitamin C | Peppers, broccoli, brussels sprouts, spinach, citrus fruits, strawberries, tomatoes, potatoes, cabbage, other fruits and vegetables | Maintenance and repair of connective tissue, bones, teeth, cartilage; promotion of healing; aid in iron absorption | Scurvy, anemia, reduced resistance to infection, loosened teeth, joint pain, poor wound healing, hair loss, poor iron absorption | Urinary stones in some people, acid stomach from ingesting supplements in pill form, nausea, diarrhea, headache, fatigue |

**SOURCES:** Food and Nutrition Board, Institute of Medicine. 2006. *Dietary Reference Intakes: The Essential Guide to Nutrient Requirements.* Washington, D.C.: National Academies Press. The complete Dietary Reference Intake reports are available from the National Academies Press (http://www.nap.edu). Shils, M. E., et al., eds. 2005. *Modern Nutrition in Health and Disease,* 10th ed. Baltimore: Lippincott Williams and Wilkins.

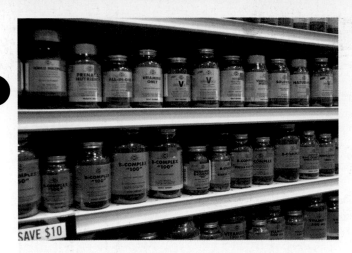
Vitamin and mineral supplements are popular, but they are not usually necessary for healthy people who eat a balanced diet.

**Functions of Vitamins** Many vitamins help chemical reactions take place. They provide no energy to the body directly but help unleash the energy stored in carbohydrates, proteins, and fats. Other vitamins are critical in the production of red blood cells and the maintenance of the nervous, skeletal, and immune systems. Some vitamins act as **antioxidants**, which help preserve the health of cells. Key vitamin antioxidants include vitamin E, vitamin C, and the vitamin A precursor beta-carotene. (Antioxidants are described later in the chapter.)

**Sources of Vitamins** The human body does not manufacture most of the vitamins it requires and must obtain them from foods. Vitamins are abundant in fruits, vegetables, and grains. In addition, many processed foods, such as flour and breakfast cereals, contain added vitamins. A few vitamins are made in certain parts of the body: The skin makes vitamin D when it is exposed to sunlight, and intestinal bacteria make vitamin K. Nonetheless, you still need to get vitamin D and vitamin K from foods (see Table 8.4).

**Vitamin Deficiencies and Excesses** If your diet lacks a particular vitamin, characteristic symptoms of deficiency can develop (see Table 8.4). For example, vitamin A deficiency can cause blindness, and vitamin B-12 deficiency can cause anemia. Vitamin deficiency diseases are most often seen in developing countries; they are relatively rare in the United States because vitamins are readily available from our food supply. However, intakes below recommended levels can have adverse effects on health even if they are not low enough to cause a deficiency disease. For example, low intake of folate increases a woman's chance of giving birth to a baby with a neural tube defect (a congenital malformation of the central nervous system). Low intake of folate and vitamins B-6 and B-12 has been linked to increased heart disease risk. A great deal of recent research has focused on vitamin D, suggesting that vitamin D supplementation can reduce the risk of cardiovascular disease and linking low vitamin D levels to an increased risk of several cancers. As important as vitamins are, however, many Americans consume less-than-recommended amounts of some vitamins.

Extra vitamins in the diet can be harmful, especially when taken as supplements. Megadoses of fat-soluble vitamins are particularly dangerous because the excess is stored in the body rather than excreted, increasing the risk of toxicity. Even when supplements are not taken in excess, relying on them for an adequate intake of vitamins can be problematic. There are many substances in foods other than vitamins and minerals, and some of these compounds may have important health effects. Later, this chapter discusses specific recommendations for vitamin intake and when a supplement is advisable. For now, keep in mind that it's best to get most of your vitamins from foods rather than supplements.

The vitamins and minerals in foods can be easily lost or destroyed during storage or cooking. To retain their value, eat or process vegetables immediately after buying them. If you can't do this, store them in a cool place, covered to retain moisture—either in the refrigerator (for a few days) or in the freezer (for a longer term). To reduce nutrient losses during food preparation, minimize the amount of water used and the total cooking time. Develop a taste for a crunchier texture in cooked vegetables. Baking, steaming, broiling, grilling, and microwaving are all good methods of preparing vegetables.

## Minerals—Inorganic Micronutrients

**Minerals** are inorganic (non-carbon-containing) elements you need in relatively small amounts to help regulate body functions, aid in the growth and maintenance of body tissues, and help release energy (Table 8.5). There are about 17 essential minerals. The major minerals, those that the body needs in amounts exceeding 100 milligrams per day, include calcium, phosphorus, magnesium, sodium, potassium, and chloride. The essential trace minerals, which you need in minute amounts, include copper, fluoride, iodine, iron, selenium, and zinc.

Characteristic symptoms develop if an essential mineral is consumed in a quantity too small or too large for good health. The minerals commonly lacking in the American diet are iron, calcium, magnesium, and potassium. Iron-deficiency **anemia** is a problem in some

**antioxidant** A substance that protects against the breakdown of food or body constituents by free radicals; antioxidants' actions include binding oxygen, donating electrons to free radicals, and repairing damage to molecules.

**minerals** Inorganic compounds needed in relatively small amounts for the regulation, growth, and maintenance of body tissues and functions.

**anemia** A deficiency in the oxygen-carrying material in the red blood cells.

KEY TERMS

**Table 8.5** Facts About Selected Minerals

| MINERAL | IMPORTANT DIETARY SOURCES | MAJOR FUNCTIONS | SIGNS OF PROLONGED DEFICIENCY | TOXIC EFFECTS OF MEGADOSES |
|---|---|---|---|---|
| Calcium | Milk and milk products, tofu, fortified orange juice and bread, green leafy vegetables, bones in fish | Formation of bones and teeth; control of nerve impulses, muscle contraction, blood clotting | Stunted growth in children, bone mineral loss in adults; urinary stones | Kidney stones, calcium deposits in soft tissues, inhibition of mineral absorption, constipation |
| Fluoride | Fluoridated water, tea, marine fish eaten with bones | Maintenance of tooth and bone structure | Higher frequency of tooth decay | Increased bone density, mottling of teeth, impaired kidney function |
| Iodine | Iodized salt, seafood, processed foods | Essential part of thyroid hormones, regulation of body metabolism | Goiter (enlarged thyroid), cretinism (birth defect) | Depression of thyroid activity, hyperthyroidism in susceptible people |
| Iron | Meat and poultry, fortified grain products, dark green vegetables, dried fruit | Component of hemoglobin, myoglobin, and enzymes | Iron-deficiency anemia, weakness, impaired immune function, gastrointestinal distress | Nausea, diarrhea, liver and kidney damage, joint pains, sterility, disruption of cardiac function, death |
| Magnesium | Widespread in foods and water (except soft water); especially found in grains, legumes, nuts, seeds, green vegetables, milk | Transmission of nerve impulses, energy transfer, activation of many enzymes | Neurological disturbances, cardiovascular problems, kidney disorders, nausea, growth failure in children | Nausea, vomiting, diarrhea, central nervous system depression, coma; death in people with impaired kidney function |
| Phosphorus | Present in nearly all foods, especially milk, cereal, peas, eggs, meat | Bone growth and maintenance, energy transfer in cells | Impaired growth, weakness, kidney disorders, cardio-respiratory and nervous system dysfunction | Drop in blood calcium levels, calcium deposits in soft tissues, bone loss |
| Potassium | Meats, milk, fruits, vegetables, grains, legumes | Nerve function and body water balance | Muscular weakness, nausea, drowsiness, paralysis, confusion, disruption of cardiac rhythm | Cardiac arrest |
| Selenium | Seafood, meat, eggs, whole grains | Defense against oxidative stress; regulation of thyroid hormone action | Muscle pain and weakness, heart disorders | Hair and nail loss, nausea and vomiting, weakness, irritability |
| Sodium | Salt, soy sauce, fast food, processed foods, especially lunch meats, canned soups and vegetables, salty snacks, processed cheese | Body water balance, acid-base balance, nerve function | Muscle weakness, loss of appetite, nausea, vomiting; deficiency rarely seen | Edema, hypertension in sensitive people |
| Zinc | Whole grains, meat, eggs, liver, seafood (especially oysters) | Synthesis of proteins, RNA, and DNA; wound healing; immune response; ability to taste | Growth failure, loss of appetite, impaired taste acuity, skin rash, impaired immune function, poor wound healing | Vomiting, impaired immune function, decline in blood HDL levels, impaired copper absorption |

**SOURCES:** Food and Nutrition Board, Institute of Medicine. 2006. *Dietary Reference Intakes: The Essential Guide to Nutrient Requirements.* Washington, D.C.: National Academies Press. The complete Dietary Reference Intake reports are available from the National Academies Press (http://www.nap.edu). Shils, M. E., et al., eds. 2005. *Modern Nutrition in Health and Disease,* 10th ed. Baltimore: Lippincott Williams and Wilkins.

age groups, and researchers fear poor calcium intakes in childhood are sowing the seeds for future **osteoporosis**, especially in women. See the box "Eating for Healthy Bones" to learn more.

## Water—Vital but Often Ignored

Water is the major component in both foods and the human body: You are composed of about 50–60% water. Your need for other nutrients, in terms of weight, is much less than your need for water. You can live up to 50 days without food but only a few days without water.

Water is distributed all over the body, among lean and other tissues and in blood and other body fluids. Water is used in the digestion and absorption of food and is the medium in which most chemical reactions take place within the body. Some water-based fluids, such as blood, transport substances around the body; other fluids serve as lubricants or cushions. Water also helps regulate body temperature.

# Eating for Healthy Bones

Osteoporosis is a condition in which the bones become dangerously thin and fragile over time. An estimated 10 million Americans over age 50 have osteoporosis, and another 34 million are at risk. Women account for about 80% of osteoporosis cases.

Most bone mass is built by age 18. After bone density peaks between ages 25 and 35, bone mass is lost over time. To prevent osteoporosis, the best strategy is to build as much bone as possible during your youth and do everything you can to maintain it as you age. Up to 50% of bone loss is determined by controllable lifestyle factors such as diet and exercise. Key nutrients for bone health include the following:

- **Calcium.** Getting enough calcium is important throughout life to build and maintain bone mass. Milk, yogurt, and calcium-fortified orange juice, bread, and cereals are all good sources.

- **Vitamin D.** Vitamin D is necessary for bones to absorb calcium; a daily intake of 600 IU is recommended for individuals age 1–70. Vitamin D can be obtained from foods and is manufactured by the skin when exposed to sunlight. Candidates for vitamin D supplements include people who don't eat many foods rich in vitamin D; those who don't expose their face, arms, and hands to the sun (without sunscreen) for 5–15 minutes a few times each week; and people who live north of an imaginary line drawn across the United States from Boston to the Oregon-California border (where the sun is weaker).

- **Vitamin K.** Vitamin K promotes the synthesis of proteins that help keep bones strong. Broccoli and leafy green vegetables are rich in vitamin K.

- **Other nutrients.** Other nutrients that may play an important role in bone health include vitamin C, magnesium, potassium, phosphorus, fluoride, manganese, zinc, copper, and boron.

Several dietary substances may have a *negative* effect on bone health, especially if consumed in excess. These include alcohol, sodium, caffeine, and retinol (a form of vitamin A). Drinking lots of soda, which often replaces milk in the diet, has been shown to increase the risk of bone fracture in teenage girls.

The effect of protein intake on bone mass depends on other nutrients: Protein helps build bone as long as calcium and vitamin D intake are adequate. But if intake of calcium and vitamin D is low, high protein intake can lead to bone loss.

Weight-bearing aerobic exercise helps maintain bone mass throughout life, and strength training improves bone density, muscle mass, strength, and balance. Drinking alcohol only in moderation, refraining from smoking, and managing depression and stress are also important for maintaining strong bones. For people who develop osteoporosis, a variety of medications are available to treat the condition.

---

Water is contained in almost all foods, particularly in liquids, fruits, and vegetables. The foods and fluids you consume provide 80–90% of your daily water intake; the remainder is generated through metabolism. You lose water each day in urine, feces, and sweat and through evaporation from your lungs.

Most people can maintain a healthy water balance by consuming beverages at meals and drinking fluids in response to thirst. The Food and Nutrition Board has set levels of adequate water intake to maintain hydration. All fluids, including those containing caffeine, can count toward your total daily fluid intake. Under these guidelines, men need to consume about 3.7 total liters of water, with 3.0 liters (about 13 cups) coming from beverages; women need 2.7 total liters, with 2.2 liters (about 9 cups) coming from beverages. About 20% of daily water intake comes from food. (See Table 1 in the Nutrition Resources section

at the end of the chapter for recommendations for specific age groups.) If you exercise vigorously or live in a hot climate, you need to consume additional fluids to maintain a balance between water consumed and water lost. Severe dehydration causes weakness and can lead to death.

## Other Substances in Food

Many substances in food are not essential nutrients but may influence health.

**Antioxidants** When the body uses oxygen or breaks down certain fats or proteins as a normal part of metabolism, it gives rise to substances called **free radicals**. Environmental factors such as cigarette smoke, exhaust fumes, radiation, excessive sunlight, certain drugs, and stress can increase free radical production. A free radical is a

---

### Fitness Tip

Drink plenty of water before, during, and after workouts, especially when the weather is warm. Proper hydration helps you avoid cramps and heat-related problems such as heat stroke.

---

**osteoporosis** A condition in which the bones become extremely thin and brittle and break easily; due largely to insufficient calcium intake.

**free radical** An electron-seeking compound that can react with fats, proteins, and DNA, damaging cell membranes and mutating genes in its search for electrons; produced through chemical reactions in the body and by exposure to environmental factors such as sunlight and tobacco smoke.

Experts say that two of the most important factors in a healthy diet are eating the "right" kinds of carbohydrates and eating the "right" kinds of fats. Based on what you've read so far in this chapter, which are the "right" carbohydrates and the "right" fats? How would you say your own diet stacks up when it comes to carbs and fats?

chemically unstable molecule that reacts with fats, proteins, and DNA, damaging cell membranes and mutating genes. Free radicals have been implicated in aging, cancer, cardiovascular disease, and other degenerative diseases like arthritis.

Antioxidants found in foods can help protect the body by blocking the formation and action of free radicals and repairing the damage they cause. Some antioxidants, such as vitamin C, vitamin E, and selenium, are also essential nutrients. Others—such as carotenoids, found in yellow, orange, and dark green leafy vegetables—are not. Researchers recently identified the top antioxidant-containing foods and beverages as blackberries, walnuts, strawberries, artichokes, cranberries, brewed coffee, raspberries, pecans, blueberries, cloves, grape juice, unsweetened baking chocolate, sour cherries, and red wine. Also high in antioxidants are brussels sprouts, kale, cauliflower, and pomegranates.

**Phytochemicals** Antioxidants fall into the broader category of **phytochemicals**, substances found in plant foods that may help prevent chronic disease. In the past 30 years, researchers have identified and studied hundreds of different compounds found in foods, and many findings are promising. For example, certain substances found in soy foods may help lower cholesterol levels. Sulforaphane, a compound isolated from broccoli and other **cruciferous vegetables**, may render some carcinogenic compounds harmless. Allyl sulfides, a group of chemicals found in garlic and onions, appear to boost the activity of cancer-fighting immune cells. Carotenoids found in green vegetables may help preserve eyesight with age. Further research on phytochemicals may extend the role of nutrition to the prevention and treatment of many chronic diseases.

To increase your intake of phytochemicals, eat a variety of fruits, vegetables, and grains rather than relying on supplements. Like many vitamins and minerals, isolated phytochemicals may be harmful if taken in high doses. In many cases, their health benefits may be the result of chemical substances working in combination. The role of phytochemicals in disease prevention is discussed further in Chapters 11 and 12.

# NUTRITIONAL GUIDELINES: PLANNING YOUR DIET

Various tools have been created by scientific and government groups to help people design healthy diets:

- The **Dietary Reference Intakes (DRIs)** are standards for nutrient intake designed to prevent nutritional deficiencies and reduce the risk of chronic diseases.
- The **Dietary Guidelines for Americans** were established to promote health and reduce the risk of major chronic diseases through diet and physical activity.
- **MyPlate** (formerly MyPyramid) provides daily food intake patterns that meet the DRIs and are consistent with the Dietary Guidelines for Americans.

## Dietary Reference Intakes (DRIs)

The Food and Nutrition Board establishes dietary standards, or recommended intake levels, for Americans of all ages. The current set of standards, called Dietary Reference Intakes (DRIs), was introduced in 1997. The DRIs are frequently reviewed and are updated as substantial new nutrition-related information becomes available. The DRIs present different categories of nutrients in easy-to-read table format. The DRIs have a broad focus, being based on research that looks not just at the prevention of nutrient deficiencies but also at the role of nutrients in promoting health and preventing chronic diseases such as cancer, osteoporosis, and heart disease.

The DRIs include standards for both recommended intakes and maximum safe intakes. The recommended intake of each nutrient is expressed as either a *Recommended Dietary Allowance (RDA)* or as *Adequate Intake (AI)*. An AI is set when there is not enough information available to set an RDA value; regardless of the type of standard used, however, the DRI represents the best available estimate of intake for optimal health. The Estimated Average Requirement (EAR) is the average daily nutrient intake level estimated to meet the requirement of half the healthy individuals in a particular life stage and gender group. The *Tolerable Upper Intake Level (UL)* is the maximum daily intake that is unlikely to cause health problems in a healthy person. For example, the RDA for calcium for an 18-year-old female is 1300 milligrams (mg) per day; the UL is 3000 milligrams per day.

Because of a lack of data, ULs have not been set for all nutrients. This does not mean that people can tolerate long-term intakes of these vitamins and minerals above recommended levels. Like all chemical agents, nutrients can produce adverse effects if intakes are excessive. There is no established benefit from consuming nutrients at levels above the RDA or AI. The DRIs can be found in the Nutrition Resources section at the end of the chapter.

**Daily Values** Because the DRIs are too cumbersome to use as a basis for food labels, the FDA developed another set of dietary standards, the **Daily Values**. The Daily Values are based on several different sets of guidelines and include standards for fat, cholesterol, carbohydrate, dietary fiber, and selected vitamins and minerals. The Daily Values represent appropriate intake levels for a 2000-calorie diet. The percent Daily Value shown on a food label shows how well that food contributes to your recommended daily intake. Food labels are described in detail later in the chapter.

**Should You Take Supplements?** The aim of the DRIs is to guide you in meeting your nutritional needs primarily with food, rather than with vitamin and mineral supplements. Supplements lack potentially beneficial phytochemicals and fiber that are found only in whole foods. Most Americans can get the vitamins and minerals they need by eating a varied, nutritionally balanced diet.

The question of whether to take supplements is a serious one. Some vitamins and minerals are dangerous when ingested in excess, as described previously in Tables 8.4 and 8.5. Large doses of particular nutrients can also cause health problems by affecting the absorption of other vitamins and minerals. For all these reasons, you should think carefully about whether to take high-dose supplements; consider consulting a physician or registered dietitian.

Over the past two decades, high-dose supplement use has been promoted as a way to prevent or delay the onset of many diseases, including heart disease and several forms of cancer. These claims remain controversial, however, and a growing body of research shows that vitamin or mineral supplements have no significant impact on the risk of developing such illnesses. For example, a 2008 study conducted as part of the Women's Health Initiative showed no differences in the levels of heart disease, cancer, or overall mortality between postmenopausal women who took multivitamin supplements and those who did not. A similar study of adult men indicated that taking vitamins C and E did not reduce the risk of heart disease or certain cancers. According to the experts behind these and other studies, the research provides further proof that a balanced diet of whole foods—not high-dose supplementation—is the best way to promote health and prevent disease.

In setting the DRIs, the Food and Nutrition Board recommended supplements of particular nutrients for the following groups:

- Women who are capable of becoming pregnant should take 400 micrograms (μg) per day of folic

acid (the synthetic form of the vitamin folate) from fortified foods and/or supplements in addition to folate from a varied diet. Research indicates that this level of folate intake will reduce the risk of neural tube defects. Enriched breads, flours, corn meals, rice, noodles, and other grain products are fortified with folic acid. Folate is found naturally in green leafy vegetables, legumes, oranges, and strawberries.

- People over age 50 should eat foods fortified with vitamin B-12, take B-12 supplements, or both to meet the majority of the DRI of 2.4 micrograms of B-12 daily. Up to 30% of people over 50 may have problems absorbing protein-bound B-12 in foods.

- Because of the oxidative stress caused by smoking, smokers should get 35 milligrams *more* vitamin C per day than the RDA set for their age and sex. However, supplements are not usually needed because this extra vitamin C can easily be found in foods. For example, an 8-ounce glass of orange juice has about 100 mg of vitamin C.

Supplements may also be recommended in other cases. Women with heavy menstrual flows may need extra iron. Older people, people with dark skin, and people exposed to little sunlight may need extra vitamin D. Some vegetarians may need supplemental calcium, iron, zinc, and vitamin B-12, depending on their food choices. Other people may benefit from supplementation based on their lifestyle, physical condition, medicines, or dietary habits.

Before deciding whether to take a vitamin or mineral supplement, consider whether you already eat a fortified breakfast cereal every day. Many breakfast cereals contain almost as many nutrients as a multivitamin pill. If you

---

---

**Wellness Tip**

If you take a supplement, *never* take more than the recommended dosage unless your doctor tells you to.

---

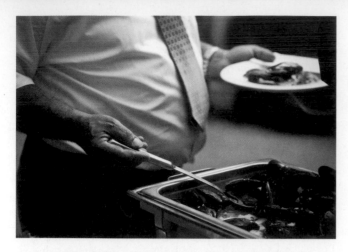

Food choices and portion control are key factors in weight management.

elect to take a supplement, choose one that contains 50–100% of the Daily Value for vitamins and minerals. Avoid supplements containing large doses of nutrients that may be harmful.

## Dietary Guidelines for Americans

To provide general guidance for choosing a healthy diet, the USDA and the U.S. Department of Health and Human Services (DHHS) jointly issue the Dietary Guidelines for Americans, updating and revising the guidelines every 5 years. The guidelines are intended for all Americans aged 2 and older. Following these guidelines promotes health and reduces the risk of chronic diseases, including heart disease, cancer, diabetes, stroke, osteoporosis, and obesity. Each of the recommendations is supported by an extensive review of scientific and medical evidence.

The 2010 Dietary Guidelines highlight four areas. First, because the majority of Americans are overweight or obese, the guidelines focus on ways to balance calorie consumption and calorie expenditure to manage weight. Second, because Americans also tend to consume too many calories without getting enough of certain nutrients, the guidelines focus on foods to reduce in the diet (the second highlighted area) and foods to increase in the diet (the third highlighted area). Finally, the guidelines focus on ways to incorporate the recommendations into overall healthy eating patterns. Specific recommendations for putting the Dietary Guidelines into practice are provided in MyPlate (discussed in the next section).

**Balancing Calories to Manage Weight** Calorie balance—the balance between calories consumed and calories expended—is the key to weight management. Current high rates of overweight and obesity can be attributed at least in part to people consuming more calories in foods and beverages than they expend in physical activity.

The guidelines recognize that many aspects of American life promote obesity, leading to an "obesogenic food environment." Factors contributing to this environment include an increase in the number of fast-food restaurants in communities, an increase in meals eaten outside the home, increased portion sizes, sedentary work and home environments, limited availability of safe outdoor walking and recreational spaces, and increased dependence on transportation and technological advances that lead to lower calorie expenditure on everyday tasks.

Still, managing body weight means that individuals need to control total calorie intake, and for people who are overweight or obese, this means consuming fewer calories from foods and beverages. The guidelines encourage people to become more conscious of what, when, why, and how much they eat; to deliberately make better choices; and to seek ways to be more physically active. Several specific behaviors and practices can help people manage their calorie balance and maintain a healthy weight. Recommendations include:

- Know what calorie level is appropriate for you at your current level of activity, and be aware of how many calories you are consuming.

- Cook at home more and eat out less, and when you do eat out, eat smaller portions and lower-calorie options.

- Limit screen time, whether watching television, playing games, or using a computer, and don't eat when watching TV.

**Foods and Food Components to Reduce** In addition to overall calories, Americans tend to consume certain foods and food components in excess—in particular, sodium, solid fats, added sugars, and refined grains. These foods often replace needed nutrients in the diet. Key recommendations include:

- Reduce daily sodium intake to less than 2300 mg, and further reduce intake to 1500 mg if you are 51 or older, are African American, or have hypertension, diabetes, or chronic kidney disease. The 1500 mg recommendation applies to about half the U.S. population, including children, and the majority of adults. The average intake of sodium for all Americans is estimated at 3400 mg; for boys and men between the ages of 12 and 50, it is estimated at more than 4000 mg. High sodium intake is associated with high blood pressure. Most salt in the diet comes from salt added during food processing.

- Limit intake of saturated fat, trans fat, and dietary cholesterol. Consume less than 10% of calories from saturated fats by replacing them with monounsaturated and polyunsaturated fats. Keep trans fatty acid consumption as low as possible, especially by limiting foods that contain synthetic sources of trans fats, such as partially hydrogenated oils. (See the

| Nutrient | Recommended Daily Intake* 2000 calories | Orange Juice 168 calories % Daily | Nutrient value | Low-Fat (1%) Milk 150 calories % Daily | Nutrient value | Regular Cola 152 calories % Daily | Nutrient value | Bottled Iced Tea 150 calories % Daily | Nutrient value |
|---|---|---|---|---|---|---|---|---|---|
| Carbohydrate | 300 g | 14% | 40.5 g | 6% | 18 g | 13% | 38 g | 13% | 37.5 g |
| Added sugars | 32 g | | | | | 119% | 38 g + | 108% | 34.5 g + |
| Fat | 65 g | | | 6% | 3.9 g | | | | |
| Protein | 55 g | | | 22% | 12 g | | | | |
| Calcium | 1000 mg | 3% | 33 mg | 45% | 450 mg | 1% | 11 mg | | |
| Potassium | 4700 mg | 15% | 710 mg | 12% | 570 mg | <1% | 4 mg | | |
| Vitamin A | 700 µg | 4% | 30 µg | 31% | 216 µg | | | | |
| Vitamin C | 75 mg | 193% | 145.5 mg + | 5% | 3.6 mg | | | | |
| Vitamin D | 5 µg | | | 74% | 3.7 µg | | | | |
| Folate | 400 µg | 40% | 160 µg | 5% | 20 µg | | | | |

Bars show percentage of recommended daily intake or limit

+ = Greater than 100% of recommended

*Recommended intakes and limits appropriate for a 20-year-old woman consuming 2000 calories per day.

**FIGURE 8.3** **Nutrient density of 12-ounce portions of selected beverages.**
Color bars represent percentage of recommended daily intake or limit for each nutrient.

box "Reducing the Saturated and Trans Fats in Your Diet" for more information.) Consume less than 300 mg per day of dietary cholesterol.

- Reduce the intake of calories from solid fats and added sugars. Together, solid fats and added sugars contribute about 35% of the calories consumed by Americans, without contributing many nutrients. Most people should consume no more than 5–15% of daily calories from foods in these categories. Suggestions include limiting the amount of solid fats and added sugars when cooking and eating; consuming smaller and fewer portions of foods and beverages with these components, such as desserts and sodas; and eating the most nutrient-dense forms of foods in all food groups. Sodas, energy drinks, and sports drinks are the biggest source of added sugars in the American diet. The differences in nutrients between soda and other beverages are shown in Figure 8.3.

- Limit the consumption of foods that contain refined grains, especially refined grain foods that contain solid fats, added sugars, and sodium.

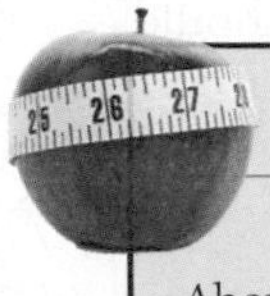

## Wellness Tip

About a dozen major American cities, and the entire state of California, have enacted laws restricting the use of trans fats in commercially prepared foods.

- If alcohol is consumed, it should be consumed in moderation.

**Foods and Nutrients to Increase** In general, Americans don't eat a wide enough variety of nutrient-dense foods to obtain all the nutrients they need for optimal health. Recommendations include:

- Eat more fruits and vegetables, and eat a variety of vegetables, especially dark green, red, and orange vegetables and beans and peas. These foods are major sources of many nutrients that are underconsumed by many Americans, and they are relatively low in calories (unless prepared with added fats and sugars).

- Consume at least half of all grains as whole grains, which are a source of important nutrients such as iron, B vitamins, and dietary fiber.

- Increase intake of fat-free and low-fat milk and milk products, such as milk, yogurt, cheese, and fortified soy beverages. These foods are important sources of calcium, potassium, magnesium, vitamin D, and vitamin A. Milk and yogurt are preferable to cheese, which has more solid fat and more calories.

- Choose a variety of protein foods, including seafood, lean meat and poultry, eggs, beans and peas, soy products, and unsalted nuts and seeds. Increase the amount and variety of seafood, and reduce protein foods that are high in solid fats and calories. In addition to protein, these foods provide B vitamins,

**TAKE CHARGE**

Your overall goal is to limit total fat intake to no more than 35% of total calories. Favor unsaturated fats over saturated and trans fats. Here are some steps that can help reduce these types of fat in your diet:

- Be moderate in your consumption of foods high in fat, including fast foods, commercially prepared baked goods and desserts, deep-fried food, meat, poultry, nuts and seeds, and regular dairy products.

- When you eat high-fat foods, limit your portion sizes, and balance your intake with other foods that are low in fat.

- Choose lean cuts of meat, and trim any visible fat from meat before and after cooking. Remove skin from poultry before or after cooking.

- Drink fat-free or low-fat milk instead of whole milk, and use lower-fat milk when cooking or baking. Substitute plain low-fat yogurt, low-fat cottage cheese, or buttermilk for sour cream.

- Use vegetable oil instead of butter or margarine. Use tub or squeeze margarine instead of stick margarine. Look for margarines that are free of trans fats. Minimize intake of coconut or palm oil.

- Season vegetables, seafood, and meats with herbs and spices rather than with creamy sauces, butter, or margarine.

- Use olive oil and lemon juice on salad, or use a yogurt-based salad dressing instead of mayonnaise or sour cream dressings.

- Steam, boil, bake, or microwave vegetables, or stir-fry them in a small amount of vegetable oil.

- Roast, bake, or broil meat, poultry, or fish so that fat drains away as the food cooks.

- Use a nonstick pan for cooking so that added fat will be unnecessary; use a vegetable spray for frying.

- Substitute egg whites for whole eggs when baking; limit the number of egg yolks when scrambling eggs.

- Choose fruits as desserts most often.

- Eat a low-fat vegetarian main dish at least once a week.

---

vitamin E, zinc, and magnesium. Seafood provides a range of nutrients, notably omega-3 fatty acids, which are associated with reduced risk of heart disease. (Seafood consumption is discussed in more detail later in the chapter.)

- Replace solid fats with oils where possible. Oils should not be added to the diet in addition to solid fats; instead, they should replace them.

- Because most Americans do not get enough potassium, dietary fiber, calcium, or vitamin D in their diet, they should consume more foods that contain these nutrients.

  - Potassium, which can help lower blood pressure, is found in many fruits, vegetables, and milk products. Recommended intake is 4700 mg per day.

  - Dietary fiber is found in beans and peas, other vegetables, fruits, nuts, and whole grains. Recommended daily intake for fiber is 25 g for women and 38 g for men; the current average daily intake is only about 15 g.

  - Calcium plays several important roles in health, including bone health. Low intake of calcium is a concern in children 9 and older, adolescent girls, adult women, and all adults age 51 and older. The chief sources of calcium in the diet are milk and milk products.

  - Vitamin D also has an important role in bone health. Chief sources are fortified foods, especially milk and yogurt.

- Other nutrients are a concern for certain special population groups, such as folic acid for women who may become pregnant.

**Building Healthy Eating Patterns** There are many different ways to incorporate the recommendations of the 2010 Dietary Guidelines into healthy eating patterns that (1) meet nutrient needs; (2) stay within calorie limits; (3) accommodate cultural, ethnic, traditional, and personal preferences; and (4) consider food cost and availability. In other words, people can eat healthfully in many different ways. Currently, however, there is a large discrepancy between the guidelines and the actual American diet.

Three eating plans that show how to put the Dietary Guidelines recommendations into action are the USDA Food Pattern (MyPlate), vegetarian adaptations of the USDA Food Pattern, and the DASH Eating Plan. (MyPlate and vegetarian diets are discussed later in the chapter, and the DASH Eating Plan is explained in the Nutrition Resources section at the end of this chapter.) A general principle in all these diets is that people should eat nutrient-dense foods—foods with little or no solid fats and added sugars. Another principle is that people should get their nutrients from foods rather than from supplements, although dietary supplements or fortification may be helpful in certain situations.

**Helping Americans Make Healthy Choices** A final area covered by the 2010 Dietary Guidelines for Americans is the environment in which people make their food choices.

To make healthy choices, individuals need *opportunities* to obtain healthy foods and engage in physical activity. Significant numbers of Americans—notably, members of racial and ethnic minorities, people with disabilities, and people with lower incomes—lack access to affordable, nutritious foods and/or opportunities for safe physical activity in their neighborhoods. The guidelines recognize the problem of *food security* in the United States—the ability to acquire adequate food to meet nutritional needs. Nearly 15% of the population is not able to obtain sufficient food to meet basic nutritional needs, and as noted above, many more Americans have diets that provide adequate calories but are deficient in essential nutrients.

The Dietary Guidelines propose the Social Ecological Model as a way to understand and address these complex problems. This model considers the interaction among individual factors (such as gender, income, and race/ethnicity), environmental settings (such as schools, workplaces, and restaurants), various sectors of influence (such as health care systems, agriculture, and media), and social and cultural norms and values (such as assumptions regarding body weight, types of foods consumed, and amount of physical activity incorporated into one's free time). All these factors play a role in a person's food and physical activity choices—and ultimately, in the person's health risks and outcomes.

The guidelines call on all elements of society, ranging from educators to communities to government policy makers, to implement strategies aimed at improving the food and activity environment in the United States. Examples of such strategies are expanding access to grocery stores, farmers markets, and other sources of healthy food; ensuring that meals and snacks served in schools are consistent with the Dietary Guidelines; encouraging physical activity in schools; developing policies to limit food and beverage marketing to children; supporting sustainable agricultural practices; and providing nutrition assistance programs. Such measures have the potential to improve the health of current and future generations by making healthy physical activity and eating choices the norm.

## USDA's MyPlate

To help consumers put the Dietary Guidelines for Americans into practice, the USDA also issues the food guidance system known as MyPlate (called MyPyramid until 2011). MyPlate is designed for individuals to take advantage of the customization made possible by the Internet (Figure 8.4).

**Key Messages of MyPlate** MyPlate was developed to remind consumers to make healthy food choices and to be active every day. Key messages include the following:

- *Personalization* is an important element of the MyPlate program and the ChooseMyPlate.gov site, which includes individualized recommendations, interactive assessments of food intake and physical

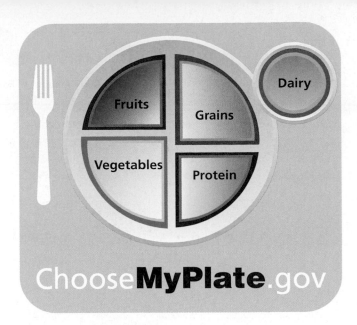

**FIGURE 8.4   USDA's MyPlate.**
The USDA food guidance system, called MyPlate, can be personalized based on an individual's sex, age, and activity level; visit www.ChooseMyPlate.gov to obtain a food plan appropriate for you.
**SOURCE:** U.S. Department of Agriculture. 2011. *MyPlate* (http://www.choosemyplate.gov; retrieved August 6, 2011).

activity, weight-management tools, and tips for success.

- *Daily physical activity* is important for maintaining a healthy weight and reducing the risk of chronic disease.

- *Moderation* of food intake is represented by advice to use smaller plates and to carefully watch portion sizes.

- *Proportionality* is represented by the different sizes of the food groups on the plate. The serving sizes provide a general guide for how much food a person should choose from each group.

- *Variety* is represented by the five food groups. Foods from all groups are needed daily for good health.

- *Gradual improvement* is a good strategy; people can benefit from taking small steps to improve their diet and activity habits each day.

The MyPlate chart in Figure 8.5 shows the food intake patterns recommended for different levels of calorie intake. Table 8.6 provides guidance for determining an appropriate calorie intake for weight maintenance. Use the table to identify an energy intake that is about right for you, and then refer to the appropriate column in Figure 8.5. You can also get a personalized version of MyPlate recommendations by visiting ChooseMyPlate.gov. Each food group is described briefly in the following sections. Many Americans have trouble identifying serving sizes, so recommended daily intakes from each group are given in terms of cups and ounces; see the box "Judging Portion Sizes" for additional advice.

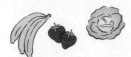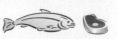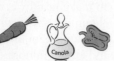

## Daily Amount of Food from Each Group
Food group amounts shown in cups (c) or ounce-equivalents (oz-eq)

| Calorie level of pattern | 1600 | 1800 | 2000 | 2200 | 2400 | 2600 | 2800 | 3000 |
|---|---|---|---|---|---|---|---|---|
| **Fruits** | 1.5 c | 1.5 c | 2 c | 2 c | 2 c | 2 c | 2.5 c | 2.5 c |
| **Vegetables** | 2 c | 2.5 c | 2.5 c | 3 c | 3 c | 3.5 c | 3.5 c | 4 c |
| Dark-green | 1.5 c/wk | 1.5 c/wk | 1.5 c/wk | 2 c/wk | 2 c/wk | 2.5 c/wk | 2.5 c/wk | 2.5 c/wk |
| Red and orange | 4 c/wk | 5.5 c/wk | 5.5 c/wk | 6 c/wk | 6 c/wk | 7 c/wk | 7 c/wk | 7.5 c/wk |
| Beans and peas (legumes) | 1 c/wk | 1.5 c/wk | 1.5 c/wk | 2 c/wk | 2 c/wk | 2.5 c/wk | 2.5 c/wk | 3 c/wk |
| Starchy | 4 c/wk | 5 c/wk | 5 c/wk | 6 c/wk | 6 c/wk | 7 c/wk | 7 c/wk | 8 c/wk |
| Other | 3.5 c/wk | 4 c/wk | 4 c/wk | 5 c/wk | 5 c/wk | 5.5 c/wk | 5.5 c/wk | 7 c/wk |
| **Grains** | 5 oz-eq | 6 oz-eq | 6 oz-eq | 7 oz-eq | 8 oz-eq | 9 oz-eq | 10 oz-eq | 10 oz-eq |
| Whole grains | 3 oz-eq | 3 oz-eq | 3 oz-eq | 3.5 oz-eq | 4 oz-eq | 4.5 oz-eq | 5 oz-eq | 5 oz-eq |
| Enriched grains | 2 oz-eq | 3 oz-eq | 3 oz-eq | 3.5 oz-eq | 4 oz-eq | 4.5 oz-eq | 5 oz-eq | 5 oz-eq |
| **Protein foods** | 5 oz-eq | 5 oz-eq | 5.5 oz-eq | 6 oz-eq | 6.5 oz-eq | 6.5 oz-eq | 7 oz-eq | 7 oz-eq |
| Seafood | 8 oz/wk | 8 oz/wk | 8 oz/wk | 9 oz/wk | 10 oz/wk | 10 oz/wk | 11 oz/wk | 11 oz/wk |
| Meat poultry, eggs | 24 oz/wk | 24 oz/wk | 26 oz/wk | 29 oz/wk | 31 oz/wk | 31 oz/wk | 34 oz/wk | 34 oz/wk |
| Nuts, seeds, soy products | 4 oz/wk | 4 oz/wk | 4 oz/wk | 4 oz/wk | 5 oz/wk | 5 oz/wk | 5 oz/wk | 5 oz/wk |
| **Dairy** | 3 c | 3 c | 3 c | 3 c | 3 c | 3 c | 3 c | 3 c |
| **Oils** | 22 g | 24 g | 27 g | 29 g | 31 g | 34 g | 36 g | 44 g |
| **Maximum SoFAS limit, calories (% of calories)** | 121 (8%) | 161 (9%) | 258 (13%) | 266 (12%) | 330 (14%) | 362 (14%) | 395 (14%) | 459 (15%) |

**FIGURE 8.5   MyPlate food intake patterns.**
To determine an appropriate amount of food from each group, find the column with your approximate daily energy intake. That column lists the daily recommended intake from each food group. Visit ChooseMyPlate.gov for a personalized intake plan and for intakes for other calorie levels.
**SOURCE:** U.S. Department of Health and Human Services and U.S. Department of Agriculture. 2011. *Dietary Guidelines for Americans, 2010, Appendix 7. USDA Food Patterns* (http://www.cnpp.usda.gov/Publications/DietaryGuidelines/2010/PolicyDoc/PolicyDoc.pdf; retrieved August 7, 2011).

**Whole and Refined Grains** Foods from this group are usually low in fat and rich in complex carbohydrates, dietary fiber (if grains are unrefined), and many vitamins and minerals. A 2000-calorie diet should include 6 ounce-equivalents each day. The following count as 1 ounce-equivalent:

- 1 slice of bread
- 1 small (2½-inch diameter) muffin
- 1 cup ready-to-eat cereal flakes

- ½ cup cooked cereal, rice, grains, or pasta
- 1 6-inch tortilla

Choose foods that are typically made with little fat or added sugar (bread, rice, pasta) over those that are high in fat and added sugar (croissants, chips, cookies, doughnuts). The key message is to make at least half your grains whole grains.

**Vegetables** Vegetables contain carbohydrates, dietary fiber, and many other nutrients, and they are naturally low in fat. A 2000-calorie diet should include 2½ cups of

# Judging Portion Sizes

Studies have shown that most people underestimate the size of their food portions, in many cases by as much as 50%. If you need to retrain your eye, try using measuring cups and spoons and an inexpensive kitchen scale when you eat at home. With a little practice, you'll learn the difference between 3 and 8 ounces of chicken or meat, and what a half-cup of rice really looks like. For quick estimates, use the following equivalents:

- 1 teaspoon of margarine = one dice

- 1 ½ ounce of cheese = your thumb, four dice stacked together

- 3 ounces of chicken or meat = a deck of cards

- ½ cup of cooked rice, pasta, or potato = ½ baseball

- 1 cup of cereal flakes = a fist

- 2 tablespoons of peanut butter = a ping-pong ball

- 1 medium potato = a computer mouse

- 1–2-ounce muffin or roll = a plum or large egg

- 2-ounce bagel = a hockey puck or yo-yo

- 1 medium fruit (apple or orange) = a baseball

- ¼ cup nuts = a golf ball

- Small cookie or cracker = a poker chip

---

vegetables daily. Each of the following counts as 1/2 cup or equivalent of vegetables:

- ½ cup raw or cooked vegetables
- 1 cup raw leafy salad greens
- ½ cup vegetable juice

Because vegetables vary in the nutrients they provide, MyPlate recommends servings from five different subgroups within the vegetables group. Choose vegetables from several subgroups each day. (For clarity, Figure 8.5 shows servings from the subgroups in terms of weekly consumption.) The key message is to fill half your plate with fruits and vegetables.

**Fruits** Fruits are rich in carbohydrates, dietary fiber, and many vitamins, especially vitamin C. A 2000-calorie diet should include 2 cups of fruits daily. Each of the following counts as ½ cup or equivalent of fruit:

- ½ cup fresh, canned, or frozen fruit
- ½ cup fruit juice (100% juice)
- ½ large (3½" diameter) whole fruit
- ¼ cup dried fruit

Choose whole fruits often; they are higher in fiber and often lower in calories than fruit juices. Fruit *juices* typically contain more nutrients and less added sugar than fruit *drinks*. Choose canned fruits packed in 100% fruit juice or water rather than in syrup. Again, MyPlate's key message for consumers is to fill half your plate with fruits and vegetables.

**Dairy** This group includes all milk and milk products, as well as lactose-free and lactose-reduced products. Those consuming 2000 calories per day should include 3 cups

of milk or the equivalent daily. Each of the following counts as the equivalent of 1 cup:

- 1 cup milk or yogurt
- ½ cup ricotta cheese
- 1½ ounces natural cheese
- 2 ounces processed cheese

Cottage cheese is lower in calcium than most other cheeses; ½ cup is equivalent to ¼ cup milk. Ice cream is also lower in calcium and higher in sugar and fat than many other dairy products; one scoop counts as ⅓ cup milk. MyPlate's key message for consumers is to switch to fat-free or low-fat (1%) milk and dairy products.

**Protein Foods (Meat and Beans)** This group includes meat, poultry, fish, dried beans and peas, eggs, nuts, and seeds. A 2000-calorie diet should include 5½ ounce-equivalents daily. Each of the following counts as equivalent to 1 ounce:

- 1 ounce cooked lean meat, poultry, or fish
- ¼ cup cooked dry beans (legumes) or tofu
- 1 egg
- 1 tablespoon peanut butter
- ½ ounce nuts or seeds

Choose lean meats and skinless poultry, and watch your serving sizes carefully. Choose at least one serving of plant proteins, such as black beans, lentils, or tofu, every day.

**Oils** Oils and soft margarines include vegetable oils and soft vegetable oil table spreads that have no trans fats. These are major sources of vitamin E and unsaturated fatty

| Table 8.6 | USDA Daily Calorie Intake Levels | | |
|---|---|---|---|
| AGE (YEARS) | SEDENTARY* | MODERATELY ACTIVE** | ACTIVE+ |
| **FEMALE** | | | |
| 2–3 | 1000 | 1000–1200 | 1000–1400 |
| 4–8 | 1200–1400 | 1400–1600 | 1400–1800 |
| 9–13 | 1400–1600 | 1600–2000 | 1800–2200 |
| 14–18 | 1800 | 2000 | 2400 |
| 19–25 | 2000 | 2200 | 2400 |
| 26–30 | 1800 | 2000 | 2400 |
| 31–50 | 1800 | 2000 | 2200 |
| 51 + | 1600 | 1800 | 2000–2200 |
| **MALE** | | | |
| 2–3 | 1000–1200 | 1000–1400 | 1000–1400 |
| 4–8 | 1200–1400 | 1400–1600 | 1600–2000 |
| 9–13 | 1600–2000 | 1800–2200 | 2000–2600 |
| 14–18 | 2000–2400 | 2400–2800 | 2800–3200 |
| 19–20 | 2600 | 2800 | 3000 |
| 21–25 | 2400 | 2800 | 3000 |
| 26–30 | 2400 | 2600 | 3000 |
| 31–35 | 2400 | 2600 | 3000 |
| 36–40 | 2400 | 2600 | 2800 |
| 41–45 | 2200 | 2600 | 2800 |
| 46–50 | 2200 | 2400 | 2800 |
| 51–55 | 2200 | 2400 | 2800 |
| 56 + | 2000–2200 | 2200–2400 | 2400–2600 |

*A lifestyle that includes only the light physical activity associated with typical day-to-day life.

**A lifestyle that includes physical activity equivalent to walking about 1.5–3 miles per day at 3–4 miles per hour (30–60 minutes a day of moderate physical activity), in addition to the light physical activity associated with typical day-to-day life.

+A lifestyle that includes physical activity equivalent to walking more than 3 miles per day at 3–4 miles per hour (60 or more minutes a day of moderate physical activity), in addition to the light physical activity associated with typical day-to-day life.

**SOURCE:** U.S. Department of Health and Human Services and U.S. Department of Agriculture. 2011. *Dietary Guidelines for Americans, 2010, Appendix 6. Estimated Calorie Needs per Day by Age, Gender, and Physical Activity Level* (http://www.cnpp.usda.gov/Publications /DietaryGuidelines/2010/PolicyDoc/PolicyDoc.pdf; retrieved August 7, 2011).

acids, including the essential fatty acids. A 2000-calorie diet should include 6 teaspoons of oils per day. One teaspoon is the equivalent of the following:

- 1 teaspoon vegetable oil or soft margarine
- 1 tablespoon salad dressing or light mayonnaise

Foods that are mostly oils include nuts, olives, avocados, and some fish. The following portions include about 1 teaspoon of oil: 4 large olives, ½ medium avocado, 2 tablespoons peanut butter, and 1 ounce roasted nuts.

Food labels can help you identify the type and amount of fat in various foods.

**Solid Fats and Added Sugars** If you consistently choose nutrient-dense foods that are fat-free or low-fat and that contain no added sugars, you can also have a small amount of additional calories in the form of solid fats and added sugars (SoFAS). Figure 8.5 shows the maximum number of SoFAS calories allowed at each calorie level in MyPlate.

People who are trying to lose weight may choose not to use SoFAS calories. For those wanting to maintain weight, these calories may be used to increase the amount of food from a food group; to consume foods that are not in the lowest-fat form or that contain added sugars; to add oil, fat, or sugars to foods; or to consume alcohol.

The current American diet includes higher levels of sugar intake and more calories per day from sugar than recommended. For teenagers age 14–18, sodas and energy and sports drinks are the top source of calories in the diet, accounting for 226 calories per beverage; teens typically drink more than one such beverage daily. In particular, experts advise consumers to be wary of products containing high-fructose corn syrup. Although this sweetener is not harmful in itself, it is high in calories and very low in nutritional value. High-fructose corn syrup is found in many products, especially soft drinks and processed foods. Research has linked high consumption of high-fructose corn syrup with obesity, diabetes, and other health problems.

**Physical Activity** Like the Dietary Guidelines and other plans, MyPlate encourages physical activity for improving health, preventing chronic diseases, and managing weight. The physical activity recommendations in MyPlate are very similar to those found in the Dietary Guidelines (described earlier in this chapter); if you meet the Department of Health and Human Services' guidelines of 150 minutes per week of moderate physical activity, you will meet the recommendations found in MyPlate.

## Other Food-Group Plans

A variety of experts have proposed other food-group plans. Some of these address perceived shortcomings in the USDA plans, and some have adapted the old MyPyramid plans to special populations. Two alternative food plans appear in the Nutrition Resources section at the end

*Fitness Tip*

Consumption of red meats, sweets, eggs, and butter is greatly reduced or eliminated entirely in most forms of the Mediterranean diet.

of the chapter: the DASH eating plan and the Harvard Healthy Eating Pyramid. The USDA Center for Nutrition Policy and Promotion (www.usda.gov/cnpp) has more on alternative food plans for special populations such as young children, older adults, and people choosing particular ethnic diets. MyPlate is available in Spanish, and there are special adaptations of MyPlate for children and for women who are pregnant or breastfeeding.

Another food plan that has received attention in recent years is the Mediterranean diet, which emphasizes vegetables, fruits, and whole grains; daily servings of beans, legumes, and nuts; moderate consumption of fish, poultry, and dairy products; and the use of olive oil over other types of fat, especially saturated fat. The Mediterranean diet has been associated with lower rates of heart disease and cancer, and recent studies have found a link between the diet and a greatly reduced risk of Parkinson's disease and Alzheimer's disease.

## The Vegetarian Alternative

**Vegetarians** choose a diet with one essential difference from the diets described previously—they eliminate or restrict foods of animal origin (meat, poultry, fish, eggs, milk). Many people choose such diets for health reasons; vegetarian diets tend to be lower in saturated fat, cholesterol, and animal protein and higher in complex carbohydrates, dietary fiber, folate, vitamins C and E, carotenoids, and phytochemicals. Some people adopt a vegetarian diet out of concern for the environment, for financial considerations, or for reasons related to ethics or religion.

**Types of Vegetarian Diets** There are various vegetarian styles. The wider the variety of the diet eaten, the easier it is to meet nutritional needs.

- *Vegans* eat only plant foods.
- *Lacto-vegetarians* eat plant foods and dairy products.
- *Lacto-ovo-vegetarians* eat plant foods, dairy products, and eggs.

Others can be categorized as partial vegetarians, semi-vegetarians, or pescovegetarians. These people eat plant foods, dairy products, eggs, and usually a small selection of poultry, fish, and other seafood. Many other people choose vegetarian meals frequently but are not strictly vegetarian. Including some animal protein (such as dairy products) in a mostly vegetarian diet makes meal planning easier, but it is not necessary.

**A Food Plan for Vegetarians** MyPlate can be adapted for use by vegetarians with only a few key modifications. For the meat and beans group, vegetarians can focus on the nonmeat choices of dry beans and peas, nuts, seeds, eggs, and soy foods like tofu. Vegans and other vegetarians who do not eat or drink any dairy products must find other rich sources of calcium (see the following list). Fruits, vegetables, and whole grains are healthy choices for people following all types of vegetarian diets.

A healthy vegetarian diet emphasizes a wide variety of plant foods. Although plant proteins are generally of a lower quality than animal proteins, choosing a variety of plant foods will supply all of the essential amino acids. Choosing minimally processed and unrefined foods will maximize nutrient value and provide ample dietary fiber. Daily consumption of a variety of plant foods in amounts that meet total energy needs can provide all needed nutrients except vitamin B-12 and possibly vitamin D. Strategies for getting these and other nutrients include the following:

- *Vitamin B-12* is found naturally only in animal foods. If dairy products and eggs are limited or avoided, B-12

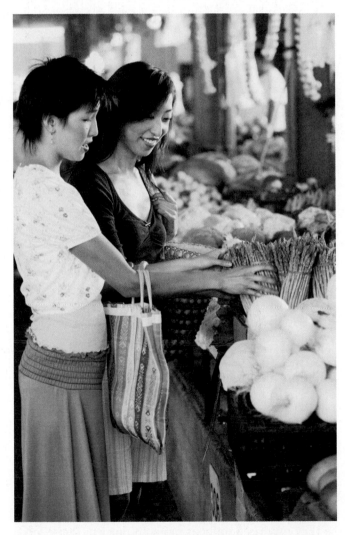

Variety is the key to maintaining a healthy, balanced vegetarian diet.

**vegetarian**  Someone who follows a diet that restricts or eliminates foods of animal origin.

KEY TERM

can be found in fortified foods such as ready-to-eat cereals, soy beverages, meat substitutes, special yeast products, and supplements.

- *Vitamin D* can be obtained by spending 5–15 minutes a day in the sun, by consuming vitamin D–fortified products like ready-to-eat cereals and soy or rice milk, or by taking a supplement.
- *Calcium* is found in legumes, tofu processed with calcium, dark-green leafy vegetables, nuts, tortillas made from lime-processed corn, fortified orange juice, soy milk, bread, and other foods.
- *Iron* is found in whole grains, fortified bread and breakfast cereals, dried fruits, leafy green vegetables, nuts and seeds, legumes, and soy foods. The iron in plant foods is more difficult for the body to absorb than the iron from animal sources. Eating or drinking a good source of vitamin C with most meals is helpful because vitamin C improves iron absorption.
- *Zinc* is found in whole grains, nuts, legumes, and soy foods.

If you are a vegetarian, remember that it's especially important to eat as wide a variety of foods as possible to ensure that all your nutritional needs are satisfied. Consulting with a registered dietitian will make your planning easier. Vegetarian diets for children, teens, and pregnant and lactating women warrant professional guidance.

## Dietary Challenges for Various Population Groups

MyPlate and the Dietary Guidelines for Americans provide a basis that nearly everyone can use to create a healthy diet. However, different population groups should be aware of special dietary challenges.

**Children and Teenagers** The best approach for parents with young children is to provide a variety of foods. For example, parents can add vegetables to casseroles and fruit to cereal, or they can offer fruit and vegetable juices or homemade yogurt or fruit shakes instead of sugary drinks. Allowing children to help prepare meals is another good way to encourage good eating habits.

**Women** Women tend to need fewer calories than men, so they may need to focus more on nutrient-dense foods to make sure they are getting enough of all the essential nutrients. Two nutrients of special concern to women are calcium and iron. Low calcium intake may be linked to the development of osteoporosis in later life. Nonfat and low-fat dairy products and fortified cereal, bread, and orange juice are good sources of calcium.

## Ask Yourself

### QUESTIONS FOR CRITICAL THINKING AND REFLECTION

What factors influence your food choices—convenience, cost, availability, habit? Do you ever consider nutritional content or nutritional recommendations like those found in MyPlate? If not, how big a change would it be for you to think of nutritional content first when choosing food? Is it something you could do easily?

Menstruating women have higher iron requirements than other groups, and a lack of iron in the diet can lead to iron-deficiency anemia. Lean red meat, leafy green vegetables, and fortified breakfast cereals are good sources of iron. As discussed earlier, all women capable of becoming pregnant should also get enough folate or folic acid from fortified foods and/or supplements.

Good nutrition is essential to a healthy pregnancy. Nutritional counseling can help a woman create a plan for healthy eating before and during pregnancy. Diet is especially important for any woman with special nutritional needs or an eating disorder, or who is overweight or obese. Physicians commonly prescribe prenatal vitamin supplements to pregnant women. The U.S. Public Health Service recommends that all women of childbearing age get 400 μg of folic acid from fortified foods and/or supplements each day to reduce the risk of neural tube defects that can arise in the fetus.

**College Students** Foods that are convenient for college students are not always the healthiest choices. However, it is possible to make healthy eating both convenient and affordable. See the tips in the box "Eating Strategies for College Students."

**Older Adults** As people age, they tend to become less active, so they require fewer calories to maintain their weight. At the same time, the absorption of nutrients tends to be lower in older adults because of age-related changes in the digestive tract. As discussed earlier, foods fortified with vitamin B-12 and/or B-12 supplements are recommended for people over age 50. Because constipation is a common problem, consuming foods high in dietary fiber and drinking enough fluids are important goals.

**Athletes** Key dietary concerns for athletes are meeting increased energy and fluid requirements for training and making healthy food choices throughout the day. For more on this topic, see the box "Do Athletes Need a Different Diet?"

**People with Special Health Concerns** Many Americans have special health concerns that affect their dietary needs. For example, women who are pregnant or breastfeeding

# Eating Strategies for College Students

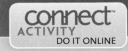

## In General

● Eat a colorful, varied diet. The more colorful your diet is, the more varied and rich in fruits and vegetables it will be. Fruits and vegetables are typically inexpensive, delicious, nutritious, and low in fat and calories.

● Eat breakfast. You'll have more energy in the morning and be less likely to grab an unhealthy snack later on.

● Choose healthy snacks—fruits, vegetables, whole grains, and cereals.

● Drink nonfat milk, water, mineral water, or 100% fruit juice more often than soft drinks or sweetened beverages.

● Pay attention to portion sizes.

● Combine physical activity with healthy eating.

## Eating in the Dining Hall

● Choose a meal plan that includes breakfast.

● Decide what you want to eat before you get in line, and stick to your choices.

● Build your meals around whole grains and vegetables. Ask for small servings of meat and high-fat main dishes.

● Choose leaner poultry, fish, or bean dishes rather than high-fat meats and fried entrees.

● Ask that gravies and sauces be served on the side; limit your intake.

● Choose broth-based or vegetable soups rather than cream soups.

● At the salad bar, load up on leafy greens, beans, and fresh vegetables. Avoid mayonnaise-coated salads, bacon, croutons, and high-fat dressings. Put dressing on the side; dip your fork into it rather than pouring it over the salad.

● Choose fruit for dessert rather than cookies or cakes.

## Eating in Fast-Food Restaurants

● Most fast-food chains can provide a brochure with the nutritional content of their menu items. Ask for it, or check the restaurant's Web site for nutritional information. Order small single burgers with no cheese instead of double burgers with many toppings. If possible, get them broiled instead of fried.

● Ask for items to be prepared without mayonnaise, tartar sauce, sour cream, or other high-fat sauces. Ketchup, mustard, and fat-free mayonnaise or sour cream are better choices and are available at many fast-food restaurants.

● Choose whole-grain buns or bread for sandwiches.

● Choose chicken items made from chicken breast, not processed chicken.

● Order vegetable pizzas without extra cheese.

● If you order french fries or onion rings, get the smallest size and/or share them with a friend. Better yet, get a salad or a fruit cup instead.

## Eating on the Run

● When you need to eat in a hurry, remember that you can carry healthy foods in your backpack or a small insulated lunch sack (with a frozen gel pack to keep fresh food from spoiling).

● Carry items that are small and convenient but nutritious, such as fresh fruits or vegetables, whole-wheat buns or muffins, snack-size cereal boxes, and water.

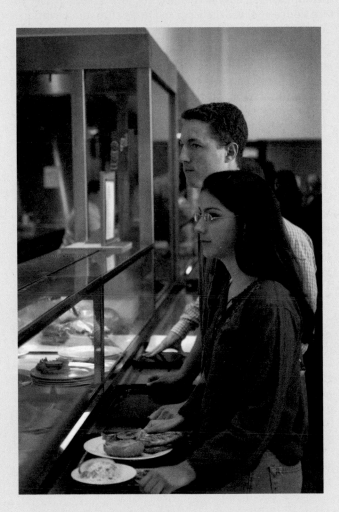

**TAKE CHARGE**

# Do Athletes Need a Different Diet?

If you exercise vigorously and frequently, or if you are an athlete in training, you likely have increased energy and fluid requirements. Research supports the following recommendations for athletes:

- **Energy intake:** Someone engaged in a vigorous training program may have energy needs as high as 6000 calories per day—far greater than the energy needs of a moderately active person. For athletes, the Academy of Nutrition and Dietetics (formerly the American Dietetic Association) recommends a diet with 60–65% of calories coming from carbohydrates, 10–15% from protein, and no more than 30% from fat.

  Athletes who need to maintain low body weight and fat (such as gymnasts, skaters, and wrestlers) need to get enough calories and nutrients while avoiding unhealthy eating patterns such as bulimia. The combination of low body fat, high physical activity, disordered eating habits—and, in women, amenorrhea—is associated with osteoporosis, stress fractures, and other injuries. If keeping your weight and body fat low for athletic reasons is important to you, seek dietary advice from a qualified dietician and make sure your physician is aware of your eating habits.

- **Carbohydrates:** Endurance athletes involved in competitive events lasting longer than 90 minutes may benefit from increasing carbohydrate intake to 65–70% of their total calories. Specifically, the American College of Sports Medicine (ACSM) recommends that athletes consume 2.7–4.5 grams per pound of body weight daily, depending on their weight, sport, and other nutritional needs. This increase should come in the form of complex carbohydrates.

  High carbohydrate intake builds and maintains glycogen stores in the muscles, resulting in greater endurance and delayed fatigue during competitive events. The ACSM recommends that before exercise an active adult or athlete eat a meal or snack that is relatively high in carbohydrates, moderate in protein, and low in fat and fiber. Eating carbohydrates 30 minutes, 2 hours, and 4 hours after exercise can help replenish glycogen stores in the liver and muscles.

- **Fat:** The ACSM recommends that all athletes get 20–35% of calories from fat in their diets. This is in line with the daily intake suggested by the Food and Nutrition Board. Reducing fat intake to less than 20% of daily calories can negatively affect performance and be harmful to health.

- **Protein:** For endurance and strength-trained athletes, the ACSM recommends eating 0.5–0.8 gram of protein per pound of body weight each day, which is considerably higher than the standard DRI of 0.36 gram per pound. This level of protein is easily obtainable from foods; in fact, most Americans eat more protein than they need every day. A balanced, moderate-protein diet can provide the protein most athletes need.

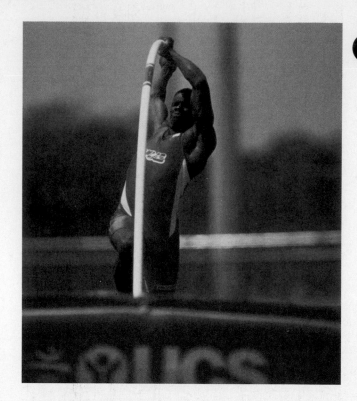

There is no evidence that consuming supplements containing vitamins, minerals, protein, or specific amino acids builds muscle or improves sports performance. Strength and muscle are built with exercise, not extra protein, and carbohydrates provide the fuel needed for muscle-building exercise.

- **Fluids:** If you exercise heavily or live in a hot climate, you should drink extra fluids to maximize performance and prevent heat illness. For a strenuous endurance event, prepare yourself the day before by drinking plenty of fluids. The ACSM recommends drinking 2–3 milliliters of fluid per pound of body weight about 4 hours before the event. During the event, take in enough fluids to compensate for fluid loss due to sweating; the amount required depends on the individual and his or her sweat rate. Afterward, drink enough to replace lost fluids— about 16–24 ounces for every pound of weight lost.

  Water is a good choice for fluid replacement for events lasting 60–90 minutes. For longer workouts or events, a sports drink can be a good choice. These contain water, electrolytes, and carbohydrates and can provide some extra energy as well as replace electrolytes like sodium lost in sweat.

**SOURCE:** American College of Sports Medicine. 2009. *American College of Sports Medicine Position Stand: Nutrition and Athletic Performance* (http://www.acsm-msse.org/pt/pt-core/template-journal/msse/media/0309nutrition.pdf; retrived April 23, 2011).

require extra calories, vitamins, and minerals. People with diabetes benefit from a well-balanced diet that is low in simple sugars, high in complex carbohydrates, and relatively rich in monounsaturated fats. People with high blood pressure need to limit their sodium consumption and control their weight. If you have a health problem or concern that may require a special diet, discuss your situation with a physician or registered dietitian.

# Using Food Labels

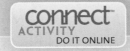

The "Nutrition Facts" section of a food label designed to help consumers make food choices based on the nutrients that are most important to good health. In addition to listing nutrient content by weight, the label puts the information in the context of a daily diet of 2000 calories that includes no more than 65 grams of fat (approximately 30% of total calories). For example, if a serving of a particular product has 13 grams of fat, the label will show that the serving represents 20% of the daily fat allowance. If your daily diet contains fewer or more than 2000 calories, you need to adjust these calculations accordingly.

Food labels contain uniform serving sizes. This means that if you look at different brands of salad dressing, for example, you can compare calories and fat content based on the serving amount. (Food label serving sizes may be larger or smaller than USDA serving size equivalents, however.) Regulations also require that foods meet strict definitions if their packaging includes the terms *light, low-fat,* or *high-fiber* (see below). Health claims such as "good source of dietary fiber" or "low in saturated fat" on packages are signals that those products can wisely be included in your diet. Overall, the food label is an important tool to help you choose a diet that conforms to MyPlate and the Dietary Guidelines.

## Selected Nutrient Claims and What They Mean

- **Healthy** A food that is low in fat, is low in saturated fat, has no more than 360–480 mg of sodium and 60 mg of cholesterol, *and* provides 10% or more of the Daily Value for vitamin A, vitamin C, protein, calcium, iron, or dietary fiber.

- **Light or lite** 33% fewer calories or 50% less fat than a similar product.

- **Reduced or fewer** At least 25% less of a nutrient than a similar product; can be applied to fat ("reduced fat"), saturated fat, cholesterol, sodium, and calories.

- **Extra or added** 10% or more of the Daily Value per serving when compared to what a similar product has.

- **Good source** 10–19% of the Daily Value for a particular nutrient per serving.

- **High, rich in, or excellent source of** 20% or more of the Daily Value for a particular nutrient per serving.

- **Low calorie** 40 calories or less per serving.

- **High fiber** 5 g or more of fiber per serving.

- **Good source of fiber** 2.5–4.9 g of fiber per serving.

- **Fat-free** Less than 0.5 g of fat per serving.

- **Low-fat** 3 g of fat or less per serving.

- **Saturated fat-free** Less than 0.5 g of saturated fat and 0.5 g of trans fatty acids per serving.

- **Low saturated fat** 1 g or less of saturated fat per serving and no more than 15% of total calories.

- **Cholesterol-free** Less than 2 mg of cholesterol and 2 g or less of saturated fat per serving.

- **Low cholesterol** 20 mg or less of cholesterol and 2 g or less of saturated fat per serving.

- **Low sodium** 140 mg or less of sodium per serving.

- **Very low sodium** 35 mg or less of sodium per serving.

- **Lean** Cooked seafood, meat, or poultry with less than 10 g of fat, 4.5 g or less of saturated fat, and less than 95 mg of cholesterol per serving.

- **Extra lean** Cooked seafood, meat, or poultry with less than 5 g of fat, 2 g of saturated fat, and 95 mg of cholesterol per serving.

NOTE: The FDA has not yet defined nutrient claims relating to carbohydrates, so foods labeled low- or reduced-carbohydrate do not conform to any approved standard.

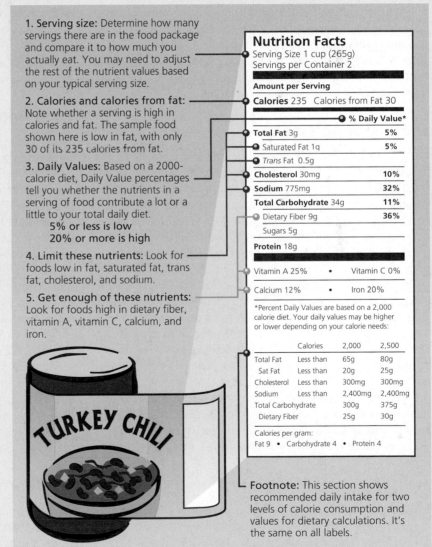

1. **Serving size:** Determine how many servings there are in the food package and compare it to how much you actually eat. You may need to adjust the rest of the nutrient values based on your typical serving size.

2. **Calories and calories from fat:** Note whether a serving is high in calories and fat. The sample food shown here is low in fat, with only 30 of its 235 calories from fat.

3. **Daily Values:** Based on a 2000-calorie diet, Daily Value percentages tell you whether the nutrients in a serving of food contribute a lot or a little to your total daily diet.
   5% or less is low
   20% or more is high

4. **Limit these nutrients:** Look for foods low in fat, saturated fat, trans fat, cholesterol, and sodium.

5. **Get enough of these nutrients:** Look for foods high in dietary fiber, vitamin A, vitamin C, calcium, and iron.

### Nutrition Facts
Serving Size 1 cup (265g)
Servings per Container 2

**Amount per Serving**

**Calories** 235   Calories from Fat 30

| | % Daily Value* |
|---|---|
| **Total Fat** 3g | **5%** |
| Saturated Fat 1g | **5%** |
| *Trans* Fat 0.5g | |
| **Cholesterol** 30mg | **10%** |
| **Sodium** 775mg | **32%** |
| **Total Carbohydrate** 34g | **11%** |
| Dietary Fiber 9g | **36%** |
| Sugars 5g | |
| **Protein** 18g | |

| | | | |
|---|---|---|---|
| Vitamin A 25% | | • | Vitamin C 0% |
| Calcium 12% | | • | Iron 20% |

*Percent Daily Values are based on a 2,000 calorie diet. Your daily values may be higher or lower depending on your calorie needs:

| | | Calories | 2,000 | 2,500 |
|---|---|---|---|---|
| Total Fat | Less than | | 65g | 80g |
| Sat Fat | Less than | | 20g | 25g |
| Cholesterol | Less than | | 300mg | 300mg |
| Sodium | Less than | | 2,400mg | 2,400mg |
| Total Carbohydrate | | | 300g | 375g |
| Dietary Fiber | | | 25g | 30g |

Calories per gram:
Fat 9 • Carbohydrate 4 • Protein 4

**Footnote:** This section shows recommended daily intake for two levels of calorie consumption and values for dietary calculations. It's the same on all labels.

# NUTRITIONAL PLANNING: MAKING INFORMED CHOICES ABOUT FOOD

Knowing about nutrition is a good start to making sound choices about food. It also helps if you can interpret food labels, understand food additives, and avoid foodborne illnesses.

## Food Labels

All processed foods regulated by either the FDA or the USDA include standardized nutrition information on their labels. Every food label shows serving sizes and the amount of fat, saturated fat, trans fat, cholesterol, protein, dietary fiber, sugars, total carbohydrate, and sodium in each serving. To make intelligent choices about food, learn to read and understand food labels (see the box "Using Food Labels").

Food labels are not required on fresh meat, poultry, fish, fruits, and vegetables (many of these products are not packaged). You can get information on the nutrient content of these items from basic nutrition books, registered dietitians, nutrient analysis computer software, the Web, and the companies that produce or distribute these foods. Also, supermarkets often have posters or pamphlets listing the nutrient contents of these foods. In Lab 8.3, you compare foods using the information on their labels.

## Dietary Supplements

Dietary supplements include vitamins, minerals, amino acids, herbs, enzymes, and other compounds. Although dietary supplements are often thought of as safe and natural, they contain powerful bioactive chemicals that have the potential for harm. About one-quarter of all pharmaceutical drugs are derived from botanical sources, and even essential vitamins and minerals can have toxic effects if consumed in excess.

In the United States, supplements are not legally considered drugs and are not regulated the way drugs are. Before they are approved by the FDA and put on the market, drugs undergo clinical studies to determine safety, effectiveness, side effects and risks, possible interactions with other substances, and appropriate dosages. The FDA does not authorize or test dietary supplements, and manufacturers are not required to demonstrate either safety or effectiveness before they are marketed. Although dosage guidelines exist for some of the compounds in dietary supplements, dosages for many are not well established.

Many ingredients in dietary supplements are classified by the FDA as "generally recognized as safe," but some have been found to be dangerous on their own or to interact with prescription or over-the-counter drugs in dangerous ways. Garlic supplements, for example, can cause bleeding if taken with anticoagulant (blood-thinning) medications. Some supplements can have side effects. St. John's wort, for example, increases the skin's sensitivity to sunlight and may decrease the effectiveness of oral contraceptives, drugs used to treat HIV infection, and many other medications.

There are also key differences in the way drugs and supplements are manufactured: FDA-approved medications are standardized for potency, and quality control and proof of purity are required. Dietary supplement manufacture is not as closely regulated, and there is no guarantee that a product contains a given ingredient at all, let alone in the appropriate amount. The potency of herbal supplements can vary widely due to differences in growing and harvesting conditions, preparation methods, and storage. Contamination and misidentification of plant compounds are also potential problems.

In an effort to provide consumers with more reliable and consistent information about supplements, the FDA has developed labeling regulations. Labels similar to those found on foods are now required for dietary supplements; for more information, see the box "Using Dietary Supplement Labels."

## Food Additives

Today, some 2800 substances are intentionally added to foods to maintain or improve nutritional quality, to maintain freshness, to help in processing or preparation, or to alter taste or appearance. Additives make up less than 1% of our food. The most widely used are sugar, salt, and corn syrup; these three, plus citric acid, baking soda, vegetable colors, mustard, and pepper, account for 98% by weight of all food additives used in the United States.

Food additives pose no significant health hazard to most people because the levels used are well below any that could produce toxic effects. Two additives of potential concern for some people are sulfites, used to keep vegetables from turning brown, and monosodium glutamate (MSG), used as a flavor enhancer. Sulfites can cause severe reactions in some people, and the FDA strictly limits their use and requires clear labeling on any food containing sulfites. MSG may cause some people to experience episodes of sweating and increased blood pressure. If you have any sensitivity to an additive, check food labels when you shop and ask questions when you eat out.

## Foodborne Illness

Many people worry about additives or pesticide residues in their food, but a greater threat comes from microorganisms that cause foodborne illnesses. Raw or

# Using Dietary Supplement Labels

Since 1999, specific types of information have been required on the labels of dietary supplements. In addition to basic information about the product, labels include a "Supplement Facts" panel, modeled after the "Nutrition Facts" panel used on food labels (see the figure). Under the Dietary Supplement Health and Education Act (DSHEA) and food labeling laws, supplement labels can make three types of health-related claims:

- *Nutrient-content claims,* such as "high in calcium," "excellent source of vitamin C," or "high potency." The claims "high in" and "excellent source of" mean the same as they do on food labels. A "high potency" single-ingredient supplement must contain 100% of its Daily Value; a "high potency" multi-ingredient product must contain 100% or more of the Daily Value of at least two-thirds of the nutrients present for which Daily Values have been established.

- *Health claims,* if they have been authorized by the FDA or another authoritative scientific body. The association between adequate calcium intake and lower risk of osteoporosis is an example of an approved health claim. The FDA also allows so-called *qualified health claims* for situations in which there is emerging but as yet inconclusive evidence for a particular claim. Such claims must include qualifying language such as "scientific evidence suggests but does not prove" the claim.

- *Structure-function claims,* such as "antioxidants maintain cellular integrity" or "this product enhances energy levels." Because these claims are not reviewed by the FDA, they must carry a disclaimer (see the sample label).

## Tips for Choosing and Using Dietary Supplements

- Check with your physician before taking a supplement. Many are not meant for children, older people, women who are pregnant or breastfeeding, people with chronic illnesses or upcoming surgery, or people taking prescription or over-the-counter medications.

- Follow the cautions, instructions for use, and dosage given on the label.

- Look for the USP verification mark on the label, indicating that the product meets minimum safety and purity standards developed under the Dietary Supplement Verification Program by the United States Pharmacopeia (USP). The USP mark means that the product (1) contains the ingredients stated on the label, (2) has the declared amount and strength of ingredients, (3) will dissolve effectively, (4) has been screened for harmful contaminants, and (5) has been manufactured using safe, sanitary, and well-controlled procedures. The National Nutritional Foods Association has a self-regulatory testing program for its members; other, smaller associations and labs, including ConsumerLab.com, also test and rate dietary supplements.

- Choose brands made by nationally known food and drug manufacturers or " house brands" from large retail chains. Due to their size and visibility, such sources are likely to have high manufacturing standards.

- If you experience side effects, stop using the product and contact your physician. Report any serious reactions to the FDA's MedWatch monitoring program (1-800-FDA-1088 or on-line at http://www.fda.gov/Safety/MedWatch/default.htm).

## For More Information About Dietary Supplements

ConsumerLab.Com: http://www.consumerlab.com

Food and Drug Administration: http://www.fda.gov/Food/DietarySupplements/default.htm

National Institutes of Health, Office of Dietary Supplements: http://ods.od.nih.gov

Natural Products Association: http://www.npainfo.org

U.S. Department of Agriculture: http://fnic.nal.usda.gov/nal_display/index.php?info_center=4&tax_level=1&tax_subject=274

U.S. Pharmacopeia: http://www.usp.org/USPVerified/DietarySupplements

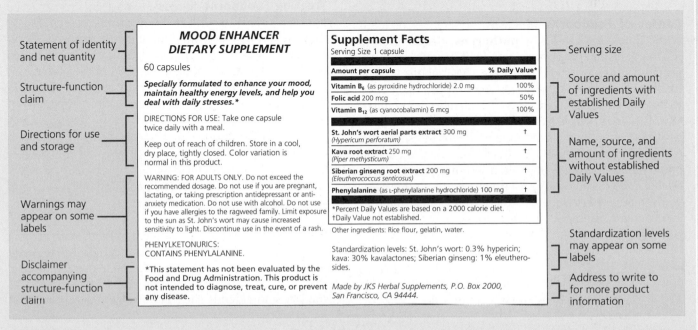

| Statement of identity and net quantity | **MOOD ENHANCER DIETARY SUPPLEMENT**<br>60 capsules | | Serving size |

**MOOD ENHANCER DIETARY SUPPLEMENT**

Statement of identity and net quantity

60 capsules

Structure-function claim

*Specially formulated to enhance your mood, maintain healthy energy levels, and help you deal with daily stresses.\**

Directions for use and storage

DIRECTIONS FOR USE: Take one capsule twice daily with a meal.

Keep out of reach of children. Store in a cool, dry place, tightly closed. Color variation is normal in this product.

Warnings may appear on some labels

WARNING: FOR ADULTS ONLY. Do not exceed the recommended dosage. Do not use if you are pregnant, lactating, or taking prescription antidepressant or anti-anxiety medication. Do not use with alcohol. Do not use if you have allergies to the ragweed family. Limit exposure to the sun as St. John's wort may cause increased sensitivity to light. Discontinue use in the event of a rash.

PHENYLKETONURICS: CONTAINS PHENYLALANINE.

Disclaimer accompanying structure-function claim

\*This statement has not been evaluated by the Food and Drug Administration. This product is not intended to diagnose, treat, cure, or prevent any disease.

### Supplement Facts
Serving Size 1 capsule

| Amount per capsule | % Daily Value* |
|---|---|
| **Vitamin B₆** (as pyroxidine hydrochloride) 2.0 mg | 100% |
| **Folic acid** 200 mcg | 50% |
| **Vitamin B₁₂** (as cyanocobalamin) 6 mcg | 100% |
| **St. John's wort aerial parts extract** 300 mg<br>*(Hypericum perforatum)* | † |
| **Kava root extract** 250 mg<br>*(Piper methysticum)* | † |
| **Siberian ginseng root extract** 200 mg<br>*(Eleutherococcus senticosus)* | † |
| **Phenylalanine** (as L-phenylalanine hydrochloride) 100 mg | † |

*Percent Daily Values are based on a 2000 calorie diet.
†Daily Value not established.

Other ingredients: Rice flour, gelatin, water.

Standardization levels: St. John's wort: 0.3% hypericin; kava: 30% kavalactones; Siberian ginseng: 1% eleutherosides.

*Made by JKS Herbal Supplements, P.O. Box 2000, San Francisco, CA 94444.*

Serving size

Source and amount of ingredients with established Daily Values

Name, source, and amount of ingredients without established Daily Values

Standardization levels may appear on some labels

Address to write to for more product information

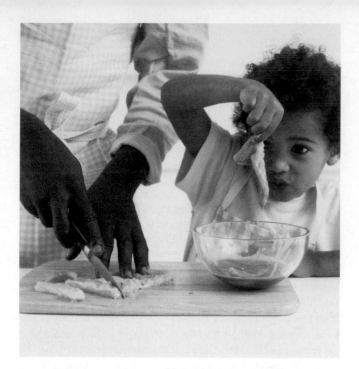

Careful food handling greatly reduces the risk of foodborne illness.

## Wellness Tip

To get produce as clean as possible, rub it with a soft brush while holding it under running water.

undercooked animal products, such as chicken, hamburger, and oysters, pose the greatest risk, although in recent years contaminated fruits and vegetables have been catching up.

The CDC estimates that 48 million illnesses, 128,000 hospitalizations, and 3000 deaths occur each year in the United States due to foodborne contaminants. Symptoms include diarrhea, vomiting, fever, pain, headache, and weakness. Although the effects of foodborne illness are usually not serious, some groups, such as children, pregnant women, and elderly people, are more at risk for severe complications such as rheumatic diseases, seizures, blood poisoning, and death.

**Causes of Foodborne Illnesses** Most cases of foodborne illness are caused by **pathogens**, disease-causing microorganisms that contaminate food, usually from improper handling. According to the CDC, about 90% of foodborne illnesses, hospitalizations, and deaths in 2010 were due to seven pathogens: *Salmonella* (most often found in eggs, on vegetables, and on poultry); norovirus (most often found in salad ingredients and shellfish); *Campylobacter jejuni* (most often found in meat and poultry); *Toxoplasma* (most often found in meat); *Escherichia coli (E. coli)* O157:H7 (most often found in meat and water); *Listeria monocytogenes* (most often found in lunch meats, sausages, and hot dogs); and *Clostridium perfringens* (most often found in meat and gravy). Salmonella was the leading cause of hospitalizations and deaths, accounting for 28% of deaths and 35% of hospitalizations. About 60% of illness, but a much smaller percentage of severe illness, was caused by norovirus.

Although pathogens are usually destroyed during cooking, the U.S. government is taking steps to bring down levels of contamination by improving national testing and surveillance. Raw meat and poultry products are now sold with safe-handling and -cooking instructions, and all packaged, unpasteurized fresh fruit and vegetable juices carry warnings about potential contamination. Although foodborne illness outbreaks associated with food-processing plants make headlines, most cases of illness trace back to poor food handling in the home or in restaurants. The 2010 Dietary Guidelines for Americans encourages people to follow four basic food safety principles:

- **Clean** hands, food contact surfaces, and vegetables and fruits.
- **Separate** raw, cooked, and read-to-eat foods while shopping, storing, and preparing foods.
- **Cook** foods to a safe temperature.
- **Chill** (refrigerate) perishable foods promptly.

The Dietary Guidelines also advise people to avoid certain high-risk foods, including raw (unpasteurized) milk, cheeses, and juices; raw or undercooked animal foods, such as seafood, meat, poultry, and eggs; and raw sprouts. These precautions are especially important for pregnant women, young children, older adults, and people with weakened immune systems or certain chronic diseases. For more information on food safety, see the box "Safe Food Handling."

**Treating Foodborne Illness** If you think you may be having a bout of foodborne illness, drink plenty of clear fluids to prevent dehydration, and rest to speed recovery. To prevent further contamination, wash your hands often and always before handling food until you recover. A fever higher than 102°F, blood in the stool, or dehydration deserves a physician's evaluation, especially if the symptoms persist for more than 2–3 days. In cases of suspected botulism—characterized by symptoms such as double vision, paralysis, dizziness, and vomiting—consult a physician immediately.

## Irradiated Foods

**Food irradiation** is the treatment of foods with gamma rays, X-rays, or high-voltage electrons to kill potentially harmful pathogens, including bacteria, parasites, insects, and fungi that cause foodborne illness. It also reduces spoilage and extends shelf life. Even though irradiation

# Safe Food Handling

## Shopping

- Don't buy food in containers that leak, bulge, or are severely dented. Refrigerated foods should be cold, and frozen foods should be solid.

- Check the food label for an expiration date and for safe-handling instructions.

- Place meat, poultry, and seafood in plastic bags, and separate foods in your grocery cart.

- Select cold and frozen food last to ensure that they stay refrigerated until just before checkout.

## Storing Food

- Store raw meat, poultry, fish, and shellfish in containers in the refrigerator so that the juices don't drip onto other foods. Keep these items away from other foods, surfaces, utensils, and serving dishes to prevent cross-contamination.

- Store eggs in the coldest part of the refrigerator, not in the door, and use them within 3–5 weeks.

- Keep hot foods hot (140°F or above) and cold foods cold (40°F or below); harmful bacteria can grow rapidly between these two temperatures. Refrigerate foods within 2 hours of purchase or preparation and within 1 hour if the air temperature is above 90°F. Freeze foods at or below 0°F. Use or freeze fresh meats within 3–5 days and fresh poultry, fish, and ground meat within 1–2 days. Use refrigerated leftovers within 3–4 days.

## Preparing Food

- Thoroughly wash your hands with warm soapy water for 20 seconds before and after handling food, especially raw meat, fish, shellfish, poultry, or eggs.

- Make sure counters, cutting boards, dishes, utensils, and other equipment are thoroughly cleaned with hot soapy water before and after use. Wash dishcloths and kitchen towels frequently.

- Use separate cutting boards for meat, poultry, and seafood and for foods that will be eaten raw, such as fruits and vegetables. Replace cutting boards once they become worn or develop hard-to-clean grooves.

- Thoroughly rinse and scrub fruits and vegetables with a brush (but not with soap or detergent), or peel off the skin.

- Don't eat raw animal products, including raw eggs in homemade hollandaise sauce, eggnog, or cookie dough.

- Thaw frozen food in the refrigerator, in cold water, or in the microwave, not on the kitchen counter. Cook foods immediately after thawing.

## Cooking

- Cook foods thoroughly, especially beef, poultry, fish, pork, and eggs; cooking kills most microorganisms. Use a food thermometer to ensure that foods are cooked to a safe temperature. Hamburgers should be cooked to 160°F. Turn or stir microwaved food to make sure it is heated evenly throughout.

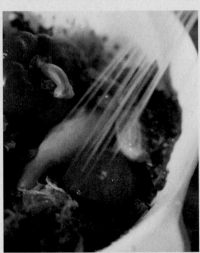

- Cook stuffing separately from poultry; or wash poultry thoroughly, stuff immediately before cooking, and transfer the stuffing to a clean bowl immediately after cooking. The temperature of cooked stuffing should reach 165°F.

- Cook eggs until they're firm, and fully cook foods containing eggs.

- To protect against *Listeria*, reheat ready-to-eat foods like hot dogs and cold cuts until steaming hot.

- Because of possible contamination with *E. coli* 0157:H7 and *Salmonella*, avoid raw sprouts.

According to the USDA, "When in doubt, throw it out." Even if a food looks and smells fine, it may not be safe. If you aren't sure that a food has been prepared, served, and stored safely, don't eat it. For more information, see the USDA's *Kitchen Companion: Your Safe Food Handbook* at http://www.fsis.usda.gov /PDF/Kitchen_Companion.pdf.

---

has been generally endorsed by agencies such as the World Health Organization, the CDC, and the American Medical Association, few irradiated foods are currently on the market due to consumer resistance and skepticism. Studies haven't conclusively identified any harmful effects of food irradiation, and newer methods of irradiation involving electricity and X-rays do not require the use of any radioactive materials. Studies indicate that

when consumers are given information about the process of irradiation and the benefits of irradiated foods, most want to purchase them.

**food irradiation** The treatment of foods with gamma rays, X-rays, or high-voltage electrons to kill potentially harmful pathogens and increase shelf life.

All primary irradiated foods (meat, vegetables, and so on) are labeled with the flowerlike radura symbol and a brief information label; spices and foods that are merely ingredients do not have to be labeled. It is important to remember that although irradiation kills most pathogens, it does not completely sterilize foods. Proper handling of irradiated foods is still critical for preventing foodborne illness.

## Environmental Contaminants and Organic Foods

Contaminants are present in the food-growing environment. Environmental contaminants include various minerals, antibiotics, hormones, pesticides, and industrial chemicals. Safety regulations attempt to keep our exposure to contaminants at safe levels, but monitoring is difficult, and many substances (such as pesticides) persist in the environment long after being banned from use.

**Organic Foods** Some people who are concerned about pesticides and other environmental contaminants choose to buy foods that are **organic.** To be certified as organic,

foods must meet strict production, processing, handling, and labeling criteria. Organic crops must meet limits on pesticide residues. For meat, milk, eggs, and other animal products to be certified organic, animals must be given organic feed and access to the outdoors and may not be given antibiotics or growth hormones. The use of genetic engineering, ionizing radiation, and sewage sludge is prohibited. Products can be labeled "100% organic" if they contain all organic ingredients and "organic" if they contain at least 95% organic ingredients; all such products may carry the USDA organic seal. A product with at least 70% organic ingredients can be labeled "made with organic ingredients" but cannot use the USDA seal.

Organic foods, however, are not necessarily free of chemicals. They may be contaminated with pesticides used on neighboring lands or on foods transported in the same train or truck. However, they tend to have lower levels of pesticide residues than conventionally grown crops. Some experts recommend that consumers who want to buy organic fruits and vegetables spend their money on those that carry lower pesticide residues than their conventional counterparts (the "dirty dozen"): apples, bell peppers, celery, cherries, imported grapes, nectarines, peaches, pears, potatoes, red raspberries, spinach, and strawberries. Experts also recommend buying organic

**KEY TERM**

> **organic**  A designation applied to foods grown and produced according to strict guidelines limiting the use of pesticides, nonorganic ingredients, hormones, antibiotics, genetic engineering, irradiation, and other practices.

## Ask Yourself

### QUESTIONS FOR CRITICAL THINKING AND REFLECTION

Have you ever taken a dietary supplement, such as St. John's wort for mild depression or echinacea or zinc for a cold? If so, who or what influenced your decision to use this product? Did you do any research before taking it? Did you read the label on the package? Do you think the product had the desired effect?

beef, poultry, eggs, dairy products, and baby food. Fruits and vegetables that carry little pesticide residue whether grown conventionally or organically include asparagus, avocadoes, bananas, broccoli, cauliflower, corn, kiwi, mangoes, onions, papaya, pineapples, and peas. All foods are subject to strict pesticide limits; the debate about the health effects of small amounts of residue is ongoing.

Whether organic foods are better for your health cannot be said for certain, but organic farming is better for the environment. It helps maintain biodiversity of crops and replenish the Earth's resources. It is less likely to degrade soil, contaminate water, or expose farm workers to toxic chemicals. As multinational food companies get into the organic food business, however, consumers who want to support environmentally friendly farming methods should look for foods that are not only organic but also locally grown.

**Guidelines for Fish Consumption** A specific area of concern has been possible mercury contamination in fish. Overall, fish and shellfish are healthy sources of protein, omega-3 fats, and other nutrients. Prudent choices can minimize the risk of any possible negative health effects. High mercury concentrations are most likely to be found in predator fish—large fish that eat smaller fish. Mercury can cause brain damage to fetuses and young children. According to FDA and Environmental Protection Agency (EPA) guidelines, women who are or who may become pregnant and nursing mothers should follow these guidelines to minimize their exposure to mercury:

- Do not eat shark, swordfish, king mackerel, or tilefish.

- Eat up to 12 ounces a week of a variety of fish and shellfish that are lower in mercury, such as shrimp, canned light tuna, salmon, pollock, and catfish. Limit consumption of albacore tuna to 6 ounces per week.

- Check advisories about the safety of recreationally caught fish from local lakes, rivers, and coastal areas. If no information is available, limit consumption to 6 ounces per week.

The same FDA/EPA guidelines apply to children, although they should consume smaller servings.

# Ethnic Foods

There is no one ethnic diet that clearly surpasses all others in providing people with healthful foods. Every diet has its advantages and disadvantages, and within each cuisine, some foods are better choices. The dietary guidelines described in this chapter can be applied to any ethnic cuisine. For additional guidance, refer to the table below.

| | Choose More Often | Choose Less Often |
|---|---|---|
| CHINESE | Dishes that are steamed, poached (jum), boiled (chu), roasted (kow), barbecued (shu), or lightly stir-fried<br>Hoisin sauce, oyster sauce, wine sauce, plum sauce, velvet sauce, or hot mustard<br>Fresh fish and seafood, skinless chicken, tofu<br>Mixed vegetables, Chinese greens<br>Steamed rice, steamed spring rolls, soft noodles | Fried wontons or egg rolls<br>Crab rangoon<br>Crispy (Peking) duck or chicken<br>Sweet-and-sour dishes made with breaded and deep-fried meat, poultry, or fish<br>Fried or crispy noodles<br>Fried rice |
| FRENCH | Dishes prepared au vapeur (steamed), en brochette (skewered and broiled), or grillé (grilled)<br>Fresh fish, shrimp, scallops, mussels, or skinless chicken, without sauces<br>Clear soups | Dishes prepared á la créme (in cream sauce), au gratin or gratinée (baked with cream and cheese), or en croûte (in pastry crust)<br>Drawn butter, hollandaise sauce, and remoulade (mayonnaise-based sauce) |
| GREEK | Dishes that are stewed, broiled, or grilled, including shish kabobs (souvlaki)<br>Dolmas (grape leaves) stuffed with rice<br>Tzatziki (yogurt, cucumbers, and garlic)<br>Tabouli (bulgur-based salad)<br>Pita bread, especially whole wheat | Moussaka, saganaki (fried cheese)<br>Vegetable pies such as spanakopita and tyropita<br>Baba ghanoush (eggplant and olive oil)<br>Deep-fried falafel (chickpea patties)<br>Gyros stuffed with ground meat<br>Baklava |
| INDIAN | Dishes prepared masala (curry), tandoori (roasted in a clay oven), or tikke (pan roasted); kabobs<br>Raita (yogurt and cucumber salad) and other yogurt-based dishes and sauces<br>Dal (lentils), pullao or pilau (basmati rice)<br>Chapati (baked bread) | Ghee (clarified butter)<br>Korma (meat in cream sauce)<br>Samosas, pakoras (fried dishes)<br>Molee and other coconut milk-based dishes<br>Poori, bhatura, or paratha (fried breads) |
| ITALIAN | Pasta primavera or pasta, polenta, risotto, or gnocchi withmarinara, red or white wine, white or red clam, or light mushroom sauce<br>Dishes that are grilled or prepared cacciatore (tomato-based sauce), marsala (broth and wine sauce), or piccata (lemon sauce)<br>Cioppino (seafood stew)<br>Vegetable soup, minestrone or fagioli (beans) | Antipasto (cheese, smoked meats)<br>Dishes that are prepared alfredo, frito (fried), crema (creamed), alla panna (with cream), or carbonara<br>Veal scaloppini<br>Chicken, veal, or eggplant parmigiana<br>Italian sausage, salami, and prosciutto<br>Buttered garlic bread<br>Cannoli |
| JAPANESE | Dishes prepared nabemono (boiled), shabu-shabu (in boiling broth), mushimono (steamed), nimono (simmered), yaki (broiled), or yakimono (grilled)<br>Sushi or domburi (mixed rice dish)<br>Steamed rice or soba (buckwheat), udon (wheat), or rice noodles | Tempura (battered and fried)<br>Agemono (deep fried)<br>Katsu (fried pork cutlet)<br>Sukiyaki<br>Fried tofu |
| MEXICAN | Soft corn or wheat tortillas<br>Burritos, fajitas, enchiladas, soft tacos, and tamales filled with beans, vegetables, or lean meats<br>Refried beans, nonfat or low-fat; rice and beans<br>Ceviche (fish marinated in lime juice)<br>Salsa, enchilada sauce, and picante sauce<br>Gazpacho, menudo, or black bean soup<br>Fruit or flan for dessert | Crispy, fried tortillas<br>Dishes that are fried, such as chile rellenos, chimichangas, flautas, and tostadas<br>Nachos and cheese, chili con queso, and other dishes made with cheese or cheese sauce<br>Guacamole, sour cream, and extra cheese<br>Refried beans made with lard<br>Fried ice cream |
| THAI | Dishes that are barbecued, sauteed, broiled, boiled, steamed, braised, or marinated<br>Sáte (skewered and grilled meats)<br>Fish sauce, basil sauce, chili or hot sauces<br>Bean thread noodles, Thai salad | Coconut milk soup<br>Peanut sauce or dishes topped with nuts<br>Mee-krob (crispy noodles)<br>Red, green, and yellow curries, which typically contain coconut milk |

Some experts have also expressed concern about the presence of toxins in farmed fish, especially farmed salmon. Although no federal guidelines have been set, some researchers suggest that consumers limit themselves to 8 ounces of farmed salmon per month. Fish should be labeled with its country of origin and whether it is wild or farmed; most canned salmon is wild.

## A PERSONAL PLAN: APPLYING NUTRITIONAL PRINCIPLES

Based on your particular nutrition and health status, there probably is an ideal diet for you, but no single type of diet provides optimal health for everyone. Many cultural dietary patterns can meet people's nutritional requirements (see the box "Ethnic Foods"). Customize your food plan based on your age, gender, weight, activity level, medical risk factors, and personal tastes.

### Assessing and Changing Your Diet

The first step in planning a healthy diet is to examine what you currently eat. Labs 8.1 and 8.2 help you analyze your current diet and compare it with optimal dietary goals. (This analysis can be completed using a nutritional analysis software program or one of several Web sites.)

To put your plan into action, use the behavioral self-management techniques and tips described in Chapter 1. If you identify several changes you want to make, focus on one at a time. You might start, for example, by substituting nonfat or low-fat milk for whole milk. When you become used to that, you can try substituting whole-wheat bread for white bread. The information on eating behavior in Lab 8.1 will help you identify and change unhealthy patterns of eating.

### Staying Committed to a Healthy Diet

Beyond knowledge and information, you also need support in difficult situations. Keeping to your plan is easiest when you choose and prepare your own food at home. Advance planning is the key: mapping out meals and shopping appropriately, cooking in advance when possible, and preparing enough food for leftovers. A tight budget does not necessarily make it more difficult to eat

## Ask Yourself

**QUESTIONS FOR CRITICAL THINKING AND REFLECTION**

What is the least healthy food you eat every day (either during meals or as a snack)? Identify at least one substitute that would be healthier but just as satisfying.

---

### TIPS FOR TODAY AND THE FUTURE

Opportunities to improve your diet present themselves every day, and small changes add up.

#### RIGHT NOW YOU CAN
- Substitute a healthy snack for an unhealthy one.
- Drink a glass of water and put a bottle of water in your backpack for tomorrow.
- Plan to make healthy selections when you eat out, such as steamed vegetables instead of french fries or salmon instead of steak.

#### IN THE FUTURE YOU CAN
- Visit the MyPlate Web site at www.choosemyplate.gov and use the online tools to create a personalized nutrition plan and begin tracking your eating habits.
- Learn to cook healthier meals. There are hundreds of free Web sites and low-cost cookbooks that provide recipes for healthy dishes.

---

healthy meals. It makes good health sense and good budget sense to use only small amounts of meat and to have a few meatless meals each week.

In restaurants, sticking to food plan goals becomes somewhat more difficult. Portion sizes in restaurants tend to be larger than MyPlate serving size equivalents, but by remaining focused on your goals, you can eat only part of your meal and take the rest home for a meal later in the week. Don't hesitate to ask questions when you're eating in a restaurant. Most restaurant personnel are glad to explain how menu selections are prepared and to make small adjustments, such as serving salad dressings and sauces on the side so they can be avoided or used sparingly.

Strategies like these are helpful, but small changes cannot change a fundamentally high-fat, high-calorie meal into a moderate, healthful one. Often, the best advice is to bypass a large steak with potatoes au gratin for a flavorful but low-fat entree. Many of the selections offered in ethnic restaurants are healthy choices (refer to the box on ethnic foods for suggestions).

### SUMMARY

- The six classes of nutrients are carbohydrates, proteins, fats, vitamins, minerals, and water.

- The nutrients essential to humans are released into the body through digestion. Nutrients in foods provide energy, measured in kilocalories (commonly called calories), build and maintain body tissues, and regulate body functions.

- Protein, an important component of body tissue, is composed of amino acids; nine are essential to good health. Foods from animal sources provide complete proteins. Plants provide incomplete proteins.

- Fats, a major source of energy, also insulate the body and cushion the organs. Just 3–4 teaspoons of vegetable oil per day supply the essential fats. For most people, dietary fat intake should be 20–35% of total calories, and unsaturated fats should be favored over saturated and trans fats.

- Carbohydrates provide energy to the brain, nervous system, and blood and to muscles during high-intensity exercise. Naturally occurring simple carbohydrates and unrefined complex carbohydrates should be favored over added sugars and refined carbohydrates.

- Fiber includes plant substances that are impossible for the human body to digest. It helps reduce cholesterol levels and promotes the passage of wastes through the intestines.

- The 13 essential vitamins are organic substances that promote specific chemical and cell processes and act as antioxidants. The 17 known essential minerals are inorganic substances that regulate body functions, aid in growth and tissue maintenance, and help in the release of energy from food. Deficiencies in vitamins and minerals can cause severe symptoms over time, but excess doses are also dangerous.

- Water aids in digestion and food absorption, allows chemical reactions to take place, serves as a lubricant or cushion, and helps regulate body temperature.

- Foods contain other substances, such as phytochemicals, that may not be essential nutrients but that may protect against chronic diseases.

- The Dietary Reference Intakes, Dietary Guidelines for Americans, and MyPlate food guidance system provide standards and recommendations for getting all essential nutrients from a varied, balanced diet and for eating in ways that protect against chronic disease.

- The Dietary Guidelines for Americans advise us to balance calorie intake and calorie expenditure to manage weight; reduce consumption of sodium, solid fats, added sugars, and refined grains; increase consumption of fruits, vegetables, and whole grains; and follow a healthy eating pattern.

- Choosing foods from each group in MyPlate every day helps ensure the appropriate amounts of necessary nutrients.

- A vegetarian diet requires special planning but can meet all human nutritional needs.

- Different population groups, such as college students and athletes, face special dietary challenges and should plan their diets to meet their particular needs.

- Consumers can get help applying nutritional principles by reading the standardized labels that appear on all packaged foods and on dietary supplements.

- Although nutritional basics are well established, no single diet provides wellness for everyone. Individuals should focus on their particular needs and adapt general dietary principles to meet them.

## FOR FURTHER EXPLORATION

### BOOKS

Byrd-Bredbenner, C., et al. 2009. *Wardlaw's Perspectives in Nutrition,* 8th ed. New York: McGraw-Hill. *An easy-to-understand review of major concepts in nutrition.*

Duyff, R. L. 2006. *ADA Complete Food and Nutrition Guide,* 3rd ed. Hoboken, N.J.: Wiley. *An excellent review of current nutrition information.*

Insel, P., D. Ross, K. McMahon, and M. Bernstein. 2011. *Nutrition,* 4th ed. Sudbury, Mass.: Jones & Bartlett. *An introductory nutrition textbook covering a variety of key topics.*

Nestle, M. 2007. *What to Eat.* New York: North Point Press. *A nutritionist examines the marketing of food and explains how to interpret food-related information while shopping.*

Selkowitz, A. 2005. *The College Student's Guide to Eating Well on Campus,* revised ed. Bethesda, Md.: Tulip Hill Press. *Provides practical advice for students, including how to make healthy choices when eating in a dorm or restaurant and how to stock a first pantry.*

Warshaw, H. 2008. *Eat Out Eat Right: The Guide to Healthier Restaurant Eating.* 3rd ed. Agate Surrey. *A registered dietitian provides realistic, informative guidelines for restaurant eating to enable diners to make healthy menu choices from a wide variety of foods and cuisines.*

### NEWSLETTERS

*Environmental Nutrition* (800-424-7887;
    http://www.environmentalnutrition.com)
*Nutrition Action Health Letter* (202-332-9110;
    http://www.cspinet.org/nah/index.htm)
*Tufts University Health & Nutrition Letter* (800-274-7581;
    http://www.tuftshealthletter.com)

### ORGANIZATIONS, HOTLINES, AND WEB SITES

*Academy of Nutrition and Dietetics.* Provides a wide variety of educational materials on nutrition.
    http://www.eatright.org
*American Heart Association: Delicious Decisions.* Provides basic information about nutrition, tips for shopping and eating out, and heart-healthy recipes.
    http://www.deliciousdecisions.org
*FDA: Food.* Offers information and interactive tools about topics such as food labeling, food additives, dietary supplements, and foodborne illness.
    http://www.fda.gov/food/default.htm
*Food Safety Hotlines.* Provide information on the safe purchase, handling, cooking, and storage of food.
    800-535-4555 (USDA)
    888-SAFEFOOD (FDA)

**Q** **Which should I eat— butter or margarine?**

**A** Both butter and margarine are concentrated sources of fat, containing about 11 grams of fat and 100 calories per tablespoon. Butter is higher in saturated fat, which raises levels of artery-clogging LDL ("bad" cholesterol). Each tablespoon of butter has about 8 grams of saturated fat; margarine has about 2. Butter also contains cholesterol, which margarine does not.

Margarine, on the other hand, contains trans fat, which not only raises LDL but lowers HDL ("good" cholesterol). A tablespoon of stick margarine contains about 2 grams of trans fat. Butter contains a small amount of trans fat as well. Although butter has a combined total of saturated and trans fats that is twice that of stick margarine, the trans fat in stick margarine may be worse for you. Clearly, you should avoid both butter and stick margarine. To solve this dilemma, remember that softer is better. The softer or more liquid a margarine or spread is, the less hydrogenated it is and the less trans fat it contains. Tub and squeeze margarines contain less trans fat than stick margarines; some margarines are modified to be low-trans or trans-fat-free and are labeled as such. Vegetable oils are an even better choice for cooking and for table use (such as olive oil for dipping bread) because most are low in saturated fat and completely free of trans fats.

**Q** **MyPlate recommends such large amounts of vegetables and fruit.**

**How can I possibly eat that many servings without gaining weight?**

**A** First, consider your typical portion sizes; you may be closer to meeting the recommendations than you think. Many people consume large servings of foods and underestimate the size of their portions. For example, a large banana may contain the equivalent of a cup of fruit, or half the recommended daily total for someone consuming 2000–2600 calories per day. Likewise, a medium baked potato (3-inch diameter) or an ear of corn (8-inch length) counts as a cup of vegetables. Use a measuring cup or a food scale for a few days to train your eye to accurately estimate food portion sizes. The ChooseMyPlate .gov Web site includes charts of portion-size equivalents for each food group.

If an analysis of your diet indicates that you need to increase your overall intake of fruits and vegetables, look for healthy substitutions. If you are like most Americans, you are consuming more than the recommended number of calories from added sugars and solid fats; trim some of these calories to make room for additional servings of fruits and vegetables. Your beverage choices may be a good place to start. Do you routinely consume regular sodas, sweetened energy or fruit drinks, or whole milk? One regular 12-ounce soda contains the equivalent of about 150 calories of added sugars; an 8-ounce glass of whole milk provides about 75 calories as discretionary fats. Substituting water or low-fat milk would free up calories for additional servings of fruits and vegetables. A half-cup of carrots, tomatoes,

apples, or melon has only about 25 calories; you could consume 6 cups of these foods for the calories in one can of regular soda. Substituting lower-fat condiments for such full-fat items as butter, mayonnaise, and salad dressing is another good way to trim calories to make room for additional servings of nutrient-rich fruits and vegetables.

Also consider your portion sizes and/or the frequency with which you consume foods high in discretionary calories: You may not need to eliminate a favorite food—instead, just cut back. For example, cut your consumption of fast-food fries from four times a week to once a week, or reduce the size of your ice cream dessert from a cup to half a cup. Treats should be consumed infrequently, and in small amounts.

For additional help on improving food choices to meet dietary recommendations, visit the ChooseMyPlate.gov Web site and the family-friendly chart of "Go, Slow, and Whoa" foods at the site for the National Heart, Lung, and Blood Institute (www.nhlbi.nih.gov/health /public/heart/ obesity/wecan/downloads /gswtips.pdf).

**Q** **What exactly are genetically modified foods? Are they safe? How can I recognize them on the shelf, and how can I know when I'm eating them?**

**A** Genetic engineering involves altering the characteristics of a plant, animal, or microorganism by adding, rearranging, or replacing genes in its

*Fruits and Veggies Matter.* Hosted by a partnership of the CDC, DHHS, and National Cancer Institute; promotes the consumption of fruits and vegetables every day.
 http://www.fruitsandveggiesmatter.gov
*Gateways to Government Nutrition Information.* Provides access to government resources relating to food safety, including consumer advice and information on specific pathogens.
 http://www.foodsafety.gov
 http://www.nutrition.gov

*Harvard School of Public Health: Nutrition Source.* Provides advice on interpreting news on nutrition; an overview of the Healthy Eating Pyramid, an alternative to the basic USDA pyramid; and suggestions for building a healthy diet.
 http://www.hsph.harvard.edu/nutritionsource
*International Food Information Council.* Provides information on food safety and nutrition for consumers, journalists, and educators.
 http://www.ific.org

DNA; the result is a genetically modified (GM) organism. New DNA may come from related species of organisms or from entirely different types of organisms. Many GM crops are already grown in the United States: About 75% of the current U.S. soybean crop has been genetically modified to be resistant to an herbicide used to kill weeds, and about a third of the U.S. corn crop carries genes for herbicide resistance or to produce a protein lethal to a destructive type of caterpillar. Products made with GM organisms include juice, soda, nuts, tuna, frozen pizza, spaghetti sauce, canola oil, chips, salad dressing, and soup.

The potential benefits of GM foods cited by supporters include improved yields overall and in difficult growing conditions, increased disease resistance, improved nutritional content, lower prices, and less use of pesticides. Critics of biotechnology argue that unexpected effects may occur: Gene manipulation could elevate levels of naturally occurring toxins or allergens, permanently change the gene pool and reduce biodiversity, and produce pesticide-resistant insects through the transfer of genes. In 2000, a form of GM corn approved for use only in animal feed was found to have commingled with other varieties of corn and to have been used in human foods; this mistake sparked fears of allergic reactions and led to recalls. Opposition to GM foods is particularly strong in Europe; in many developing nations that face food shortages, responses to GM crops have tended to be more positive.

In April 2000, the National Academy of Sciences released a report stating that there is no proof that GM food on the market is unsafe but that changes are needed to better coordinate regulation of GM foods and to assess potential problems.

Labeling has been another major concern. Surveys indicate that the majority of Americans want to know if their foods contain GM organisms. However, under current rules, the FDA requires special labeling only when a food's composition is changed significantly or when a known allergen is introduced. For example, soybeans that contain a gene from a peanut would have to be labeled because peanuts are a common allergen. The only foods guaranteed not to contain GM ingredients are those certified as organic.

## Q How can I tell if I'm allergic to a food?

**A** A true food allergy is a reaction of the body's immune system to a food or food ingredient, usually a protein. This immune reaction can occur within minutes of ingesting the food, resulting in symptoms such as hives, diarrhea, difficulty breathing, or swelling of the lips or tongue. The most severe response is a systemic reaction called anaphylaxis, which involves a potentially life-threatening drop in blood pressure. Food allergies affect only about 1.5% of the adult population and 4% of children. Between 1997 and 2007, the food allergy rate among American children increased 18%. People with food allergies, especially children, are more likely to have asthma or other allergic conditions.

Just eight foods account for more than 90% of the food allergies in the United States: cow's milk, eggs, peanuts, tree nuts (walnuts, cashews, and so on), soy, wheat, fish, and shellfish. Food manufacturers are now required to state the presence of these eight allergens in plain language in the list of ingredients on food labels.

Many people who believe they have food allergies may actually suffer from a food intolerance, a much more common source of adverse food reactions that typically involves problems with metabolism rather than with the immune system. The body may not be able to adequately digest a food or the body may react to a particular food compound. Food intolerances have been attributed to lactose (milk sugar), gluten (a protein in some grains), tartrazine (yellow food coloring), sulfite (a food additive), MSG, and the sweetener aspartame. Although symptoms of a food intolerance may be similar to those of a food allergy, they are typically more localized and not life-threatening. Many people with food intolerance can safely and comfortably consume small amounts of the food that affects them.

If you suspect you have a food allergy or intolerance, a good first step is to keep a food diary. Note everything you eat or drink, any symptoms you develop, and how long after eating the symptoms appear. Then make an appointment with your physician to go over your diary and determine if any additional tests are needed. People at risk for severe allergic reactions must diligently avoid trigger foods and carry medications to treat anaphylaxis.

*For more **Common Questions Answered** about nutrition, visit the Online Learning Center at www.mhhe.com/fahey.*

*MedlinePlus: Nutrition.* Provides links to information from government agencies and major medical associations on a variety of nutrition topics.

http://www.nlm.nih.gov/medlineplus/nutrition.html

*MyPlate.* Provides personalized dietary plans and interactive food and activity tracking tools.

http://www.choosemyplate.gov

*National Academies' Food and Nutrition Board.* Provides information about the Dietary Reference Intakes and related guidelines.

http://www.iom.edu/CMS/3788.aspx

*National Institutes of Health: Osteoporosis and Related Bone Diseases' National Resource Center.* Provides information about osteoporosis prevention and treatment; includes a special section on men and osteoporosis.

http://www.osteo.org

*National Osteoporosis Foundation.* Provides information on the causes, prevention, detection, and treatment of osteoporosis.

    http://www.nof.org

*USDA Center for Nutrition Policy and Promotion.* Includes information on the Dietary Guidelines and the Food Guide Pyramid.

    http://www.cnpp.usda.gov

*USDA Food and Nutrition Information Center.* Provides a variety of materials relating to the Dietary Guidelines, food labels, Food Guide Pyramid, MyPlate, and many other topics.

    http://www.nal.usda.gov/fnic

*Vegetarian Resource Group.* Provides information and links for vegetarians and people interested in learning more about vegetarian diets.

    http://www.vrg.org

You can find nutrient breakdowns of individual food items at the following sites:

*Nutrition Analysis Tool, University of Illinois, Urbana/Champaign*
    http://www.nat.uiuc.edu

*USDA Nutrient Data Laboratory*
    http://www.ars.usda.gov/ba/bhnrc/ndl

See also the resources listed in Chapters 9, 11, and 12.

## SELECTED BIBLIOGRAPHY

A guide to the best and worst drinks. 2006. *Consumer Reports on Health*, July, 8–9.

American Heart Association. 2010. *Diet and Lifestyle Recommendations* (http://www.americanheart.org/presenter.jhtml?identifier=851; retrieved September 15, 2010).

American Heart Association. 2010. *Fish, Levels of Mercury and Omega-3 Fatty Acids* (http://www.americanheart.org/presenter.jhtml?identifier=3013797; retrieved September 15, 2010).

American Heart Association. 2010. Trans Fats (http://www.americanheart.org/presenter.jhtml?identifier=3045792; retrieved September 15, 2010).

Bleich, S. N., et al. 2009. Increasing consumption of sugar-sweetened beverages among U.S. adults: 1988–1994 to 1999–2004. *American Journal of Clinical Nutrition* 89(1): 372–381.

Centers for Disease Control and Prevention. 2009. Application of lower sodium intake recommendations to adults—United States, 1999–2006. *Morbidity and Mortality Weekly Report* 58(11): 281–283.

Centers for Disease Control and Prevention. 2009. *Listeriosis* (http://www.cdc.gov/nczved/divisions/dfbmd/diseases/listeriosis; retrieved September 15, 2010).

Centers for Disease Control and Prevention. 2010. *Foodborne Illness* (http://www.cdc.gov/ncidod/dbmd/diseaseinfo/foodborneinfections_g.htm; retrieved September 15, 2010).

Council for Responsible Nutrition. 2009. *Dietary Supplements: Safe, Regulated and Beneficial* (http://www.crnusa.org/pdfs/CRN_FACT_DSSafeRegulatedBeneficial_09.pdf; retrieved September 15, 2010).

Food and Agriculture Organization of the United Nations. 2009. 1.02 billion people hungry (http://www.fao.org/news/story/en/item/20568/icode: retrieved September 15, 2010).

Food and Nutrition Board, Institute of Medicine. 2005. *Dietary Reference Intakes for Energy, Carbohydrate, Fiber, Fat, Fatty Acids, Cholesterol, Protein, and Amino Acids.* Washington, D.C.: National Academy Press.

Food and Nutrition Board, Institute of Medicine. 2005. *Dietary Reference Intakes for Water, Potassium, Sodium, Chloride, and Sulfate.* Washington, D.C.: National Academy Press.

Grisenbeck, J. S., et al. 2010. Maternal characteristics associated with the dietary intake of nitrates, nitrites, and nitrosamines in women of childbearing age: A cross-sectional study. *Environmental Health* 9(1): 10.

Harris, W. S., et al. 2009. Omega-6 fatty acids and risk for cardiovascular disease: A science advisory from the American Heart Association Nutrition Subcommittee of the Council on Nutrition, Physical Activity, and Metabolism; Council on Cardiovascular Nursing; and Council on Epidemiology and Prevention. *Circulation* 119(6): 902–907

Harvard School of Public Health, Department of Nutrition. 2010. *The Nutrition Source: Knowledge for Healthy Eating* (http://www.hsph.harvard.edu/nutritionsource; retrieved September 15, 2010).

Hasler, C. M., et al. 2009. Position of the American Dietetic Association: Functional foods. *Journal of the American Dietetic Association* 109(4): 735–736.

Johnson, R. K., et al. 2009. Dietary sugars intake and cardiovascular health: A scientific statement from the American Heart Association. *Circulation* 120(11): 1011–1020.

Lichtenstein, A. H., et al. 2006. Diet and Lifestyle Recommendations, Revision 2006. A Scientific Statement from the American Heart Association Nutrition Committee. *Circulation* 114(1): 82–96.

Liebman, B. 2006. Whole Grains: The Inside Story. *Nutrition Action Health Letter* 33(4): 1–5.

Maki, K. C., et al. 2010. Whole-grain ready-to-eat oat cereal, as part of a dietary program for weight loss, reduces low-density lipoprotein cholesterol in adults with overweight and obesity more than a dietary program including low-fiber control foods. *Journal of the American Dietetic Association* 110(2): 205–214.

Mayo Clinic. 2010. *Food Pyramids: Explore These Healthy Diet Options* (http://www.mayoclinic.com/health/healthy-diet/NU00190; retrieved September 15, 2010).

Mosaffarian, D., et al. 2006. Trans fatty acids and cardiovascular disease. *New England Journal of Medicine* 354(15): 1601–1613.

Nicholls, S. J., et al. 2006. Consumption of saturated fat impairs the anti-inflammatory properties of high-density lipoproteins and endothelial function. *Journal of the American College of Cardiology* 48(4): 715–720.

Siri-Tarino, P. W., et al. 2010. Meta-analysis of prospective cohort studies evaluating the association of saturated fat with cardiovascular disease. *American Journal of Clinical Nutrition* 91(3): 535–546.

Trump, D. L., et al. 2010. Vitamin D: Considerations in the continued development as an agent for cancer prevention and therapy. *Cancer Journal* 16(1): 1–9.

Tucker, K. L. 2009. Osteoporosis prevention and nutrition. *Current Osteoporosis Reports* 7(4): 111–117.

U.S. Department of Agriculture and Centers for Disease Control and Prevention. 2010. *What We Eat in America* (http://www.ars.usda.gov/Services/docs.htm?docid=15044; retrieved September 15, 2010).

U.S. Department of Health and Human Services and U.S. Department of Agriculture. 2010. *Dietary Guidelines for Americans 2010* (http://www.cnpp.usda.gov/DGAs2010-PolicyDocument.htm; retrieved April 1, 2011).

U.S. Food and Drug Administration. 2009. *Food Allergies* (http://www.fda.gov/Food/FoodSafety/FoodAllergens/default.htm; retrieved September 15, 2010).

Varraso R, et al. 2010. Prospective study of dietary fiber and risk of chronic obstructive pulmonary disease among U.S. women and men. *American Journal of Epidemiology* (Published online Feb. 19).

Wang, Y. C., et al. 2008. Increasing caloric contribution from sugar-sweetened beverages and 100% fruit juices among U.S. children and adolescents, 1988–2004. *Pediatrics* 121(6): e1604–e1614.

## Table 1 — Dietary Reference Intakes (DRIs): Recommended Levels for Individual Intake

| Life Stage | Group | BIOTIN (µg/day) | CHOLINE (mg/day)[a] | FOLATE (µg/day)[b] | NIACIN (mg/day)[c] | PANTOTHENIC ACID (mg/day) | RIBOFLAVIN (mg/day) | THIAMIN (mg/day) | VITAMIN A (µg/day)[d] | VITAMIN B-6 (mg/day) | VITAMIN B-12 (µg/day) | VITAMIN C (mg/day)[e] | VITAMIN D (IU/day)[f] | VITAMIN E (mg/day)[g] |
|---|---|---|---|---|---|---|---|---|---|---|---|---|---|---|
| Infants | 0–6 months | 5 | 125 | 65 | 2 | 1.7 | 0.3 | 0.2 | 400 | 0.1 | 0.4 | 40 | 400 | 4 |
|  | 7–12 months | 6 | 150 | 80 | 4 | 1.8 | 0.4 | 0.3 | 500 | 0.3 | 0.5 | 50 | 400 | 5 |
| Children | 1–3 years | 8 | 200 | 150 | 6 | 2 | 0.5 | 0.5 | 300 | 0.5 | 0.9 | 15 | 600 | 6 |
|  | 4–8 years | 12 | 250 | 200 | 8 | 3 | 0.6 | 0.6 | 400 | 0.6 | 1.2 | 25 | 600 | 7 |
| Males | 9–13 years | 20 | 375 | 300 | 12 | 4 | 0.9 | 0.9 | 600 | 1.0 | 1.8 | 45 | 600 | 11 |
|  | 14–18 years | 25 | 550 | 400 | 16 | 5 | 1.3 | 1.2 | 900 | 1.3 | 2.4 | 75 | 600 | 15 |
|  | 19–30 years | 30 | 550 | 400 | 16 | 5 | 1.3 | 1.2 | 900 | 1.3 | 2.4 | 90 | 600 | 15 |
|  | 31–50 years | 30 | 550 | 400 | 16 | 5 | 1.3 | 1.2 | 900 | 1.3 | 2.4 | 90 | 600 | 15 |
|  | 51–70 years | 30 | 550 | 400 | 16 | 5 | 1.3 | 1.2 | 900 | 1.7 | 2.4[h] | 90 | 600 | 15 |
|  | >70 years | 30 | 550 | 400 | 16 | 5 | 1.3 | 1.2 | 900 | 1.7 | 2.4[h] | 90 | 600 | 15 |
| Females | 9–13 years | 20 | 375 | 300 | 12 | 4 | 0.9 | 0.9 | 600 | 1.0 | 1.8 | 45 | 600 | 11 |
|  | 14–18 years | 25 | 400 | 400[i] | 14 | 5 | 1.0 | 1.0 | 700 | 1.2 | 2.4 | 65 | 600 | 15 |
|  | 19–30 years | 30 | 425 | 400[i] | 14 | 5 | 1.1 | 1.1 | 700 | 1.3 | 2.4 | 75 | 600 | 15 |
|  | 31–50 years | 30 | 425 | 400[i] | 14 | 5 | 1.1 | 1.1 | 700 | 1.3 | 2.4 | 75 | 600 | 15 |
|  | 51–70 years | 30 | 425 | 400[i] | 14 | 5 | 1.1 | 1.1 | 700 | 1.5 | 2.4[h] | 75 | 600 | 15 |
|  | >70 years | 30 | 425 | 400 | 14 | 5 | 1.1 | 1.1 | 700 | 1.5 | 2.4[h] | 75 | 600 | 15 |
| Pregnancy | ≤18 years | 30 | 450 | 600[j] | 18 | 6 | 1.4 | 1.4 | 750 | 1.9 | 2.6 | 80 | 800 | 15 |
|  | 19–30 years | 30 | 450 | 600[j] | 18 | 6 | 1.4 | 1.4 | 770 | 1.9 | 2.6 | 85 | 600 | 15 |
|  | 31–50 years | 30 | 450 | 600[j] | 18 | 6 | 1.4 | 1.4 | 770 | 1.9 | 2.6 | 85 | 600 | 15 |
| Lactation | ≤18 years | 35 | 550 | 500 | 17 | 7 | 1.6 | 1.4 | 1200 | 2.0 | 2.8 | 115 | 600 | 19 |
|  | 19–30 years | 35 | 550 | 500 | 17 | 7 | 1.6 | 1.4 | 1300 | 2.0 | 2.8 | 120 | 600 | 19 |
|  | 31–50 years | 35 | 550 | 500 | 17 | 7 | 1.6 | 1.4 | 1300 | 2.0 | 2.8 | 120 | 600 | 19 |
| Tolerable Upper Intake Levels for Adults (19–70) |  | 3500 | 1000[k] | 35[k] | 3000 |  |  |  | 3000 | 100 | 2000 |  | 4000[k] | 1000 |

NOTE: The table includes values for the type of DRI standard—Adequate Intake (AI) or Recommended Dietary Allowance (RDA)—that has been established for that particular nutrient and life stage; RDAs are shown in **bold type**. The final row of the table shows the Tolerable Upper Intake Levels (ULs) for adults; refer to the full DRI report for information on other ages and life stages. A UL is the maximum level of daily nutrient intake that is likely to pose no risk of adverse effects. There is insufficient data to set ULs for all nutrients, but this does not mean that there is no potential for adverse effects; source of intake should be from food only to prevent high levels of intake of nutrients without established ULs. In healthy individuals, there is no established benefit from nutrient intakes above the RDA or AI.

a Although AIs have been set for choline, there are few data to assess whether a dietary supply of choline is needed at all stages of the life cycle, and it may be that the choline requirement can be met by endogenous synthesis at some of these stages.

b As dietary folate equivalents (DFE): 1 DFE = 1 µg food folate = 0.6 µg folate from fortified food or as a supplement consumed with food = 0.5 µg of a supplement taken on an empty stomach.

c As niacin equivalents (NE): 1 mg niacin = 60 mg tryptophan.

## Table 1    Dietary Reference Intakes (DRIs): Recommended Levels for Individual Intake (continued)

| Life Stage | Group | VITAMIN K (µg/day) | CALCIUM (mg/day) | CHROMIUM (µg/day) | COPPER (µg/day) | FLUORIDE (mg/day) | IODINE (mg/day) | IRON (mg/day)[l] | MAGNESIUM (mg/day) | MANGANESE (mg/day) | MOLYBDENUM (µg/day) | PHOSPHORUS (mg/day) | SELENIUM (µg/day) | ZINC (mg/day)[m] |
|---|---|---|---|---|---|---|---|---|---|---|---|---|---|---|
| Infants | 0–6 months | 2.0 | 200 | 0.2 | 200 | 0.01 | 110 | 0.27 | 30 | 0.003 | 2 | 100 | 15 | 2 |
|  | 7–12 months | 2.5 | 260 | 5.5 | 220 | 0.5 | 130 | 11 | 75 | 0.6 | 3 | 275 | 20 | 3 |
| Children | 1–3 years | 30 | 700 | 11 | 340 | 0.7 | 90 | 7 | 80 | 1.2 | 17 | 460 | 20 | 3 |
|  | 4–8 years | 55 | 1000 | 15 | 440 | 1 | 90 | 10 | 130 | 1.5 | 22 | 500 | 30 | 5 |
| Males | 9–13 years | 60 | 1300 | 25 | 700 | 2 | 120 | 8 | 240 | 1.9 | 34 | 1250 | 40 | 8 |
|  | 14–18 years | 75 | 1300 | 35 | 890 | 3 | 150 | 11 | 410 | 2.2 | 43 | 1250 | 55 | 11 |
|  | 19–30 years | 120 | 1000 | 35 | 900 | 4 | 150 | 8 | 400 | 2.3 | 45 | 700 | 55 | 11 |
|  | 31–50 years | 120 | 1000 | 35 | 900 | 4 | 150 | 8 | 420 | 2.3 | 45 | 700 | 55 | 11 |
|  | 51–70 years | 120 | 1000 | 30 | 900 | 4 | 150 | 8 | 420 | 2.3 | 45 | 700 | 55 | 11 |
|  | >70 years | 120 | 1200 | 30 | 900 | 4 | 150 | 8 | 420 | 2.3 | 45 | 700 | 55 | 11 |
| Females | 9–13 years | 60 | 1300 | 21 | 700 | 2 | 120 | 8 | 240 | 1.6 | 34 | 1250 | 40 | 8 |
|  | 14–18 years | 75 | 1300 | 24 | 890 | 3 | 150 | 15 | 360 | 1.6 | 43 | 1250 | 55 | 9 |
|  | 19–30 years | 90 | 1000 | 25 | 900 | 3 | 150 | 18 | 310 | 1.8 | 45 | 700 | 55 | 8 |
|  | 31–50 years | 90 | 1000 | 25 | 900 | 3 | 150 | 18 | 320 | 1.8 | 45 | 700 | 55 | 8 |
|  | 51–70 years | 90 | 1200 | 20 | 900 | 3 | 150 | 8 | 320 | 1.8 | 45 | 700 | 55 | 8 |
|  | >70 years | 90 | 1200 | 20 | 900 | 3 | 150 | 8 | 320 | 1.8 | 45 | 700 | 55 | 8 |
| Pregnancy | ≤18 years | 75 | 3000 | 29 | 1000 | 3 | 220 | 27 | 400 | 2.0 | 50 | 1250 | 60 | 13 |
|  | 19–30 years | 90 | 2500 | 30 | 1000 | 3 | 220 | 27 | 350 | 2.0 | 50 | 700 | 60 | 11 |
|  | 31–50 years | 90 | 2500 | 30 | 1000 | 3 | 220 | 27 | 360 | 2.0 | 50 | 700 | 60 | 11 |
| Lactation | ≤18 years | 75 | 3000 | 44 | 1300 | 3 | 290 | 10 | 360 | 2.6 | 50 | 1250 | 70 | 14 |
|  | 19–30 years | 90 | 2500 | 45 | 1300 | 3 | 290 | 9 | 310 | 2.6 | 50 | 700 | 70 | 12 |
|  | 31–50 years | 90 | 2500 | 45 | 1300 | 3 | 290 | 9 | 320 | 2.6 | 50 | 700 | 70 | 12 |
| Tolerable Upper Intake Levels for Adults (19–70) | |  | 2500 |  | 10,000 | 10 | 1100 | 45 | 350[k] | 11 | 2000 | 4000 | 400 | 40 |

[a]As retinol activity equivalents (RAEs): 1 RAE = 1 µg retinol, 12 µg β-carotene, or 24 µg α-carotene or β-cryptoxanthin. Preformed vitamin A (retinol) is abundant in animal-derived foods; provitamin A carotenoids are abundant in some dark yellow, orange, red, and deep-green fruits and vegetables. For preformed vitamin A and for provitamin A carotenoids in supplements, IRE = 1 RAE; for provitamin A carotenoids in foods, divide the REs by 2 to obtain RAEs. The UL applies only to preformed vitamin A.

[b]Individuals who smoke require an additional 35 mg/day of vitamin C over that needed by nonsmokers; nonsmokers regularly exposed to tobacco smoke should ensure they meet the RDA for vitamin C.

[c]IU = International Unit.

[d]As α-tocopherol. Includes naturally occurring RRR-α-tocopherol and the 2R-stereoisomeric forms from supplements; does not include the 2S-stereoisomeric forms from supplements.

[e]Because 10–30% of older people may malabsorb food-bound B-12, those over age 50 should meet their RDA mainly with supplements or foods fortified with B-12.

[f]In view of evidence linking folate intake with neural tube defects in the fetus it is recommended that all women capable of becoming pregnant consume 400 µg from supplements or fortified foods in addition to consuming folate from a varied diet.

[g]It is assumed that women will continue consuming 400 µg from supplements or fortified food until their pregnancy is confirmed and they enter prenatal care, which ordinarily occurs after the end of the periconceptional period—the critical time for formation of the neural tube.

[h]The UL applies only to intake from supplements, fortified foods, and/or pharmacological agents and not to intake from foods.

[i]Because the absorption of iron from plant foods is low compared to that from animal foods, the RDA for strict vegetarians is approximately 1.8 times higher than the values established for omnivores (14 mg/day for adult male vegetarians; 33 mg/day for premenopausal female vegetarians). Oral contraceptives (OCs) reduce menstrual blood losses, so women taking them need less daily iron; the RDA for premenopausal women taking OCs is 10.9 mg/day. For more on iron requirements for other special situations, refer to Dietary Reference Intakes for Vitamin A, Vitamin K, Arsenic, Boron, Chromium, Copper, Iodine, Iron, Manganese, Molybdenum, Nickel, Silicon, Vanadium, and Zinc (visit http://www.nap.edu for the complete report).

[m]Zinc absorption is lower for those consuming vegetarian diets, so the zinc requirement for vegetarians is approximately twofold greater than for those consuming a nonvegetarian diet.

## Table 1 — Dietary Reference Intakes (DRIs): Recommended Levels for Individual Intake (continued)

| Life Stage | Group | POTASSIUM (g/day) | SODIUM (g/day) | CHLORIDE (g/day) | CARBOHYDRATE RDA/AI (g/day) | CARBOHYDRATE AMDR[n] (%) | TOTAL FIBER RDA/AI (g/day) | TOTAL FAT AMDR[o] (%) | LINOLEIC ACID RDA/AI (g/day) | LINOLEIC ACID AMDR[o] (%) | ALPHA-LINOLENIC ACID RDA/AI (g/day) | ALPHA-LINOLENIC ACID AMDR[o] (%) | PROTEIN RDA/AI (g/day) | PROTEIN AMDR[o] (%) | WATER[p] (L/day) |
|---|---|---|---|---|---|---|---|---|---|---|---|---|---|---|---|
| Infants | 0–6 months | 0.4 | 0.12 | 0.18 | 60 | ND[c] | ND | r | 4.4 | ND[q] | 0.5 | ND[q] | 9.1 | ND[q] | 0.7 |
|  | 7–12 months | 0.7 | 0.37 | 0.57 | 95 | ND[c] | ND | r | 4.6 | ND[q] | 0.5 | ND[q] | 13.5 | ND[q] | 0.8 |
| Children | 1–3 years | 3.0 | 1.0 | 1.5 | 130 | 45–65 | 19 | 30–40 | 7 | 5–10 | 0.7 | 0.6–1.2 | 13 | 5–20 | 1.3 |
|  | 4–8 years | 3.8 | 1.2 | 1.9 | 130 | 45–65 | 25 | 25–35 | 10 | 5–10 | 0.9 | 0.6–1.2 | 19 | 10–30 | 1.7 |
| Males | 9–13 years | 4.5 | 1.5 | 2.3 | 130 | 45–65 | 31 | 25–35 | 12 | 5–10 | 1.2 | 0.6–1.2 | 34 | 10–30 | 2.4 |
|  | 14–18 years | 4.7 | 1.5 | 2.3 | 130 | 45–65 | 38 | 25–35 | 16 | 5–10 | 1.6 | 0.6–1.2 | 52 | 10–30 | 3.3 |
|  | 19–30 years | 4.7 | 1.5 | 2.3 | 130 | 45–65 | 38 | 20–35 | 17 | 5–10 | 1.6 | 0.6–1.2 | 56 | 10–35 | 3.7 |
|  | 31–50 years | 4.7 | 1.5 | 2.3 | 130 | 45–65 | 38 | 20–35 | 17 | 5–10 | 1.6 | 0.6–1.2 | 56 | 10–35 | 3.7 |
|  | 51–70 years | 4.7 | 1.3 | 2.0 | 130 | 45–65 | 30 | 20–35 | 14 | 5–10 | 1.6 | 0.6–1.2 | 56 | 10–35 | 3.7 |
|  | >70 years | 4.7 | 1.2 | 1.8 | 130 | 45–65 | 30 | 20–35 | 14 | 5–10 | 1.6 | 0.6–1.2 | 56 | 10–35 | 3.7 |
| Females | 9–13 years | 4.5 | 1.5 | 2.3 | 130 | 45–65 | 26 | 25–35 | 10 | 5–10 | 1.0 | 0.6–1.2 | 34 | 10–30 | 2.1 |
|  | 14–18 years | 4.7 | 1.5 | 2.3 | 130 | 45–65 | 26 | 25–35 | 11 | 5–10 | 1.1 | 0.6–1.2 | 46 | 10–30 | 2.3 |
|  | 19–30 years | 4.7 | 1.5 | 2.3 | 130 | 45–65 | 25 | 20–35 | 12 | 5–10 | 1.1 | 0.6–1.2 | 46 | 10–35 | 2.7 |
|  | 31–50 years | 4.7 | 1.5 | 2.3 | 130 | 45–65 | 25 | 20–35 | 12 | 5–10 | 1.1 | 0.6–1.2 | 46 | 10–35 | 2.7 |
|  | 51–70 years | 4.7 | 1.3 | 2.0 | 130 | 45–65 | 21 | 20–35 | 11 | 5–10 | 1.1 | 0.6–1.2 | 46 | 10–35 | 2.7 |
|  | >70 years | 4.7 | 1.2 | 1.8 | 130 | 45–65 | 21 | 20–35 | 11 | 5–10 | 1.1 | 0.6–1.2 | 46 | 10–35 | 2.7 |
| Pregnancy | ≤18 years | 4.7 | 1.5 | 2.3 | 175 | 45–65 | 28 | 20–35 | 13 | 5–10 | 1.4 | 0.6–1.2 | 71 | 10–35 | 3.0 |
|  | 19–30 years | 4.7 | 1.5 | 2.3 | 175 | 45–55 | 28 | 20–35 | 13 | 5–10 | 1.4 | 0.6–1.2 | 71 | 10–35 | 3.0 |
|  | 31–50 years | 4.7 | 1.5 | 2.3 | 175 | 45–55 | 28 | 20–35 | 13 | 5–10 | 1.4 | 0.6–1.2 | 71 | 10–35 | 3.0 |
| Lactation | ≤18 years | 5.1 | 1.5 | 2.3 | 210 | 45–65 | 29 | 20–35 | 13 | 5–10 | 1.3 | 0.6–1.2 | 71 | 10–35 | 3.8 |
|  | 19–30 years | 5.1 | 1.5 | 2.3 | 210 | 45–65 | 29 | 20–35 | 13 | 5–10 | 1.3 | 0.6–1.2 | 71 | 10–35 | 3.8 |
|  | 31–50 years | 5.1 | 1.5 | 2.3 | 210 | 45–65 | 29 | 20–35 | 13 | 5–10 | 1.3 | 0.6–1.2 | 71 | 10–35 | 3.8 |
| *Tolerable Upper Intake Level for Adults (19–70)* |  |  | 2.3 | 3.6 |  |  |  |  |  |  |  |  |  |  |  |

[n]Daily protein recommendations are based on body weight for reference body weights. To calculate for a specific body weight, use the following values: 1.5 g/kg for infants, 1.1 g/kg for 1–3 years, 0.95 g/kg for 4–13 years, 0.85 g/kg for 14–18 years, 0.8 g/kg for adults, and 1.1 g/kg for pregnant (using prepregnancy weight) and lactating women.

[o]Acceptable Macronutrient Distribution Range (AMDR), expressed as a percent of total daily calories, is the range of intake for a particular energy source that is associated with reduced risk of chronic disease while providing intakes of essential nutrients. If an individual consumes in excess of the AMDR, there is a potential for increasing the risk of chronic diseases and/or insufficient intakes of essential nutrients.

[p]Total water intake from fluids and food.

[q]Not determinable due to lack of data of adverse effects in this age group and concern with regard to lack of ability to handle excess amounts. Source of intake should be from food only to prevent high levels of intake.

[r]For infants, Adequate Intake of total fat is 31 grams/day (0–6 months) and 30 grams per day (7–12 months) from breast milk and, for infants 7–12 months, complementary food and beverages.

**SOURCE:** Food and Nutrition Board, Institute of Medicine, National Academies. 2004. *Dietary Reference Intakes Tables.* Washington, D.C.: National Academies Press. The complete Dietary Reference Intake reports are available from the National Academy Press (http://www.nap.edu).

*Reprinted with permission from *Dietary Reference Intakes Applications in Dietary Planning.* Copyright © 2004 by the National Academy of Sciences. Reprinted with permission from the National Academies Press, Washington, D.C.

# Nutrition Resources

**Number of servings per day (or per week, as noted)**

| Food groups | 1600 calories | 2000 calories | 2600 calories | 3100 calories | Serving sizes and notes |
|---|---|---|---|---|---|
| Grains | 6 | 6–8 | 10–11 | 12–13 | 1 slice bread, 1 oz dry cereal, 1/2 cup cooked rice, pasta, or cereal; choose whole grains |
| Vegetables | 3–4 | 4–5 | 5–6 | 6 | 1 cup raw leafy vegetables, 1/2 cup cooked vegetables, 1/2 cup vegetable juice |
| Fruits | 4 | 4–5 | 5–6 | 6 | 1/2 cup fruit juice, 1 medium fruit, 1/4 cup dried fruit, 1/2 cup fresh, frozen, or canned fruit |
| Low-fat or fat-free dairy foods | 2–3 | 2–3 | 3 | 3–4 | 1 cup milk; 1 cup yogurt, 1 1/2 oz cheese; choose fat-free or low-fat types |
| Meat, poultry, fish | 3–6 | 6 or less | 6 | 6–9 | 1 oz cooked meats, poultry, or fish: select only lean; trim away visible fats; broil, roast, or boil instead of frying; remove skin from poultry |
| Nuts, seeds, legumes | 3 servings per week | 4–5 servings per week | 1 | 1 | 1/3 cup or 1 1/2 oz nuts, 2 Tbsp or 1/2 oz seeds, 1/2 cup cooked dry beans/peas, 2 Tbsp peanut butter |
| Fats and oils | 2 | 2–3 | 3 | 4 | 1 tsp soft margarine, 1 Tbsp low-fat mayonnaise, 2 Tbsp light salad dressing, 1 tsp vegetable oil; DASH has 27% of calories as fat (low in saturated fat) |
| Sweets | 0 | 5 servings/ week or less | 2 | 2 | 1 Tbsp sugar, 1 Tbsp jelly or jam, 1/2 cup sorbet, 1 cup lemonade; sweets should be low in fat |

**FIGURE 1** **The DASH Eating Plan.**

SOURCE: National Institutes of Health, National Heart, Lung, and Blood Institute. 2006. *Your Guide to Lowering Your Blood Pressure with DASH: How Do I Make the Dash?* (http://www.nhlbi.nih.gov/health/public/heart/hbp/dash/how_make_dash html; retrieved April 30, 2009).

**FIGURE 2** **Healthy Eating Pyramid.** The Healthy Eating Pyramid is an alternative food-group plan developed by researchers at the Harvard School of Public Health. This pyramid reflects many major research studies that have looked at the relationship between diet and long-term health. The Healthy Eating Pyramid differentiates between the various dietary sources of fat, protein, and carbohydrates, and it emphasizes whole grains, vegetable oils, fruits and vegetables, nuts, and dried peas and beans.

SOURCE: Reprinted by permission of Simon & Schuster Inc., from *Eat, Drink, and Be Healthy: The Harvard Medical School Guide to Healthy Eating* by Walter C. Willett, M.D. Copyright © 2001, 2005 by President and Fellows of Harvard College. All rights reserved.

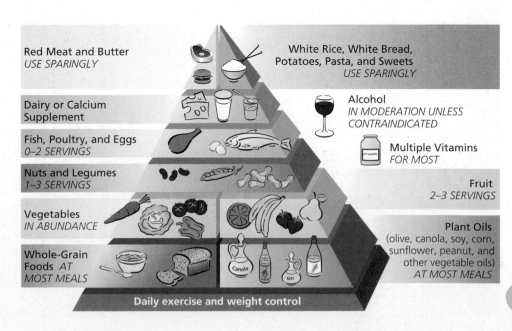

Red Meat and Butter
*USE SPARINGLY*

White Rice, White Bread, Potatoes, Pasta, and Sweets
*USE SPARINGLY*

Dairy or Calcium Supplement

Alcohol
*IN MODERATION UNLESS CONTRAINDICATED*

Fish, Poultry, and Eggs
*0–2 SERVINGS*

Multiple Vitamins
*FOR MOST*

Nuts and Legumes
*1–3 SERVINGS*

Fruit
*2–3 SERVINGS*

Vegetables
*IN ABUNDANCE*

Plant Oils
(olive, canola, soy, corn, sunflower, peanut, and other vegetable oils)
*AT MOST MEALS*

Whole-Grain Foods *AT MOST MEALS*

**Daily exercise and weight control**

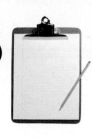

# LAB 8.1  Your Daily Diet Versus MyPlate

Make three photocopies of the worksheet in this lab and use them to keep track of everything you eat for 3 consecutive days. Break down each food item into its component parts, and list them separately in the column labeled "Food." Then enter the portion size you consumed in the correct food-group column. For example, a turkey sandwich might be listed as follows: whole-wheat bread, 2 oz-equiv of whole grains; turkey, 2 oz-equiv of meat/beans; tomato, $\frac{1}{3}$ cup other vegetables; romaine lettuce, $\frac{1}{4}$ cup dark green vegetables; 1 tablespoon mayonnaise dressing, 1 teaspoon oils. It can be challenging to track values for added sugars and oils and fats, but use food labels to be as accurate as you can. ChooseMyPlate.gov has additional guidelines for counting discretionary calories.

For vegetables, enter your portion sizes in both the "Total" column and the column corresponding to the correct subgroup; for example, the spinach in a spinach salad would be entered under "Dark Green" and carrots would be entered under "Orange." For the purpose of this 3-day activity, you will compare only your total vegetable consumption against MyPlate guidelines; as described in the chapter, vegetable subgroup recommendations are based on weekly consumption. However, it is important to note which vegetable subgroups are represented in your diet; over a 3-day period, you should consume several servings from each of the subgroups.

Date: _____

| Food | Grains (oz-eq) | | Vegetable (cups) | | | | | | Fruits (cups) | Milk (cups) | Meat/ Beans (oz-eq) | Oils (tsp) | Discretionary Calories | |
|---|---|---|---|---|---|---|---|---|---|---|---|---|---|---|
| | Whole | Other | Total | Dark Green | Orange | Legume | Starchy | Other | | | | | Solid Fats (g) | Added Sugars (g/tsp) |
| | | | | | | | | | | | | | | |
| | | | | | | | | | | | | | | |
| | | | | | | | | | | | | | | |
| | | | | | | | | | | | | | | |
| | | | | | | | | | | | | | | |
| | | | | | | | | | | | | | | |
| | | | | | | | | | | | | | | |
| | | | | | | | | | | | | | | |
| | | | | | | | | | | | | | | |
| | | | | | | | | | | | | | | |
| | | | | | | | | | | | | | | |
| | | | | | | | | | | | | | | |
| | | | | | | | | | | | | | | |
| | | | | | | | | | | | | | | |
| | | | | | | | | | | | | | | |
| | | | | | | | | | | | | | | |
| | | | | | | | | | | | | | | |
| Daily Total | | | | | | | | | | | | | | |

Next, average your daily intake totals for the 3 days and enter them in the chart below. For example, if your three daily totals for the fruit group were 1 cup, 1½ cups, and 2 cups, your average daily intake would be 1½ cups. Fill in the recommended intake totals that apply to you from Figure 8.5 and Table 8.6.

| MyPlate Food Group | Recommended Daily Amounts or Limits | Your Actual Average Daily Intake |
|---|---|---|
| **Grains (total)** | oz-eq | oz-eq |
| *Whole grains* | oz-eq | oz-eq |
| *Other grains* | oz-eq | oz-eq |
| **Vegetables (total)** | cups | cups |
| **Fruits** | cups | cups |
| **Milk** | cups | cups |
| **Meat and beans** | oz-eq | oz-eq |
| **Oils** | tsp | tsp |
| **Solid fats** | g | g |
| **Added sugars** | g/tsp | g/tsp |

## Using Your Results

*How did you score?* How close is your diet to that recommended by MyPlate? Are you surprised by the amount of food you are consuming from each food group or from added sugars and solid fats?

*What should you do next?* If the results of the assessment indicate that you could boost your level of wellness by improving your diet, set realistic goals for change. Do you need to increase or decrease your consumption of any food groups? List any areas of concern below, along with a goal for change and strategies for achieving the goal you've set. If you see that you are falling short in one food group, such as fruits or vegetables, but have many foods that are rich in discretionary calories from solid fats and added sugars, you might try decreasing those items in favor of an apple, a bunch of grapes, or some baby carrots. Think carefully about the reasons behind your food choices. For example, if you eat doughnuts for breakfast every morning because you feel rushed, make a list of ways to save time to allow for a healthier breakfast.

Problem: _____

Goal: _____

Strategies for change: _____

_____

_____

Problem: _____

Goal: _____

Strategies for change: _____

_____

_____

Problem: _____

Goal: _____

Strategies for change: _____

_____

_____

Enter the results of this lab in the Preprogram Assessment column in Appendix C. If you've set goals and identified strategies for change, begin putting your plan into action. After several weeks of your program, complete this lab again and enter the results in the Postprogram Assessment column of Appendix C. How do the results compare?

**Name** _____ **Section** _____ **Date** _____

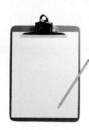

## LAB 8.2 Dietary Analysis

You can complete this activity using either a nutrition analysis software program or information about the nutrient content of foods available online; see the For Further Exploration section and page A–1 for recommended Web sites. (This lab asks you to analyze 1 day's diet. For a more complete and accurate assessment of your diet, analyze the results from several different days, including a weekday and a weekend day.)

| Food | Amount | Calories | Protein (g) | Carbohydrate (g) | Dietary fiber (g) | Fat, total (g) | Saturated fat (g) | Cholesterol (mg) | Sodium (mg) | Vitamin A (RE) | Vitamin C (mg) | Calcium (mg) | Iron (mg) |
|---|---|---|---|---|---|---|---|---|---|---|---|---|---|
| | | | | | | | | | | | | | |
| | | | | | | | | | | | | | |
| | | | | | | | | | | | | | |
| | | | | | | | | | | | | | |
| | | | | | | | | | | | | | |
| | | | | | | | | | | | | | |
| | | | | | | | | | | | | | |
| | | | | | | | | | | | | | |
| | | | | | | | | | | | | | |
| | | | | | | | | | | | | | |
| | | | | | | | | | | | | | |
| | | | | | | | | | | | | | |
| | | | | | | | | | | | | | |
| | | | | | | | | | | | | | |
| | | | | | | | | | | | | | |
| | | | | | | | | | | | | | |
| | | | | | | | | | | | | | |
| **Recommended totals*** | | | 10–35% | 45–65% | 25–38 g | 20–35% | <10% | ≤300 mg | ≤2300 mg | RE | mg | mg | mg |
| **Actual totals**** | | cal | g / % | g / % | g | g / % | g / % | mg | mg | RE | mg | mg | mg |

DATE _____  DAY: M  Tu  W  Th  F  Sa  Su

*Fill in the appropriate DRI values for vitamin A, vitamin C, calcium, and iron from Table 1 in the Nutrition Resources section.

**Total the values in each column. Protein and carbohydrate provide 4 calories per gram; fat provides 9 calories per gram. For example, if you consume a total of 270 grams of carbohydrates and 2000 calories, your percentage of total calories from carbohydrates would be (270 g × 4 cal/g) ÷ 2000 cal = 54%. Do not include data for alcoholic beverages in your calculations. Percentages may not total 100% due to rounding.

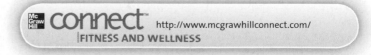

FITNESS AND WELLNESS  http://www.mcgrawhillconnect.com/

*How did you score?* How close is your diet to that recommended in this chapter? Are you surprised by any of the results of this assessment?

*What should you do next?* Enter the results of this lab in the Preprogram Assessment column in Appendix C. If your daily diet meets all the recommended intakes, congratulations—and keep up the good work. If the results of the assessment pinpoint areas of concern, then work with your food record on the previous page to determine what changes you could make to meet all the guidelines. Make changes, additions, and deletions until it conforms to all or most of the guidelines. Or, if you prefer, start from scratch to create a day's diet that meets the guidelines. Use the chart below to experiment and record your final, healthy sample diet for 1 day. Then put what you learned from this exercise into practice in your daily life. After several weeks of your program, complete this lab again and enter the results in the Postprogram Assessment column of Appendix C. How do the results compare?

DATE _____     DAY:  M  Tu  W  Th  F  Sa  Su

| Food | Amount | Calories | Protein (g) | Carbohydrate (g) | Dietary fiber (g) | Fat, total (g) | Saturated fat (g) | Cholesterol (mg) | Sodium (mg) | Vitamin A (RE) | Vitamin C (mg) | Calcium (mg) | Iron (mg) |
|---|---|---|---|---|---|---|---|---|---|---|---|---|---|
|  |  |  |  |  |  |  |  |  |  |  |  |  |  |
| Recommended totals |  |  | 10–35% | 45–65% | 25–38 g | 20–38% | < 10% | ≤300 mg | ≤2300 mg | RE | mg | mg | mg |
| Actual totals |  | cal | g / % | g / % | g | g / % | g / % | mg | mg | RE | mg | mg | mg |

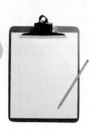

## LAB 8.3 Informed Food Choices

### Part I  Using Food Labels

Choose three food items to evaluate. You might want to select three similar items, such as regular, low-fat, and nonfat salad dressing, or three very different items. Record the information from their food labels in the table below.

| Food Items | | | |
| --- | --- | --- | --- |
| Serving size | | | |
| Total calories | cal | cal | cal |
| Total fat—grams | g | g | g |
| —% Daily Value | % | % | % |
| Saturated fat—grams | g | g | g |
| —% Daily Value | % | % | % |
| Trans fat—grams | g | g | g |
| Cholesterol—milligrams | mg | mg | mg |
| —% Daily Value | % | % | % |
| Sodium—milligrams | mg | mg | mg |
| —% Daily Value | % | % | % |
| Carbohydrates (total)—gram | g | g | g |
| —% Daily Value | % | % | % |
| Dietary fiber—grams | g | g | g |
| —% Daily Value | % | % | % |
| Sugars—grams | g | g | g |
| Protein—grams | g | g | g |
| Vitamin A—% Daily Value | % | % | % |
| Vitamin C—% Daily Value | % | % | % |
| Calcium—% Daily Value | % | % | % |
| Iron—% Daily Value | % | % | % |

How do the items you chose compare? You can do a quick nutrient check by totaling the Daily Value percentages for nutrients you should limit (total fat, cholesterol, sodium) and the nutrients you should favor (dietary fiber, vitamin A, vitamin C, calcium, iron) for each food. Which food has the largest percent Daily Value sum for nutrients to limit? For nutrients to favor?

| Food Items | | | |
| --- | --- | --- | --- |
| Calories | cal | cal | cal |
| % Daily Value total for nutrients to limit (total fat, cholesterol, sodium) | % | % | % |
| % Daily Value total for nutrients to favor (fiber, vitamin A, vitamin C, calcium, iron) | % | % | % |

## Part II   Evaluating Fast Food

Use the nutritional information available from fast-food restaurants to complete the chart on this page for the last fast-food meal you ate. Add up your totals for the meal. Compare the values for fat, protein, carbohydrate, cholesterol, and sodium content for each food item and for the meal as a whole with the levels suggested by the Dietary Guidelines for Americans. Calculate the percent of total calories derived from fat, saturated fat, protein, and carbohydrate using the formulas given.

To get fast-food nutritional information, ask for a nutrition information brochure when you visit the restaurant, or visit restaurant Web sites: Arby's (http://www.arbysrestaurant.com), Burger King (http://www.burgerking.com), Domino's Pizza (http://www.dominos.com), Jack in the Box (http://www.jackinthebox.com), KFC (http://www.kfc.com), McDonald's (http://www.mcdonalds.com), Subway (http://www.subway.com), Taco Bell (http://www.tacobell.com), Wendy's (http://www.wendys.com).

If you haven't recently been to a fast-food restaurant, fill in the chart for any sample meal you might eat.

### FOOD ITEMS

| | Dietary Guidelines | | | | | | | Total** |
|---|---|---|---|---|---|---|---|---|
| Serving size (g) | | g | g | g | g | g | g | g |
| Calories | | cal | cal | cal | cal | cal | cal | cal |
| Total fat—grams | | g | g | g | g | g | g | g |
| —% calories* | 20–35% | % | % | % | % | % | % | % |
| Saturated fat—grams | | g | g | g | g | g | g | g |
| —% calories* | <10% | % | % | % | % | % | % | % |
| Protein—grams | | g | g | g | g | g | g | g |
| —% calories* | 10–35% | % | % | % | % | % | % | % |
| Carbohydrate—grams | | g | g | g | g | g | g | g |
| —% calories* | 45–65% | % | % | % | % | % | % | % |
| Cholesterol† | 100 mg | mg | mg | mg | mg | mg | mg | mg |
| Sodium† | 800 mg | mg | mg | mg | mg | mg | mg | mg |

*To calculate the percent of total calories from each food energy source (fat, carbohydrate, protein), use the following formula:

$$\frac{(\text{number of grams of energy source}) \times (\text{number of calories per gram of energy source})}{(\text{total calories in serving of food item})}$$

(*Note:* Fat and saturated fat provide 9 calories per gram; protein and carbohydrate provide 4 calories per gram.) For example, the percent of total calories from protein in a 150-calorie dish containing 10 grams of protein is

$$\frac{(10 \text{ grams of protein}) \times (4 \text{ calories per gram})}{(150 \text{ calories})} = \frac{40}{150} - 0.27, \text{ or } 27\% \text{ of total calories from protein}$$

**For the Total column, add up the total grams of fat, carbohydrate, and protein contained in your sample meal and calculate the percentages based on the total calories in the meal. (Percentages may not total 100% due to rounding.) For cholesterol and sodium values, add up the total number of milligrams.

†Recommended daily limits of cholesterol and sodium are divided by 3 here to give an approximate recommended limit for a single meal.

SOURCE: Insel, P. M., and W. T. Roth. 2010. Wellness Worksheet 66. *Core Concepts in Health*, 11th ed. Copyright © 2010 The McGraw-Hill Companies, Inc. Reprinted with permission.

# CHAPTER 9

# Weight Management

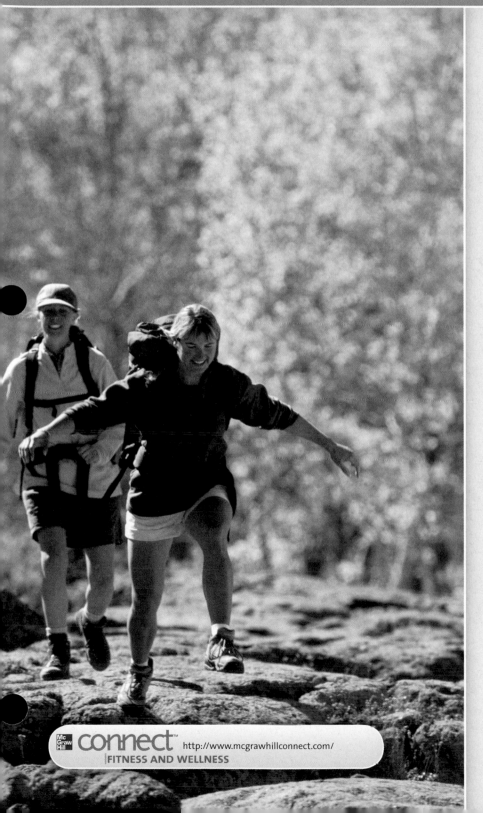

## LOOKING AHEAD...

After reading this chapter, you should be able to:

- Explain the health risks associated with overweight and obesity

- Explain the factors that may contribute to a weight problem, including genetic, physiological, lifestyle, and psychosocial factors

- Describe lifestyle factors that contribute to weight gain and loss, including the role of diet, exercise, and emotional factors

- Identify and describe the symptoms of eating disorders and the health risks associated with them

- Design a personal plan for successfully managing body weight

## TEST YOUR KNOWLEDGE

1. About what percentage of American adults are overweight?
   a. 15%
   b. 35%
   c. 65%

2. The consumption of low-calorie sweeteners has helped Americans control their weight. True or false?

3. Approximately how many female high school and college students have either anorexia or bulimia?
   a. 0%
   b. 1%
   c. 2%

**Answers**

1. **c.** About 68% of American adults are overweight, including 32.2% of adult men and 35.5% of adult women who are obese.

2. **False.** Since the introduction of low-calorie sweeteners, both total calorie and sugar intake have increased, as has the proportion of Americans who are overweight.

3. **c.** About 2–4% of female students suffer from bulimia or anorexia, and many more occasionally engage in behaviors associated with these eating disorders.

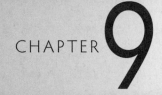

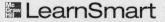

chieving and maintaining a healthy body weight is a serious public health challenge in the United States and a source of distress for many Americans. Under standards developed by the National Institutes of Health, about 68% of American adults are overweight, including more than 33.8% who are obese (Table 9.1 and Figure 9.1). In 2007–2008, 32.2% of adult men and 35.5% of adult women were obese. The problems of overweight and obesity affect Americans of all ages. According to the National Center for Health Statistics, 24% of Americans age 18–29 are obese. The American Medical Association says that one-third of American children are at risk of becoming overweight. And while millions struggle to lose weight, others fall into dangerous eating patterns such as binge eating or self-starvation.

| Table 9.1 | Vital Statistics: Weight of Americans Age 20 and Older: 2007–2008 | |
|---|---|---|
| GROUP | PERCENT OVERWEIGHT* | PERCENT OBESE |
| Both sexes | 68.0 | 33.8 |
| All races, male | 72.3 | 32.2 |
| All races, female | 64.1 | 35.5 |
| White, male | 72.6 | 31.9 |
| White, female | 61.2 | 33.0 |
| African American, male | 68.5 | 37.3 |
| African American, female | 78.2 | 49.6 |
| Latino, male | 79.3 | 34.3 |
| Latino, female | 76.1 | 43.0 |

*Includes obesity

SOURCE: Flegal, K. M., et al. 2010. Prevalence and Trends in Obesity Among US Adults, 1999–2008. *Journal of the American Medical Association* 303(3): 235–241.

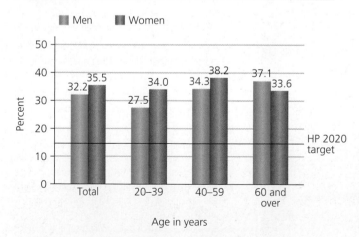

**FIGURE 9.1 Obesity pevalence, by age and sex of American adults, 2007–2008.**
*Healthy People 2020* sets a target obesity prevalence of not greater than 15% for all adults.
SOURCE: Flegal, K. M., et al. 2010. Prevalence and Trends in Obesity Among US Adults, 1999–2008. *Journal of the American Medical Association* 303(3): 235–241.

Controlling body weight is a matter of controlling body fat. As explained in Chapter 6, the most important consideration for health is not total weight but body composition—the proportion of fat to fat-free mass. Many people who are "overweight" are also "overfat," and the health risks they face are due to the latter condition. Although this chapter uses the common terms *weight management* and *weight loss,* the goal for wellness is to adopt healthy behaviors and achieve an appropriate body composition, not to conform to rigid standards of total body weight.

Although not completely understood, managing body weight is not a mysterious process. The "secret" is balancing calories consumed with calories expended in daily activities—in other words, eating a moderate diet and getting regular physical activity.

This chapter explores the factors that contribute to the development of overweight and obesity as well as to eating disorders. It also takes a closer look at weight management through lifestyle and suggests specific strategies for reaching and maintaining a healthy weight.

## HEALTH IMPLICATIONS OF OVERWEIGHT AND OBESITY

As rates of overweight and obesity have risen in the United States, so has the prevalence of the health conditions associated with overweight—including a more than 33% rise in the rate of type 2 diabetes in just the past decade. It is estimated that inactivity and overweight account for more than 100,000 premature deaths annually in the United States, second only to tobacco-related deaths. More than $75 billion per year is spent treating obesity-related health problems.

Obesity is one of six major controllable risk factors for heart disease; it also increases the risk for other forms of cardiovascular disease (CVD), hypertension, certain forms of cancer, diabetes, gallbladder disease, respiratory problems, joint diseases, skin problems, impaired immune function, and sleep disorders. Obesity doubles mortality rates and can reduce life expectancy by 10–20 years. In fact, if current trends in overweight and obesity (and their related health problems) continue, some experts predict that the average American's life expectancy will soon decline by 5 years.

Gaining weight over the years also has been found to be dangerous. A recent study showed that women who gained more than 22 pounds since they were 18 years old had a sevenfold increase in the risk of heart disease. Many studies have confirmed that obesity and—to a lesser extent—overweight shorten lives.

At the same time, even modest weight loss can have a significant positive impact on health. A weight loss of just 5–10% in obese individuals can reduce the risk of weight-related health conditions and increase life expectancy.

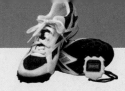

# Beating the "Freshman 15"

How much weight have you put on since you started going to college? It isn't unusual for first-year college students to gain some weight (often called the "Freshman 15"), and many students continue gaining weight throughout their college years.

If you've gained weight since starting college, write down the number of pounds you've gained: _____ pounds

Next, think of five reasons why you have gained this weight, and list them below:

1: _____

2: _____

3: _____

4: _____

5: _____

Now, think of five things you can start doing right now either to stop gaining weight or start losing weight:

1: _____

2: _____

3: _____

4: _____

5: _____

Keep these lists in mind as you work through this chapter, its labs, and the Behavior Change Workbook at the end of the text. The lists may become the starting point for creating a personal weight-management plan, should you decide you need one.

## FACTORS CONTRIBUTING TO EXCESS BODY FAT

Several factors determine body weight and composition. These factors can be grouped into genetic, physiological, lifestyle, and psychosocial factors.

### Genetic Factors

Estimates of the genetic contribution to obesity vary widely, from about 25–40% of an individual's body fat. More than 600 genes have been linked to obesity, but their actions are still under study. Genes influence body size and shape, body fat distribution, and metabolic rate. Genetic factors also affect the ease with which weight is gained as a result of overeating and where on the body extra weight is added.

If both parents are obese, their children have an 80% risk of being obese; children with one obese parent face a 40% risk of becoming obese. In studies that compared adoptees and their biological parents, the weights of the adoptees were found to be more like those of the biological parents than the adoptive parents, indicating a strong genetic link.

Hereditary influences, however, must be balanced against the contribution of environmental factors. Not all children of obese parents become obese, and normal-weight parents can have overweight children. Environmental factors like diet and exercise are probably responsible for such differences. Thus, the *tendency* to develop obesity may be inherited, but the expression of this tendency is affected by environmental influences.

### Physiological Factors

Metabolism is a key physiological factor in the regulation of body fat and body weight. Hormones also play a role. A few other physiological factors have been proposed as causes for weight gain, such as carbohydrate craving due to low levels of the neurotransmitter serotonin, but research on this and other theories has so far been inconclusive.

**Metabolism and Energy Balance** Metabolism is the sum of all the vital processes by which food energy and nutrients are made available to and used by the body. The largest component of metabolism, **resting metabolic rate (RMR)**, is the energy required to maintain vital body functions, including respiration, heart rate, body temperature,

---

> **resting metabolic rate (RMR)** The energy required (in calories) to maintain vital body functions, including respiration, heart rate, body temperature, and blood pressure, while the body is at rest.
>

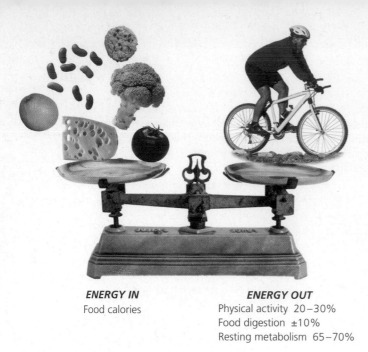

**ENERGY IN**
Food calories

**ENERGY OUT**
Physical activity 20–30%
Food digestion ±10%
Resting metabolism 65–70%

**FIGURE 9.2  The energy-balance equation**

and blood pressure, while the body is at rest. As shown in Figure 9.2, RMR accounts for about 65–70% of daily energy expenditure. The energy required to digest food accounts for an additional ±10% of daily energy expenditure. The remaining 20–30% is expended during physical activity.

Both heredity and behavior affect metabolic rate. Men, who have a higher proportion of muscle mass than women, have a higher RMR (muscle tissue is more metabolically active than fat). Also, some individuals inherit a higher or lower RMR than others. A higher RMR means that a person burns more calories while at rest and can therefore take in more calories without gaining weight.

Weight loss or gain also affects metabolic rate. When a person loses weight, both RMR and the energy required to perform physical tasks decrease. The reverse occurs when weight is gained. One reason exercise is so important during a weight-loss program is that exercise, especially resistance training, helps maintain muscle mass and metabolic rate.

Exercise has a positive effect on metabolism. When people exercise, they slightly increase their RMR—the number of calories their bodies burn at rest. In fact, a 2011 study of college-age men showed that following 45 minutes of vigorous exercise, the participants' resting metabolic rate remained elevated for 14 hours—during which the men burned an additional 200 calories while at rest or performing normal, everyday activities. People who regularly exercise also increase their muscle mass, which is associated with a higher metabolic rate. The exercise itself also burns calories, raising total energy expenditure. The higher the energy expenditure, the more the person can eat without gaining weight.

The energy-balance equation is the key to weight management. If you burn the same amount of energy as you take in (a *neutral* energy balance), your weight remains constant. If you consume more calories than you expend (a *positive* energy balance), your weight increases. If you burn more calories than you consume (a *negative* energy balance), your weight decreases.

To create a negative energy balance and lose weight and body fat, you can increase the amount of energy you burn by increasing your level of physical activity and/or decrease the amount of energy you take in by consuming fewer calories.

**Hormones**  Hormones clearly play a role in the accumulation of body fat, especially for women. Hormonal changes at puberty, during pregnancy, and at menopause contribute to the amount and location of fat accumulation. For example, during puberty, hormones cause the development of secondary sex characteristics, including larger breasts, wider hips, and a fat layer under the skin. This addition of body fat at puberty is normal and healthy.

One hormone thought to be linked to obesity is *leptin*. Secreted by the body's fat cells, leptin is carried to the brain, where it appears to let the brain know how big or small the body's fat stores are. With this information, the brain can regulate appetite and metabolic rate accordingly. Researchers hope to use leptin and other hormones to develop treatments for obesity based on appetite control. As most of us will admit, however, hunger is often *not* the primary reason we overeat. Cases of obesity based solely or primarily on hormone abnormalities do exist, but they are rare.

## Lifestyle Factors

Genetic and physiological factors may increase the risk for excess body fat, but they are not sufficient to explain the increasingly high rate of obesity in the United States. The gene pool has not changed dramatically in the past 40 years, but the rate of obesity among Americans has more than doubled. Clearly, other factors are at work—particularly lifestyle factors such as increased energy intake and decreased physical activity.

**Eating**  Americans have access to plenty of calorie-dense foods, and many have eating habits that contribute to weight gain. Most overweight adults will admit to eating more than they should of high-fat, high-sugar, high-calorie foods. Americans eat out more frequently now than in the past, and we rely more heavily on fast food and packaged convenience foods. Restaurant and convenience food portion sizes tend to be large, and the foods themselves are likely to be high in fat, sugar, and calories and low in nutrients.

Studies have consistently found that people underestimate portion sizes by as much as 25%. When participants in one study were asked to report their food intake over the previous 24 hours, the majority underestimated their actual intake by about 600 calories. Many Americans are unaware of how many calories they actually consume each day.

Americans' average calorie intake has increased by 18% since 1983. Many of those extra calories come from carbohydrates, such as refined sugars. The popularity of sugar-free soft drinks does not appear to be helping people lose weight. The result has been a substantial increase in the number of overweight and obese Americans.

**Physical Activity** Activity levels among Americans are declining, beginning in childhood and continuing throughout life. Many schools have cut back on physical education classes and even recess. Most adults drive to work, sit all day, and then relax in front of the TV (or continue working) at night. One study found that 60% of the incidence of overweight can be linked to excessive television viewing. On average, Americans exercise 15 minutes per day and watch 170 minutes of TV and movies.

**Psychosocial Factors** Many people have learned to use food as a means of coping with stress and negative emotions. Eating can provide a powerful distraction from difficult feelings—loneliness, anger, boredom, anxiety, shame, sadness, inadequacy. It can be used to combat low moods, low energy levels, and low self-esteem. When eating becomes the primary means of regulating emotions, **binge eating** or other unhealthy eating patterns can develop.

Obesity is strongly associated with socioeconomic status. The prevalence of obesity goes down as income level goes up. More women than men are obese at lower income levels, but men are somewhat more obese at higher levels. These differences may reflect the greater sensitivity and concern for a slim physical appearance among upper-income women, as well as greater access to information about nutrition and to low-fat and low-calorie foods. It may also reflect the greater acceptance of obesity among certain ethnic groups, as well as different cultural values related to food choices.

In some families and cultures, food is used as a symbol of love and caring. It is an integral part of social gatherings and celebrations. In such cases, it may be difficult

to change established eating patterns because they are linked to cultural and family values.

## ADOPTING A HEALTHY LIFESTYLE FOR SUCCESSFUL WEIGHT MANAGEMENT

When all the research is assessed, it becomes clear that most weight problems are lifestyle problems. Even though more and more young people are developing weight problems, most arrive at early adulthood with the advantage of having a normal body weight—neither too fat nor too thin. In fact, many young adults get away with very poor eating and exercise habits and don't develop a weight problem. But as the rapid growth of adolescence slows and family and career obligations increase, maintaining a healthy weight becomes a greater challenge. Slow weight gain is a major cause of overweight and obesity, so weight management is important for everyone, not just for people who are currently overweight. A good time to develop a lifestyle for successful weight management is during early adulthood, when healthy behavior patterns have a better chance of taking hold.

Permanent weight loss is not something you start and stop. You need to adopt healthy behaviors that you can maintain throughout your life, including eating habits, physical activity and exercise, an ability to think positively and manage your emotions effectively, and the coping strategies you use to deal with the stresses and challenges in your life.

### Diet and Eating Habits

In contrast to dieting, which involves some form of food restriction, the term *diet* refers to your daily food choices. Everyone has a diet, but not everyone is dieting. It's important to develop a diet that you enjoy and that enables you to maintain a healthy body composition.

Use MyPlate or DASH as the basis for planning a healthy diet (Chapter 8), and choose the healthiest

**binge eating**    A pattern of eating in which normal food consumption is interrupted by episodes of high consumption.

KEY TERM

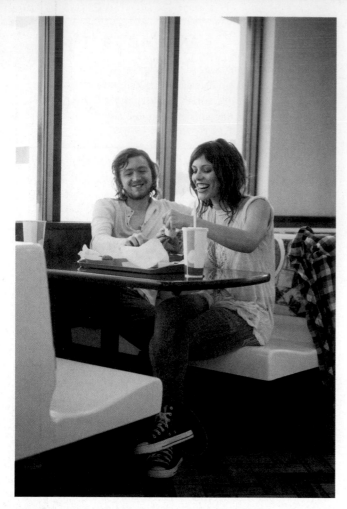

When fast food is the only available option, it can be difficult to make healthy lifestyle changes.

options within each food group. For weight management, you may need to pay special attention to total calories, portion sizes, energy density, fat and carbohydrate intake, and eating habits.

**Total Calories** The USDA suggests approximate daily energy intakes based on gender, age, and activity level. However, the precise number of calories needed to maintain weight will vary from one person to another based on heredity, fitness status, level of physical activity, and other factors. It may be more important to focus on individual energy balance than on a general recommendation for daily calorie intake. To calculate your approximate daily caloric needs, complete Lab 9.1.

The best approach for weight loss is combining an increase in physical activity with moderate calorie restriction. Don't go on a crash diet. You need to eat and drink enough to meet your need for essential nutrients. To maintain weight loss, you will probably have to maintain some degree of the calorie restriction you used to lose the weight. Therefore, it is important that you adopt a level of food intake that you can live with over the long term. For most people, maintaining weight loss is more

difficult than losing the weight in the first place. To identify weight-loss goals and ways to meet them, complete Lab 9.2.

**Portion Sizes** Overconsumption of total calories is closely tied to portion sizes. Many Americans are unaware that the portion sizes of packaged foods and of foods served at restaurants have increased in size, and most of us significantly underestimate the amount of food we eat. Studies have found that the larger the meal, the greater the underestimation of calories. Limiting portion sizes is critical for weight management. For many people, concentrating on portion sizes is easier than counting calories. See Chapter 8 for more information and hints on choosing appropriate portion sizes.

**Energy (Calorie) Density** Experts also recommend that you pay attention to *energy density*—the number of calories per ounce or gram of weight in a food. Studies suggest that it isn't consumption of a certain amount of fat or calories in food that reduces hunger and leads to feelings of fullness and satisfaction. Rather, it is consumption of a certain weight of food. Foods that are low in energy density have more volume and bulk; that is, they are relatively heavy but have few calories (Table 9.2). For example, for the same 100 calories, you could eat 20 baby carrots or four pretzel twists. You are more likely to feel full after eating the serving of carrots because it weighs ten times as much as the serving of pretzels (10 ounces versus 1 ounce).

Fresh fruits and vegetables, with their high water and fiber content, are low in energy density, as are whole-grain foods. Fresh fruits contain fewer calories and more fiber than fruit juices or drinks. Meat, ice cream, potato chips, croissants, crackers, and cakes and cookies are examples of foods high in energy density. Strategies

| Table 9.2 | Examples of Foods Low in Energy Density | |
|---|---|---|
| FOOD | AMOUNT | CALORIES |
| Carrot, raw | 1 medium | 25 |
| Popcorn, air popped | 2 cups | 62 |
| Apple | 1 medium | 72 |
| Vegetable soup | 1 cup | 72 |
| Plain instant oatmeal | ½ cup | 80 |
| Fresh blueberries | 1 cup | 80 |
| Corn on the cob (plain) | 1 ear | 80 |
| Cantaloupe | ½ melon | 95 |
| Light (fat-free) yogurt with fruit | 6 oz. | 100 |
| Unsweetened apple sauce | 1 cup | 100 |
| Pear | 1 medium | 100 |
| Corn flakes | 1 cup | 101 |
| Sweet potato, baked | 1 medium | 120 |

# Evaluating Fat and Sugar Substitutes

Foods made with fat and sugar substitutes are often promoted for weight loss. But what are fat and sugar substitutes? And can they really contribute to weight management?

## Fat Substitutes

A variety of substances are used to replace fats in processed foods and other products. Some contribute calories, protein, fiber, and/or other nutrients; others do not. Fat replacers can be classified into three general categories:

- *Carbohydrate-based fat replacers* include starch, fibers, gums, cellulose, polydextrose, and fruit purees. They are found in dairy and meat products, baked goods, salad dressing, and many other prepared foods. Newer types such as Oatrim, Z-trim, and Nu-trim are made from types of dietary fiber that may actually lower cholesterol levels. Carbohydrate-based fat replacers contribute up to 4 calories per gram.

- *Protein-based fat replacers* are typically made from milk, egg whites, soy, or whey; trade names include Simplesse, Dairy-lo, and Supro. They are used in cheese, sour cream, mayonnaise, margarine spreads, frozen desserts, salad dressings, and baked goods. These substances contribute 1–4 calories per gram.

- *Fat-based fat replacers* include glycerides, olestra, and other types of fatty acids. Some of these compounds are not absorbed well by the body and so provide fewer calories per gram (5 calories compared with the standard 9 for fats); others are impossible for the body to digest and so contribute no calories at all. Olestra, marketed under the trade name Olean and used in fried snack foods, is an example of the latter type of compound. Concerns have been raised about the safety of olestra because it reduces the absorption of fat-soluble nutrients and certain antioxidants and because it causes gastrointestinal distress in some people.

## Nonnutritive Sweeteners and Sugar Alcohols

Sugar substitutes are often referred to as nonnutritive sweeteners because they provide no calories or essential nutrients. The Food and Drug Administration (FDA) has approved five types of non-nutritive sweeteners for use in the United States: acesulfame-K (Sunett, Sweet One), aspartame (NutraSweet, Equal, NatraTaste), saccharin (Sweet 'N Low), sucralose (Splenda), and neotame. They are used in beverages, desserts, baked goods, yogurt, chewing gum, and products such as toothpaste, mouthwash, and cough

syrup. Another sweetener, stevia, is an extract of a South American shrub. The FDA has not objected to the use of stevia or sweeteners made from a highly processed component of stevia, called rebaudioside-A. Several such products are available.

Sugar alcohols are made by altering the chemical form of sugars extracted from fruits and other plant sources; they include erythritol, isomalt, lactitol, maltitol, mannitol, sorbitol, and zylitol. Sugar alcohols provide 0.2–2.5 calories per gram, compared to 4 calories per gram in standard sugar. They have typically been used to sweeten sugar-free candies but are now being added to many sweet foods (candy, cookies, and so on) promoted as low-carbohydrate products, often combined with other sweeteners. Sugar alcohols are digested in a way that can create gas, cramps, and diarrhea if they are consumed in large amounts—more than about 10 grams in one meal.

## Fat and Sugar Substitutes in Weight Management

Whether fat and sugar substitutes help you achieve and maintain a healthy weight depends on your eating and activity habits. The increase in the availability of fat-free and sugar-free foods in the United States has *not* been associated with a drop in calorie consumption. When evaluating foods containing fat and sugar substitutes, consider these issues:

- *Is the food lower in calories or just lower in fat?* Reduced-fat foods often contain extra sugar to improve the taste and texture lost when fat is removed, so such foods may be as high or even higher in total calories than their fattier counterparts.

- *Are you choosing foods with fat and/or sugar substitutes instead of foods you typically eat or in addition to foods you typically eat?* If you consume low-fat, no-sugar-added ice cream instead of regular ice cream, you may save calories. But if you add such ice cream to your daily diet simply because it is lower in fat and sugar, your overall calorie consumption—and your weight—may increase.

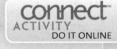
connect ACTIVITY DO IT ONLINE

- *Is an even healthier choice available?* Many of the foods containing fat and sugar substitutes are low-nutrient snack foods. Fruits, vegetables, and whole grains are healthier snack choices.

CRITICAL CONSUMER

---

for lowering the energy density of your diet include the following:

- Eat fruit with breakfast and for dessert.
- Add extra vegetables to sandwiches, casseroles, stir-fry dishes, pizza, pasta dishes, and fajitas.
- Start meals with a bowl of broth-based soup; include a green salad or fruit salad.
- Snack on fresh fruits and vegetables rather than crackers, chips, or other energy-dense snack foods.
- Limit serving sizes of energy-dense foods such as butter, mayonnaise, cheese, chocolate, fatty meats,

croissants, and snack foods that are fried, are high in added sugars (including reduced-fat products), or contain trans fat.

- Avoid processed foods, which can be high in fat and sodium. Even processed foods labeled "fat-free" or "reduced fat" may be high in calories. Such products may contain sugar and fat substitutes (see the box "Evaluating Fat and Sugar Substitutes").

**Eating Habits** Equally important to weight management is eating small, frequent meals—four to five meals per day, including breakfast and snacks—on a regular schedule.

## Nutrition Facts

Serving Size 1 cup (59g)
Servings per Container about 10

| Amount per Serving | Cereal | Cereal with 1/2 cup Fat Free Milk |
|---|---|---|
| Calories | 190 | 230 |
| Calories from Fat | 10 | 10 |
| | % Daily Value** | |
| Total Fat 1g* | 2% | 2% |
| Saturated Fat 0g | 0% | 0% |
| Trans Fat 0g | | |
| Polyunsaturated Fat 0.5g | | |
| Monounsaturated Fat 0g | | |
| Cholesterol 0mg | 0% | 0% |
| Sodium 775mg | 13% | 32% |
| Potassium 330mg | 9% | 15% |
| Total Carbohydrate 32g | 15% | 11% |
| Dietary Fiber 8g | 32% | 32% |
| Soluble Fiber 1g | | |
| Sugars 4g | | |
| Other Carbohydrate 19g | | |
| Protein 4g | | |

| | Cereal | Cereal with Milk |
|---|---|---|
| Vitamin A | 15% | 20% |
| Vitamin C | 2% | 2% |
| Calcium | 2% | 15% |
| Iron | 60% | 60% |
| Vitamin D | 10% | 25% |
| Thiamin | 25% | 30% |
| Riboflavin | 25% | 35% |
| Niacin | 25% | 25% |
| Vitamin B6 | 25% | 25% |
| Folic Acid | 50% | 50% |
| Vitamin B12 | 25% | 35% |
| Phosphorus | 20% | 30% |
| Magnesium | 25% | 30% |
| Zinc | 15% | 20% |
| Copper | 15% | 15% |

*Amount in Cereal. One half cup fat free milk contributes an additional 40 calories, 65mg sodium, 200mg potassium, 6g total carbohydrate (6g sugars), and 4g protein.
*Percent Daily Values are based on a 2,000 calorie diet. Your daily values may be higher or lower depending on your calorie needs:

| | | Calories | 2,000 | 2,500 |
|---|---|---|---|---|
| Total Fat | Less than | | 65g | 80g |
| Sat Fat | Less than | | 20g | 25g |
| Cholesterol | Less than | | 300mg | 300mg |
| Sodium | Less than | | 2,400mg | 2,400mg |
| Potassium | | | 3,500mg | 3,500mg |
| Total Carbohydrate | | | 300g | 375g |
| Dietary Fiber | | | 25g | 30g |

**INGREDIENTS:** WHOLE WHEAT FLOUR, RAISINS, CORN SYRUP, SALT, MALTED BARLEY FLOUR.
**VITAMINS AND MINERALS:** REDUCED IRON, NIACINAMIDE, ZINC OXIDE (SOURCE OF ZINC), VITAMIN B6, VITAMIN A PALMITATE, RIBOFLAVIN (VITAMIN B2), THIAMIN MONONITRATE (VITAMIN B1), FOLIC ACID, VITAMIN B12, VITAMIN D.
**MAY CONTAIN TRACES OF SOY.**

**FIGURE 9.3  High-fiber, low-calorie breakfast cereal.**
Many breakfast cereals are excellent sources of fiber, complex carbohydrates, and essential nutrients and are low in fat and cholesterol.

Skipping meals leads to excessive hunger, feelings of deprivation, and increased vulnerability to binge eating or snacking. Establish a regular pattern of eating, and set some rules governing food choices. Rules governing breakfast might be these, for example: Choose a low-sugar, high-fiber cereal (Figure 9.3) with nonfat milk and fruit most of the time; have a hard-boiled egg no more than three times a week; save pancakes and waffles for special occasions. For effective weight management, it is better to consume the majority of calories during the day rather than in the evening.

Decreeing some foods off-limits generally sets up a rule to be broken. A more sensible rule is "everything in moderation." No foods need to be entirely off-limits, though some should be eaten judiciously.

## PHYSICAL ACTIVITY AND EXERCISE

Regular physical activity is another important lifestyle factor in weight management. Physical activity and exercise burn calories and keep the metabolism geared to using food for energy instead of storing it as fat. Making significant cuts in food intake in order to lose weight is a difficult strategy to maintain; increasing your physical activity is a much better approach. Regular physical activity also protects against weight gain and is essential for maintaining weight loss.

**Physical Activity**  All physical activity will help you manage your weight. The first step in becoming more active is to incorporate more physical activity into your daily life. If you are currently sedentary, start by accumulating short bouts of moderate-intensity physical activity—walking, gardening, doing housework, and so on—for a total of 150 minutes or more per week. Even a small increase in activity level can help maintain your current weight or help you lose a moderate amount of weight. In fact, research suggests that fidgeting—stretching, squirming, standing up, and so on—may help prevent weight gain in some people. Short bouts of activity spread throughout the day can produce many of the same health benefits as continuous physical activity.

If you are overweight and want to lose weight, or if you are trying to maintain a lower weight following weight loss, a greater amount of physical activity can help. Researchers have found that people who lose weight and don't regain it typically burn about 2800 calories per week in physical activity—the equivalent of about 1 hour of brisk walking per day.

**Exercise**  Once you become more active every day, begin a formal exercise program that includes cardiorespiratory endurance exercise, resistance training, and stretching exercises (see the box "What Is the Best Way to Exercise for Weight Loss?"). Moderate-intensity endurance exercise, if performed frequently for a relatively long duration, can burn a significant number of calories. Endurance training also increases the rate at which your body uses calories after your exercise session is over—burning an additional 5–180 extra calories, depending on the intensity of exercise. Resistance training builds muscle mass, and more muscle translates into a higher metabolic rate. Resistance training can also help you maintain your muscle mass during a period of weight loss, helping you avoid the significant drop in RMR associated with weight loss.

Regular physical activity, maintained throughout life, makes weight management easier. The sooner you establish good habits, the better. The key to success is making exercise an integral part of a lifestyle you can enjoy now and will enjoy in the future.

### Fitness Tip

When you watch TV, turn commercial breaks into exercise breaks. When commercials come on, get off the couch and move: Do jumping jacks, push-ups, curl-ups, run in place, or just walk around. During a 2-hour program, you can accumulate about 30 minutes of physical activity this way!

# What Is the Best Way to Exercise for Weight Loss?

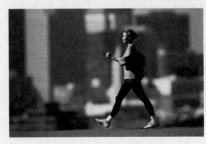

If weight loss is your primary goal, the guidelines for planning a fitness program can vary depending on your weight, body composition, and current level of fitness. For example, there is some dispute among fitness experts about the best target heart rate (THR) zone to use when exercising for weight loss. Some experts recommend exercising at a moderate THR (55–69% of maximum heart rate) because the body burns fat at a slightly more efficient rate at this level of exertion. Others recommend exercising vigorously (70–90% of maximum heart rate) because exercise at this intensity burns more calories overall. According to some estimates, for example, a 30-minute workout at 80–85% of maximum heart rate burns about 30% more calories overall than a 30-minute workout at 60–65% maximum heart rate—but the lower-intensity workout burns roughly 20% more fat calories than the higher-intensity workout.

Regardless, if you are obese or your fitness level is very low, start with a lower-intensity workout (55% of maximum heart rate), and stick with it until your cardiorespiratory fitness level improves enough to support short bouts of higher-intensity exercise. This way, you will burn more fat, reduce the risk of injury and strain on your heart, and improve your chances of staying with your program. Even if your primary goal is to lose weight, you are also improving your cardiorespiratory fitness. Any amount of exercise, even at low to moderate intensity, will help you achieve both goals. But patience is required, especially if you need to lose a great deal of weight.

For weight loss to occur, exercise at lower intensities has to be offset by longer and/or more frequent exercise sessions. Experts recommend 60–90 minutes of daily exercise for anyone who needs to lose weight or maintain weight loss. If you cannot fit such a large block of activity into your daily schedule, break your workouts into short segments—as little as 10–15 minutes each. This approach is probably best for someone who has been sedentary, because it allows the body to become accustomed to exercise at a gradual pace while preventing injury and avoiding strain on the heart.

Many research studies have shown that walking is an ideal form of exercise for losing weight and avoiding weight gain. A landmark 15–year study by the University of North Carolina at Charlotte showed that, over time, people who walked only 30 minutes per day gained 18 pounds less than people who did not walk. Those who regularly walked farther were better able to lose or maintain weight. Other studies found that people who walked 30 minutes five times per week lost an average of 5 pounds in 6–12 months, without dieting, watching what they ate, or exercising intensely. You can lose even more weight if you eat sensibly and walk farther and faster.

A 165-pound adult who walks at a speed of 3 miles per hour for 60 minutes a day, 5 days a week, can lose about one-half pound of body weight per week. Regular walking is the simplest and most effective health habit for controlling body weight and promoting health. Even if you're sedentary, a few months of walking can increase your fitness level to the point where more vigorous types of exercise—and even greater health benefits—are possible.

SOURCES: Gordon-Larsen, P., et al. 2009. Fifteen-year longitudinal trends in walking patterns and their impact on weight change. *American Journal of Clinical Nutrition* 89(1): 19–26. Levine, J. A., et al. 2008. The role of free-living daily walking in human weight gain and obesity. *Diabetes* 57(3): 548–554. Nelson, M. E., and S. C. Folta. 2009. Further evidence for the benefits of walking. *American Journal of Clinical Nutrition* 89(1): 15–16. Physical Activity Guidelines Advisory Committee. 2008. *Physical Activity Guidelines Advisory Committee Report, 2008.* Washington, D.C.: U.S. Department of Health and Human Services.

## THOUGHTS AND EMOTIONS

The way you think about yourself and your world influences, and is influenced by, how you feel and how you act. In fact, research on people who have a weight problem indicates that low self-esteem and the negative emotions that accompany it are significant problems. People with low self-esteem mentally compare the actual self to an internally held picture of the "ideal self," an image based on perfectionist goals and beliefs about how they and others should be. The more these two pictures differ, the larger the impact on self-esteem and the more likely the presence of negative emotions.

Besides the internal picture we carry of ourselves, all of us carry on an internal dialogue about events happening to us and around us. This *self-talk* can be either self-deprecating or positively motivating, depending on our beliefs and attitudes. Having realistic beliefs and goals and engaging in positive self-talk and problem solving support a healthy lifestyle. (Chapter 10 and Activity 11 in the Behavior Change Workbook at the end of the text include strategies for developing realistic self-talk.)

## Coping Strategies

Appropriate coping strategies help you deal with the stresses of life; they are also an important lifestyle factor

### Ask Yourself

QUESTIONS FOR CRITICAL THINKING AND REFLECTION

Have you ever used food as an escape when you were stressed out or distraught? Were you aware of what you were doing at the time? How can you avoid using food as a coping mechanism in the future?

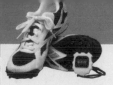
If you're trying to lose weight or maintain your current weight, it's a good idea to write down everything you eat, including how many calories it contains. Researchers have found that writing down the food choices you make every day increases your commitment and helps you stick to your diet, especially during high-risk times such as holidays, parties, and family gatherings.

Writing every day also serves as a reminder to you that losing weight is important. In a multicenter study conducted over 6 months in 2008, dieters who kept a daily food journal lost twice as much weight as those who didn't track what they ate.

Besides tracking what you eat, keep track of your formal exercise program and other daily physical activities so you can begin increasing either their intensity or duration. People who succeed in their health program expend lots of energy in physical activity—according to one study, an average of 2700 calories a week. Tracking your physical activities and daily exercise routines provides all the same benefits as tracking your eating habits. Your log will help you see your progress, track fitness improvements and weight loss, and maintain a positive perspective on your efforts. All this will help you take your program seriously over the long term.

in weight management. Many people use eating as a way to cope; others may use drugs, alcohol, smoking, or gambling. Those who overeat might use food to alleviate loneliness or to serve as a pickup for fatigue, as an antidote to boredom, or as a distraction from problems. Some people even overeat to punish themselves for real or imagined transgressions.

Those who recognize that they are misusing food in such ways can analyze their eating habits with fresh eyes. They can consciously attempt to find new coping strategies and begin to use food appropriately—to fuel life's activities, to foster growth, and to bring pleasure, but *not* to manage stress. For a summary of the components of weight management through healthy lifestyle choices, see the box "Lifestyle Strategies for Successful Weight Management."

## APPROACHES TO OVERCOMING A WEIGHT PROBLEM

Each year, Americans spend more than $40 billion on various weight-loss plans and products. If you are overweight, you may already be creating a plan to lose weight and keep it off. You have many options.

### Doing It Yourself

If you need to lose weight, focus on adopting the healthy lifestyle described throughout this book. The "right" weight for you will evolve naturally, and you won't have to diet. Combine modest cuts in energy intake with exercise, and avoid very-low-calorie diets. (In general, a low-calorie diet should provide 1200–1500 calories per day.) By achieving a negative energy balance of 250–1000 calories

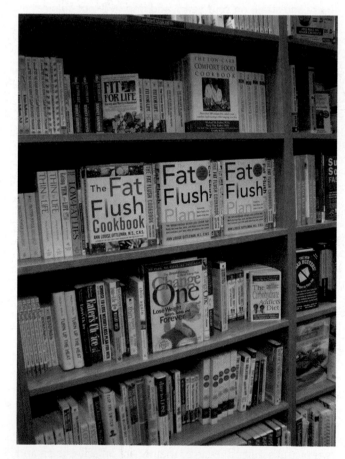

There are many plans and supplements promoted for weight loss, but few have any research supporting their effectiveness for long-term weight management.

per day, you'll produce the recommended weight loss of ½–2 pounds per week.

Most low-calorie diets cause a rapid loss of body water at first. When this phase passes, weight loss declines. As

# Lifestyle Strategies for Successful Weight Management

## Food Choices

- Focus on making good choices from each food group.

- Favor foods with a *low energy (calorie) density* and a *high nutrient density*.

- Check labels for serving sizes, calories, and nutrients.

- Watch for hidden calories. Reduced-fat foods often have as many calories as their full-fat versions.

- Drink fewer calories in the form of soda, fruit drinks, sports drinks, alcohol, and specialty coffees and teas.

## Planning and Serving

- Keep a log of what you eat, as described earlier in the text.

- Eat four to five meals/snacks daily, *including breakfast,* to distribute calories throughout your day.

- Fix more meals yourself and eat out less often.

- Keep low-calorie snacks on hand to combat the "munchies." Fresh fruits and vegetables are good choices.

- When shopping, make a list and stick to it. Don't shop when you're hungry. Avoid aisles that contain problem foods.

- Consume the majority of your daily calories during the day, not in the evening.

- Pay attention to portion sizes. Use measuring cups and spoons and a food scale to become familiar with portion sizes.

- Serve meals on small plates and in small bowls to help you eat smaller portions without feeling deprived.

- Eat only in specifically designated spots. Remove food from other areas of your home.

- When you eat, just eat. Don't do anything else.

- Avoid late-night eating, a behavior specifically associated with weight gain among college students.

- Eat slowly. It takes time for your brain to get the message that your stomach is full. Take small bites and chew food thoroughly. Pay attention to every bite, and enjoy your food.

## Special Occasions

- When you eat out, choose a restaurant where you can make healthy food choices. Ask the server not to put bread and butter on the table before the meal, and request that sauces and salad dressings be served on the side. If portion sizes are large, take half your food home for a meal later in the week. Don't choose supersized meals.

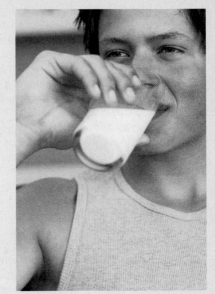

- If you cook a large meal for friends, send leftovers home with your guests.

- If you're eating at a friend's home, eat a little and leave the rest. Don't eat to be polite.

## Physical Activity and Stress Management

- Increase your level of daily physical activity, as slowly as necessary based on your current fitness level.

- Begin an exercise program that includes cardiorespiratory endurance exercise, strength training, and stretching.

- Develop techniques for handling stress. See Chapter 10 for more on stress management.

- Develop strategies for coping with nonhunger cues to eat, such as boredom, sleepiness, or anxiety. Try calling a friend, taking a shower, or reading a magazine.

- Tell family members and friends that you're changing your eating and exercise habits. Ask them to be supportive.

Visit the Small Steps site for more tips (www.smallstep.gov).

---

a result, dieters are often misled into believing that their efforts are not working. They give up, not realizing that smaller losses later in the diet are actually more significant than the initial big losses, because later loss is mostly fat loss, whereas initial loss is primarily fluid. For someone who is overweight, reasonable weight loss is 8–10% of body weight over 6 months.

For many Americans, maintaining weight loss is a bigger challenge than losing weight. Most weight lost during a period of dieting is regained. When planning a weight-management program, you need to include strategies that you can maintain over the long term, both for food choices and for physical activity. Weight management is a lifelong project. A registered dietitian or nutritionist can recommend an appropriate plan for you when you want to lose weight on your own. For more tips on losing weight on your own, refer to the section later in the chapter on creating an individual weight-management plan.

## Diet Books

Many people who try to lose weight by themselves fall prey to one or more of the dozens of diet books on the market. Although some books contain useful advice and

# High-Tech Weight Management

Technology is making inroads into the area of weight management at an ever-quickening pace. Once the domain of clinical weight-loss programs, digital tools are now available for consumers who want to lose weight or keep it off.

At the clinical level, new research shows that overweight patients who are equipped with high-tech monitoring devices (which monitor their energy intake and output) lose at least as much weight as patients who participate only in in-person weight-management counseling sessions. When person-to-person counseling is added to the use of digital monitors, patients lose even more weight and manage to keep it off longer.

At the consumer level, a wide and ever-growing range of portable devices and weight-loss applications are also available to consumers. There are dozens of "apps" that run on smart phones, for example, which can help you keep a nutrition journal and calculate your daily intake of calories and nutrients. Such apps often pair with other programs that can help you track your physical activity level and calculate the number of calories you burn throughout the day. Some of these apps can upload your daily data to a Web site that lets you track energy intake and output over the course of time. Many such programs can also help with goal-setting, provide dietary or exercise advice, or let you join communities of users who are also trying to manage their weight.

Internet-based weight-loss programs have proliferated over the last decade. Most such Web sites offer a cross between self-help and group support through chat rooms, bulletin boards, and e-newsletters. Many sites offer online self-assessment for diet and physical activity habits as well as a meal plan; some provide access to a staff professional for individualized help. Many are free, but some charge a weekly or monthly fee.

Research suggests that this type of program provides an alternative to in-person diet counseling and can lead to weight loss for some people. Studies found that people who logged on more frequently tended to lose more weight; weekly online contact in terms of behavior therapy proved most successful for weight loss. The criteria used to evaluate commercial programs can also be applied to Internet-based programs. If you're interested in joining an online weight-loss program, make sure the service offers member-to-member support and access to staff professionals.

An example of a particularly successful online weight-management program is the National Weight Control

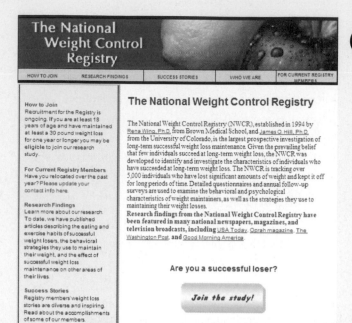

Registry. This site is part of an ongoing study of people who have lost significant amounts of weight and kept it off. The average participant in the registry has lost 71 pounds and kept the weight off for more than 5 years. Nearly all participants use a combination of diet and exercise to manage their weight. Most follow moderate-calorie diets that are relatively low in fat and fried foods; users monitor their body weight and their food intake frequently. Participants engage in an average of 60 minutes of moderate physical activity daily. The National Weight Control Registry study illustrates that to lose weight and keep it off, you must decrease daily calorie intake and/or increase daily physical activity—and continue to do so over your lifetime. And this fact is an important lesson: Even with the help of digital devices and programs, weight management is still primarily a matter of personal effort, perseverance, and a commitment to lifestyle changes that last for life.

**SOURCE:** The National Weight Control Registry, www.nwcr.ws. Screen reprinted by permission.

**connect** ACTIVITY DO IT ONLINE

---

motivational tips, most make empty promises. Accept books that advocate a balanced approach to diet plus exercise and sound nutritional advice, but reject any book that:

- Advocates an unbalanced way of eating, such as a high-carbohydrate-only diet or a low-carbohydrate, high-protein diet, or that promotes a single food, such as cabbage or grapefruit.
- Claims to be based on a "scientific breakthrough" or to have the "secret to success."

- Uses gimmicks, such as matching eating to blood type, hyping insulin resistance as the cause of obesity, or combining foods in special ways to achieve weight loss.
- Promises quick weight loss or limits the selection of foods.

Many diets cause weight loss if maintained. The real difficulty is finding a safe and healthy pattern of food choices and physical activity that results in long-term maintenance of a healthy body weight and reduced risk of chronic disease (see the box "High-Tech Weight Management").

## Dietary Supplements and Diet Aids

The number of dietary supplements and other weight-loss aids on the market has also increased in recent years. Promoted in advertisements, magazines, direct mail campaigns, infomercials, and on Web sites, these products typically promise a quick and easy path to weight loss. Most of these products are marketed as dietary supplements and so are subject to fewer regulations than over the counter (OTC) medications. A 2002 report from the Federal Trade Commission stated that more than half of advertisements for weight-loss products made representations that are likely to be false.

In late 2008, the FDA identified more than 25 weight-loss pill products that consumers should not purchase or use and ordered the products recalled from stores. Such recalls are becoming more common. Studies revealed that some of the recalled supplements contained prescription medications, including sibutramine (a weight-loss medication sold under the brand name Meridia) and phenytoin, an antiseizure medication. In its consumer alert, the FDA noted that a number of the recalled supplements contained pharmaceuticals in amounts far exceeding FDA-recommended levels. Some of the supplements contained substances that are not approved for sale in the United States, including rimonabant (a prescription weight-loss drug sold in Europe) and phenolphthalein, which is thought to be a carcinogen. The use of these drugs could lead to complications such as heart attack, stroke, suicide, and even cancer. The prescription medications were not listed on any of the supplements' labels, meaning consumers could be taking lethal doses of prescription drugs without knowing it.

The following sections describe some commonly marketed OTC products for weight loss.

**Formula Drinks and Food Bars** Canned diet drinks, powders used to make shakes, and diet food bars and snacks are designed to achieve weight loss by substituting for some or all of a person's daily food intake. However, most people find it difficult to use these products for long periods, and muscle loss and other serious health problems may result if they are used as the sole source of nutrition for an extended period. Use of such products sometimes results in rapid short-term weight loss, but the weight is typically regained because users don't learn to change their eating and lifestyle behaviors.

---

**Wellness Tip**

If you're tempted to start taking an OTC weight-loss supplement, do your homework first. Ask for your doctor's opinion, and check the FDA's supplement Web page at http://www.fda.gov/Food/DietarySupplements/default.htm.

---

**Herbal Supplements** As described in Chapter 8, herbs are marketed as dietary supplements, so there is little information about effectiveness, proper dosage, drug interactions, and side effects. In addition, labels may not accurately reflect the ingredients and dosages present, and safe manufacturing practices are not guaranteed. For example, the substitution of a toxic herb for another compound during the manufacture of a Chinese herbal weight-loss preparation caused more than 100 cases of kidney damage and cancer among users in Europe.

The FDA has banned the sale of ephedra (*ma huang*), stating that it presented a significant and unreasonable risk to human health. Ephedrine, the active ingredient in ephedra, is structurally similar to amphetamine and was widely used in weight-loss supplements. It may suppress appetite, but adverse effects have included elevated blood pressure, panic attacks, seizures, insomnia, and increased risk of heart attack or stroke, particularly when combined with another stimulant, such as caffeine. The FDA banned the synthetic stimulant phenylpropanolamine for similar reasons. Other herbal stimulants still on the market are described in Table 9.3.

**Other Supplements** Fiber is another common ingredient in OTC diet aids, promoted for appetite control. However, dietary fiber acts as a bulking agent in the large intestine, not the stomach, so it doesn't have a pronounced effect on appetite. In addition, many diet aids contain only 3 or fewer grams of fiber, which does not contribute much toward the recommended daily intake of 25–38 grams.

Other popular dietary supplements include conjugated linoleic acid, carnitine, chromium, pyruvate, calcium, B vitamins, chitosan, and a number of products labeled "fat absorbers," "fat blockers," or "starch blockers." Research has not found these products to be effective, and many have potentially adverse side effects.

## Weight-Loss Programs

Weight-loss programs come in a variety of types, including noncommercial support organizations, commercial programs, Web sites, and clinical programs.

A study lasting from 2008 to 2011 revealed an interesting phenomenon regarding weight-loss interventions among college students: Groups of students who shared certain characteristics did better at losing and managing weight than groups of dissimilar students. The study grouped students according to common eating habits or common psychosocial characteristics, both of which contribute to weight gain. These "clusters" of similar students were able to lose more weight and keep more weight off than were "nonclustered" groups of students who did not share common dietary or psychosocial characteristics. The findings of this study may help shape group-oriented weight-loss programs in the future, whether such programs are commercial, noncommercial, or clinical.

## Table 9.3    Ingredients Commonly Found in Weight-Loss Products

| COMMON NAME | USE/CLAIM | EVIDENCE/EFFICACY | SAFETY ISSUES |
|---|---|---|---|
| Bitter orange extract (*Citrus aurantium*) | CNS stimulant | Limited evidence | Highly concentrated extracts may increase blood pressure; should not be used by people with cardiac problems |
| Caffeine | CNS stimulant; increases fat metabolism | Amplifies effects of ephedra | Generally considered safe; caution advised in caffeine-sensitive individuals |
| *Garcinia cambogia* | May interfere with fat metabolism or suppress appetite | Inconclusive evidence | Short-term use (<12 weeks) generally considered safe when used as directed |
| Green tea extract | Diuretic; increases metabolism | Limited evidence | Generally considered safe |
| Guarana | CNS stimulant; diuretic | Few clinical trials | Same as for caffeine; overdose can cause painful urination, abdominal spasms, and vomiting |
| Senna, cascara, aloe, buckthorn berries | Stimulant, laxative | Not effective for weight loss | Chronic use decreases muscle tone in large intestine, causes electrolyte imbalances, and leads to dependence on laxatives |
| Tea, kola, dandelion, bucho, uva-ursi, damiana, juniper | Diuretic | Not effective for weight loss | Chronic use can cause possible electrolyte imbalance in some people |
| Yerba mate | Stimulant, laxative, diuretic | Limited evidence | Long-term use as a beverage may increase the risk of oral cancer |

**SOURCE:** Adapted from Leslie, K. K. 2003. Herbal weight-loss products: Effective and appropriate? *Today's Dietician* 5(8).

**Noncommercial Weight-Loss Programs** Noncommercial programs such as TOPS (Take Off Pounds Sensibly) and Overeaters Anonymous (OA) mainly provide group support. They do not advocate any particular diet, but they do recommend seeking professional advice for creating an individualized diet and exercise plan. Like Alcoholics Anonymous, OA is a 12-step program with a spiritual orientation that promotes abstinence from compulsive overeating. These types of programs are generally free. Your physician or a registered dietitian can also provide information and support for weight loss.

**Commercial Weight-Loss Programs** Commercial weight-loss programs typically provide group support, nutrition education, physical activity recommendations, and behavior modification advice. Some also make packaged foods available to assist in following dietary advice.

A responsible and safe weight-loss program should have the following features:

- The recommended diet should be safe and balanced, include all the food groups, and meet the Dietary Reference Intakes (DRIs) for all nutrients. Physical activity and exercise should be strongly encouraged.

- The program should promote slow, steady weight loss averaging ½–2 pounds per week. (There may be rapid weight loss initially due to fluid loss.)

- If a participant plans to lose more than 20 pounds, has any health problems, or is taking medication on a regular basis, the program should offer physician evaluation and monitoring. The program's staff should include qualified counselors and health professionals.

- The program should include plans for weight maintenance after the weight-loss phase is over.

- The program should provide information on all fees and costs, including those of supplements and prepackaged foods, as well as data on risks and expected outcomes of participating in the program.

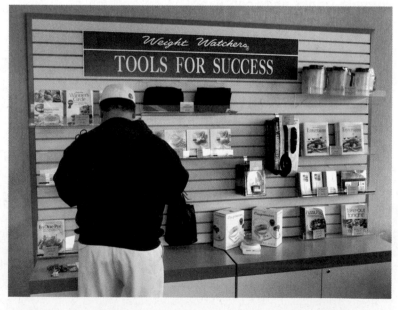

A variety of commercial weight-loss programs are available. These programs yield mixed results, but most provide nutritional counseling and support for people who are serious about losing weight.

You should also consider whether a program fits your lifestyle and whether you are truly ready to make a commitment to it. A strong commitment and a plan for maintenance are especially important because only 10–15% of program participants maintain their weight loss; the rest gain back all or more than they had lost. One study of participants found that regular exercise was the best predictor of maintaining weight loss, and frequent television viewing was the best predictor of weight gain.

**Clinical Weight-Loss Programs** Medically supervised clinical programs are usually located in a hospital or other medical setting. Designed to help those who are severely obese, these programs typically involve a closely monitored very-low-calorie diet. The cost of a clinical program is usually high, but insurance often covers part of the fee.

## Prescription Drugs

For a medicine to cause weight loss, it must reduce energy consumption, increase energy expenditure, and/or interfere with energy absorption. The medications most often prescribed for weight loss are appetite suppressants that reduce feelings of hunger or increase feelings of fullness. Appetite suppressants usually work by increasing levels of catecholamine or serotonin, two brain chemicals that affect mood and appetite.

All prescription weight-loss drugs have potential side effects. Those that affect catecholamine levels, including phentermine (Ionamin, Obenix, Fastin, and Adipex-P), diethylpropion (Tenuate), and mazindol (Sanorex), may cause sleeplessness, nervousness, and euphoria.

Most appetite suppressants are approved by the FDA only for short-term use. One drug—orlistat (Xenical)—is approved for longer-term use. Orlistat lowers calorie consumption by blocking fat absorption in the intestines; it prevents about 30% of the fat in food from being digested. Similar to the fat substitute olestra, orlistat also reduces the absorption of fat-soluble vitamins and antioxidants.

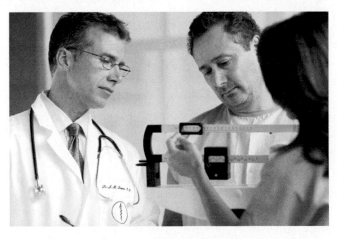

Very obese people may get the most benefit from a clinical weight-loss program, where diet and activity are monitored closely by health professionals.

Therefore, taking a vitamin supplement is highly recommended if taking orlistat. Side effects include diarrhea, cramping, and other gastrointestinal problems if users do not follow a low-fat diet. In 2007, the FDA approved Alli, a lower-dose version of orlistat that is sold over the counter.

All of these medications work best in conjunction with behavior modification. Appetite suppressants produce modest weight loss—about 5–22 pounds above the loss expected with nondrug obesity treatments. Individuals respond differently, however, and some experience more weight loss than others. Weight loss tends to level off or reverse after 4–6 months on a medication, and many people regain the weight they've lost when they stop taking the drug.

Prescription weight-loss drugs are not for people who just want to lose a few pounds. The latest federal guidelines advise people to try lifestyle modification for at least 6 months before trying drug therapy. Prescription drugs are recommended only in certain cases: for people who have been unable to lose weight with nondrug options and who have a body mass index (BMI) over 30 (or over 27 if two or more additional risk factors such as diabetes and high blood pressure are present). For severely obese people who have been unable to lose weight by other methods, prescription drugs may provide a good option.

## Surgery

It is estimated that 5.7% of adult Americans have a BMI grreater than 40, qualifying them as severely or "morbidly" obese. The number of severely obese people has nearly doubled in the last two decades. Severe obesity is a serious medical condition that is often complicated by other health problems such as diabetes, sleep disorders, heart disease, and arthritis. Surgical intervention—known as *bariatric surgery*—may be necessary as a treatment of last resort. Bariatric surgery may be recommended for patients with a BMI greater than 40, or greater than 35 with obesity-related illnesses.

Due to the increasing prevalence of severe obesity, surgical treatment of obesity is growing worldwide. Obesity-related health conditions, as well as risk of premature death, generally improve after surgical weight loss. Surgery, however, is not without risks. A 2006 study found that patients with poor cardiorespiratory fitness prior to surgery experienced more postoperative complications, including stroke, kidney failure, and even death, than patients with higher fitness levels.

Bariatric surgery modifies the gastrointestinal tract by changing the size of the stomach by partitioning the stomach with staples or a band, or by modifying the way the stomach drains (gastric bypass). In either type of surgical intervention, the goal is to promote weight loss by reducing the amount of food the patient can eat. The two most common surgeries are the Roux-en-Y gastric bypass and the vertical banded gastroplasty (VGB/Lap-Band). Potential complications from surgery include nutritional deficiencies, fat intolerance, nausea,

## Ask Yourself

### QUESTIONS FOR CRITICAL THINKING AND REFLECTION

Why do you think people continue to buy into fad diets and weight-loss gimmicks, even though they are constantly reminded that the key to weight management is lifestyle change? Have you ever tried a fad diet or dietary supplement? If so, what were your reasons for trying it? What were the results?

## Fitness Tip

It may not be possible to be "too fit," but it is possible to exercise too much. This is a common problem among people who are obsessed with their weight or body image. Track your exercise habits for a week; if they seem excessive and you can't seem to cut back, talk to a professional counselor or your doctor to find out if you have a body image problem.

vomiting, and reflux. As many as 10–20% of patients may require follow-up surgery to address complications. According to a 2009 study by the Agency for Healthcare Research and Quality, however, the rate of complications in bariatric surgery patients fell more than 20% from 2002–2006. This drop in complications has reduced the number of rehospitalizations for bariatric surgery patients, and has also helped bring down the overall cost of these procedures.

Weight loss from surgery generally ranges between 40% and 70% of total body weight over the course of a year. The key to success is to have adequate follow-up and to stay motivated so that life behaviors and eating patterns are changed permanently.

The surgical technique of liposuction involves the removal of small amounts of fat from specific locations. Liposuction is not a method for treating obesity.

## Psychological Help

When concerns about body weight and shape have developed into an eating disorder, professional help is recommended. Therapists who help people with these disorders should have experience in weight management, body image issues, eating disorders, addictions, and abuse issues.

## BODY IMAGE

The collective picture of the body as seen through the mind's eye, **body image** consists of perceptions, images, thoughts, attitudes, and emotions. A negative body image is characterized by dissatisfaction with the body in general or some part of the body in particular.

More and more people are becoming unhappy with their bodies and obsessed with their weight. In recent surveys, more than half of Americans have stated that they are dissatisfied with their weight; only about 10% report being completely satisfied with their bodies. Dissatisfaction with body weight and shape is associated with dangerous eating patterns, such as binge eating or self-starvation, and with eating disorders.

## Severe Body Image Problems

Poor body image can cause significant psychological distress. A person can become preoccupied by a perceived defect in appearance, thereby damaging self-esteem and interfering with relationships. Adolescents and adults who have a negative body image are more likely to diet restrictively, eat compulsively, or develop some other form of disordered eating.

When dissatisfaction becomes extreme, the condition is called *body dysmorphic disorder (BDD)*. BDD affects about 2% of Americans, males and females in equal numbers. BDD usually begins before age 18 but can begin in adulthood. Sufferers are overly concerned with physical appearance, often focusing on slight flaws that are not obvious to others. Individuals with BDD may spend hours every day thinking about their flaws and looking at themselves in mirrors; they may desire and seek repeated cosmetic surgeries. BDD is related to obsessive-compulsive disorder and can lead to depression, social phobia, and suicide if left untreated. Medication and therapy can help people with BDD.

In some cases, body image may bear little resemblance to fact. A person with the eating disorder anorexia nervosa typically has a severely distorted body image, believing herself to be fat even when she has become emaciated (see the next section for more on anorexia). Distorted body image is also a hallmark of *muscle dysmorphia*, a disorder experienced by some bodybuilders and other active people who see themselves as small and out of shape despite being very muscular. People with muscle dysmorphia may let obsessive weight training interfere with their work and relationships. They may also use potentially dangerous muscle-building drugs.

To assess your body image, complete the body image self-test in Lab 9.3.

## Acceptance and Change

There are limits to the changes that can be made to body weight and body shape, both of which are influenced by heredity. Knowing when the limits to healthy change have been reached—and learning to accept those limits—is crucial for overall wellness. Women in particular tend to measure self-worth in terms of their appearance. When they don't measure up to an unrealistic cultural ideal,

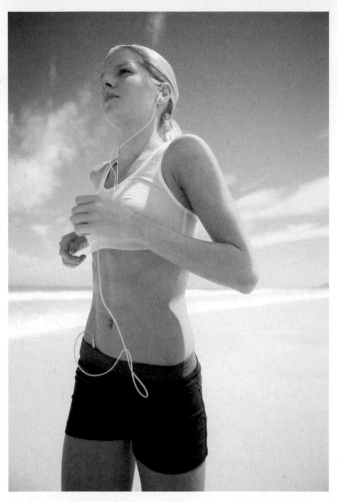

Exercise is a healthy practice, but people with eating disorders sometimes exercise compulsively, building their lives around their workouts. Compulsive exercise can lead to injuries, low body fat, and other health problems.

they see themselves as defective, and their self-esteem falls. The result can be negative body image, disordered eating, or even a full-blown eating disorder (see the box "Gender, Ethnicity, and Body Image").

Weight management needs to take place in a positive and realistic atmosphere. For an obese person, losing as few as 10 pounds can reduce blood pressure and improve mood. The hazards of excessive dieting and overconcern about body weight need to be countered by a change in attitude. A reasonable weight must take into account a person's weight history, social circumstances, metabolic profile, and psychological well-being.

## EATING DISORDERS

Problems with body weight and weight control are not limited to excessive body fat. A growing number of people, especially adolescent girls and young women, experience **eating disorders**, characterized by severe disturbances in body image, eating patterns, and eating-related behavior.

The major eating disorders are anorexia nervosa, bulimia nervosa, and binge-eating disorder. Eating disorders affect about 10 million American females and 1 million males. Many more people have abnormal eating habits and attitudes about food that, although not meeting the criteria for a major eating disorder, do disrupt their lives. To assess your eating habits, complete Lab 9.3.

Although many different explanations for the development of eating disorders have been proposed, they share one central feature: a dissatisfaction with body image and body weight. Such dissatisfaction is created by distorted thinking, including perfectionist beliefs, unreasonable demands for self-control, and excessive self-criticism. Dissatisfaction with body weight leads to dysfunctional attitudes about eating, such as fear of fat, preoccupation with food, and problematic eating behaviors. Eating disorders are classified as mental disorders.

### Anorexia Nervosa

A person with **anorexia nervosa** does not eat enough food to maintain a reasonable body weight. Anorexia affects 1% of Americans, or about 3 million people, 95% of them female. Although it can occur later, anorexia typically develops between ages 12 and 18.

People with anorexia have an intense fear of gaining weight or becoming fat. Their body image is distorted so that, even when emaciated, they think they are fat. People with anorexia may engage in compulsive behaviors or rituals that help them keep from eating. They also commonly use vigorous and prolonged physical activity to reduce body weight. Although they may express a great interest in food, their diet becomes more and more extreme.

People with anorexia are typically introverted, emotionally reserved, and socially insecure. Their entire sense of self-esteem may be tied up in their evaluation of their body shape and weight.

Anorexia nervosa has been linked to a variety of medical complications, including disorders of the cardiovascular, gastrointestinal, and endocrine systems. Because of extreme weight loss, females with anorexia often stop menstruating. When body fat is virtually gone and muscles are severely wasted, the body turns to its organs in a desperate search for protein. Death can occur from heart failure caused by electrolyte imbalances. About one in ten

**body image**  The mental representation a person holds about her or his body at any given moment in time, consisting of perceptions, images, thoughts, attitudes, and emotions about the body.

**eating disorder**  A serious disturbance in eating patterns or eating-related behavior, characterized by a negative body image and concerns about body weight or body fat.

**anorexia nervosa**  An eating disorder characterized by a refusal to maintain body weight at a minimally healthy level and an intense fear of gaining weight or becoming fat; self-starvation.

KEY TERMS

# Gender, Ethnicity, and Body Image

## Body Image and Gender

Women are much more likely than men to be dissatisfied with their bodies, often wanting to be thinner than they are. In one study, only 30% of eighth-grade girls reported being content with their bodies, while 70% of their male classmates expressed satisfaction with their looks. Girls and women are much more likely than boys and men to diet, develop eating disorders, and be obese.

The image of the ideal woman presented in the media is often unrealistic and even unhealthy. In a review of BMI data for Miss America pageant winners since 1922, researchers noted a significant decline in BMI over time, with an increasing number of recent winners having BMIs in the "underweight" category. The average fashion model is 4–7 inches taller and almost 50 pounds lighter than the average American woman. Most fashion models are thinner than 98% of American women.

Our culture may be promoting an unattainable masculine ideal as well. Researchers have found that media consumption is positively associated with a desire for thinness and muscularity. Researchers studying male action figures note that they have become increasingly muscular. Such media messages can be demoralizing; although not as commonly as girls and women, boys and men also suffer from body image problems.

## Body Image and Ethnicity

Although some groups espouse thinness as an ideal body type, others do not. In many traditional African societies, for example, full-figured women's bodies are seen as symbols of health, prosperity, and fertility. African American teenage girls have a more positive body image than white girls; in one survey, two-thirds of them defined beauty as "the right attitude," whereas white girls were more preoccupied with weight and body shape.

Nevertheless, recent evidence indicates that African American women are as likely to engage in disordered eating behavior—especially binge eating and vomiting—as their Latina, Native American, and white counterparts. This finding underscores the complex nature of eating disorders and body image.

## Avoiding Body-Image Problems

To minimize your risk of developing a body-image problem, keep the following strategies in mind:

- Focus on healthy habits and good physical health.

- Put concerns about physical appearance in perspective. Your worth as a human being does not depend on how you look.

- Practice body acceptance. You can influence your body size and type through lifestyle to some degree, but the fact is that some people are genetically designed to be bigger or heavier than others.

- Find things to appreciate in yourself besides an idealized body image. People who can learn to value other aspects of themselves are more accepting of the physical changes that occur naturally with age.

- View eating as a morally neutral activity—eating dessert isn't "bad" and doesn't make you a bad person.

- See the beauty and fitness industries for what they are. Realize that their goal is to prompt dissatisfaction with yourself so that you will buy their products.

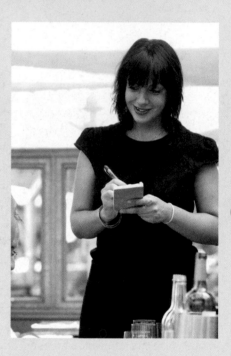

---

women with anorexia dies of starvation, cardiac arrest, or other medical complications—one of the highest death rates for any psychiatric disorder. Depression is also a serious risk, and about half the fatalities relating to anorexia are suicides.

## Bulimia Nervosa

A person with **bulimia nervosa** engages in recurrent episodes of binge eating followed by **purging**. Although bulimia usually begins in adolescence or young adulthood, it has recently begun to emerge at increasingly younger (11–12 years) and older (40–60 years) ages. Research suggests that about 5% of college-age women have bulimia.

During a binge, a bulimic person may rapidly consume thousands of calories. This is followed by an attempt to get rid of the food by purging, usually by vomiting or using laxatives or diuretics. During a binge, bulimics feel as though they have lost control and cannot stop or limit how much they eat. Some binge and purge only occasionally; others do so many times every day. Binges may be triggered by a major life change or other stressful event. Binge eating and purging may become a way of dealing with difficult feelings such as anger and disappointment.

The binge-purge cycle of bulimia places a tremendous strain on the body and can have serious health effects, including tooth decay, esophageal damage and chronic hoarseness, menstrual irregularities, depression, liver

**Ask Yourself**

QUESTIONS FOR CRITICAL THINKING AND REFLECTION

Do you know someone you suspect may be suffering from an eating disorder? Does the advice in this chapter seem helpful to you? Do you think you could follow it? Why or why not? Have you ever experienced disordered eating patterns yourself? If so, can you identify your reasons for it?

and kidney damage, and cardiac arrhythmia. Bulimia is often difficult to recognize because bulimics conceal their eating habits and usually maintain a normal weight, although they may experience fluctuations of 10–15 pounds.

## Binge-Eating Disorder

**Binge-eating disorder** affects about 2% of American adults. It is characterized by uncontrollable eating without any compensatory purging behaviors. Common eating patterns are eating more rapidly than normal, eating until uncomfortably full, eating when not hungry, and preferring to eat alone. Uncontrolled eating is usually followed by weight gain and feelings of guilt, shame, and depression. Many people with binge-eating disorder mistakenly see rigid dieting as the only solution to their problem, but this usually causes feelings of deprivation and a return to overeating.

Compulsive overeaters rarely eat because of hunger. Instead, they use food to cope with stress, conflict, and other difficult emotions or to provide solace or entertainment. Binge eaters are almost always obese, so they face all the health risks associated with obesity. In addition, binge eaters may have higher-than-average rates of depression and anxiety.

## Borderline Disordered Eating

People with *borderline disordered eating* have some symptoms of eating disorders—for example, excessive dieting or occasional bingeing or purging—but do not meet the full diagnostic criteria for anorexia, bulimia, or binge-eating disorder. Some experts estimate, however, that as many as one-quarter of people with borderline disordered eating will eventually develop a full eating disorder.

Meaningful statistics about borderline disordered eating are hard to come by, in part because it is difficult to define exactly when eating habits cross the line between normal and disordered. However, many experts feel that the majority of Americans, particularly women, have at least some unhealthy attitudes and behaviors in relation to food and self-image. Concerns about weight and dieting are so common as to be considered culturally normal for many Americans.

Ideally, our relationship to food should be a happy one. The biological urge to satisfy hunger is one of our most basic drives, and eating is associated with many pleasurable sensations. For some of us, food triggers pleasant memories of good times, family, holidays, and fun. But for too many people, food is a source of anguish rather than pleasure. Eating results in feelings of guilt and self-loathing rather than satisfaction, causing tremendous disruption in the lives of affected individuals.

How do you know if you have disordered eating habits? When thoughts about weight and food dominate your life, you have a problem. If you're convinced that your worth as a person hinges on how you look and how much you weigh, it's time to get help. Self-induced vomiting or laxative use after meals, even if only once in a while, is reason for concern. Do you feel compelled to overexercise to compensate for what you've eaten? Do you routinely restrict your food intake and sometimes eat nothing in an effort to feel more in control? These are all danger signs and could mean that you are developing a serious problem. Lab 9.3 can help you determine whether you are at risk for an eating disorder.

## Treating Eating Disorders

The treatment of eating disorders must address both problematic eating behaviors and the misuse of food to manage stress and emotions. Treatment for anorexia nervosa first involves averting a medical crisis by restoring adequate body weight; then the psychological aspects of the disorder can be addressed. The treatment of bulimia nervosa or binge-eating disorder involves first stabilizing the eating patterns, then identifying and changing the patterns of thinking that lead to disordered eating. Treatment usually involves a combination of psychotherapy, medication, and medical management. Friends and family members often want to know what they can do to help; for suggestions, see the box "If Someone You Know Has an Eating Disorder."

People with milder patterns of disordered eating may benefit from getting a nutrition checkup with a registered dietitian. A professional can help determine appropriate body weight and calorie intake and offer advice on how to budget calories into a balanced, healthy diet.

**bulimia nervosa** An eating disorder characterized by recurrent episodes of binge eating and then purging to prevent weight gain.

**purging** The use of vomiting, laxatives, excessive exercise, restrictive dieting, enemas, diuretics, or diet pills to compensate for food that has been eaten and that the person fears will produce weight gain.

**binge-eating disorder** An eating disorder characterized by binge eating and a lack of control over eating behavior in general.

# If Someone You Know Has an Eating Disorder . . .

Secrecy and denial are two hallmarks of eating disorders, so it can be hard to know if someone has anorexia or bulimia. Signs that someone may have anorexia include sudden weight loss, excessive dieting or exercise, guilt or preoccupation with food or eating, frequent weighing, fear of becoming fat despite being thin, and baggy or layered clothes to conceal weight loss. Signs that someone may have bulimia include excessive eating without weight gain, secretiveness about food (stealing, hiding, or hoarding food), self-induced vomiting (bathroom visits during or after a meal), swollen glands or puffy face, erosion of tooth enamel, and use of laxatives, diuretics, or diet pills to control weight.

If you decide to approach a friend with your concerns, here are some tips to follow:

- Find out about treatment resources in your community (see the For Further Exploration section for suggestions). You may want to consult a professional at your school clinic or counseling center about the best way to approach the situation.

- Arrange to speak with your friend in a private place, and allow enough time to talk.

- Express your concerns, with specific observations of your friend's behavior. Expect him or her to deny or minimize the problem and possibly to become angry with you. Stay calm and nonjudgmental, and continue to express your concern.

- Avoid giving simplistic advice about eating habits. Listen if your friend wants to talk, and offer your support and understanding. Give your friend the information you found about where he or she can get help, and offer to go along.

- If the situation is an emergency—if your friend has fainted, for example, or attempted suicide—call 911 for help immediately.

- If you are upset about the situation, consider talking to someone yourself. The professionals at the clinic or counseling center are there to help you. Remember, you are not to blame for another person's eating disorder.

---

## ✱ TIPS FOR TODAY AND THE FUTURE

Many approaches work, but the simplest formula for weight management is moderate food intake coupled with regular exercise.

### RIGHT NOW YOU CAN

- Assess your weight-management needs. Do you need to gain weight, lose weight, or stay at your current weight?
- List five things you can do to add more physical activity (not exercise) to your daily routine.
- Identify the foods you regularly eat that may be sabotaging your ability to manage your weight.

### IN THE FUTURE YOU CAN

- Make an honest assessment of your body image. Is it accurate and fair, or is it unduly negative and unhealthy? If your body image presents a problem, consider getting professional advice on how to view yourself realistically.
- Keep track of your energy needs to determine whether your energy-balance equation is correct. Use this information as part of your long-term weight-management efforts.

## SUMMARY

- Excess body weight increases the risk of numerous diseases, particularly cardiovascular disease, cancer, and diabetes.

- Although genetic factors help determine a person's weight, the influence of heredity can be overcome to an extent.

- Physiological factors involved in the regulation of body weight and body fat include metabolic rate and hormones.

- Energy-balance components that an individual can control are calories taken in and calories expended in physical activity.

- Nutritional guidelines for weight management and wellness include controlling consumption of total calories, unhealthy fats and carbohydrates, and protein; monitoring portion sizes and calorie density; increasing consumption of whole grains, fruits, and vegetables; and developing an eating schedule based on rules.

- Activity guidelines for weight control emphasize engaging in moderate-intensity physical activity for 60–90 minutes or more per day; regular, prolonged endurance exercise and weight training can burn a significant number of calories while maintaining muscle mass.

- The sense of well-being that results from a well-balanced diet can reinforce commitment to weight control; improve self-esteem; and lead to realistic, as opposed to negative, self-talk. Successful weight management results in not using food as a way to cope with stress.

- In cases of extreme obesity, weight loss requires medical supervision; in less extreme cases, people can set up individual programs, perhaps getting guidance from reliable books or by joining a formal weight-loss program.

- Dissatisfaction with body image and body weight can lead to physical problems and serious eating disorders, including anorexia nervosa, bulimia nervosa, and binge-eating disorder.

## Q How can I safely gain weight?

**A** Just as for losing weight, a program for weight gain should be gradual and should include both exercise and dietary changes. The foundation of a successful and healthy program for weight gain is a combination of strength training and a high-carbohydrate, high-calorie diet. Strength training will help you add weight as muscle rather than fat.

Energy balance is also important in a program for gaining weight. You need to consume more calories than your body requires in order to gain weight, but you need to choose those extra calories wisely. Fatty, high-calorie foods may seem like an obvious choice, but consuming additional calories as fat can jeopardize your health and your weight-management program. A diet high in fat carries health risks, and your body is more likely to convert dietary fat into fat tissue than into muscle mass. A better strategy is to consume additional calories as complex carbohydrates from whole grains, fruits, and vegetables.

A diet for weight gain should contain about 60–65% of total daily calories from carbohydrates. You probably do not need to be concerned with protein. Although protein requirements increase when you exercise, the protein consumption of most Americans is already well above the DRI.

In order to gain primarily muscle weight instead of fat, a gradual program of weight gain is your best bet. Try these strategies for consuming extra calories:

- Don't skip any meals.
- Add two or three snacks to your daily eating routine.
- Try a sports drink or supplement that has at least 60% of calories from carbohydrates, as well as significant amounts of protein, vitamins, and minerals. (But don't use supplements to replace meals, because they don't contain all of the components of food.)

## Q How can I achieve a "perfect" body?

**A** The current cultural ideal of an ultratoned, ultrafit body is impossible for most people to achieve. A reasonable goal for body weight and body shape must take into account your heredity, weight history, social circumstances, metabolic rate, and psychological well-being. Don't set goals based on movie stars or fashion models. Modern photographic techniques can make people look much different on film or in magazines than they do in person. Many of these people are also genetically endowed with body shapes that are impossible for most of us to emulate. The best approach is to work with what you've got. Adopting a wellness lifestyle that includes regular exercise and a healthy diet will naturally result in the best possible body shape for you. Obsessively trying to achieve unreasonable goals can lead to problems such as eating disorders, overtraining, and injuries.

*For more Common Questions Answered about weight management, visit the Online Learning Center at www.mhhe.com /fahey.*

---

## FOR FURTHER EXPLORATION

### BOOKS

American Heart Association. 2011. *American Heart Association No-Fad Diet, 2nd Edition: A Personal Plan for Healthy Weight Loss.* New York: Clarkson Potter. *Provides guidelines for successful weight management.*

Dillon, E. 2009. *Issues That Concern You: Obesity.* New York: Greenhaven Press. *A collection of perspectives on the causes of obesity, its management, and its impact on individuals and society .*

Gaesser, G. A., and K. Katrina. 2006. *It's the Calories, Not the Carbs.* Victoria, B.C.: Trafford. *Provides a detailed look at the facts behind successful weight loss by shunning fad diets and practicing sound energy balance .*

Hochstrasser, A., and S. R. Fox. 2010. *The Patient's Guide to Weight Loss Surgery, Revised ed.* New York: Hatherleigh. *An easy-to-read guide to the benefits and risks of weight-loss surgery.*

Mayo Clinic. 2009. *Mayo Clinic's Essential Diabetes Book.* Rochester, Minn.: Mayo Clinic. *A user-friendly guide to diabetes.*

Smolin, L. A., and M. B. Grosvenor. 2010. *Nutrition and Eating Disorders.* New York: Chelsea House Publications. *An easy-to-understand guide to eating disorders.*

### ORGANIZATIONS AND WEB SITES

*Calorie Control Council.* Includes a variety of interactive calculators, including an Exercise Calculator that estimates the calories burned from various forms of physical activity.
http://www.caloriecontrol.org

*Frontline: Fat.* Information from a PBS Frontline special that looked at how society, genetics, and biology have influenced our relationship with food and at current problems with obesity and eating disorders.
http://www.pbs.org/wgbh/pages/frontline/shows/fat

*MedlinePlus: Obesity and Weight Loss.* Provides reliable information from government agencies and key professional associations.
http://www.nlm.nih.gov/medlineplus/obesity.html
http://www.nlm.nih.gov/medlineplus/weightcontrol.html

*National Heart, Lung, and Blood Institute (NHLBI): Aim for a Healthy Weight.* Provides information and tips on diet and physical activity, as well as a BMI calculator.
http://www.nhlbi.nih.gov/health/public/heart/obesity/lose_wt

*SmallStep.gov.* Provides resources for increasing activity and improving diet through small changes in daily habits.
http://www.smallstep.gov

*Weight-control Information Network (WIN).* A service of the National Institute of Diabetes and Digestive and Kidney Diseases, serves as an online clearinghouse of weight-management information.
http://win.niddk.nih.gov/

*WHO: Obesity and Overweight.* Provides information on WHO's global strategy on diet and physical activity.
  http://www.who.int/dietphysicalactivity/en

There are also many resources for people concerned about body image and eating disorders:

*Something Fishy Website on Eating Disorders*
  http://www.something-fishy.org

*MedlinePlus:Eating Disorders*
  http://www.nlm.nih.gov/medlineplus/eatingdisorders.html

*National Association of Anorexia Nervosa and Associated Eating Disorders*
  http://www.anad.org

*National Eating Disorders Association*
  http://www.nationaleatingdisorders.org

*Women's Body Image and Health*
  http://www.womenshealth.gov/bodyimage

See also the listings in Chapters 1, 6, and 8.

## SELECTED BIBLIOGRAPHY

Anton, S. D., et al. 2010. Effects of stevia, aspartame, and sucrose on food intake, satiety, and postprandial glucose and insulin levels. *Appetite* 55(1): 37–43.

Balkon, N., et al. 2001. Overweight and obesity: Pharmacotherapeutic considerations. *Journal of the American Academy of Nurse Practitioners* 23(2): 61–66.

Basen-Engquist, K., and M. Chang. 2011. Obesity risk and cancer: Recent review and evidence. *Current Oncology Reports* 13(1): 71–76.

Beverages total 22% of US calories—but who's counting? 2007. T*ufts Health & Nutrition Letter,* March.

Chandon, P., and B. Wansink. 2007. The biasing health halos of fast-food restaurant health claims: Lower calorie estimates and higher side-dish consumption intentions. *Journal of Consumer Research* 34(3): 301–304.

Dahlman, I., and P. Arner. 2007. Obesity and polymorphisms in genes regulating human adipose tissue. *International Journal of Obesity* 31(11): 1629–1641.

Dhingra, R., et al. 2007. Soft drink consumption and risk of developing cardiometabolic risk factors and the metabolic syndrome in middle-aged adults in the community. *Circulation* 116(5): 480–488.

Donnelly, J. E., et al. 2009. American College of Sports Medicine Position Stand: Appropriate physical activity intervention strategies for weight loss and prevention of weight regain for adults. *Medicine and Science in Sports and Medicine* 41(2): 459–471.

Drewnowski, A., and F. Bellisle. 2007. Liquid calories, sugar and body weight. *American Journal of Clinical Nutrition* 85(3): 651–661.

Greene, G. W., et al. 2011. Identifying clusters of college students at elevated health risk based on eating and exercise behaviors and psychosocial determinants of body weight. *Journal of the American Dietetic Association* 111(3): 394–400.

Hamilton, M., et al. 2007. Role of low energy expenditure and sitting in obesity, metabolic syndrome, type 2 diabetes, and cardiovascular disease. *Diabetes* 56(11): 2655–2667.

Hollis, J. F., et al. 2008. Weight loss during the intensive intervention phase of the Weight-Loss Maintenance Trial. *American Journal of Preventive Medicine* 35(2): 18–126.

Hudson, J. I., et al. 2007. The prevalence and correlates of eating disorders in the National Comorbidity Survey Replication. *Biological Psychiatry* 61(3): 348–358.

Huizinga, M. M., et al. 2009. Literacy, numeracy, and portion-size estimation skills. *American Journal of Preventive Medicine* 36(4): 324–328.

Hutchinson, D. M., and R. M. Rapee. 2007. Do friends share similar body image and eating problems? The role of social networks and peer influences in early adolescence. *Behavior Research and Therapy* 45(7): 1557–1577.

Idelevich, E., et al. 2009. Current pharmacotherapeutic concepts for the treatment of obesity in adults. *Therapeutic Advances in Cardiovascular Disease* 3(1): 75–90.

Janiszewski, P. M., and R. Ross. 2007. Physical activity in the treatment of obesity: Beyond body weight reduction. *Applied Physiology, Nutrition and Metabolism* 32(3): 512–522.

Kirk, E. P., et al. 2009. Minimal resistance training improves daily energy expenditure and fat oxidation. *Medicine and Science in Sports and Exercise,* April (published online).

Knab, A. M., et al. 2011. A 45-minute vigorous exercise bout increases metabolic rate for 14 hours. *Medicine and Science in Sports and Exercise,* February (published online).

Kulie, T., et al. 2011. Obesity and women's health: An evidence-based review. *Journal of the American Board of Family Medicine* 24(1): 75–85.

Kumanyika, S. K., et al. 2008. Population-based prevention of obesity: The need for comprehensive promotion of healthful eating, physical activity, and energy balance: A scientific statement from the American Heart Association Council on Epidemiology and Prevention, Interdisciplinary Committee for Prevention (formerly the Expert Panel on Population and Prevention Science). *Circulation* 118(4): 428–464.

Leone, J. E., and J. V. Fetro. 2007. Perceptions and attitudes toward androgenic-anabolic steroid use among two age categories: A qualitative study. *Journal of Strength and Conditioning Research* 21(2): 532–537.

Moore, S. C., et al. 2008. Past body mass index and risk of mortality among women. *International Journal of Obesity* 32(5): 730–739.

Narayan, K. M., et al. 2007. Effect of BMI on lifetime risk for diabetes in the U.S. *Diabetes Care* 30(6): 1562–1566.

Ogden, C. L., et al. 2007. Obesity among adults in the United States: No statistically significant change since 2003–2004. *National Center for Health Statistics Data Brief* 1: 1–8.

Ogden, C. L., et al. 2007. The epidemiology of obesity. *Gastroenterology* 132(6): 2087–2102.

Pellegrini, C. A., et al. 2011. The comparison of a technology-based system and an in-person behavioral weight loss intervention. *Obesity,* February (published online).

Pereira, M. A., et al. 2005. Fast-food habits, weight gain, and insulin resistance (the CARDIA study): 15–year prospective analysis. *Lancet* 365(9453): 36–42.

Ritchie, S. A., and J. M. Connell. 2007. The link between abdominal obesity, metabolic syndrome and cardiovascular disease. *Nutrition, Metabolism, and Cardiovascular Diseases* 17(4): 319–326.

Schroder, K. E. 2011. Computer-assisted dieting: Effects of a randomized nutrition intervention. *American Journal of Health Behavior* 35(2): 175–188.

U.S. Department of Health and Human Services. 2011. *Dietary Guidelines for Americans, 2010* (http://health.gov/dietaryguidelines/2010.asp; retrieved February 26, 2011).

Whitlock, G. et al. 2009. Body-mass index and cause-specific mortality in 900,000 adults: Collaborative analysis of 57 prospective studies. *Lancet* 373(9669): 1083–1096).

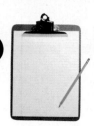

## LAB 9.1  Calculating Daily Energy Needs

### Part I  Estimating Current Energy Intake from a Food Record

If your weight is stable, your current daily energy intake is the number of calories you need to consume to maintain your weight at your current activity level. If you completed Lab 8.2, you should have a record of your current energy intake; if you didn't complete the lab, keep a careful and complete record of everything you eat for one day, and then total the calories in all the foods and beverages you consumed. Record your total energy intake below:

**Current energy intake (from food record):** _____ **calories per day**

### Part II  Estimating Daily Energy Requirements Using Food and Nutrition Board Formulas

Many people underestimate the size of their food portions, and so energy goals based on estimates of current calorie intake from food records can be inaccurate. You can also estimate your daily energy needs using the formulas listed below. To use the appropriate formula for your sex, you'll need to plug in the following:

- Age (in years)
- Height (in inches)
- Weight (in pounds)
- Physical activity coefficient (PA) from the table below.

   To help estimate your physical activity level, consider the following guidelines: Someone who typically engages in 30 minutes of moderate-intensity activity, equivalent to walking 2 miles in 30 minutes, in addition to the activities involved in maintaining a sedentary lifestyle, is considered "low active"; someone who typically engages in the equivalent of 90 minutes of moderate-intensity activity is rated as "active." You might find it helpful to refer back to Lab 2.2 to estimate your physical activity level.

| Physical Activity Level | Physical Activity Coefficient (PA) | |
|---|---|---|
| | *Men* | *Women* |
| Sedentary | 1.00 | 1.00 |
| Low active | 1.12 | 1.14 |
| Active | 1.27 | 1.27 |
| Very active | 1.54 | 1.45 |

*Estimated Daily Energy Requirement for Weight Maintenance in Men*

$$864 - (9.72 \times age) + (PA \times [(6.39 \times weight) + (12.78 \times height)])$$

1.  $9.72 \times$ _____ age (years) = _____
2.  $864 -$ _____ result from step 1 = _____ [*result may be a negative number*]
3.  $6.39 \times$ _____ weight (pounds) = _____
4.  $12.78 \times$ _____ height (inches) = _____
5.  _____ result from step 3 + _____ result from step 4 = _____
6.  _____ PA (from table) $\times$ _____ result from step 5 = _____
7.  _____ result from step 2 + _____ result from step 6 = _____ calories per day

*Estimated Daily Energy Requirement for Weight Maintenance in Women*

$$387 - (7.31 \times age) + (PA \times [(4.91 \times weight) + (16.78 \times height)])$$

1.  $7.31 \times$ _____ age (years) = _____
2.  $387 -$ _____ result from step 1 = _____ [*result may be a negative number*]
3.  $4.91 \times$ _____ weight (pounds) = _____
4.  $16.78 \times$ _____ height (inches) = _____

Mc Graw Hill **connect**  http://www.mcgrawhillconnect.com/
**FITNESS AND WELLNESS**

5. _____ result from step 3 + _____ result from step 4 = _____

6. _____ PA (from table) × _____ result from step 5 = _____

7. _____ result from step 2 + _____ result from step 6 = _____ calories per day

**Daily energy needs for weight maintenance (from formula):** _____ calories/day

## Part III   Determining an Individual Daily Energy Goal for Weight Maintenance

If you calculated values for daily energy needs based on both methods, examine the two values. Some difference is likely—people tend to underestimate their food intake and overestimate their level of physical activity—but if the two values are very far off, check your food record and your physical activity estimate for accuracy, and make any necessary adjustments. For an individualized estimate of daily calorie needs, average the two values:

**Daily energy needs = (food record result _____ calories/day + formula result _____ calories/day)**
        **÷ 2 _____ calories/day**

## Using Your Results

*How did you score?* Are you surprised by the value you calculated for your approximate daily energy needs? If so, is the value higher or lower than you expected?

*What should you do next?* Enter the results of this lab in the Preprogram Assessment column in Appendix C. If you want to change your energy balance to lose weight, complete Lab 9.2 to set goals and develop specific strategies for change. (If your goal is weight gain, see p. 293 for basic guidelines.) One of the best ways to tip your energy balance toward weight loss is to increase your daily physical activity. If you include increases in activity as part of your program, then you can use the results of this lab to chart changes in your daily energy expenditure (and needs). Look for ways to increase the amount of time you spend in physical activity, thus increasing your physical activity coefficient. After several weeks of your program, complete this lab again, and enter the results in the Postprogram Assessment column of Appendix C. How do the results compare? Did your program for increasing physical activity show up as an increase in your daily energy expenditure and need?

**SOURCE:** Estimating Daily Energy Requirements Using Food and Nutrition Board Formulas Part II: Reprinted with permission from *Dietary Reference Intakes for Energy, Carbohydrate, Fiber, Fat, Fatty Acids, Cholesterol, Protein, and Amino Acids (Macronutrients)*. Reprinted with permission from the National Academies Press, Copyright 2005, National Academy of Sciences.

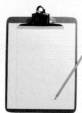

## LAB 9.2  Identifying Weight-Loss Goals

### Negative Calorie Balance

Complete the following calculations to determine your weekly and daily negative calorie balance goals and the number of weeks to achieve your target weight.

Current weight _____ lb − target weight (from Lab 6.2) _____ lb

  = total weight to lose _____ lb

Total weight to lose _____ lb ÷ weight to lose each week _____ lb

  = time to achieve target weight _____ weeks

Weight to lose each week _____ lb × 3500 cal/lb = weekly negative calorie balance _____ cal/week

Weekly negative calorie balance _____ cal/week ÷ 7 days/week

  = daily negative calorie balance _____ cal/day

To keep your weight-loss program on schedule, you must achieve the daily negative calorie balance by either decreasing your calorie consumption (eating less) or increasing your calorie expenditure (being more active). Combining the two strategies may be most successful.

### Changes in Activity Level

Adding a few minutes of exercise every day is a good way of expending calories. Use the calorie costs for different activities listed in the following table.

| Activity | Cal/lb/min | × | Body weight | × | min | = | Total calories |
|---|---|---|---|---|---|---|---|
| Aerobic dance | .046 | | _____ | | ____ | | _____ |
| Basketball (half ct.) | .045 | | _____ | | ____ | | _____ |
| Bicycling (casual) | .049 | | _____ | | ____ | | _____ |
| Bicycling (13 mph) | .071 | | _____ | | ____ | | _____ |
| Elliptical exercise | .049 | | _____ | | ____ | | _____ |
| Football (touch) | .049 | | _____ | | ____ | | _____ |
| Hiking | .051 | | _____ | | ____ | | _____ |
| Housework | .029 | | _____ | | ____ | | _____ |
| Jogging | .060 | | _____ | | ____ | | _____ |
| Rope skipping | .071 | | _____ | | ____ | | _____ |
| Rowing | .032 | | _____ | | ____ | | _____ |
| Skating | .049 | | _____ | | ____ | | _____ |
| Soccer | .052 | | _____ | | ____ | | _____ |
| Swimming | .032 | | _____ | | ____ | | _____ |
| Walking (normal pace) | .029 | | _____ | | ____ | | _____ |
| Walking (briskly) | .048 | | _____ | | ____ | | _____ |

| Activity | Duration | Calories Used |
|---|---|---|
| _____ | _____ | _____ |
| _____ | _____ | _____ |
| _____ | _____ | _____ |

Total calories expended: _____

Mc Graw Hill **connect** http://www.mcgrawhillconnect.com/
FITNESS AND WELLNESS

## Changes in Diet

Look closely at your diet from one day, as recorded in Lab 8.2. Identify ways to cut calorie consumption by eliminating certain items or substituting lower-calorie choices. Be realistic in your cuts and substitutions; you need to develop a plan you can live with.

Food Item            Substitute Food Item            Calorie Savings

_____    _____    _____

_____    _____    _____

_____    _____

Total calories cut: _____

Total calories expended _____ + total calories cut _____ = total negative calorie balance _____

## Common Problem Eating Behaviors

For each of the groups of statements that appear below, check those that are true for you. If you check several statements for a given pattern or problem, it will probably be a significant factor in your weight-management program. One possible strategy for dealing with each type of problem is given. For those eating problems you identify as important, add your own ideas to the strategies listed.

1. _____ I often skip meals.

   _____ I often eat a number of snacks in place of a meal.

   _____ I don't have a regular schedule of meal and snack times.

   _____ I make up for missed meals and snacks by eating more at the next meal.

Problem: Irregular eating habits

Possible solutions:

- Write out a plan for each day's meals in advance. Carry it with you and stick to it.
- _____
- _____

2. _____ I eat more than one sweet dessert or snack each day.

   _____ I usually snack on foods high in calories and fat (chips, cookies, ice cream).

   _____ I drink regular (not sugar-free) soft drinks.

   _____ I choose types of meat that are high in fat.

   _____ I consume more than one alcoholic beverage a day.

Problem: Poor food choices

Possible solutions:

- Keep a supply of raw fruits and vegetables handy for snacks.
- _____
- _____

3. _____ I always eat everything on my plate.

   _____ I often go back for seconds and thirds.

   _____ I take larger helpings than most people.

   _____ I eat up leftovers instead of putting them away.

Problem: Portion sizes too large

Possible solutions:

- Measure all portions with a scale or measuring cup.
- _____
- _____

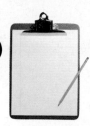

**LAB 9.3** **Checking for Body Image Problems and Eating Disorders**

## Assessing Your Body Image

| | Never | Sometimes | Often | Always |
|---|---|---|---|---|
| 1. I dislike seeing myself in mirrors. | 0 | 1 | 2 | 3 |
| 2. When I shop for clothing, I am more aware of my weight problem, and consequently I find shopping for clothes somewhat unpleasant. | 0 | 1 | 2 | 3 |
| 3. I'm ashamed to be seen in public. | 0 | 1 | 2 | 3 |
| 4. I prefer to avoid engaging in sports or public exercise because of my appearance. | 0 | 1 | 2 | 3 |
| 5. I feel somewhat embarrassed about my body in the presence of someone of the other sex. | 0 | 1 | 2 | 3 |
| 6. I think my body is ugly. | 0 | 1 | 2 | 3 |
| 7. I feel that other people must think my body is unattractive. | 0 | 1 | 2 | 3 |
| 8. I feel that my family or friends may be embarrassed to be seen with me. | 0 | 1 | 2 | 3 |
| 9. I find myself comparing myself with other people to see if they are heavier than I am. | 0 | 1 | 2 | 3 |
| 10. I find it difficult to enjoy activities because I am self-conscious about my physical appearance. | 0 | 1 | 2 | 3 |
| 11. Feeling guilty about my weight problem occupies most of my thinking. | 0 | 1 | 2 | 3 |
| 12. My thoughts about my body and physical appearance are negative and self-critical. | 0 | 1 | 2 | 3 |

Now add up the number of points you have circled in each column: _____  0  + _____  + _____  + _____

## Score Interpretation

The lowest possible score is 0, and this indicates a positive body image. The highest possible score is 36, and this indicates an unhealthy body image. A score higher than 14 suggests a need to develop a healthier body image.

**SOURCE:** Nash, J. D. 1997. *The New Maximize Your Body Potential.* Palo Alto, Calif.: Bull Publishing. Reprinted with permission from Bull Publishing. All rights reserved.

## Eating Disorder Checklist

| | Always | Very Often | Often | Sometimes | Rarely | Never |
|---|---|---|---|---|---|---|
| 1. I like eating with other people. | 0 | 0 | 0 | 1 | 2 | 3 |
| 2. I like my clothes to fit tightly. | 0 | 0 | 0 | 1 | 2 | 3 |
| 3. I enjoy eating meat. | 0 | 0 | 0 | 1 | 2 | 3 |
| 4. I have regular menstrual periods. | 0 | 0 | 0 | 1 | 2 | 3 |
| 5. I enjoy eating at restaurants. | 0 | 0 | 0 | 1 | 2 | 3 |
| 6. I enjoy trying new rich foods. | 0 | 0 | 0 | 1 | 2 | 3 |
| 7. I prepare foods for others, but do not eat what I cook. | 3 | 2 | 1 | 0 | 0 | 0 |
| 8. I become anxious prior to eating. | 3 | 2 | 1 | 0 | 0 | 0 |
| 9. I am terrified about being overweight. | 3 | 2 | 1 | 0 | 0 | 0 |
| 10. I avoid eating when I am hungry. | 3 | 2 | 1 | 0 | 0 | 0 |
| 11. I find myself preoccupied with food. | 3 | 2 | 1 | 0 | 0 | 0 |

connect http://www.mcgrawhillconnect.com/
FITNESS AND WELLNESS

| | Always | Very Often | Often | Sometimes | Rarely | Never |
|---|---|---|---|---|---|---|
| 12. I have gone on eating binges where I feel that I may not be able to stop. | 3 | 2 | 1 | 0 | 0 | 0 |
| 13. I cut my food into small pieces. | 3 | 2 | 1 | 0 | 0 | 0 |
| 14. I am aware of the calorie content of foods that I eat. | 3 | 2 | 1 | 0 | 0 | 0 |
| 15. I particularly avoid foods with a high carbohydrate content (bread, potatoes, rice, etc.). | 3 | 2 | 1 | 0 | 0 | 0 |
| 16. I feel bloated after meals. | 3 | 2 | 1 | 0 | 0 | 0 |
| 17. I feel others would prefer me to eat more. | 3 | 2 | 1 | 0 | 0 | 0 |
| 18. I vomit after I have eaten. | 3 | 2 | 1 | 0 | 0 | 0 |
| 19. I feel extremely guilty after eating. | 3 | 2 | 1 | 0 | 0 | 0 |
| 20. I am preoccupied with a desire to be thinner. | 3 | 2 | 1 | 0 | 0 | 0 |
| 21. I exercise strenuously to burn off calories. | 3 | 2 | 1 | 0 | 0 | 0 |
| 22. I weigh myself several times a day. | 3 | 2 | 1 | 0 | 0 | 0 |
| 23. I wake up early in the morning. | 3 | 2 | 1 | 0 | 0 | 0 |
| 24. I eat the same foods day after day. | 3 | 2 | 1 | 0 | 0 | 0 |
| 25. I think about burning up calories when I exercise. | 3 | 2 | 1 | 0 | 0 | 0 |
| 26. Other people think I am too thin. | 3 | 2 | 1 | 0 | 0 | 0 |
| 27. I am preoccupied with the thought of having fat on my body. | 3 | 2 | 1 | 0 | 0 | 0 |
| 28. I take longer than others to eat my meals. | 3 | 2 | 1 | 0 | 0 | 0 |
| 29. I take laxatives. | 3 | 2 | 1 | 0 | 0 | 0 |
| 30. I avoid foods with sugar in them. | 3 | 2 | 1 | 0 | 0 | 0 |
| 31. I eat diet foods. | 3 | 2 | 1 | 0 | 0 | 0 |
| 32. I feel that food controls my life. | 3 | 2 | 1 | 0 | 0 | 0 |
| 33. I display self-control around foods. | 3 | 2 | 1 | 0 | 0 | 0 |
| 34. I feel that others pressure me to eat. | 3 | 2 | 1 | 0 | 0 | 0 |
| 35. I give too much time and thought to food. | 3 | 2 | 1 | 0 | 0 | 0 |
| 36. I suffer from constipation. | 3 | 2 | 1 | 0 | 0 | 0 |
| 37. I feel uncomfortable after eating sweets. | 3 | 2 | 1 | 0 | 0 | 0 |
| 38. I engage in dieting behavior | 3 | 2 | 1 | 0 | 0 | 0 |
| 39. I like my stomach to be empty. | 3 | 2 | 1 | 0 | 0 | 0 |
| 40. I have the impulse to vomit after meals. | 3 | 2 | 1 | 0 | 0 | 0 |

Now add up the number of points in each column for statements 1 through 40: _____

_____ + _____ + _____ + _____ + _____ + _____

## Score Interpretation

The possible range is 0–120. A score higher than 50 suggests an eating disorder. A score between 30 and 50 suggests a borderline eating disorder. A score less than 30 is within the normal range. Among those with normal eating habits, the average score is 15.4.

SOURCE: Garner, D. M., Olmstead, M., Polivy, J., Development and Validation of a Multidimensional Eating Disorder Inventory for Anorexia Nervosa and Bulimia. *International Journal of Eating Disorders* 2: 15–33, 1983. Copyright © 1983 John Wiley & Sons. Reprinted by permission of John Wiley & Sons, Inc.

## Using Your Results

*How did you score?* Are you surprised by your scores? Do the results of either assessment indicate that you may have a problem with body image or disordered eating?

*What should you do next?* If your results are borderline, consider trying some of the self-help strategies suggested in the chapter. If body image or disordered eating is a significant problem for you, get professional advice; a physician, therapist, and/or registered dietitian can help. Make an appointment today.

# CHAPTER 10

# Stress

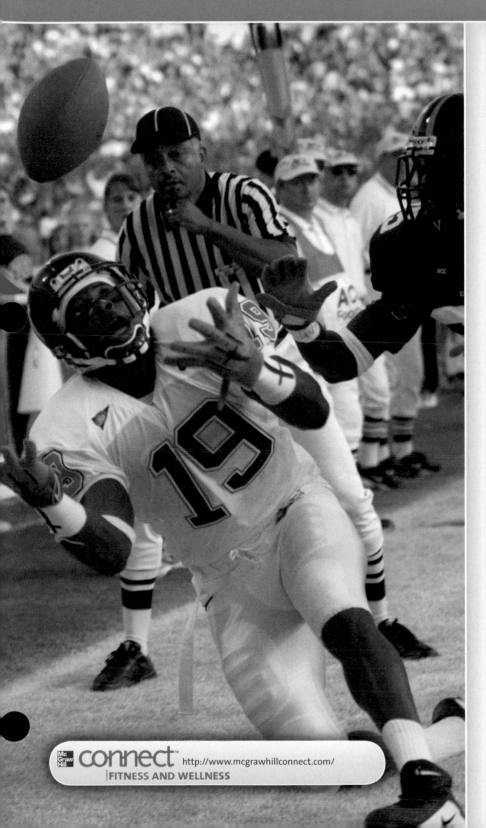

## LOOKING AHEAD...

After reading this chapter, you should be able to:

- Explain what stress is and how people react to it—physically, emotionally, and behaviorally
- Describe the relationship between stress and disease
- List common sources of stress
- Describe techniques for preventing and managing stress
- Put together a plan for successfully managing the stress in your life

## TEST YOUR KNOWLEDGE

1. Which of the following events can cause stress?
   a. taking out a loan
   b. failing a test
   c. graduating from college

2. Exercise stimulates which of the following?
   a. analgesia (pain relief)
   b. birth of new brain cells
   c. relaxation

3. Which of the following can be a result of chronic stress?
   a. violence
   b. heart attack
   c. stroke

**Answers**

1. **All three.** Stress-producing factors can be pleasant or unpleasant and can include physical challenges, goal achievement, and events that are perceived as negative.
2. **All three.** Regular exercise is linked to improvements in many dimensions of wellness.
3. **All three.** Chronic—or ongoing— stress can last for years. People who suffer from long-term stress may ultimately become violent toward themselves or others. They also run a greater-than-normal risk for certain ailments, especially cardiovascular disease.

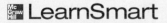

Like the term *fitness*, *stress* is a word many people use without really understanding its precise meaning. Stress is popularly viewed as an uncomfortable response to a negative event, which probably describes *nervous tension* more than the cluster of physical and psychological responses that actually constitute stress. In fact, stress is not limited to negative situations; it is also a response to pleasurable physical challenges and the achievement of personal goals.

Whether stress is experienced as pleasant or unpleasant depends largely on the situation and the individual. Because learning effective responses to stress can enhance psychological health and help prevent a number of serious diseases, stress management can be an important part of daily life.

This chapter explains the physiological and psychological reactions that make up the stress response and describes how these reactions can be risks to good health. The chapter also presents methods of managing stress.

## WHAT IS STRESS?

In common usage, the term *stress* refers to two different things: situations that trigger physical and emotional reactions *and* the reactions themselves. This text uses the more precise term **stressor** for a situation that triggers physical and emotional reactions and the term **stress response** for those reactions. A first date and a final exam are examples of stressors; sweaty palms and a pounding heart are symptoms of the stress response. We'll use the term **stress** to describe the general physical and emotional state that accompanies the stress response. So, a person taking a final exam experiences stress.

## Physical Responses to Stressors

Imagine a near miss: As you step off the curb, a car speeds toward you. With just a fraction of a second to spare, you leap safely out of harm's way. In that split second of danger and in the moments following it, you experience a predictable series of physical reactions. Your body goes from a relaxed state to one prepared for physical action to cope with a threat to your life.

Two systems in your body are responsible for your physical response to stressors: the nervous system and the endocrine system. Through rapid chemical reactions affecting almost every part of your body, you are primed to act quickly and appropriately in time of danger.

**Actions of the Nervous System**  The nervous system consists of the brain, spinal cord, and nerves. Part of the nervous system is under voluntary control, as when you tell your arm to reach for a chocolate. The part that is not under conscious supervision—for example, the part that controls the digestion of the chocolate—is the **autonomic nervous system**. In addition to digestion, it controls your heart rate, breathing, blood pressure, and hundreds of other involuntary functions.

The autonomic nervous system consists of two divisions:

- The **parasympathetic division** is in control when you are relaxed. It aids in digesting food, storing energy, and promoting growth.
- The **sympathetic division** is activated during times of arousal, including exercise, and when there is an emergency, such as severe pain, anger, or fear.

Sympathetic nerves use the neurotransmitter **norepinephrine** (or *noradrenaline*) to exert their actions on nearly every organ, sweat gland, blood vessel, and muscle to enable your body to handle an emergency. In general, the sympathetic division commands your body to stop storing energy and to use it in response to a crisis.

**Actions of the Endocrine System**  During stress, the sympathetic nervous system triggers the **endocrine system**. This system of glands, tissues, and cells helps control body functions by releasing **hormones** and other chemical messengers into the bloodstream to influence metabolism and other body processes. These chemicals act on a variety of targets throughout the body. Along with the nervous system, the endocrine system prepares the body to respond to a stressor.

**The Two Systems Together**  How do both systems work together in an emergency? Let's go back to your near-collision with a car. Both reflexes and higher cognitive (thinking) areas in your brain quickly make the decision that you are facing a threat, and your body prepares to meet the danger. Chemical messages and actions of sympathetic nerves cause the release of key hormones,

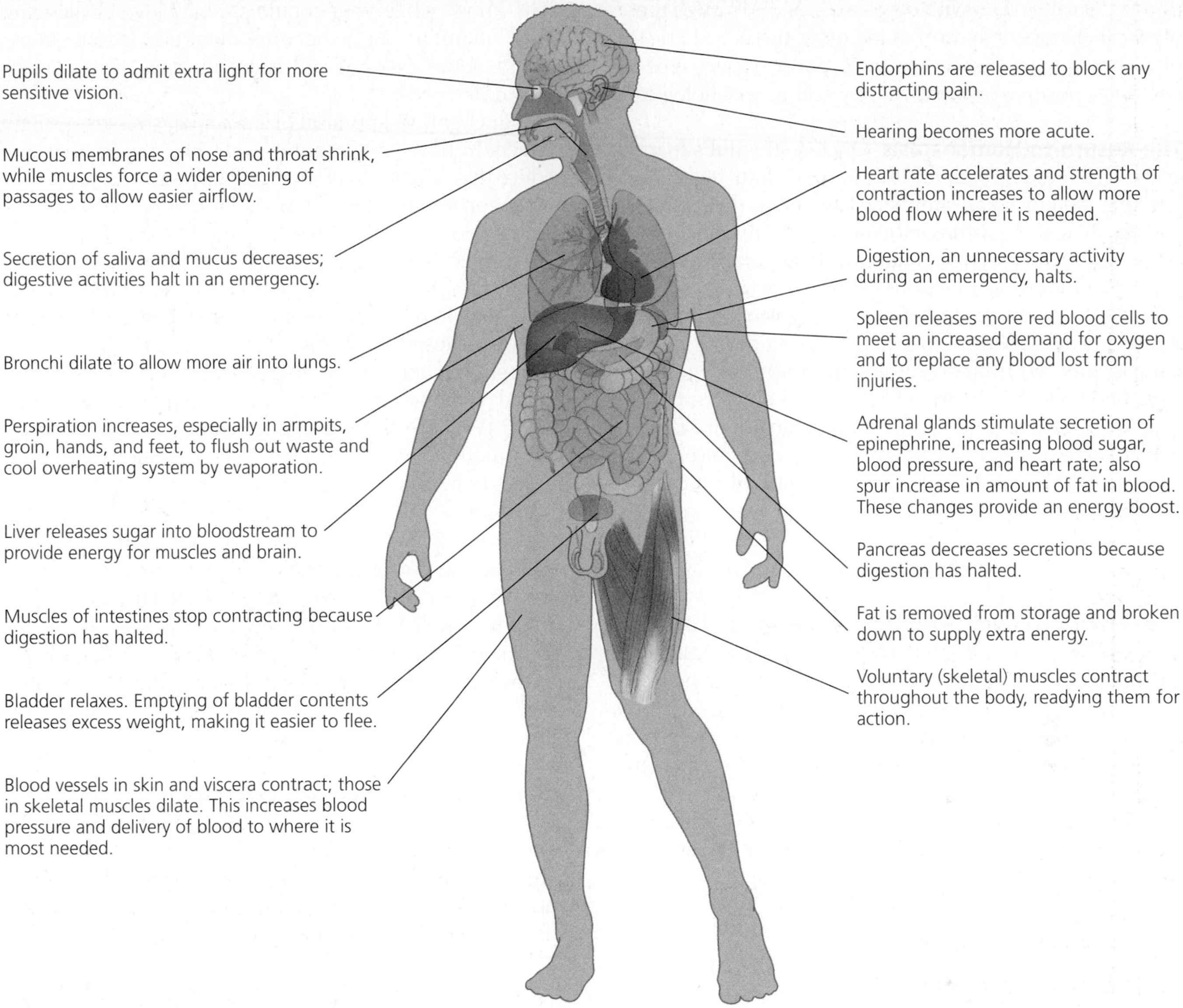

Pupils dilate to admit extra light for more sensitive vision.

Mucous membranes of nose and throat shrink, while muscles force a wider opening of passages to allow easier airflow.

Secretion of saliva and mucus decreases; digestive activities halt in an emergency.

Bronchi dilate to allow more air into lungs.

Perspiration increases, especially in armpits, groin, hands, and feet, to flush out waste and cool overheating system by evaporation.

Liver releases sugar into bloodstream to provide energy for muscles and brain.

Muscles of intestines stop contracting because digestion has halted.

Bladder relaxes. Emptying of bladder contents releases excess weight, making it easier to flee.

Blood vessels in skin and viscera contract; those in skeletal muscles dilate. This increases blood pressure and delivery of blood to where it is most needed.

Endorphins are released to block any distracting pain.

Hearing becomes more acute.

Heart rate accelerates and strength of contraction increases to allow more blood flow where it is needed.

Digestion, an unnecessary activity during an emergency, halts.

Spleen releases more red blood cells to meet an increased demand for oxygen and to replace any blood lost from injuries.

Adrenal glands stimulate secretion of epinephrine, increasing blood sugar, blood pressure, and heart rate; also spur increase in amount of fat in blood. These changes provide an energy boost.

Pancreas decreases secretions because digestion has halted.

Fat is removed from storage and broken down to supply extra energy.

Voluntary (skeletal) muscles contract throughout the body, readying them for action.

**FIGURE 10.1   The fight-or-flight reaction.**

including **cortisol** and **epinephrine**. These hormones trigger the physiological changes shown in Figure 10.1, including these:

- Heart and respiration rates accelerate to speed oxygen through the body.
- Hearing and vision become more acute.
- The liver releases extra sugar into the bloodstream to boost energy.
- Perspiration increases to cool the skin.
- The brain releases **endorphins**—chemicals that can inhibit or block sensations of pain—in case you are injured.

Taken together, these almost-instantaneous physical changes are called the **fight-or-flight reaction.** They give you the heightened reflexes and strength you need to

**KEY TERMS**

**endocrine system**   The system of glands, tissues, and cells that secretes hormones into the bloodstream to influence metabolism and other body processes.

**hormone**   A chemical messenger produced in the body and transported in the bloodstream to targeted cells or organs for specific regulation of their activities.

**cortisol**   A steroid hormone secreted by the cortex (outer layer) of the adrenal gland; also called *hydrocortisone*.

**epinephrine**   A hormone secreted by the medulla (inner core) of the adrenal gland that affects the functioning of organs involved in responding to a stressor; also called *adrenaline*.

**endorphins**   Brain secretions that have pain-inhibiting effects.

**fight-or-flight reaction**   A defense reaction that prepares a person for conflict or escape by triggering hormonal, cardiovascular, metabolic, and other changes.

dodge the car or deal with other stressors. Although these physical changes may vary in intensity, the same basic set of physical reactions occurs in response to any type of stressor—positive or negative, physical or psychological.

**The Return to Homeostasis** Once a stressful situation ends, the parasympathetic division of your autonomic nervous system takes command and halts the stress response. It restores **homeostasis**, a state in which your body maintains blood pressure, heart rate, hormone levels, and other vital functions within a narrow range of normal. Your parasympathetic nervous system calms your body down, slowing a rapid heartbeat, drying sweaty palms, and returning breathing to normal. Gradually, your body resumes its normal "housekeeping" functions, such as digestion and temperature regulation. Damage that may have been sustained during the fight-or-flight reaction is repaired. The day after you narrowly dodge the car, you wake up feeling fine. In this way, your body can grow, repair itself, and build energy reserves. When the next crisis comes, you'll be ready to respond again.

**The Fight-or-Flight Reaction in Modern Life** The fight-or-flight reaction is a part of our biological heritage, and it's a survival mechanism that has served both humans and animals well. In modern life, however, it is often absurdly inappropriate. Many stressors we face in everyday life—such as an exam, a mess left by a roommate, or a stop light—do not require a physical response. The fight-or-flight reaction prepares the body for physical action regardless of whether such action is a necessary or appropriate response to a particular stressor.

## Emotional and Behavioral Responses to Stressors

We all experience a similar set of physical responses to stressors, which make up the fight-or-flight reaction. These responses, however, vary from person to person and from one situation to another. People's perceptions of potential stressors—and their reactions to such stressors—also vary greatly. For example, you may feel confident about taking exams but be nervous about talking to people you don't know, while your roommate may love challenging social situations but be nervous about taking tests. Many factors, some external and some internal, help explain these differences.

Your cognitive appraisal of a potential stressor strongly influences how you respond to it. Two factors that can reduce the magnitude of the stress response are successful prediction and the perception of control. For instance, receiving course syllabi at the beginning of the term allows you to predict the timing of major deadlines and exams. Having this predictive knowledge also allows you to exert some control over your study plans and can help reduce the stress caused by exams.

Cognitive appraisal is highly individual and strongly related to emotions. The facts of a situation—Who? What? Where? When?—typically are evaluated fairly consistently from person to person. Evaluation with respect to personal outcome, however, varies: What does this mean for me? Can I do anything about it? Will it improve or worsen? If an individual perceives a situation as exceeding her or his ability to cope, the result can be negative emotions and an inappropriate stress response. If, on the other hand, a person perceives a situation as a challenge that is within her or his ability to manage, more positive and appropriate responses are likely. A moderate level of stress, if coped with appropriately, can help promote optimal performance (Figure 10.2).

**Effective and Ineffective Responses** Common emotional responses to stressors include anxiety, depression, and fear. Although emotional responses are determined in part by inborn personality or temperament, we often can moderate or learn to control them. Coping techniques are discussed later in the chapter.

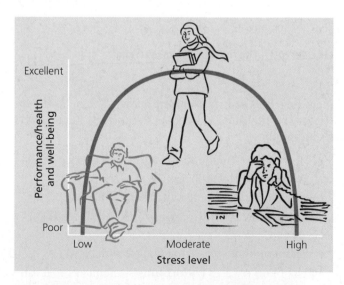

**FIGURE 10.2 Stress level, performance, and well-being.** A moderate level of stress challenges individuals in a way that promotes optimal performance and well-being. Too little stress, and people are not challenged enough to improve; too much stress, and the challenges become stressors that can impair physical and emotional health.

---

### Wellness Tip

Chronic stress not only harms your health, it can make you age faster. A study of women who were long-term caregivers to very sick children revealed that, over time, the women's bodies lost their ability to create new red blood cells. On average, these women were physically 10 years older than their actual chronological age. This is one reason it pays to learn to manage stress, especially when you're young!

Behavioral responses to stressors—controlled by the **somatic nervous system**, which manages our conscious actions—are entirely under our control. Effective behavioral responses such as talking, laughing, exercising, meditating, learning time-management skills, and becoming more assertive can promote wellness and enable us to function at our best. Ineffective behavioral responses to stressors include overeating, expressing hostility, and using tobacco, alcohol, or other drugs.

**Personality and Stress** Some people seem to be nervous, irritable, and easily upset by minor annoyances; others are calm and composed even in difficult situations. Scientists remain unsure just why this is or how the brain's complex emotional mechanisms work. But **personality**—the sum of behavioral, cognitive, and emotional tendencies—clearly affects how people perceive and react to stressors. To investigate the links among personality, stress, and wellness, researchers have looked at different clusters of characteristics, or "personality types."

- *Type A.* People with Type A personality are described as ultracompetitive, controlling, impatient, aggressive, and even hostile. Type A people have a higher perceived stress level and more problems coping with stress. They react explosively to stressors and are upset by events that others would consider only annoyances. Studies indicate that certain characteristics of the Type A pattern—anger, cynicism, and hostility—increase the risk of heart disease.
- *Type B.* The Type B personality is relaxed and contemplative. Type B people are less frustrated by daily events and more tolerant of the behavior of others.
- *Type C.* The Type C personality is characterized by anger suppression, difficulty expressing emotions, feelings of hopelessness and despair, and an exaggerated response to minor stressors. This heightened response may impair immune functions.

Studies of Type A and C personalities suggest that expressing your emotions is beneficial but that habitually expressing exaggerated stress responses or hostility is unhealthy.

Researchers have also looked for personality traits that enable people to deal more successfully with stress. One such trait is *hardiness,* a particular form of optimism. People with a hardy personality view potential stressors as challenges and opportunities for growth and learning, rather than as burdens. Hardy people perceive fewer situations as stressful, and their reaction to stressors tends to be less intense. They are committed to their activities, have a sense of inner purpose and an inner locus of control, and feel at least partly in control of their lives.

You probably can't change your basic personality, but you can change your typical behaviors and patterns of

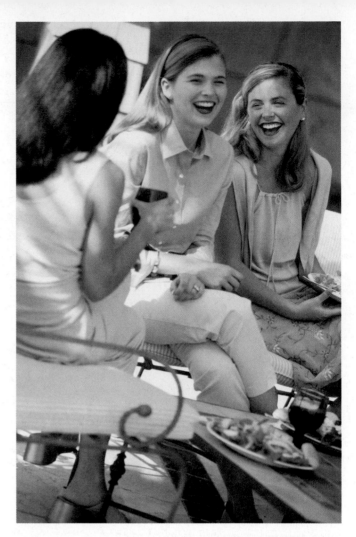

A person's emotional and behavioral responses to stressors depend on many different factors, including personality, gender, and cultural background. Research suggests that women are more likely than men to respond to stressors by seeking social contact and support.

thinking, and you can use positive stress-management techniques like those described later in the chapter.

**Gender and Stress** Our gender role—the activities, abilities, and behaviors our culture expects of us based on our sex—can affect our experience of stress. Some behavioral responses to stressors, such as crying or openly expressing anger, may be deemed more appropriate for one gender than the other.

Strict adherence to gender roles can limit one's response to stress and can itself become a source of stress. Adherence

**homeostasis** A state of stability and consistency in a person's physiological functioning.

**somatic nervous system** The branch of the peripheral nervous system that governs motor functions and sensory information, largely under conscious control.

**personality** The sum of behavioral, cognitive, and emotional tendencies.

KEY TERMS

## Table 10.1 — Symptoms of Excess Stress

| PHYSICAL SYMPTOMS | EMOTIONAL SYMPTOMS | BEHAVIORAL SYMPTOMS |
|---|---|---|
| Dry mouth | Anxiety | Crying |
| Excessive perspiration | Depression | Disrupted eating habits |
| Frequent illnesses | Edginess | Disrupted sleeping habits |
| Gastrointestinal problems | Fatigue | Harsh treatment of others |
| Grinding of teeth | Hypervigilance | Problems communicating |
| Headaches | Impulsiveness | Sexual problems |
| High blood pressure | Inability to concentrate | Social isolation |
| Pounding heart | Irritability | Increased use of tobacco, alcohol, or other drugs |
| Stiff neck or aching lower back | Trouble remembering things | |

## Ask Yourself

### QUESTIONS FOR CRITICAL THINKING AND REFLECTION

Think of the last time you faced a significant stressor. How did you respond? List the physical, emotional, and behavioral reactions you felt. Did these responses help you deal with the stress, or did they interfere with your efforts to handle it?

to traditional gender roles can also affect the perception of a stressor. For example, if a man derives most of his sense of self-worth from his work, retirement may be a more stressful life change for him than for a woman whose self-image is based on several different roles.

Although both men and women experience the fight-or-flight response to stress, women are more likely to respond with a behavioral pattern known as "tend-and-befriend"—nurturing friends and family and seeking social support and social contacts. Rather than becoming aggressive or withdrawing from difficult situations, women are more likely to create or enhance their social networks in ways that reduce stress.

**Experience** Past experiences can profoundly influence the way you evaluate a potential stressor. Someone who has had a bad experience giving a speech in the past is much more likely to perceive an upcoming speech as stressful than someone who has had positive public speaking experiences. Effective behavioral responses, such as preparing carefully and visualizing success, can help overcome the effects of negative past experiences.

### The Stress Experience as a Whole

As Table 10.1 shows, the physical, emotional, and behavioral symptoms of excess negative stress are distinct. But they are also intimately interrelated. The more intense the emotional response, the stronger the physical response.

Effective behavioral responses can lessen stress; ineffective ones only worsen it. Sometimes people have such intense responses to stressors or such ineffective coping techniques that they need professional help to overcome the stress in their lives. More often, however, people can learn to handle stressors on their own.

## STRESS AND WELLNESS

According to the American Psychological Association, 43% of adult Americans suffer from stress-related health problems. The role of stress in health is complex, but evidence suggests that stress can increase vulnerability to many ailments. Several theories have been proposed to explain the relationship between stress and disease.

### The General Adaptation Syndrome

Biologist Hans Selye was one of the first scientists to develop a comprehensive theory of stress and disease. Based on his work in the 1930s and 1940s, Selye coined the term **general adaptation syndrome (GAS)** to describe what he believed to be a universal and predictable response pattern to all stressors. Some stressors are pleasant, such as attending a party, or unpleasant, such as a bad grade. In the GAS theory, stress triggered by a pleasant stressor is called **eustress**; stress triggered by an unpleasant stressor is called **distress**. The sequence of physical responses associated with GAS (Figure 10.3) is the same for both eustress and distress and occurs in three stages:

- *Alarm.* The alarm stage includes the complex sequence of events brought on by the fight-or-flight reaction. At this stage, the body is more susceptible to disease or injury because it is geared up to deal with a crisis. Someone in this phase may experience headaches, indigestion, anxiety, and disrupted sleeping and eating patterns.

- *Resistance.* With continued stress, the body develops a new level of homeostasis in which it is more

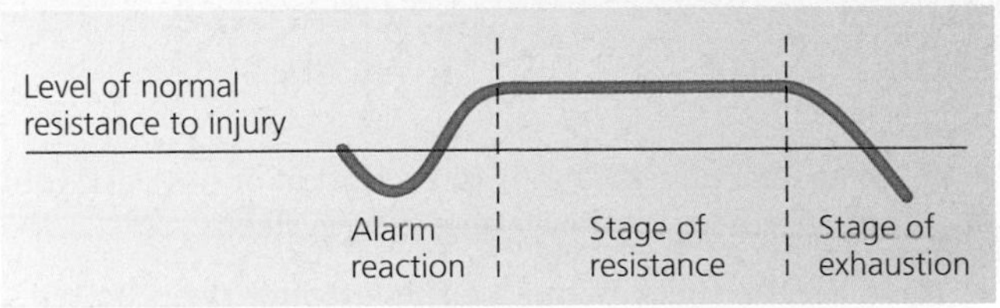

**FIGURE 10.3 The general adaptation syndrome.**
During the alarm stage, a lower resistance to injury is evident. With continued stress, resistance to injury is actually enhanced. With prolonged exposure to repeated stressors, exhaustion sets in, with a return of low resistance levels seen during acute stress.

resistant to disease and injury than normal. In this stage, a person can cope with normal life and added stress.

- **Exhaustion.** The first two stages of GAS require a great deal of energy. If a stressor persists, or if several stressors occur in succession, general exhaustion results. This is not the sort of exhaustion you feel after a long, busy day. Rather, it's a life-threatening type of physiological exhaustion.

## Allostatic Load

Although GAS is still viewed as a key conceptual contribution to the understanding of stress, some aspects of it are considered outdated. For example, increased susceptibility to disease after repeated or prolonged stress is now thought to be due to the effects of the stress response itself rather than to a depletion of resources (the exhaustion stage). In particular, long-term overexposure to stress hormones such as cortisol has been linked with health problems. Further, although physical stress reactions promote homeostasis (resistance stage), they also have negative effects on the body.

The long-term wear and tear of the stress response is called the **allostatic load.** A person's allostatic load depends on many factors, including genetics, life experiences, and emotional and behavioral responses to stressors. A high allostatic load may be due to frequent stressors, poor adaptation to common stressors, an inability to shut down the stress response, or imbalances in the stress responses of different body systems. High allostatic load is linked to heart disease, hypertension, obesity, and reduced brain and immune system functioning. In other words, when your allostatic load exceeds your ability to cope, you are more likely to get sick.

## Psychoneuroimmunology

One of the most fruitful areas of current research into the relationship between stress and disease is **psychoneuroimmunology (PNI).** PNI is the study of the interactions among the nervous system, the endocrine system, and the immune system. The underlying premise of PNI is that stress, through the actions of the nervous and endocrine systems, impairs the immune system and thereby affects health.

A complex network of nerve and chemical connections exists between the nervous, endocrine, and immune systems. In general, increased levels of stress hormones are linked to a decreased number of immune system cells, or lymphocytes. Epinephrine appears to promote the release of lymphocytes but at the same time reduces their efficiency. Scientists have identified hormone-like substances called *neuropeptides* that appear to translate emotions into biochemical events, some of which impact the immune system, providing a physical link between emotions and immune function.

Different types of stress may affect immunity in different ways. For example, during acute stress (typically lasting less than 100 minutes), white blood cells move into the skin, where they enhance the immune response. During a stressful sequence of events, such as a personal trauma and the events that follow, however, there are typically no overall significant immune changes. Chronic (ongoing) stressors such as unemployment have negative effects on almost all functional measures of immunity. Chronic stress may cause prolonged secretion of cortisol and may accelerate the course of diseases that involve inflammation, including multiple sclerosis, heart disease, and type 2 diabetes.

Mood, personality, behavior, and immune functioning are intertwined. For example, people who are generally pessimistic may neglect the basics of health care, become

## Fitness Tip

Stressed out? Then walk away—literally. Walking is a proven countermeasure against stress, and it contributes to your health in many other ways. A brisk, 10-minute walk may be enough to help you put things in perspective and get back to your normal routine. If not, just keep walking until you feel better. As you walk, try not to think too much about anything specific; the idea is to clear your head!

**general adaptation syndrome (GAS)** A pattern of stress responses consisting of three stages: alarm, resistance, and exhaustion.

**eustress** Stress resulting from a pleasant stressor.

**distress** Stress resulting from an unpleasant stressor.

**allostatic load** The long-term negative impact of the stress response on the body.

**psychoneuroimmunology (PNI)** The study of the interactions among the nervous, endocrine, and immune systems.

KEY TERMS

# Overcoming Insomnia

Most people can overcome insomnia by discovering the cause of poor sleep and taking steps to remedy it. Insomnia that lasts for more than 6 months and interferes with daytime functioning requires consultation with a physician. Sleeping pills are not recommended for chronic insomnia because they can be habit-forming; they also lose their effectiveness over time.

If you're bothered by insomnia, try the following:

- Determine how much sleep you need to feel refreshed the next day, and don't sleep longer than that.

- Go to bed at the same time every night, and, more important, get up at the same time every morning, 7 days a week, regardless of how much sleep you got.

- Don't nap more than 30 minutes per day.

- Exercise regularly, but not too close to bedtime. Your metabolism needs at least 6 hours to slow down after exercise.

- Avoid tobacco and caffeine late in the day, and alcohol before bedtime (it causes disturbed, fragmented sleep).

- If you take any medications (prescription or not), ask your doctor or pharmacist if they interfere with sleep.

- Have a light snack before bedtime; you'll sleep better if you're not hungry.

- Use your bed only for sleep. Don't eat, read, study, or watch television in bed.

- Establish a relaxing bedtime routine that helps you unwind and lets your brain know it's time to go to sleep. Read, listen to music, or practice a relaxation technique. Don't lie down in bed until you're sleepy.

- If you don't fall asleep in 15–20 minutes, or if you wake up and can't fall asleep again, get out of bed, leave the room if possible, and do something monotonous until you feel sleepy. Try distracting yourself with imagery instead of counting sheep; imagine yourself on a pleasant vacation or enjoying some beautiful scenery.

- If sleep problems persist, ask your doctor for a referral to a sleep specialist in your area. You may be a candidate for a sleep study—an overnight evaluation of your sleep pattern that can uncover many sleep-related disorders.

## Ask Yourself

### QUESTIONS FOR CRITICAL THINKING AND REFLECTION

Have you ever been so stressed that you felt ill in some way? If so, what were your symptoms? How did you handle them? Did the experience affect the way you reacted to other stressful events?

passive when ill, and fail to engage in health-promoting behaviors. People who are depressed may reduce physical activity and social interaction, which may in turn affect the immune system and the cognitive appraisal of a stressor. Optimism, successful coping, and positive problem solving, on the other hand, may positively influence immunity.

## Links Between Stress and Specific Conditions

Although much remains to be learned, it is clear that people who have unresolved chronic stress in their lives or who handle stressors poorly are at risk for a wide range of health problems. In the short term, the problem might just be a cold, a stiff neck, or a stomachache. Over the long term, the problems can be more severe, such as cardiovascular disease or impairment of the immune system.

**Cardiovascular Disease** The stress response profoundly affects the cardiovascular system. During the stress response, heart rate increases and blood vessels constrict, causing blood pressure to rise. Chronic high blood pressure is a major cause of *atherosclerosis*, a disease in which the lining of the blood vessels becomes damaged and caked with fatty deposits. These deposits can block arteries, causing heart attacks and strokes (see Chapter 11).

Certain types of emotional responses increase a person's risk of cardiovascular disease. People who exhibit extreme increases in heart rate and blood pressure in response to emotional stressors may face an increased risk of cardiovascular problems.

**Altered Immune Function** PNI research helps explain how stress affects the immune system. Some of the health problems linked to stress-related changes in immune function include vulnerability to colds and other infections, asthma and allergy attacks, susceptibility to cancer, and flare-ups of chronic diseases such as genital herpes and HIV infection.

**Other Health Problems** Many other health problems may be caused or worsened by excessive stress, including the following:

- Digestive problems such as stomachaches, diarrhea, constipation, irritable bowel syndrome, and ulcers

- Tension headaches and migraines

- Insomnia and fatigue (see the box "Overcoming Insomnia")
- Injuries, including on-the-job injuries caused by repetitive strain
- Menstrual irregularities, impotence, and pregnancy complications
- Psychological problems, including depression, anxiety, panic attacks, eating disorders, and post-traumatic stress disorder (PTSD), which afflicts people who have suffered or witnessed severe trauma

## COMMON SOURCES OF STRESS

Recognizing potential sources of stress is an important step in successfully managing the stress in your life.

### Major Life Changes

Any major change in your life that requires adjustment and accommodation can be a source of stress. Early adulthood

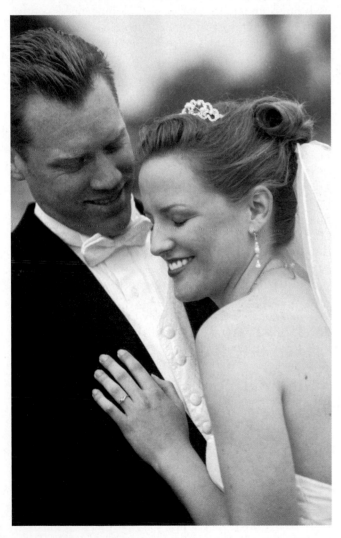

Even a joyful occasion can be a source of stress, especially if it involves a major life change.

and the college years are associated with many significant changes, such as moving out of the family home. Even changes typically thought of as positive—such as graduation, job promotion, or marriage—can be stressful.

Clusters of life changes, particularly those that are perceived negatively, may be linked to health problems in some people. Personality and coping skills, however, are important moderating influences. People with a strong support network and a stress-resistant personality are less likely to become ill in response to life changes than people with fewer resources.

### Daily Hassles

Although major life changes are undoubtedly stressful, they seldom occur regularly. Researchers have proposed that minor problems—life's daily hassles, such as losing your keys or wallet—can be an even greater source of stress because they occur much more often.

People who perceive hassles negatively are likely to experience a moderate stress response every time they are faced with one. Over time, this can take a significant toll on health. Studies indicate that for some people, daily hassles contribute to a general decrease in overall wellness.

### College Stressors

College is a time of major changes and minor hassles. For many students, college means being away from home and family for the first time. Nearly all students share stresses like the following:

- *Academic stress.* Exams, grades, and an endless workload await every college student but can be especially troublesome for young students just out of high school.
- *Interpersonal stress.* Most students are more than just students; they are also friends, children, employees, spouses, parents, and so on. Managing relationships while juggling the rigors of college life can be daunting, especially if some friends or family are less than supportive.
- *Time pressures.* Class schedules, assignments, and deadlines are an inescapable part of college life. But these time pressures can be drastically compounded for students who also have a job and/or family responsibilities.
- *Financial concerns.* The majority of college students need financial aid not just to cover the cost of tuition but to survive from day to day while in school. For many, college life isn't possible without a job, and the pressure to stay afloat financially competes with academic and other stressors.
- *Worries about the future.* As college life comes to an end, students face the reality of life after college. This means thinking about a career, choosing a place to live, and leaving the friends and routines of school behind.

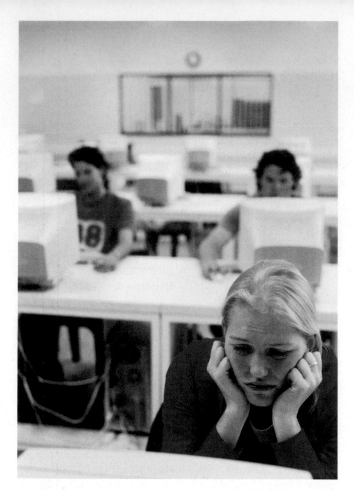

College students face a host of stressors, not the least of which is the pressure to perform academically.

## Job-Related Stressors

Americans rate their jobs as a key source of stress in their lives. According to the 2010 *Stress in America* survey, 70% of working Americans say their job is a key source of stress in their life. Tight schedules and overtime leave less time for exercising, socializing, and other stress-proofing activities. Worries about job performance, salary, job security, and interactions with others can contribute to stress. High levels of job stress are also common for people who are left out of important decisions relating to their jobs. When workers are given the opportunity to shape their job descriptions and responsibilities, job satisfaction goes up and stress levels go down.

If job-related (or college-related) stress is severe or chronic, the result can be *burnout*, a state of physical, mental, and emotional exhaustion. Burnout occurs most often in highly motivated and driven individuals who come to feel that their work is not recognized or that they are not accomplishing their goals. People in the helping professions—teachers, social workers, caregivers, police officers, and so on—are also prone to burnout. For some people who suffer from burnout, a vacation or leave of absence may be appropriate. For others, a reduced work schedule, better communication with superiors, or a change in job goals may be necessary. Improving time-management skills can also help.

## Relationships and Stress

Human beings need social relationships; we cannot thrive as solitary creatures. Simply put, people need people. Even so, our interpersonal relationships—even our deepest, most intimate ones—can be one of the most significant sources of stress in our life.

The first relationships we form outside the family are friendships. With members of either the same or the other sex, friendships give people the opportunity to share themselves and discover others. Friendships are often more stable and longer lasting than intimate partnerships. Friends are often more accepting and less critical than lovers, probably because their expectations are different. Friendships provide people with emotional support and buffer them from stress. Friendships tend to weather conflict and stressful events better than intimate relationships do. During times of stress, in fact, many people initially turn to their friends for comfort, rather than family members or lovers.

Intimate love relationships are among the most profound human experiences. When two people fall in love, their relationship at first is likely to be characterized by high levels of passion and rapidly increasing intimacy. In time, passion decreases as the partners become familiar with each other. The diminishing of passionate love often creates stress between partners (usually affecting one partner more than the other) and can be experienced as a crisis in the relationship. If a quieter, more lasting love fails to emerge, the relationship will likely break up, and each person will search for another who will once again ignite his or her passion.

The key to developing and maintaining any type of friendship or intimate relationship is good communication. Miscommunication creates frustration and distances us from our friends and partners. (For more information, see the section "Communication" later in this chapter.)

# Counterproductive Strategies for Coping with Stress

College students develop a variety of habits in response to stress—some of them ineffective and even unhealthy. Here are a few unhealthy coping techniques to avoid:

● *Alcohol.* A few drinks might make you feel at ease, and getting drunk may help you forget the stress in your life—but any relief alcohol provides is temporary. Binge drinking and excessive alcohol consumption are not effective ways to handle stress, and using alcohol to deal with stress puts you at risk for all the short- and long-term problems associated with alcohol abuse.

● *Tobacco.* The nicotine in cigarettes and other tobacco products can make you feel relaxed and may even increase your ability to concentrate. Tobacco, however, is highly addictive, and smoking causes cancer, heart disease, sexual problems, and many other health problems. Tobacco use is the leading preventable cause of death in the United States.

● *Other drugs.* Altering your body chemistry to cope with stress is a strategy with many pitfalls. Caffeine, for example, raises cortisol levels and blood pressure and can disrupt sleep. Marijuana can elicit panic attacks with repeated use, and some research suggests that it heightens the body's stress response.

● *Binge eating.* Eating can induce relaxation, which reduces stress. Eating as a means of coping with stress, however, may lead to weight gain and to binge eating, a risky behavior associated with eating disorders.

There is one other problem with these methods of fighting stress: None of them addresses the actual cause of the stress in your life. To combat stress in a healthy way, learn some of the stress-management techniques described in this chapter.

---

## Ask Yourself

**QUESTIONS FOR CRITICAL THINKING AND REFLECTION**

What are the top two or three stressors in your life right now? Are they new to your life—as part of your college experience—or are they stressors you've experienced in the past? Do they include both positive and negative experiences (eustress and distress)?

## Other Stressors

Environmental stressors—external conditions or events that cause stress—include loud noises, unpleasant smells, industrial accidents, violence, and natural disasters. (See Appendix A for preparation and coping strategies for large-scale disasters.) Internal stressors are found within ourselves. We put pressure on ourselves to reach personal goals and then evaluate our progress and performance. Physical and emotional states such as illness and exhaustion are also internal stressors.

## MANAGING STRESS

What can you do about all this stress? A great deal. By pursuing a wellness lifestyle—being physically active, eating well, getting enough sleep, and so on—and by learning simple ways to identify and moderate individual stressors, you can control the stress in your life. (There are also some stress-management practices you should avoid; see the box "Counterproductive Strategies for Coping with Stress.")

## Exercise

Researchers have found that people who exercise regularly react with milder physical stress responses before, during, and after exposure to stressors and that their overall sense of well-being increases as well (see the box "Does Exercise Improve Mental Health?"). Although even light exercise can have a beneficial effect, an integrated fitness program can have a significant impact on stress.

For some people, however, exercise can become just one more stressor in an already-stressful life. People who exercise compulsively risk overtraining, a condition characterized by fatigue, irritability, depression, and diminished athletic performance. An overly strenuous exercise program can even make a person sick by compromising immune function. (For information on creating a safe and effective exercise program, refer to Chapter 7.)

## Nutrition

A healthy, balanced diet can help you cope with stress. In addition, eating wisely will enhance your feelings of self-control and self-esteem. Avoiding or limiting caffeine is also important in stress management. Although one or two cups of coffee a day probably won't hurt you, caffeine is a mildly addictive stimulant that leaves some people jittery, irritable, and unable to sleep. Consuming caffeine during stressful situations can raise blood pressure and increase levels of cortisol. (For more on sound nutrition and for advice on evaluating dietary supplements, many of which are marketed for stress, see Chapter 8.)

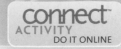

## THE EVIDENCE FOR EXERCISE

# Does Exercise Improve Mental Health?

Since 1995, more than 30 major population-based studies (involving 175,000 Americans) have been published on the association between physical activity and mental health. The overall conclusion is that exercise—even modest activity such as taking a daily walk—can help combat a variety of mental health problems. For example, studies found that regular physical activity protects against depression and the onset of major depressive disorder; it can also reduce symptoms of depression in otherwise healthy people. Other studies found that physical activity protects against anxiety and the onset of anxiety disorders (such as specific phobia, social phobia, generalized anxiety, and panic disorder); it also helps reduce symptoms in people affected with anxiety disorders.

Physical activity can enhance feelings of well-being in some people, which may provide some protection against psychological distress. Overall, physically active people are about 25–30% less likely to feel distressed than inactive people. Regardless of the number, age, or health status of the people being studied, those who were active managed stress better than their inactive counterparts.

Researchers have also looked at specific aspects of the activity-stress association. For example, one study found that taking a long walk can be effective at reducing anxiety and blood pressure. Another showed that a brisk walk of as little as 10 minutes' duration can leave people feeling more relaxed and energetic for up to 2 hours. People who took three brisk 45-minute walks each week for 3 months reported that they perceived fewer daily hassles and had a greater sense of general wellness.

The findings are not surprising. The stress response mobilizes energy resources and readies the body for physical emergencies. If you experience stress and do not exert yourself physically, you are not completing the energy cycle. You may not be able to exercise while your daily stressors are occurring, but you can be active later in the day. Such activity allows you to expend the nervous energy you have built up and trains your body to return more readily to homeostasis after stressful situations.

Physical activity also helps you sleep better, and consistently sound sleep is critical to managing stress. According to the National Sleep Foundation, about two-thirds of Americans have trouble sleeping at least a few nights a week, and about 40% say they have difficulty sleeping virtually every night. There are about 70 known sleep disorders, and disordered sleep is associated with a variety of physical and neurological problems, including health problems relating to stress. Although only a few small-scale studies have been done on the relationship between physical activity and sleep, most experts have concluded that regular activity promotes better sleep and provides some protection against sleep interruptions such as insomnia and sleep apnea. Consistent, restful sleep is now regarded as a protective factor in disorders such as depression, anxiety, obesity, and heart disease.

**SOURCES:** Physical Activity Guidelines Advisory Committee. 2008. *Physical Activity Guidelines Advisory Committee Report, 2008.* Washington, D.C.: U.S. Department of Health and Human Services. National Sleep Foundation. 2011. *2011 Sleep in America Poll: Summary of Findings.* Washington, D.C.: National Sleep Foundation.

## Sleep

Most adults need 7–9 hours of sleep every night to stay healthy and perform their best. Getting enough sleep isn't just good for you physically; adequate sleep also improves mood, fosters feelings of competence and self-worth, enhances mental functioning, and supports emotional functioning.

**Sleep and Stress** Stress hormone levels in the bloodstream vary throughout the day and are related to sleep patterns. Peak concentrations of these hormones occur in the early morning, followed by a slow decline during the day and evening. Concentrations return to peak levels during the final stages of sleep and in the early morning hours.

Even though stress hormones are released during sleep, it is the lack of sleep that has the greatest impact on stress. In someone who is suffering from sleep deprivation (not getting enough sleep over time), mental and physical processes deteriorate steadily. A sleep-deprived person experiences headaches, feels irritable, is unable to concentrate, and is more prone to forgetfulness. Poor-quality sleep has long been associated with stress and

depression. A small 2008 study of female college students further associated sleep deprivation with an increased risk of suicide.

Acute sleep deprivation slows the daytime decline in stress hormones, so evening levels are higher than normal. A decrease in total sleep time also causes an increase in the level of stress hormones. Together, these changes may cause an increase in stress hormone levels throughout the day and may contribute to physical and mental exhaustion. Extreme sleep deprivation can lead to hallucinations and other psychotic symptoms, as well as to a significant increase in heart attack risk.

**Sleep Disorders** According to the National Sleep Foundation's 2011 *Sleep in America Poll,* adults sleep just under 7 hours per night during the week, on average. (Compare this to the recommended 7–9 hours per night.) Many Americans cope with lack of sleep by trying to get extra sleep on the weekends, by napping, and by consuming lots of caffeine during the day. As many as 70 million Americans suffer from chronic sleep disorders—medical conditions that prevent them from sleeping well.

## Building Social Support

Meaningful connections with others can play a key role in stress management and overall wellness. A sense of isolation can lead to chronic stress, which in turn can increase one's susceptibility to temporary illnesses like colds and to chronic illnesses like heart disease. Although the mechanism isn't clear, social isolation can be as significant to mortality rates as factors like smoking, high blood pressure, and obesity.

There is no single best pattern of social support that works for everyone. However, research suggests that having a variety of types of relationships may be important for wellness. Here are some tips for strengthening your social ties:

- **Foster friendships.** Keep in regular contact with your friends. Offer respect, trust, and acceptance, and provide help and support in times of need. Express appreciation for your friends.

- **Keep your family ties strong**. Stay in touch with the family members you feel close to. If your family doesn't function well as a support system for its members, create a second "family" of people with whom you have built meaningful ties.

- **Get involved with a group**. Do volunteer work, take a class, attend a lecture series, or join a religious group. These types of activities can give you a sense of security, a place to talk about your feelings or concerns, and a way to build new friendships. Choose activities that are meaningful to you and that include direct involvement with other people.

- **Build your communication skills**. The more you share your feelings with others, the closer the bonds between you will become. When others are speaking, be a considerate and attentive listener.

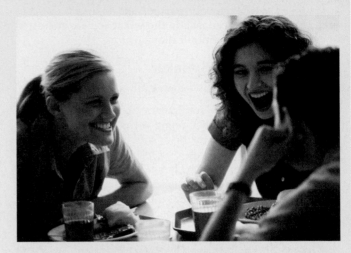

**SOURCE:** Friends Can Be Good Medicine. 1998. As found in the *Mind/Body Newsletter* 7(1): 3–6.

---

According to the Institute of Medicine, more than 50% of adults suffer from *insomnia*—trouble falling asleep or staying asleep. The most common causes of insomnia are lifestyle factors, such as high caffeine or alcohol intake before bedtime; medical problems, such as a breathing disorder; and stress. About 75% of people who suffer from chronic insomnia report some stressful life event at the onset of their sleeping problems.

Another type of chronic sleep problem, called *sleep apnea*, occurs when a person stops breathing while asleep (Figure 10.4). Apnea can be caused by a number of factors, but it typically results when the soft tissue at the back of the mouth (such as the tongue or soft palate) "collapses" during sleep, blocking the airway. When breathing is interrupted, so is sleep, as the sleeper awakens repeatedly throughout the night to begin breathing again. In most cases, this occurs without the sleeper even being aware of it. However, the disruption to sleep can be significant, and over time acute sleep deprivation can result from apnea. There are several treatments for apnea, including medications, special devices that help keep the airway open during sleep, and surgery.

## Social Support

Sharing fears, frustrations, and joys makes life richer and seems to contribute to the well-being of body and mind.

One study of college students living in overcrowded apartments, for example, found that those with a strong social support system were less distressed by their cramped quarters than were the loners who navigated life's challenges on their own. Other studies have shown that married people live longer than single people and have lower death rates from a wide range of conditions. And people infected with HIV remain symptom-free longer if they have a strong social support network. For more on developing and maintaining your social network, see the box "Building Social Support."

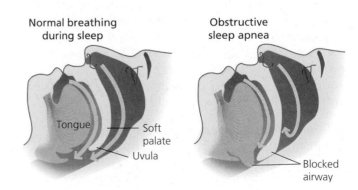

**FIGURE 10.4 Sleep apnea.**
Sleep apnea occurs when soft tissues surrounding the airway relax, "collapsing" the airway and restricting airflow.

# Guidelines for Effective Communication

## Getting Started

● When you want to have a serious discussion with your partner, choose an appropriate time and place. Find a private place and a time when you will not be interrupted.

● Face your partner and maintain eye contact. Use nonverbal feedback to show that you are interested and involved in the communication process.

## Being an Effective Speaker

● State your concern or issue as clearly as you can.

● Use "I" statements—statements about how *you* feel—rather than statements beginning with "You," which tell another person how you think he or she feels. When you use "I" statements, you are taking responsibility for your feelings. "You" statements are often blaming or accusatory and will probably get a defensive or resentful response. The statement "I feel unloved," for example, sends a clearer, less blaming message than the statement "You don't love me."

● Focus on a specific behavior rather than on the whole person. Be specific about the behavior you like or don't like. Avoid generalizations beginning with "You always" or "You never." Such statements make people feel defensive.

● Make constructive requests. Opening your request with "I would like" keeps the focus on your needs rather than your partner's supposed deficiencies.

● Avoid blaming, accusing, and belittling. Even if you are right, you have little to gain by putting your partner down. Studies have shown that when people feel criticized or attacked, they are less able to think rationally or solve problems constructively.

● Ask for action ahead of time. Tell your partner what you would like to have happen in the future; don't wait for him or her to blow it and then express anger or disappointment.

## Being an Effective Listener

● Provide appropriate nonverbal feedback (nodding, smiling, and so on).

● Don't interrupt.

● Develop the skill of reflective listening. Don't judge, evaluate, analyze, or offer solutions (unless asked to do so). Your partner may just need to have you there in order to sort out feelings. By jumping in right away to "fix" the problem, you may be cutting off communication.

● Don't give unsolicited advice. Giving advice implies that you know more about what a person needs to do than he or she does; therefore, it often evokes anger or resentment.

● Clarify your understanding of what your partner is saying by restating it in your own words and asking if your understanding is correct.

● Be sure you are really listening, not off somewhere in your mind rehearsing your reply. Try to tune in to your partner's feelings as well as the words.

● Let your partner know that you value what she or he is saying and want to understand. Respect for the other person is the cornerstone of effective communication.

# Communication

Good communication skills can help everyone form and maintain healthy relationships. Communicating in an assertive way that respects the rights of others—as well as your own—can prevent potentially stressful situations from getting out of control. When friends or partners communicate effectively, they can reduce the stresses in their relationship and spend more time focusing on the positive aspects of being together.

Three keys to good communication in relationships are self-disclosure, listening, and feedback.

● *Self-disclosure* involves revealing personal information that we ordinarily wouldn't reveal because of the risk involved. It usually increases feelings of closeness and moves the relationship to a deeper level of intimacy.

● *Listening* is a rare skill. Good listening skills require that we spend more time and energy trying to fully understand another person's "story" and less time judging, evaluating, blaming, advising, analyzing, or trying to control. Empathy, warmth, respect, and genuineness are qualities of skillful listeners. Attentive listening encourages friends or partners to share more and, in turn, to be attentive listeners. To connect with other people and develop real emotional intimacy, listening is essential.

● *Feedback,* a constructive response to another's self-disclosure, is the third key to good communication. Giving positive feedback means acknowledging that the friend's or partner's feelings are valid—no matter how upsetting or troubling—and offering self-disclosure in response. Self-disclosure and feedback can open the door to change, whereas other responses block communication and change.

For tips on improving your skills, see the box "Guidelines for Effective Communication."

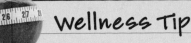
Some people have trouble either telling others what they need or saying no to the needs of others. They may suppress their feelings of anger, frustration, and resentment, and they may end up feeling taken advantage of or suffering in unhealthy relationships. At the other extreme are people who express anger openly and directly by being verbally or physically aggressive or indirectly by making critical, hurtful comments to others. Their abusive behavior pushes other people away, so they also have problems with relationships.

If you typically suppress your feelings, you might want to take an assertiveness training course that can help you identify and change your patterns of communication. If you have trouble controlling your anger, you can benefit from learning anger management strategies; see the box "Dealing with Anger."

## Conflict Resolution

Conflict is natural in any relationship, and it can become a key source of stress for friends, coworkers, family members, and intimate partners. No matter how close two people become, they still remain separate individuals with their own needs, desires, past experiences, and ways of seeing the world. Conflict itself isn't dangerous to a relationship; it may simply indicate that the relationship is growing. But if it isn't handled in a constructive way, conflict can damage—and ultimately destroy—a relationship.

Conflict is often accompanied by anger—a natural emotion, but one that can be difficult to handle. When angry, both parties should back off until they calm down and then come back to the issue later and try to resolve it rationally. Negotiation will help dissipate the anger so the conflict can be resolved. Some basic strategies are useful in successfully negotiating with a friend, family member, colleague, or intimate partner:

1. *Clarify the issue.* Take responsibility for thinking through your feelings and discovering what's really bothering you. Agree that one of you will speak first and have the chance to speak fully while the other listens. Then reverse the roles. Try to understand the other person's position fully by repeating what you've heard and asking questions to clarify or elicit more information.

2. *Find out what each person wants.* Ask the other person to express her or his desires. Don't assume you already know what those desires are, and don't try to speak for your friend or partner.

3. *Determine how you both can get what you want.* Brainstorm to generate a variety of options.

4. *Decide how to negotiate.* Work out a plan for change. For example, agree that one of you will do one task and the other will do another task or that one of you will do a task in exchange for something she or he wants.

5. *Solidify the agreements.* Go over the plan verbally and write it down, if necessary, to ensure that you both understand and agree to it.

6. *Review and renegotiate.* Decide on a time frame for trying out the new plan and set a time to discuss how it's working. Make adjustments as needed.

## Striving for Spiritual Wellness

Spiritual wellness is associated with greater coping skills and higher levels of overall wellness. It is a very personal wellness component, and there are many ways to develop it. Researchers have linked spiritual wellness to longer life expectancy, reduced risk of disease, faster recovery, and improved emotional health. Although spirituality is difficult to study, and researchers aren't sure how or why spirituality seems to improve health, several explanations have been offered. Lab 10.3 includes exercises designed to help you build spiritual wellness.

## Confiding in Yourself Through Writing

Keeping a diary is like confiding in someone else, except that you are confiding in yourself. This form of coping with severe stress may be especially helpful for those who are shy or introverted and find it difficult to open up to others. Although writing about traumatic and stressful events may have a short-term negative effect on mood, over the long term, stress is reduced and positive changes in health occur. A key to promoting health and well-being through journaling is to write about your emotional responses to stressful events. Set aside a special time each day or week to write down your feelings about stressful events in your life.

## Time Management

Learning to manage your time can be crucial to coping with everyday stressors. Overcommitment, procrastination, and even boredom are significant stressors for many people. Along with gaining control of nutrition and exercise to maintain a healthy energy balance, time management is an

# Dealing with Anger

Anger is a natural response to something we perceive as an injustice, a betrayal, an insult, or some other wrong—whether real or imagined. We may respond physically with faster heart and breathing rates, muscle tension, trembling, a knot in the stomach, or a red face. When anger alerts us that something is wrong, it is a useful emotion that can lead to constructive change. When anger leads to loss of control and to aggression, it causes problems.

According to current popular wisdom, it's healthy to express your feelings, including anger. However, research has shown that people who are overtly hostile are at higher risk for heart disease and heart attacks than calmer people. In addition, expressing anger in thoughtless or out-of-control ways can damage personal and professional relationships.

People who experience rage or explosive anger are particularly at risk for negative repercussions. Some of these people may have *intermittent explosive disorder,* characterized by aggressiveness that is impulsive and out of proportion to the stimulus. Explosive anger renders people temporarily unable to think straight or act in their own best interests. Counseling can help very angry people learn how to manage their anger.

In dealing with anger, it is important to distinguish between a reasonable degree of self-assertiveness and a gratuitous expression of aggression. When you are *assertive,* you stand up for your own rights at the same time that you respect the rights of others. When you are *aggressive,* you violate the rights of others.

## Managing Your Own Anger

What are the best ways to handle anger? If you find yourself in a situation where you are getting angry, answer these questions:

- Is the situation important enough to get angry about?
- Are you truly justified in getting angry?
- Is expressing your anger going to make a positive difference?

If the answer to all these questions is yes, then calm, assertive communication may be appropriate. Use "I" statements to express your feelings ("I would like . . .," "I feel . . ."), and listen respectfully to the other person's point of view. Don't attack verbally or make demands; try to negotiate a constructive, mutually satisfying solution.

If you answer no to any of the questions, try to calm yourself. First, reframe the situation by thinking about it differently. Try these strategies:

- Don't take it personally—maybe the driver who cut you off simply didn't see you.
- Look for mitigating factors—maybe the classmate who didn't say hello was preoccupied with money concerns.
- Practice empathy—try to see the situation from the other person's point of view.
- Ask questions—clarify the situation by asking what the other person meant. Avoid defensiveness.
- Focus on the present—don't let this situation trigger thoughts of past incidents that you perceive as similar.

Second, calm your body down.

- Use the old trick of counting to 10 before you respond.
- Concentrate on your breathing, and take long, slow breaths.
- Imagine yourself in a beautiful, peaceful place.
- If needed, take a longer cooling-off period by leaving the situation until your anger has subsided.

## Dealing with Other People's Anger

If someone you are with becomes very angry, try these strategies:

- Respond asymmetrically—remain calm. Don't get angry in response.
- Apologize if you think you are to blame. (Don't apologize if you don't think you are to blame.)
- Validate the other person by acknowledging that he or she has some reason to be angry. However, don't accept verbal abuse.
- Focus on the problem and ask what can be done to alleviate the situation.
- If the person cannot be calmed, disengage from the situation, at least temporarily. After a time-out, attempts at rational problem solving may be more successful.

## Warning Signs of Violence

Violence is never acceptable. The following behaviors over a period of time suggest the potential for violence:

- A history of making threats and engaging in aggressive behavior
- Drug or alcohol abuse
- Gang membership
- Access to or fascination with weapons
- Feelings of rejection or aloneness; the feeling of constantly being disrespected; victimization by bullies
- Withdrawal from usual activities and friends; poor school performance
- Failure to acknowledge the rights of others

The following are immediate warning signs of violence:

- Daily loss of temper or frequent physical fighting
- Significant vandalism or property damage
- Increased risk-taking behavior; increased drug or alcohol abuse
- Threats or detailed plans to commit acts of violence
- Pleasure in hurting animals
- The presence of weapons

Don't spend time with someone who shows these warning signs of violence. Don't carry a weapon or resort to violence to protect yourself. Ask someone in authority or an experienced professional for help.

important element in a wellness program. Try these strategies for improving your time-management skills:

- **Set priorities.** Divide your tasks into three groups: essential, important, and trivial. Focus on the first two, and ignore the third.

- **Schedule tasks for peak efficiency.** You probably know that you're most productive at certain times of the day (or night). Schedule as many of your tasks for those hours as you can, and stick to your schedule.

- **Set realistic goals and write them down.** Attainable goals spur you on. Impossible goals, by definition, cause frustration and failure. Fully commit yourself to achieving your goals by putting them in writing.

- **Budget enough time.** For each project you undertake, calculate how much time you will need to finish it. Then tack on another 10–15%, or even 25%, as a buffer.

- **Break up long-term goals into short-term ones.** Instead of waiting for large blocks of time, use short amounts of time to start a project or keep it moving.

- **Visualize achieving your goal.** By mentally rehearsing a task, you will be able to do it more smoothly.

- **Keep track of the tasks you put off.** Analyze the reasons you procrastinate. If the task is difficult or unpleasant, look for ways to make it easier or more fun. For example, if you find the readings for one of your classes particularly difficult, choose an especially nice setting for your reading, and then reward yourself each time you complete a section or chapter.

- **Consider doing your least favorite tasks first.** Once you have the most unpleasant ones out of the way, you can work on the tasks you enjoy more.

- **Consolidate tasks when possible.** For example, try walking to the store so that you run your errands and exercise in the same block of time.

- **Identify quick transitional tasks.** Keep a list of 5- to 10-minute tasks you can do while waiting or between other tasks, such as watering your plants, doing the dishes, or checking a homework assignment.

- **Delegate responsibility.** Asking for help when you have too much to do is no cop-out; it's good time management. Just don't delegate the jobs you know you should do yourself.

- **Say no when necessary.** If the demands made on you don't seem reasonable, say no—tactfully, but without guilt or apology.

- **Give yourself a break.** Allow time for play—free, unstructured time when you can ignore

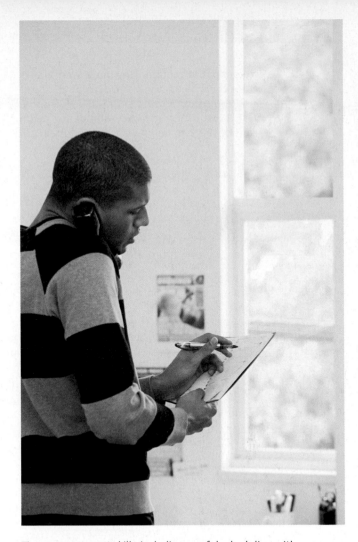

Time-management skills, including careful scheduling with a datebook or computer, can help people cope with busy days.

the clock. Don't consider this a waste of time. Play renews you and enables you to work more efficiently.

- **Avoid your personal "time sinks."** You can probably identify your own time sinks—activities like watching television, surfing the Internet, or talking on the phone that consistently use up more time than you anticipate and put you behind schedule. Some days, it may be best to avoid problematic activities altogether; for example, if you have a big paper due, don't sit down for a 5-minute TV break if it is likely to turn into a 2-hour break. Try a 5-minute walk if you need to clear your head.

- **Stop thinking or talking about what you're going to do, and just do it!** Sometimes the best solution for procrastination is to stop waiting for the right moment and just get started. You will probably find that things are not as bad as you feared, and your momentum will keep you going.

## Realistic Self-Talk

Do your patterns of thinking make events seem worse than they truly are? Do negative beliefs about yourself become self-fulfilling prophecies? Substituting realistic self-talk for negative self-talk can help you build and maintain self-esteem and cope better with the challenges in your life. Here are some examples of common types of distorted, negative self-talk, along with suggestions for more accurate and rational responses.

| COGNITIVE DISTORTION | NEGATIVE SELF-TALK | REALISTIC SELF-TALK |
|---|---|---|
| Focusing on negatives | School is so discouraging—nothing but one hassle after another. | School is pretty challenging and has its difficulties, but there certainly are rewards. It's really a mixture of good and bad. |
| Expecting the worst | Why would my boss want to meet with me this afternoon if not to fire me? | I wonder why my boss wants to meet with me? I guess I'll just have to wait and see. |
| Overgeneralizing | [*After getting a poor grade on a paper*] Just as I thought—I'm incompetent at everything. | I'll start working on the next paper earlier. That way, if I run into problems I'll have time to talk to the TA. |
| Minimizing | I won the speech contest, but none of the other speakers was very good. I wouldn't have done as well against stiffer competition. | It may not have been the best speech I'll ever give, but it was good enough to win the contest. |
| Blaming others | I wouldn't have eaten so much last night if my friends hadn't insisted on going to that restaurant. | I overdid it last night. Next time I'll make different choices. |
| Expecting perfection | I should have scored 100% on this test. I can't believe I missed that one problem through a careless mistake. | Too bad I missed one problem through carelessness, but overall I did very well on this test. Next time I'll be more careful. |

**SOURCE:** Based on W. Schafer. 1999. *Stress Management for Wellness,* 4th ed. Copyright © 2000 Wadsworth, a part of Cengage Learning, Inc. Reproduced by permission. www.cengage.com/permissions.

For more help with time management, complete Activity 10 in the Behavior Change Workbook.

## Cognitive Techniques

Certain thought patterns and ways of thinking, including ideas, beliefs, and perceptions, can contribute to stress and have a negative impact on health. But other habits of mind, if practiced with patience and consistency, can help break unhealthy thought patterns. Below are some suggestions for changing destructive thinking:

- Monitor your self-talk and try to minimize hostile, critical, suspicious, and self-deprecating thoughts (see the box "Realistic Self-Talk").

- Modify your expectations. They often restrict experience and lead to disappointment. Try to accept life as it comes.

- Live in the present. Clear your mind of old debris and fears so you can enjoy life as it is now.

- Go with the flow. Accept what you can't change, forgive others for their faults, and be flexible.

Cultivating your sense of humor is another key cognitive stress-management technique. Even a fleeting smile produces changes in your autonomic nervous system that can lift your spirits. Hearty laughter triggers the release of endorphins, and after a good laugh, your muscles go slack and your pulse and blood pressure dip below normal; you are relaxed.

## Relaxation Techniques

The **relaxation response** is a physiological state characterized by a feeling of warmth and quiet mental alertness. This state is the opposite of the fight-or-flight response. When you induce the relaxation response by using a relaxation technique, your heart rate, breathing, and metabolism slow down. Blood pressure and oxygen consumption decrease. At the same time, blood flow to the brain and skin increases, and brain waves shift from an alert beta rhythm to a relaxed alpha rhythm.

The techniques described in this section are among the most popular techniques and the easiest to learn; also, see

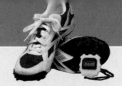

# Solving Problems

Got a problem that's stressing you out? Solve it! Problem solving is a skill—one that requires practice and patience, but one that can pay off in a more balanced, less stressful life. Think of a problem that's bugging you right now, and take the following steps to solve it:

1. Define the problem in a sentence or two. Write it down.
2. List the problem's cause. There may be more than one.
3. List some potential solutions. Don't stop with one or the most obvious one. Write down several options.
4. For each solution, list the potential positive and negative consequences. Be thorough.
5. Choose the solution you think will work best, or will have the fewest negative consequences.
6. List the steps you'll need to take to carry out your solution.
7. Get started with the list of steps you just made. Don't delay unless you have to.
8. As you work on solving the problem, pause occasionally and reevaluate. Revise your approach, if necessary.

If you can't seem to solve a problem on your own, get help. Talk to someone who knows you well, or get help from a counselor, and work through these steps again. Any problem can be solved, but some may just be too big to handle on your own.

the box "Relaxing Through Meditation." All these techniques take practice, so it may be several weeks before the benefits become noticeable in everyday life.

**Progressive Relaxation** In this simple relaxation technique, you tense and then relax the muscles of the body one group at a time. Also known as deep muscle relaxation, this technique addresses the muscle tension that occurs when the body is experiencing stress. Consciously relaxing tensed muscles sends a message to other body systems to reduce the stress response.

To practice progressive relaxation, begin by inhaling as you contract your right fist. Then exhale as you release your fist. Repeat. Contract and relax your right bicep. Repeat. Do the same using your left arm. Then, working from forehead to feet, contract and relax other muscles. Repeat each contraction at least once, inhaling as you tense and exhaling as you relax. To speed up the process, tense and relax more muscles at one time—for example, both arms simultaneously. With practice, you'll

be able to relax quickly just by clenching and releasing only your fists.

**Visualization** Also known as imagery, visualization is so effective in enhancing sports performance that it has become part of the curriculum at training camps for U.S. Olympic athletes. This same technique can be used to induce relaxation, to help change habits, and to improve performance on an exam, on stage, or on a playing field.

To practice visualization, imagine yourself floating on a cloud, sitting on a mountaintop, or lying in a meadow. Try to identify all the perceptible qualities of the environment—sight, sound, temperature, smell, and so on. Your body will respond as if your imagery were real.

An alternative is to close your eyes and imagine a deep purple light filling your body. Then change the color to a soothing gold. As the color lightens, so should your distress. Imagery can also enhance performance: Visualize yourself succeeding at a task that worries you.

**Deep Breathing** Your breathing pattern is closely tied to your stress level. Deep, slow breathing is associated with relaxation. Rapid, shallow, often irregular breathing occurs during the stress response. With practice, you can learn to slow and quiet your breathing pattern, thereby

## Fitness Tip

Activities like yoga and tai chi are well known for their relaxing, meditative aspects. But they're great workouts, too. If you're looking for a way to improve your flexibility and muscle tone while exercising in a quiet, pressure-free environment, check out a local yoga or tai chi class. Be sure the class is led by a qualified professional.

**relaxation response** A physiological state characterized by a feeling of warmth and quiet mental alertness. KEY TERM

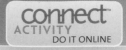
Techniques for managing stress by inducing the relaxation response have been developed in many cultures over the centuries. One such technique is yoga, described in Chapter 5. Another technique that has become popular in the United States is meditation.

At its most basic level, meditation, or self-reflective thought, involves quieting or emptying the mind to achieve deep relaxation. Some practitioners of meditation view it on a deeper level as a means of focusing concentration, increasing self-awareness, and bringing enlightenment to their lives. Meditation has been integrated into the practices of several religions—Buddhism, Hinduism, Confucianism, Taoism—but it is not a religion itself, nor does its practice require any special knowledge, belief, or background.

There are many styles of meditation, based on different ways of quieting the mind. Here is a simple, practical technique for eliciting the relaxation response using one style:

1. Pick a word, a phrase, or an object to focus on. You can choose a word or phrase that has a deep meaning for you, but any word or phrase will work. Some meditators prefer to focus on their breathing.

2. Sit comfortably in a quiet place. Close your eyes if you're not focusing on an object.

3. Relax your muscles.

4. Breathe slowly and naturally. If you're using a focus word or phrase, silently repeat it each time you exhale. If you're using an object, focus on it as you breathe.

5. Keep your attitude passive. Disregard thoughts that drift in.

6. Continue for 10–20 minutes once or twice a day.

7. After you've finished, sit quietly for a few minutes with your eyes closed, then open. Then stand up.

Allow relaxation to occur at its own pace; don't force it. Don't be surprised if you can't tune your mind out for more than a few seconds at a time. It's nothing to get angry about. The more you ignore the intrusions, the easier it will become. If you want to time your session, peek at a watch or clock occasionally, but don't set a jarring alarm.

Although you'll feel refreshed even after the first session, it may take a month or more to get noticeable results. Be patient. Eventually, the relaxation response becomes so natural that it occurs spontaneously or on demand when you sit quietly for a few moments.

---

also quieting your mind and relaxing your body. Try one of the breathing techniques described in the box "Breathing for Relaxation" for on-the-spot tension relief, as well as for long-term stress reduction.

**Listening to Music** Music can relax us. It influences pulse, blood pressure, and the electrical activity of muscles. Listening to soothing, lyrical music can lessen depression, anxiety, and stress levels. To experience the stress-management benefits of music, set aside a period of at least 15 minutes to listen quietly. Choose music you enjoy and selections that make you feel relaxed.

### Other Stress-Management Techniques

Techniques such as biofeedback, hypnosis and self-hypnosis, and massage require a partner or professional training or assistance. As with the relaxation techniques presented, all take practice, and it may be several weeks before the benefits are noticeable.

Biofeedback helps people reduce their response to stress by enabling them to become more aware of their level of physiological arousal. In biofeedback, some measure of stress—perspiration, heart rate, skin temperature, or muscle tension—is electronically monitored, and feedback is given using sound (a tone or music), light, or a meter or dial. With practice, people begin to exercise conscious control over their physiological stress responses. The point of biofeedback training is to develop the ability

to transfer the skill to daily life without the use of electronic equipment.

### GETTING HELP

You can use the principles of behavioral self-management described in Chapter 1 to create a stress-management program tailored specifically to your needs. The starting point of a successful program is to listen to your body. When you learn to recognize the stress response and the emotions and thoughts that accompany it, you'll be in a position to begin handling stress. Labs 10.1 and 10.2 can guide you in identifying and finding ways to cope with stress-inducing situations.

If you feel you need guidance beyond the information in this text, excellent self-help guides can be found in bookstores or the library; helpful Web sites are listed in For Further Exploration at the end of the chapter. Some people also find it helpful to express their feelings in a journal. Grappling with a painful experience in this way provides an emotional release and can help you develop more constructive ways of dealing with similar situations in the future.

### Peer Counseling and Support Groups

If you still feel overwhelmed despite efforts to manage your stress, you may want to seek outside help. Peer counseling, often available through the student health

# Breathing for Relaxation

Controlled breathing can do more than just help you relax. It can also help control pain, anxiety, and other conditions that lead to or are related to stress. There are many methods of controlled breathing. Two of the most popular are belly breathing and tension-release breathing.

## Belly Breathing

1. Lie on your back and relax.

2. Place one hand on your chest and the other on your abdomen. Your hands will help you gauge your breathing.

3. Take in a slow, deep breath through your nose and into your belly. Your abdomen should rise significantly (check with your hand); your chest should rise only slightly. Focus on filling your abdomen with air.

4. Exhale through your mouth, gently pushing out the air from your abdomen.

## Tension-Release Breathing

1. Lie down or sit in a chair and get comfortable.

2. Take a slow, deep breath into your abdomen. Inhale through your nose. Try to visualize the air moving to every part of your body. As you breathe in, say to yourself, "Breathe in relaxation."

3. Exhale through your mouth. Visualize tension leaving your body. Say to yourself, "Breathe out tension."

These techniques have many variations. For example, sit in a chair and raise your arms, shoulders, and chin as you inhale; lower them as you exhale. Or slowly count to 4 as you inhale, then again as you exhale.

Many yoga experts suggest breathing rhythmically, in time with your own heartbeat. Relax and listen closely for the sensation of your heart beating, or monitor your pulse while you breathe. As you inhale, count to 4 or 8 in time with your heartbeat, then repeat the count as you exhale. Breathing in time with soothing music can work well, too.

Experts suggest inhaling through the nose and exhaling through the mouth. Breathe slowly, deeply, and gently. To focus on breathing gently, imagine a candle burning a few inches in front of you. Try to exhale softly enough to make the candle's flame flicker, not hard enough to blow it out.

Practice is important, too. Perform your chosen breathing exercise two or more times daily, for 5–10 minutes per session.

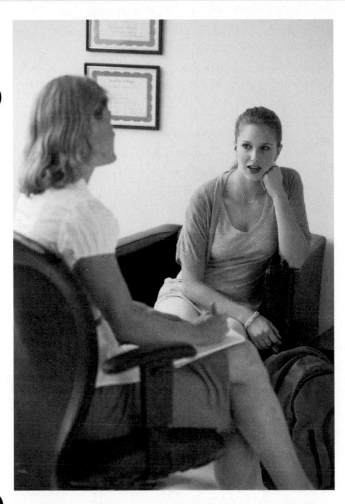

Many people seek help from professional therapists when dealing with stress-related problems.

center or counseling center, is usually staffed by volunteer students with special training that emphasizes maintaining confidentiality. Peer counselors can steer those seeking help to appropriate campus and community resources or just offer sympathetic listening.

Support groups are typically organized around a particular issue or problem: All group members might be entering a new school, reentering school after an interruption, struggling with single parenting, experiencing eating disorders, or coping with particular kinds of trauma. Simply voicing concerns that others share can relieve stress.

## Professional Help

Psychotherapy, especially a short-term course of sessions, can also be tremendously helpful in dealing with stress-related problems. Not all therapists are right for all people, so it's a good idea to shop around for a compatible psychotherapist with reasonable fees. (See the box "Choosing and Evaluating Mental Health Professionals.")

## Is It Stress or Something More Serious?

Most of us have periods of feeling down when we become pessimistic, anxious, less energetic, and less able to enjoy life. Such feelings and thoughts can be normal responses to the ordinary challenges of life. Symptoms that may indicate a more serious problem include the following:

• Depression, anxiety, or other emotional problems begin to interfere seriously with school or work performance or in getting along with others.

# Choosing and Evaluating Mental Health Professionals

College students are usually in a good position to find convenient, affordable mental health care. Larger schools typically have health services that employ psychiatrists and psychologists as well as counseling centers staffed by professionals and peer counselors. Resources in the community may include a school of medicine, a hospital, and a variety of professionals who work independently. It's a good idea to get recommendations from physicians, friends who have been in therapy, or community agencies, rather than to pick a counselor or therapist at random.

Financial considerations are also important. Find out the cost of different services and what your health insurance will cover. If you're not adequately covered by a health plan, don't let that stop you from getting help; investigate low-cost alternatives on campus and in your community. The cost of treatment is linked to how many therapy sessions will be needed, which in turn depends on the type of therapy and the nature of the problem. Psychological therapies focusing on specific problems may require eight or ten sessions at weekly intervals. Therapies aiming for psychological awareness and personality change can last months or years.

Deciding whether a therapist is right for you requires meeting the therapist in person. Before or during your first meeting, find out about the therapist's background and training:

- Does she or he have a degree from an appropriate professional school and a state license to practice?

- Has she or he had experience treating people with problems similar to yours?

- How much will therapy cost?

You have a right to know the answers to these questions and should not hesitate to ask them. After your initial meeting, evaluate your impressions:

- Does the therapist seem like a warm, intelligent person who would be able to help you and is interested in doing so?

- Are you comfortable with the personality, values, and beliefs of the therapist?

- Is the therapist willing to talk about the techniques he or she will use? Do these techniques make sense to you?

If you answer yes to these questions, this therapist may be satisfactory for you. If you feel uncomfortable—and if you are not in need of emergency care—it's worthwhile to set up one-time consultations with one or two others before you make up your mind. Take the time to find someone who feels right for you.

Later in your treatment, evaluate your progress:

- Are you being helped by the treatment?

- If you are displeased, is it because you aren't making progress or because therapy is raising difficult, painful issues you don't want to deal with?

- Can you express dissatisfaction to your therapist? Such feedback can improve your treatment.

If you're convinced your therapy isn't working or is harmful, thank your therapist for her or his efforts and find another.

---

- Suicide is attempted or is seriously considered.
- Symptoms such as hallucinations, delusions, incoherent speech, or loss of memory occur.
- Alcohol or drugs are used to the extent that they impair normal functioning, finding or taking drugs occupies much of the week, or reducing the dosage leads to psychological or physical withdrawal symptoms.

**Depression** is of particular concern because severe depression is linked to suicide, one of the leading causes of death among college students. In some cases, depression, like severe stress, is a clear-cut reaction to a specific event, such as losing a loved one or failing in school or work. In other cases, no trigger event is obvious. Symptoms of depression include the following:

- Negative self-concept
- Pervasive feelings of sadness and hopelessness

- Loss of pleasure in usual activities
- Poor appetite and weight loss
- Insomnia or disturbed sleep
- Restlessness or fatigue
- Thoughts of worthlessness and guilt
- Trouble concentrating or making decisions
- Thoughts of death or suicide

Not all of these symptoms are present in everyone who is depressed, but most experience a loss of interest or pleasure in their usual activities. Warning signs of suicide include expressing the wish to be dead, revealing contemplated suicide methods, increasing social withdrawal and isolation, and exhibiting a sudden, inexplicable lightening of mood (which can indicate the person has finally decided to commit suicide).

If you are severely depressed or know someone who is, expert help from a mental health professional is essential. Most communities and many colleges have hotlines and/or health services and counseling centers that can provide help. The National Suicide Prevention Lifeline can be reached at 1-800-273-TALK. Treatments for depression and many other psychological disorders are highly effective.

> **KEY TERM**
>
> **depression** A mood disorder characterized by loss of interest, sadness, hopelessness, loss of appetite, disturbed sleep, and other physical symptoms.

# Ask Yourself

## QUESTIONS FOR CRITICAL THINKING AND REFLECTION

What percentage of your daily stress is time related? How effective are your time-management skills? Identify one thing you can start doing right now to manage your time better, and describe how you can apply it to one aspect of your daily routine.

## TIPS FOR TODAY AND THE FUTURE

For the stress you can't avoid, develop a range of stress-management techniques and strategies.

### RIGHT NOW YOU CAN

- Practice deep breathing for 5–10 minutes.
- Visualize a relaxing, peaceful place and imagine yourself experiencing it as vividly as possible. Stay there as long as you can.
- Do some stretching exercises.
- Get out your datebook and schedule what you'll be doing the rest of today and tomorrow. Pencil in a short walk and a conversation with a friend.

### IN THE FUTURE YOU CAN

- Take a class or workshop, such as one in assertiveness training or time management, that can help you overcome a source of stress.
- Find a way to build relaxing time into every day. Just 15 minutes of meditation, stretching, or deep breathing can induce the relaxation response.

## SUMMARY

- Stress is the collective physiological and emotional response to any stressor. Physiological responses to stressors are the same for everyone.

- The autonomic nervous system and the endocrine system are responsible for the body's physical response to stressors. The sympathetic nervous system mobilizes the body and activates key hormones of the endocrine system, causing the fight-or-flight reaction. The parasympathetic system returns the body to homeostasis.

- Behavioral responses to stress are controlled by the somatic nervous system and fall under a person's conscious control.

- The general adaptation syndrome model and research in psychoneuroimmunology contribute to our understanding of the links between stress and disease. People who have many stressors in their lives or who handle stress poorly are at risk for cardiovascular disease, impairment of the immune system, and many other problems.

- Potential sources of stress include major life changes, daily hassles, college- and job-related stressors, and interpersonal and social stressors.

- Positive ways of managing stress include regular exercise, good nutrition, support from other people, clear communication, spiritual wellness, effective time management, cognitive techniques, and relaxation techniques.

- If a personal program for stress management doesn't work, peer counseling, support groups, and psychotherapy are available.

## FOR FURTHER EXPLORATION

### BOOKS

Greenberg, J. 2010. *Comprehensive Stress Management,* 12th ed. New York: McGraw-Hill. *Provides a clear explanation of the physical, psychological, sociological, and spiritual aspects of stress and offers numerous stress-management techniques.*

Kabat-Zinn, J. 2006. *Coming to Our Senses: Healing Ourselves and the World Through Mindfulness.* New York: Hyperion. *Explores the connections among mindfulness, health, and physical and spiritual well-being.*

Pennebaker, J. W. 2004. *Writing to Heal: A Guided Journal for Recovering from Trauma and Emotional Upheaval.* Oakland, Calif.: New Harbinger Press. *Provides information about using journaling to cope with stress.*

Seaward, B. L. 2009. *Managing Stress: Principles and Strategies for Health and Well-Being,* 6th ed. Boston: Jones and Bartlett. *A comprehensive textbook for college students.*

### ORGANIZATIONS AND WEB SITES

*American Headache Society* Provides information for consumers and clinicians about different types of headaches, their causes, and their treatment.
http://www.americanheadachesociety.org/

*The American Institute of Stress.* A resource of in-depth information on stress, its causes, and its treatments.
http://www.stress.org

*American Psychiatric Association: Healthy Minds, Healthy Lives.* Provides information on mental wellness especially for college students.
http://www.healthyminds.org

*American Psychological Association.* Provides information on stress management and psychological disorders.
http://www.apa.org
http://apa.org/helpcenter

*Association for Applied Psychophysiology and Biofeedback.* Provides information about biofeedback and referrals to certified biofeedback practitioners.
http://www.aapb.org

*Benson-Henry Institute for Mind Body Medicine.* Provides information about stress-management and relaxation techniques.
http://www.massgeneral.org/bhi

*National Institute of Mental Health (NIMH).* Publishes informative brochures about stress and stress management as well as other aspects of mental health.
http://www.nimh.nih.gov

*National Sleep Foundation.* Provides information about sleep and how to overcome sleep problems such as insomnia, apnea, and jet lag.
http://www.sleepfoundation.org

## Q Are there any relaxation techniques I can use in response to an immediate stressor?

**A** Yes. Try the deep breathing techniques described in the chapter, and try some of the following to see which work best for you:

- Do a full-body stretch while standing or sitting. Stretch your arms out to the sides and then reach them as far as possible over your head. Rotate your body from the waist. Bend over as far as is comfortable for you.
- Do a partial session of progressive muscle relaxation. Tense and then relax some of the muscles in your body. Focus on the muscles that are stiff or tense. Shake out your arms and legs.
- Take a short, brisk walk (3–5 minutes). Breathe deeply.
- Engage in realistic self-talk about the stressor. Mentally rehearse dealing successfully with the stressor. As an alternative, focus your mind on some other activity.
- Briefly reflect on something personally meaningful. In one study of college students, researchers found that self-reflection on important personal values prior to a stressful task reduces the hormonal response to the stressor.

## Q Can stress cause headaches?

**A** Stress is one possible cause of the most common type of headache, the tension headache. About 90% of headaches are tension headaches, characterized by a dull, steady pain, usually on both sides of the head. It may feel as though a band of pressure is tightening around the head, and the pain may extend to the neck and shoulders. Acute tension headaches may last from hours to days, while chronic tension headaches may occur almost every day for months or even years. Stress, poor posture, and immobility are leading causes of tension headaches. There is no cure, but the pain can be relieved with over-the-counter painkillers; many people also try such therapies as massage, relaxation, hot or cold showers, and rest. Stress is also one possible trigger of migraine headaches, which are typically characterized by throbbing pain (often on one side of the head), heightened sensitivity to light and noise, visual disturbances such as flashing lights, nausea, and fatigue.

If your headaches are frequent, keep a journal with details about the events surrounding each one. Are your tension headaches associated with late nights, academic deadlines, or long periods spent sitting at a computer? Are migraines associated with certain foods, stress, fatigue, specific sounds or odors, or (in women) menstruation? If you can identify the stressors or other factors that are consistently associated with your headaches, you can begin to gain more control over the situation. If you suffer persistent tension or migraine headaches, consult your physician.

*For more Common Questions Answered about stress, visit the Online Learning Center at www.mhhe.com/fahey.*

## SELECTED BIBLIOGRAPHY

American College Health Association. 2010. *American College Health Association–National College Health Assessment II Reference Group Executive Summary, Spring 2010.* Linthicum, Md.: American College Health Association.

American Psychological Association. 2010. *How Does Stress Affect Us?* (http://www.apa.org/helpcenter/stress-effects.aspx; retrieved March 20, 2011).

American Psychological Association. 2010. *Learning to Deal with Stress* (http://www.apa.org/helpcenter/stress-learning.aspx; retrieved March 20, 2011).

American Psychological Association. 2010. *Mind/Body Health: Stress* (http://www.apa.org/helpcenter/stress.aspx; retrieved March 20, 2011).

American Psychological Association. 2010. *Stress in America 2010.* Washington, D.C.: American Psychological Association.

Caldwell, K., et al. 2010. Developing mindfulness in college students through movement-based courses: Effects on self-regulatory self-efficacy, mood, stress, and sleep quality. *Journal of American College Health* 58(5): 433–442.

Centers for Disease Control and Prevention. 2010. *Coping with a Disaster or Traumatic Event: Information for Individuals and Families* (http://emergency.cdc.gov/mentalhealth/general.asp; retrieved March 20, 2011).

Cohen, S., W. J. Doyle, and A. Baum. 2006. Socioeconomic status is associated with stress hormones. *Psychosomatic Medicine* 68(3): 414–420.

Freedman, N. 2010. Treatment of obstructive sleep apnea syndrome. *Clinics in Chest Medicine* 31(2): 187–201.

Hefner, J., and D. Eisenberg. 2009. Social support and mental health among college students. *American Journal of Orthopsychiatry* 79(4): 491–499.

Hook, J. N., et al. 2010. Empirically supported religious and spiritual therapies. *Journal of Clinical Psychology* 66(1): 46–72.

Institute of Medicine Committee on Sleep Medicine and Research. 2006. *Sleep Disorders and Sleep Deprivation: An Unmet Public Health Problem,* ed. H. R. Colton and B. M. Altevogt. Washington, D.C.: National Academies Press.

Mayo Foundation for Medical Education and Research. 2008. *Stress: Win Control over the Stress in Your Life* (http://www.mayoclinic.com/health/stress/SR00001; retrieved March 20, 2011).

National Sleep Foundation. 2011. *2011 Sleep in America Poll.* Washington, D.C.: National Sleep Foundation.

Nordboe, D. J., et al. 2007. Immediate behavioral health response to the Virginia Tech shootings. *Disaster Medicine and Public Health Preparedness* 1(Suppl. 1.): S31–S32.

Roddenberry, A., and K. Renk. 2010. Locus of control and self-efficacy: Potential mediators of stress, illness, and utilization of health services in college students. *Child Psychiatry and Human Development* 41(4): 353–370.

Telles, S., et al. 2009. Effect of a yoga practice session and a yoga theory session on state anxiety. *Perceptual and Motor Skills* 109(3): 924–930.

The New York Times. 2010 Update. *Times Topics: School Shootings* (http://topics.nytimes.com/top/reference/timestopics/subjects/s/school_shootings/index.html; retrieved March 20, 2011).

Torpy, J. M. 2008. Chronic stress and the heart. *Journal of the American Medical Association* 298(14): 1722.

U.S. Department of Health and Human Services, National Institutes of Health. 2009. *Stress* (http://www.nlm.nih.gov/medlineplus/stress.html; retrieved March 20, 2011).

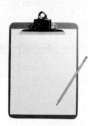

**LAB 10.1  Identifying Your Stress Level and Key Stressors**

## How Stressed Are You?

To help determine how much stress you experience on a daily basis, answer the following questions.
How many of the symptoms of excess stress in the list below do you experience frequently? _____

### Symptoms of Excess Stress

| *Physical Symptoms* | *Emotional Symptoms* | *Behavioral Symptoms* |
|---|---|---|
| Dry mouth | Anxiety | Crying |
| Excessive perspiration | Depression | Disrupted eating habits |
| Frequent illnesses | Edginess | Disrupted sleeping habits |
| Gastrointestinal problems | Fatigue | Harsh treatment of others |
| Grinding of teeth | Hypervigilance | Increased use of tobacco, |
| Headaches | Impulsiveness |    alcohol, or other drugs |
| High blood pressure | Inability to concentrate | Problems communicating |
| Pounding heart | Irritability | Sexual problems |
| Stiff neck or aching lower back | Trouble remembering things | Social isolation |

**Yes     No**

_____  _____  1.  Are you easily startled or irritated?

_____  _____  2.  Are you increasingly forgetful?

_____  _____  3.  Do you have trouble falling or staying asleep?

_____  _____  4.  Do you continually worry about events in your future?

_____  _____  5.  Do you feel as if you are constantly under pressure to produce?

_____  _____  6.  Do you frequently use tobacco, alcohol, or other drugs to help you relax?

_____  _____  7.  Do you often feel as if you have less energy than you need to finish the day?

_____  _____  8.  Do you have recurrent stomachaches or headaches?

_____  _____  9.  Is it difficult for you to find satisfaction in simple life pleasures?

_____  _____  10.  Are you often disappointed in yourself and others?

_____  _____  11.  Are you overly concerned with being liked or accepted by others?

_____  _____  12.  Have you lost interest in intimacy or sex?

_____  _____  13.  Are you concerned that you do not have enough money?

Experiencing some stress-related symptoms or answering yes to a few questions is normal. However, if you experience a large number of stress symptoms or you answered yes to a majority of the questions, you may be experiencing a high level of stress. Take time out to develop effective stress-management techniques. Many coping strategies that can aid you in dealing with college stressors are described in this chapter. Additionally, your school's counseling center can provide valuable support.

McGraw Hill **connect**  http://www.mcgrawhillconnect.com/
|FITNESS AND WELLNESS

LABORATORY ACTIVITIES

## Weekly Stress Log

Now that you are familiar with the signals of stress, complete the weekly stress log to map patterns in your stress levels and identify sources of stress. Enter a score for each hour of each day according to the ratings listed below.

| | A.M. | | | | | | | P.M. | | | | | | | | | | | | Average |
|---|---|---|---|---|---|---|---|---|---|---|---|---|---|---|---|---|---|---|---|---|
| | 6 | 7 | 8 | 9 | 10 | 11 | 12 | 1 | 2 | 3 | 4 | 5 | 6 | 7 | 8 | 9 | 10 | 11 | 12 | |
| Monday | | | | | | | | | | | | | | | | | | | | |
| Tuesday | | | | | | | | | | | | | | | | | | | | |
| Wednesday | | | | | | | | | | | | | | | | | | | | |
| Thursday | | | | | | | | | | | | | | | | | | | | |
| Friday | | | | | | | | | | | | | | | | | | | | |
| Saturday | | | | | | | | | | | | | | | | | | | | |
| Sunday | | | | | | | | | | | | | | | | | | | | |
| Average | | | | | | | | | | | | | | | | | | | | |

**Ratings:**  1 = No anxiety; general feeling of well-being
2 = Mild anxiety; no interference with activity
3 = Moderate anxiety; specific signal(s) of stress present
4 = High anxiety; interference with activity
5 = Very high anxiety and panic reactions; general inability to engage in activity

To identify daily or weekly patterns in your stress level, average your stress rating for each hour and each day. For example, if your scores for 6:00 A.M. are 3, 3, 4, 3, and 4, with blanks for Saturday and Sunday, your 6:00 A.M. rating would be 17 ÷ 5, or 3.4 (moderate to high anxiety). Then calculate an average weekly stress score by averaging your daily average stress scores. Your weekly average will give you a sense of your overall level of stress.

## Using Your Results

*How did you score?* How high are your daily and weekly stress scores?

Are you satisfied with your stress rating? If not, set a specific goal:

*What should you do next?* Enter the results of this lab in the Preprogram Assessment column in Appendix C. If you've set a goal for improvement, begin by using your log to look for patterns and significant time periods in order to identify key stressors in your life. Below, list any stressors that caused you a significant amount of discomfort this week; these can be people, places, events, or recurring thoughts or worries. For each, enter one strategy that would help you deal more successfully with the stressor. Examples of strategies might include practicing an oral presentation in front of a friend or engaging in positive self-talk.

Next, begin to put your strategies into action. In addition, complete Lab 10.2 to help you incorporate lifestyle stress-management techniques into your daily routine.

Name _____ Section _____ Date _____

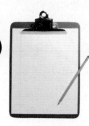

**LAB 10.2  Stress-Management Techniques**

## Part I Lifestyle Stress Management

For each of the areas listed in the table below, describe your current lifestyle as it relates to stress management. For example, do you have enough social support? How are your exercise and nutrition habits? Is time management a problem for you? For each area, list two ways that you could change your current habits to help you manage your stress. Sample strategies might include calling a friend before a challenging class, taking a short walk before lunch, and buying and using a datebook to track your time.

|  | **Current lifestyle** | **Lifestyle change #1** | **Lifestyle change #2** |
|---|---|---|---|
| Social support system |  |  |  |
| Exercise habits |  |  |  |
| Nutrition habits |  |  |  |
| Time-management techniques |  |  |  |
| Self-talk patterns |  |  |  |
| Sleep habits |  |  |  |

McGraw Hill **connect** http://www.mcgrawhillconnect.com/
FITNESS AND WELLNESS

## Part II Relaxation Techniques

Choose two relaxation techniques described in this chapter (progressive relaxation, visualization, deep breathing, meditation, listening to music). If a recording is available for progressive relaxation or visualization, these techniques can be performed by your entire class as a group.

List the techniques you tried.

1. _____

2. _____

How did you feel before you tried these techniques?

_____

_____

_____

What did you think or how did you feel during each of the techniques you tried?

1. _____

_____

_____

2. _____

_____

_____

How did you feel after you tried these techniques?

_____

_____

_____

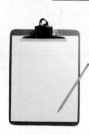

## LAB 10.3  Developing Spiritual Wellness

To develop spiritual wellness, it is important to take time out to think about what gives meaning and purpose to your life and what actions you can take to support the spiritual dimension of your life.

### Look Inward

This week, spend some quiet time alone with your thoughts and feelings. Slow the pace of your day, remove your watch, turn your phone off, and focus on your immediate experience. Try one of the following activities or develop another that is meaningful to you and that contributes to your sense of spiritual well-being.

- *Spend time in nature.* Experience continuity with the natural world by spending solitary time in a natural setting. Watch the sky (day or night), a sunrise, or a sunset; listen to waves on a shore or wind in the trees; feel the breeze on your face or raindrops on your skin; smell the grass, brush, trees, or flowers. Open all your senses to the beauty of nature.
- *Experience art, architecture, or music.* Spend time with a work of art or architecture or a piece of music. Choose one that will awaken your senses, engage your emotions, and challenge your understanding. Take a break and then repeat the experience to see how your responses change the second time.
- *Express your creativity.* Set aside time for a favorite activity, one that allows you to express your creative side. Sing, draw, paint, play a musical instrument, sculpt, build, dance, cook, garden—choose an activity in which you will be so engaged that you will lose track of time. Strive for feelings of joy and exhilaration.
- *Engage in a personal spiritual practice.* Pray, meditate, do yoga, chant. Choose a spiritual practice that is familiar to you or try one that is new. Tune out the outside world and turn your attention inward, focusing on the experience.

In the space below, describe the personal spiritual activity you tried and how it made you feel—both during the activity and after.

## Reach Out

Spiritual wellness can be a bond among people and can promote values such as altruism, forgiveness, and compassion. Try one of the following spiritual activities that involve reaching out to others.

- *Share writings that inspire you.* Find two writings that inspire, guide, and comfort you—passages from sacred works, poems, quotations from literature, songs. Share them with someone else by reading them aloud and explaining what they mean to you.
- *Practice kindness.* Spend a day practicing small acts of personal kindness for people you know as well as for strangers. Compliment a friend, send a card, let someone go ahead of you in line, pick up litter, do someone else's chores, help someone with packages, say please and thank you, smile.
- *Perform community service.* Foster a sense of community by becoming a volunteer. Find a local nonprofit group and offer your time and talent. Mentor a youth, work at a food bank, support a literacy project, help build low-cost housing, visit seniors in a nursing home. You can also work on national or international issues by writing letters to your elected representatives and other officials.

In the space below, describe the spiritual activity you performed and how it made you feel—during the activity and after. Include details about the writings you chose or the acts of kindness or community service you performed.

## Keep a Journal

One strategy for continuing on the path toward spiritual wellness is to keep a journal. Use a journal to record your thoughts, feelings, and experiences; to jot down quotes that engage you; to sketch pictures and write poetry about what is meaningful to you. Begin your spiritual journal today.

# CHAPTER 11

# Cardiovascular Health

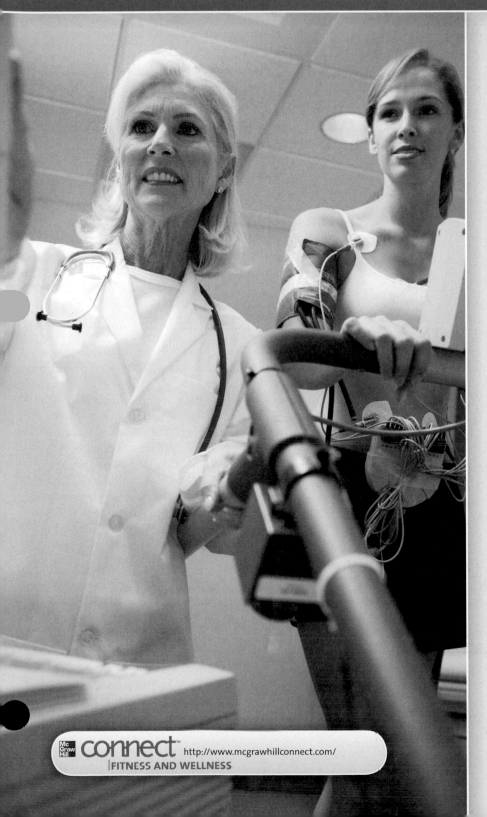

## LOOKING AHEAD...

After reading this chapter, you should be able to:

- Describe the controllable and uncontrollable risk factors associated with cardiovascular disease
- Discuss the major forms of cardiovascular disease and how they develop
- List the steps you can take now to lower your personal risk of developing cardiovascular disease

## TEST YOUR KNOWLEDGE

1. Women are about as likely to die of cardiovascular disease as they are to die of breast cancer. True or false?

2. On average, how much earlier does heart disease develop in people who don't exercise regularly than in people who do?
   a. 6 months
   b. 2 years
   c. 6 years

3. Which of the following foods would be a good choice for promoting heart health?
   a. whole grains
   b. salmon
   c. bananas

**Answers**

1. **False.** Cardiovascular disease kills far more. Among American women, nearly 1 in 3 deaths is due to cardiovascular disease and about 1 in 30 is due to breast cancer.

2. **c.** Both aerobic exercise and strength training significantly improve cardiovascular health.

3. **All three.** Whole grains (whole wheat, oatmeal, rye, barley, and brown rice), foods with omega-3 fatty acids (salmon), and foods high in potassium and low in sodium (bananas) all improve cardiovascular health.

**C**ardiovascular disease (CVD) affects nearly 83 million Americans and is the leading cause of death in the United States. CVD claims one life every 39 seconds—more than 2200 Americans every day. CVD is often thought to affect primarily men and older adults, but heart disease is the number-one killer of American women, and more than 18% of CVD-related deaths occur in people under age 65.

CVD is largely due to our way of life. Millions of Americans are overweight and sedentary, smoke, manage stress ineffectively, have uncontrolled high blood pressure or high cholesterol levels, and don't know the signs of CVD. Not all risk factors for CVD are controllable—some people have an inherited tendency toward high cholesterol levels, for example—but many are within your control.

This chapter explains the major forms of CVD, including hypertension, atherosclerosis, and stroke. It also considers the factors that put people at risk for CVD. Most important, it explains the steps you can take to protect your heart and promote cardiovascular health throughout your life.

## RISK FACTORS FOR CARDIOVASCULAR DISEASE

Researchers have identified a variety of factors associated with an increased risk of developing CVD. They are grouped into two categories: major risk factors and contributing risk factors. Some risk factors are linked to controllable aspects of lifestyle and can therefore be changed. Others are beyond your control. (You can evaluate your personal CVD risk factors in Part I of Lab 11.1.)

### Major Risk Factors That Can Be Changed

The American Heart Association (AHA) has identified six major risk factors for CVD that can be changed: tobacco use, high blood pressure, unhealthy blood cholesterol levels, physical inactivity, overweight and obesity, and diabetes. Most Americans, including young adults, have major risk factors for CVD.

**Tobacco Use** Nearly 1 in 5 deaths is attributable to smoking. In 2008, an estimated 71 million Americans were tobacco users, including 13.6 million college students. Smoking remains the number-one preventable cause of CVD in the United States. People who smoke a pack of cigarettes a day have twice the risk of heart attack as nonsmokers; smoking two or more packs a day triples the risk. When smokers have heart attacks, they are 2 to 3 times more likely than nonsmokers to die from them. Cigarette smoking also doubles the risk of stroke.

Smoking harms the cardiovascular system in several ways:

- It damages the lining of arteries.
- It reduces the level of *high-density lipoproteins* (*HDL*), or "good" cholesterol.
- It raises the levels of triglycerides and *low-density lipoproteins* (*LDL*), or "bad" cholesterol.
- Nicotine increases blood pressure and heart rate.
- The carbon monoxide in cigarette smoke displaces oxygen in the blood, reducing the oxygen available to the body.
- Smoking causes **platelets** to stick together in the bloodstream, leading to clotting.
- Smoking speeds the development of fatty deposits in the arteries.

You don't have to smoke to be affected. The risk of developing heart disease increases up to 30% among people exposed to environmental tobacco smoke (ETS)—also known as "secondhand smoke." Researchers estimate that about 49,000 nonsmokers die from heart disease each year as a result of exposure to ETS.

**High Blood Pressure** In addition to being a form of CVD in itself, high blood pressure, or **hypertension,** is a risk factor for other forms of cardiovascular disease, including heart attacks and strokes.

Blood pressure, the force exerted by the blood on the vessel walls, is created by the pumping action of the heart. High blood pressure occurs when too much force is exerted against the walls of the arteries. Short periods of high blood pressure—such as in response to excitement or exertion—are normal, but chronic high blood pressure is a health risk.

Health care professionals measure blood pressure with a stethoscope and an instrument called a *sphygmomanometer.* At home, you can track your own blood pressure by using an inexpensive blood pressure monitor (see the box "Digital Tools for Heart Health"). Blood pressure is expressed as two numbers—for example, 120 over 80—and measured in millimeters of mercury (mm Hg). The first number is systolic blood pressure; the second is diastolic blood pressure. A normal blood pressure reading for a healthy adult is below 120 systolic over 80 diastolic; CVD risk increases when blood pressure rises above this

*Wellness Tip*

Always relax a few minutes before checking your blood pressure; doing so will help your blood pressure settle to its normal level. You may get a false reading if you take your blood pressure when you're agitated or moving around.

# Digital Tools for Heart Health

Do you ever check your own heart rate or blood pressure? For people who have heart disease or certain risk factors, tracking these vital signs can become routine. Fortunately, there are plenty of electronic devices available that make it easy to check your heart rate and blood pressure.

## Heart Rate Monitors

As described in Chapter 3, there are many kinds of commercially available heart rate monitors. Although these devices are typically meant for use while exercising, they can also give you an accurate count of your resting heart rate. Knowing your resting heart rate can be important for several reasons. For example, a consistently high resting heart rate can be a sign of trouble or indicate that you need to improve your level of cardiorespiratory fitness.

Heart rate monitors usually feature a strap that goes around the user's chest and a watch-like device worn on the arm. The strap contains one or more sensors that gauge the wearer's heartbeat and transmit the information to the wrist device. Smaller, one-piece monitors are also available; some of these devices are worn on the wrist and measure the pulse in the wrist, and even smaller monitors can be worn on a finger (your index finger, for example, has its own measurable pulse).

Simple heart rate monitors display only your current heart rate, but more full-featured models can display other types of information and recall previous readings for comparison.

## Blood Pressure Monitors

A home blood pressure monitor is an electronic version of the sphygmomanometer you've seen in doctors' offices. A home monitor features an inflatable arm strap, an inflating bulb, and a monitoring device. These parts are interconnected by flexible air hoses. You place the strap around your upper arm, squeeze the bulb a few times to inflate the strap, and then wait. As the strap slowly releases air, the device checks your pulse and your blood pressure. The monitor displays your diastolic/systolic blood pressure reading on a screen, in the familiar "120/80" format, along with your pulse rate in beats per minute.

Though relatively inexpensive, home blood pressure monitors are typically accurate and widely recommended by doctors for patients with hypertension or prehypertension. If you purchase a blood pressure monitor, take it to your doctor to make sure it provides the same readings as his or her professionally calibrated equipment.

In fact, it's a good idea to talk to your doctor before monitoring your heart rate or blood pressure. Your doctor can tell if it's necessary (and it may not be if you're in overall good health); if your doctor thinks it's a good idea, he or she can give you baseline readings and advice on the proper way to monitor yourself. Your doctor will also tell you when you should be concerned about a reading, and what to do when you are concerned.

---

| Table 11.1 | Blood Pressure Classification for Healthy Adults | | |
|---|---|---|---|
| CATEGORY* | SYSTOLIC (mm Hg) | | DIASTOLIC (mm Hg) |
| Normal** | below 120 | and | below 80 |
| Prehypertension | 120–139 | or | 80–89 |
| Hypertension⁺ | | | |
| Stage 1 | 140–159 | or | 90–99 |
| Stage 2 | 160 and above | or | 100 and above |

*When systolic and diastolic pressure fall into different categories, the higher category should be used to classify blood pressure status.

**The risk of death from heart attack and stroke begins to rise when blood pressure is above 115/75.

⁺Based on the average of two or more readings taken at different physician visits. In persons over 50, systolic blood pressure greater than 140 is a much more significant CVD risk factor than diastolic blood pressure.

**SOURCE:** *The Seventh Report of the Joint National Committee on Prevention, Detection, Evaluation, and Treatment of High Blood Pressure.* 2003. Bethesda, Md.: National Heart, Lung, and Blood Institute. National Institutes of Health (NIH Publication No. 03-5233).

level. High blood pressure in adults is defined as equal to or greater than 140 over 90 (Table 11.1).

High blood pressure results from an increased output of blood by the heart or from increased resistance to blood flow in the arteries. The latter condition can be caused by the constriction of smooth muscle surrounding the arteries or by **atherosclerosis,** a disease process that causes arteries to become clogged and narrowed. High blood pressure also scars and hardens arteries, making them less elastic and further increasing blood pressure. When a person has high blood pressure, the heart must work harder than normal to force blood through the

**cardiovascular disease (CVD)** A collective term for various diseases of the heart and blood vessels.

**platelets** Cell fragments in the blood that are necessary for the formation of blood clots.

**hypertension** Sustained abnormally high blood pressure.

**atherosclerosis** A form of CVD in which the inner layers of artery walls are made thick and irregular by plaque deposits; arteries become narrowed, and blood supply is reduced.

KEY TERMS

narrowed and stiffened arteries, straining both the heart and the arteries. Eventually, the strained heart weakens and tends to enlarge, which weakens it even more.

High blood pressure is often called a silent killer, because it usually has no symptoms. A person may have high blood pressure for years without realizing it. But during that time, it damages vital organs and increases the risk of heart attack, congestive heart failure, stroke, kidney failure, and blindness.

Recent research has shed new light on the importance of lowering blood pressure to improve cardiovascular health. The risk of death from heart attack or stroke begins to rise when blood pressure is above 115 over 75, well below the traditional 140 over 90 cutoff for hypertension. People with blood pressures in the prehypertension range are at increased risk of heart attack and stroke as well as at significant risk of developing full-blown hypertension.

Hypertension is common. About 33% of adults have hypertension and 30% have prehypertension (defined as systolic pressure of 120–139 and diastolic pressure of 80–89). The incidence of high blood pressure rises dramatically with increasing age, but it can occur among children and young adults. In most cases, hypertension cannot be cured, but it can be controlled. The key to avoiding complications is to have your blood pressure tested at least once every 2 years (more often if you have other CVD risk factors).

Lifestyle changes are recommended for everyone with prehypertension and hypertension. These changes include weight reduction, regular physical activity, a healthy diet, and moderation of alcohol use. The DASH diet (see Chapter 8), is recommended specifically for people with high blood pressure; it emphasizes fruits, vegetables, and whole grains—foods that are rich in potassium and fiber, both of which may reduce blood pressure. Sodium restriction is also helpful. The 2010 Dietary Guidelines for Americans recommend restricting sodium consumption to less than 1500 mg per day. This recommendation applies to all Americans, but is particularly important for people with hypertension, African Americans, and middle-aged and older adults. Adequate potassium intake is also important. For people whose blood pressure isn't controlled adequately with lifestyle changes, medication is prescribed.

**Unhealthy Cholesterol Levels** *Cholesterol* is a fatty, waxlike substance that circulates through the bloodstream and is an important component of cell membranes, sex hormones, vitamin D, the fluid that coats the lungs, and the protective sheaths around nerves. Adequate cholesterol is essential for the proper functioning of the body. Excess cholesterol, however, can clog arteries and increase the risk of CVD (Figure 11.1). Your liver manufactures cholesterol; you also get cholesterol from foods.

**GOOD VERSUS BAD CHOLESTEROL** Cholesterol is carried in the blood by protein-lipid packages called **lipoproteins.**

**Low-density lipoproteins (LDLs)** shuttle cholesterol from the liver to the organs and tissues that require it. LDL is known as "bad" cholesterol because if there is more than the body can use, the excess is deposited in the blood vessels. LDL that accumulates and becomes trapped in artery walls may be oxidized by free radicals, speeding inflammation and damage to artery walls and increasing the likelihood that an artery will become blocked, causing a heart attack or stroke. **High-density lipoproteins (HDLs),** or "good" cholesterol, shuttle unused cholesterol back to the liver for recycling. By removing cholesterol from blood vessels, HDL helps protect against atherosclerosis.

**RECOMMENDED BLOOD CHOLESTEROL LEVELS** The risk for CVD increases with higher blood cholesterol levels, especially LDL. The National Cholesterol Education Program (NCEP) recommends lipoprotein testing at least once every 5 years for all adults, beginning at age 20. The recommended test measures total cholesterol, LDL cholesterol, HDL cholesterol, and triglycerides (another type of blood fat). In general, high LDL, total cholesterol, and triglyceride levels, combined with low HDL levels, are associated with a higher risk for CVD. You can reduce this risk by lowering LDL, total cholesterol, and triglycerides. Raising HDL is important because a high HDL level seems to offer protection from CVD even in cases where total cholesterol is high. This seems to be especially true for women.

As shown in Table 11.2, LDL levels below 100 mg/dl (milligrams per deciliter) and total cholesterol levels below 200 mg/dl are desirable. An estimated 33.5 million American adults (age 20 and over) have total cholesterol levels of 240 mg/dl or higher.

The CVD risk associated with elevated cholesterol levels also depends on other factors. For example, an above-optimal level of LDL would be of more concern for someone who also smokes and has high blood pressure than for someone without these additional CVD risk factors, and it is especially a concern for diabetics.

**IMPROVING CHOLESTEROL LEVELS** Your primary goal should be to reduce your LDL to healthy levels. Important dietary changes for reducing LDL levels include choosing unsaturated fats instead of saturated and trans fats and increasing fiber intake. Decreasing saturated and trans fats is particularly important because they promote the production and excretion of cholesterol by the liver. Exercising regularly and eating more fruits, vegetables, fish, and whole grains also help. Many experts believe that cholesterol-lowering foods may be most effective when eaten in combination rather than separately. You can raise your HDL levels by exercising regularly, losing weight if you are overweight, quitting smoking, and altering the amount and type of fat you consume.

**Physical Inactivity** An estimated 40–60 million Americans are so sedentary that they are at high risk

**FIGURE 11.1 Travels with cholesterol.**

The figure illustrates the following steps:

1. The liver regulates the body's production of cholesterol, based on the amount of fat and cholesterol that is consumed.

2. Saturated and trans fats in the diet act on the liver to increase the amount of LDL circulating in the blood. Thus saturated and trans fats are more important than dietary cholesterol for raising blood cholesterol to unhealthy levels.

3. The liver packages cholesterol with triglycerides (fat) and sends it into the bloodstream as very low-density lipoproteins (VLDLs).

4. As VLDLs travel through the bloodstream, they are broken down into triglycerides (fat) and cholesterol-rich low-density lipoproteins (LDLs). Triglycerides are used for energy or are stored as fat.

5. LDLs deliver cholesterol to cells throughout the body. High LDL levels cause an excess of cholesterol to be delivered to cells.

6. Cholesterol not used by the cells spills out and collects on artery walls. The resulting plaque buildup inhibits blood flow and may result in a heart attack.

7. High-density lipoproteins (HDLs) seek out excess cholesterol, reducing the amount available for buildup on artery walls. High HDL levels can help reverse heart disease.

8. HDLs return cholesterol to the liver, where it is converted into bile acids for elimination or recycling.

Labels in figure: Circulatory system, Cholestrol, Tryglycerides (fat), Liver, VLDL, Energy, Fat, LDL, HDL

for developing CVD. Exercise is thought to be the closest thing we have to a magic bullet against heart disease. It lowers CVD risk by helping to decrease blood pressure and resting heart rate, increase HDL levels, maintain desirable weight, improve the condition of the blood vessels, and prevent or control diabetes. One study found that women who accumulated at least 3 hours of brisk walking each week cut their risk of heart attack and stroke by more than half. (See Chapter 3 for more information on the benefits of cardiorespiratory exercise.)

**Obesity** The risk of death from CVD is 2 to 3 times higher in obese people (BMI $\geq$ 30) than it is in lean people (BMI 18.5–24.9), and for every 5-unit increment of BMI, a person's risk of death from coronary heart disease

## Fitness Tip

Weight training should be part of any fitness program, but it can raise your blood pressure, at least temporarily. Be sure to balance weight training with aerobic exercise, which can lower blood pressure over the long term.

Table 11.2 Cholesterol Guidelines

| TOTAL CHOLESTEROL (mg/dl) | |
|---|---|
| Less than 200 | Desirable |
| 200–239 | Borderline high |
| 240 or more | High |
| LDL CHOLESTEROL (mg/dl) | |
| Less than 100 | Optimal |
| 100–129 | Near optimal/above optimal |
| 130–159 | Borderline high |
| 160–189 | High |
| 190 or more | Very high |
| HDL CHOLESTEROL (mg/dl) | |
| Less than 40 | Low (undesirable) |
| 60 or more | High (desirable) |
| TRIGLYCERIDES (mg/dl) | |
| Less than 150 | Normal |
| 150–199 | Borderline high |
| 200–499 | High |
| 500 or more | Very high |

**SOURCE:** Expert Panel on Detection, Evaluation, and Treatment of High Blood Cholesterol in Adults. 2001. Executive Summary of the Third Report of the National Cholesterol Education Program (NCEP) (Adult Treatment Panel III). *Journal of the American Medical Association* 285(19).

## Contributing Risk Factors That Can Be Changed

Other CVD risk factors can be changed, including triglyceride levels, psychological and social factors, and drug use.

**High Triglyceride Levels** *Triglycerides* are blood fats that are absorbed from food and manufactured by the body. High triglyceride levels are a reliable predictor of heart disease, especially if associated with other risk factors, such as low HDL levels, obesity, and diabetes. Factors contributing to elevated triglyceride levels include excess body fat, physical inactivity, cigarette smoking, type 2 diabetes, excess alcohol intake, very-high-carbohydrate diets, and certain diseases and medications. A full lipid profile should include testing and evaluation of triglyceride levels (see Table 11.2).

For people with borderline high triglyceride levels, increased physical activity, reduced intake of sugars, and weight reduction can help bring levels down into the healthy range. For people with high triglycerides, drug therapy may be needed. Limiting alcohol use and quitting smoking are also helpful.

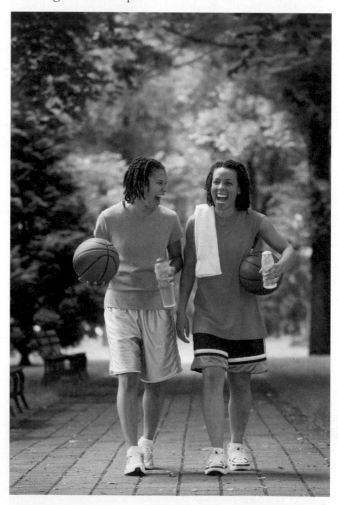

Stress and social isolation increase the risk of cardiovascular disease. A strong social support network improves both health and overall wellness.

increases by 30%. Excess weight increases the strain on the heart by contributing to high blood pressure and high cholesterol. It can also lead to diabetes, another CVD risk factor (see the next section). As discussed in Chapter 6, distribution of body fat is also significant: Fat that collects in the abdomen is more dangerous than fat that collects around the hips. Obesity in general, and abdominal obesity in particular, is significantly associated with narrowing of the coronary arteries, even in young adults in their 20s.

A sensible diet and regular exercise are the best ways to achieve and maintain a healthy body weight. For someone who is overweight, even modest weight reduction can reduce CVD risk by lowering blood pressure, improving cholesterol levels, and reducing diabetes risk.

**Diabetes** As described in Chapter 6, *diabetes* is a disorder in which the metabolism of glucose is disrupted, causing a buildup of glucose in the bloodstream. People with diabetes are at increased risk for CVD, partly because elevated blood glucose levels can damage the lining of arteries, making them more vulnerable to atherosclerosis. Diabetics also often have other risk factors, including hypertension, obesity, unhealthy cholesterol and triglyceride levels, and platelet and blood coagulation abnormalities. Even people whose diabetes is under control face an increased risk of CVD. Therefore, careful control of other risk factors is critical for people with diabetes. People with pre-diabetes also face a significantly increased risk of CVD.

**Psychological and Social Factors** Many of the psychological and social factors that influence other areas of wellness are also important risk factors for CVD. They include chronic stress, chronic hostility and anger, lack of social support, and others. The cardiovascular system is affected by both sudden, acute episodes of mental stress and the more chronic, underlying emotions of anger, anxiety, and depression.

**Alcohol and Drugs** Drinking too much alcohol raises blood pressure and can increase the risk of stroke and heart failure. Stimulant drugs, particularly cocaine, can also cause serious cardiac problems, including heart attack, stroke, and sudden cardiac death. Injection drug use can cause infection of the heart and stroke.

## Major Risk Factors That Can't Be Changed

A number of major risk factors for CVD cannot be changed. They include heredity, aging, being male, and ethnicity.

**Heredity** Multiple genes contribute to the development of CVD and its risk factors. Having an unfavorable set of genes increases your risk, but risk is modifiable by lifestyle factors such as whether you smoke, exercise, or eat a healthy diet. People who inherit a tendency for CVD are not destined to develop it, but they may have to work harder than other people to prevent it.

**Aging** About 70% of all heart attack victims are age 65 or older, and about 75% who suffer fatal heart attacks are over 65. For people over 55, the incidence of stroke more than doubles in each successive decade. However, even people in their 30s and 40s, especially men, can have heart attacks.

**Being Male** Although CVD is the leading killer of both men and women in the United States, men face a greater risk of heart attack than women, especially earlier in life. Until age 55, men also have a greater risk of hypertension than women. The incidence of stroke is higher for males than females until age 65. Estrogen production, which is highest during the childbearing years, may protect premenopausal women against CVD (see the box "Gender, Ethnicity, and CVD"). By age 75, the gender gap nearly disappears.

### Wellness Tip

Some medications can raise your blood pressure, especially if you take them every day. This includes a variety of over-the-counter medications, such as acetaminophen.

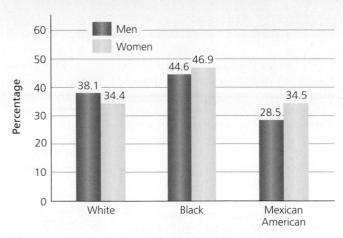

**FIGURE 11.2   Percentage of adult Americans with cardiovascular disease.**
**SOURCE:** American Heart Association. 2010. *Heart Disease and Stroke Statistics—2010 Update.* Dallas, Texas: American Heart Association.

**Ethnicity** Rates of heart disease vary among ethnic groups in the United States, with African Americans having much higher rates of hypertension, heart disease, and stroke than other groups. Figure 11.2 shows how rates of CVD compare among non-Hispanic whites, blacks, and Mexican Americans in the United States. Puerto Rican Americans, Cuban Americans, and Mexican Americans are more likely to suffer from high blood pressure and angina (a warning sign of heart disease) than non-Hispanic white Americans. Asian Americans historically have had far lower rates of CVD than white Americans.

**C-Reactive Protein** Inflammation plays a key role in the development of CVD. When an artery is injured by smoking, cholesterol, hypertension, or other factors, the body's response is to produce inflammation. A substance called C-reactive protein (CRP) is released into the bloodstream during the inflammatory response, and high levels of CRP indicate a substantially elevated risk of heart atack and stroke. CRP may also be harmful to the coronary arteries themselves.

Lifestyle changes and certain drugs can reduce CRP levels. Statin drugs, widely prescribed to lower cholesterol, also decrease inflammation; this may be one reason that statin drugs seem to lower CVD risk even in people with normal blood lipid levels.

## Possible Risk Factors Currently Being Studied

In recent years, several other possible risk factors for cardiovascular disease have been identified.

Elevated blood levels of homocysteine, an amino acid that may damage the lining of blood vessels, are associated with an increased risk of CVD. Men generally have higher homocysteine levels than women, as do individuals with diets low in folic acid, vitamin B-12, and vitamin B-6. Most

# Gender, Ethnicity, and CVD

CVD is the leading cause of death for all Americans, but significant differences exist between men and women and between white Americans and African Americans in the incidence, diagnosis, and treatment of this deadly disease.

## CVD in Women

CVD has been thought of as a "man's disease," but it actually kills more women than men. Polls indicate that women vastly underestimate their risk of dying of a heart attack and overestimate their risk of dying of breast cancer. In reality, nearly 1 in 3 women dies of CVD, while 1 in 30 dies of breast cancer. For women, CVD typically does not develop until after age 50.

The hormone estrogen, produced naturally by a woman's ovaries until menopause, improves blood lipid concentrations and reduces other CVD risk factors. For several decades, many physicians encouraged menopausal women to take hormone replacement therapy (HT) to relieve menopause symptoms and presumably to reduce their risk of CVD. However, some studies found that HT may actually *increase* a woman's risk for heart disease and other health problems, including breast cancer. Some newer studies have found that the increased risk of CVD in women who start HT may be age-dependent; women in the early stages of menopause or ages 50–59 did not appear to have excess risk. This suggests that outcomes may depend on several factors, including the timing of hormone use. The U.S. Preventive Services Task Force and the American Heart Association recommend that HT not be used to protect against CVD.

When women have heart attacks, they are more likely than men to die within a year. One reason is that because they develop heart disease at older ages, women are more likely to have other health problems that complicate treatment. Women have smaller hearts and arteries than men, possibly making diagnosis and treatment more difficult.

Women presenting with CVD are just as likely as men to report chest pain, but are also likely to report non-chest-pain symptoms, which may obscure their diagnosis. These additional symptoms include fatigue, weakness, shortness of breath, nausea, vomiting, and pain in the abdomen, neck, jaw, and back. Women are also more likely to have pain at rest, during sleep, or with mental stress. A woman who experiences these symptoms should be persistent in seeking accurate diagnosis and appropriate treatment.

Careful diagnosis of cardiac symptoms is also key in avoiding unnecessary invasive procedures in cases of stress cardiomyopathy ("broken heart syndrome"), which occurs much more commonly in women than in men. In this condition, hormones and neurotransmitters associated with a severe stress response stun the heart, producing heart-attack-like symptoms and decreased pumping function of the heart, but no damage to the heart muscle. Typically, the condition reverses quickly.

Women should be aware of their CVD risk factors and consult with a physician to assess their risk and determine the best way to prevent CVD.

## CVD in African Americans

African Americans are at substantially higher risk for death from CVD than members of other ethnic groups. The rate of hypertension among African Americans is among the highest of any group in the world. Blacks tend to develop hypertension at an earlier age than whites, and their average blood pressure is much higher. They also have a higher risk of stroke, have strokes at younger ages, and have more significant stroke-related disabilities. Some experts recommend that blacks be treated with antihypertensive drugs at an earlier stage—when blood pressure reaches 130/80 rather than the typical 140/90 cutoff for hypertension.

A number of genetic and biological factors may contribute to CVD in African Americans. For example, blacks may be

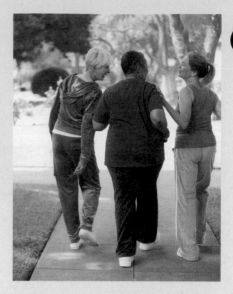

more sensitive to salt and have a physiologically different response to stress, which can lead to high blood pressure and other CVD risk factors. Low income is another factor in CVD risk and is associated with reduced access to adequate health care, insurance, and information about prevention. Discrimination may also play a role, both by increasing stress and by affecting treatment by physicians and hospitals.

Although these factors are important, some evidence favors lifestyle explanations for the higher CVD rate among African Americans. For example, black New Yorkers born in the South have a much higher CVD risk than those born in the Northeast. (Researchers speculate that some lifestyle risk factors for CVD, including smoking and a high-fat diet, may be more common in the South.) People with low incomes, who are disproportionately black, tend to smoke more, use more salt, and exercise less than those with higher incomes.

The general preventive strategies recommended for all Americans may be particularly critical for African Americans. Tailoring your lifestyle to your particular ethnic risk may also be helpful in some cases. Discuss your particular risk profile with your physician to help identify lifestyle changes most appropriate for you.

people can lower homocysteine levels easily by adopting a healthy diet rich in fruits, vegetables, and grains. Severe vitamin D deficiency has also been associated with heart dysfunction, independent of homocysteine levels.

High levels of a specific type of LDL called lipoprotein(a), or Lp(a), may be a risk factor for coronary heart disease (CHD), especially when associated with high LDL or low HDL levels. Lp(a) levels have a strong genetic component and are difficult to treat. About 25% of the U.S. population has elevated lipoprotein(a) levels.

LDL particles differ in size and density, and people with a high proportion of small, dense LDL particles—a condition called LDL pattern B—also appear to be at greater risk for CVD. Exercise, a low-fat diet, and certain lipid-lowering drugs may help lower CVD risk in people with LDL pattern B.

Several infectious agents, including *Chlamydia pneumoniae, cytomegalovirus,* and *Helicobacter pylori,* have also been identified as possible risk factors for cardiovascular disease. Infections may damage arteries and lead to chronic inflammation.

Certain CVD risk factors are often found in a cluster referred to as *metabolic syndrome* or *insulin resistance syndrome.* It is estimated that about 34% of the adult U.S. population has metabolic syndrome. As described in Chapter 6, symptoms of metabolic syndrome include abdominal obesity, high triglycerides, low HDL cholesterol, high blood pressure, and high blood glucose levels (Table 11.3). Metabolic syndrome significantly increases the risk of CVD—more so in women than in men. Weight control, physical activity, and a diet rich in unsaturated fats and fiber are recommended for people with metabolic syndrome. Exercise is especially important because it increases insulin sensitivity even if it doesn't produce weight loss.

| Table 11.3 | Defining Characteristics of Metabolic Syndrome* |
|---|---|
| Abdominal obesity (waist circumference) | |
| Men | >40 in (>102 cm) |
| Women | >35 in (>88 cm) |
| Triglycerides | ≥150 mg/dl |
| HDL cholesterol | |
| Men | <40 mg/dl or drug-treated |
| Women | <50 mg/dl or drug-treated |
| Blood pressure | ≥130/ ≥ 85 mm Hg or drug-treated |
| Fasting glucose | ≥110 mg/dl or drug-treated |

*A person is diagnosed with metabolic syndrome if he or she has three or more of the risk factors listed here.

**SOURCE:** Grundy, S. M., et al. 2005. Diagnosis and management of the metabolic syndrome: An American Heart Association/National Heart, Lung, and Blood Institute Scientific Statement. *Circulation* 112: 2735.

# MAJOR FORMS OF CARDIOVASCULAR DISEASE

Although deaths from CVD have declined drastically over the past 60 years, it remains the leading cause of death in America. According to the National Center for Health Statistics, heart disease killed nearly 600,000 Americans in 2009. The financial burden of CVD, including the costs of medical treatments and lost productivity, exceeds $286 billion annually. Although the main forms of CVD are interrelated and have elements in common, we treat them separately here for the sake of clarity. Hypertension, which is both a major risk factor and a form of CVD, was described earlier in the chapter.

## Atherosclerosis

Atherosclerosis is a form of arteriosclerosis, or thickening and hardening of the arteries. In atherosclerosis, arteries become narrowed by deposits of fat, cholesterol, and other substances. The process begins when endothelial cells (the cells lining the arteries) become damaged, most likely through a combination of factors such as smoking, high blood pressure, high insulin or glucose levels, and deposits of oxidized LDL particles. The body's response to this damage results in inflammation and changes in the artery lining. Deposits, called **plaques,** accumulate on artery walls; the arteries lose their elasticity and their ability to expand and contract, restricting blood flow. Once narrowed by a plaque, an artery is vulnerable to blockage by blood clots. (See page T3-4 of the color transparency insert "Touring the Cardiorespiratory System" in Chapter 3.) The risk of life-threatening clots and heart attacks increases if the fibrous cap covering a plaque ruptures.

If the heart, brain, and/or other organs are deprived of blood and the oxygen it carries, the effects of atherosclerosis can be deadly. Coronary arteries, which supply the heart with blood, are particularly susceptible to plaque buildup, a condition called **coronary heart disease (CHD),** or *coronary artery disease* (*CAD*). The blockage of a coronary artery causes a heart attack. If a cerebral artery (leading to the brain) is blocked, the result is a stroke. The main risk factors for atherosclerosis are cigarette smoking, physical inactivity, high levels of blood cholesterol, high blood pressure, and diabetes.

## Heart Disease and Heart Attacks

The American Heart Association estimates that 785,000 Americans have a first heart attack each year, and 470,000

**plaque** A deposit of fatty (and other) substances on the inner wall of an artery.

**coronary heart disease (CHD)** Heart disease caused by atherosclerosis in the arteries that supply blood to the heart muscle; also called *coronary artery disease* (*CAD*).

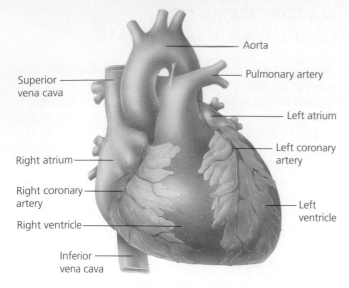

**FIGURE 11.3  Blood supply to the heart.**
Blood is supplied to the heart from the right and left coronary arteries, which branch off the aorta. If a coronary artery becomes blocked by plaque buildup or a blood clot, a heart attack occurs; part of the heart muscle may die due to lack of oxygen.

*Labels:* Superior vena cava · Aorta · Pulmonary artery · Left atrium · Left coronary artery · Right atrium · Right coronary artery · Right ventricle · Left ventricle · Inferior vena cava

suffer a recurrent attack. About 195,000 people suffer a symptomless, or "silent," heart attack each year. Although a **heart attack,** or *myocardial infarction (MI),* may come without warning, it is usually the end result of a long-term disease process. The heart requires a steady supply of oxygen-rich blood to function properly (Figure 11.3). If one of the coronary arteries that supplies blood to the heart becomes blocked, a heart attack results. A heart attack caused by a blood clot is called a *coronary thrombosis.* During a heart attack, part of the heart muscle (myocardium) may die from lack of blood flow.

Chest pain, called **angina pectoris,** is a signal that the heart isn't getting enough oxygen to supply its needs. Although not actually a heart attack, angina—felt as an extreme tightness in the chest and heavy pressure behind the breastbone or in the shoulder, neck, arm, hand, or back—is a warning that the heart is overloaded.

If the electrical impulses that control heartbeat are disrupted, the heart may beat too quickly, too slowly,

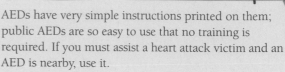

or in an irregular fashion, a condition known as **arrhythmia.** The symptoms of arrhythmia range from imperceptible to severe and even fatal. **Sudden cardiac death,** also called *cardiac arrest,* is most often caused by an arrythmia called *ventricular fibrillation,* a kind of "quivering" of the ventricle that makes it ineffective in pumping blood. If ventricular fibrillation continues for more than a few minutes, it is generally fatal. Cardiac defibrillation, in which an electrical shock is delivered to the heart, can jolt the heart into a more efficient rhythm. This shock can be administered with an automated external defibrillator (AED), a first-aid device that is available in many public places in case someone experiences a heart attack.

Heart attack symptoms may include pain or pressure in the chest; pain in the arm, neck, or jaw; difficulty breathing; excessive sweating; nausea and vomiting; and loss of consciousness. But not all heart attacks involve sharp chest pain. Women, in particular, are more likely to have different symptoms—shortness of breath, weakness, unusual fatigue, cold sweat, and dizziness.

If symptoms of heart trouble occur, it is critical to contact an emergency medical service or go immediately to the nearest hospital or clinic (see the box "What to Do in Case of a Heart Attack, Stroke, or Cardiac Arrest"). Many experts also suggest that the heart attack victim chew and swallow one adult aspirin tablet (325 mg); aspirin has an immediate anticlotting effect. If someone having a heart attack gets to the emergency department quickly enough, a clot-dissolving agent can be injected to dissolve a clot in the coronary artery, reducing the amount of damage to the heart muscle.

Physicians have a variety of diagnostic tools and treatments for heart disease. A patient may undergo a stress or exercise test, in which he or she runs on a treadmill or pedals a stationary cycle while being monitored with an electrocardiogram (ECG or EKG). Certain characteristic changes in the heart's electrical activity while it is under stress can reveal particular heart problems, such as restricted blood flow to the heart muscle. Tools that allow the physician to visualize a patient's heart and arteries include magnetic resonance imaging (MRI), electron-beam computed tomography (EBCT), echocardiograms, and others.

If tests indicate a problem or if a person has already had a heart attack, several treatments are possible. Along with a low-fat diet, regular exercise, and smoking cessation, many patients are also advised to take a low-dose aspirin tablet daily. Aspirin has an anticlotting effect, discouraging

**KEY TERMS**

**heart attack**  Damage to, or death of, heart muscle, resulting from a failure of the coronary arteries to deliver enough blood to the heart; also known as *myocardial infarction (MI).*

**angina pectoris**  A condition in which the heart muscle does not receive enough blood, causing severe pain in the chest and often in the arm and shoulder.

**arrhythmia**  A change in the normal pattern of the heartbeat.

**sudden cardiac death**  A nontraumatic, unexpected death from sudden cardiac arrest, most often due to arrhythmia; in most instances, victims have underlying heart disease.

**stroke**  An impeded blood supply to some part of the brain resulting in the destruction of brain cells; also called *cerebrovascular accident (CVA).*

# What to Do in Case of a Heart Attack, Stroke, or Cardiac Arrest

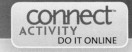

## Warning Signs of Heart Attack

Some heart attacks are sudden and intense—the "movie heart attack," where no one doubts what's happening. But most heart attacks start slowly, with mild pain or discomfort. Often people affected aren't sure what's wrong and wait too long before getting help. Here are signs that can mean a heart attack is happening:

- *Chest discomfort.* Heart attacks often involve discomfort in the chest that lasts more than a few minutes, or that goes away and comes back. It can feel like uncomfortable pressure, squeezing, fullness, or pain.

- *Discomfort in other areas of the upper body.* Symptoms can include pain or discomfort in one or both arms, the back, neck, jaw, or stomach.

- *Shortness of breath.* May occur with or without chest discomfort.

- *Other signs.* These may include breaking out in a cold sweat, nausea, vomiting, or lightheadedness.

Not all of the signs occur in every heart attack. As with men, women's most common heart attack symptom is chest pain or discomfort, but women are somewhat more likely than men to experience some of the other symptoms, particularly shortness of breath, nausea/vomiting, and back or jaw pain.

If you or someone you're with has chest discomfort, especially with one or more of the other signs, don't wait longer than a few minutes (no more than 5) before calling for help.

Calling 9-1-1 is almost always the fastest way to get life-saving treatment. Emergency medical services staff can begin treatment when they arrive—up to an hour sooner than if someone gets to the hospital by car. The staff are also trained to revive someone whose heart has stopped. Patients with chest pain who arrive by ambulance usually receive faster treatment at the hospital, too. Today, medications and treatments are available that weren't available in the past, but they must be given relatively quickly after the heart attack to be effective.

If you can't access the emergency medical services (EMS), have someone drive you to the hospital right away. If you're the one having symptoms, don't drive yourself, unless you have absolutely no other option.

## Warning Signs of Stroke

- Sudden numbness or weakness of the face, arm, or leg, especially on one side of the body

- Sudden confusion, trouble speaking or understanding

- Sudden trouble seeing in one or both eyes

- Sudden trouble walking, dizziness, or loss of balance or coordination

- Sudden, severe headache with no known cause

If you or someone with you has one or more of these signs, don't delay! Immediately call 9-1-1 or the EMS number so an ambulance (ideally with advanced life support) can be sent for you. Also, check the time so you'll know when the first symptoms appeared. It's very important to take immediate action. If given within 3 hours of the start of symptoms, a clot-busting drug called tissue plasminogen activator (tPA) can reduce long-term disability from the most common type of stroke. tPA is the only FDA-approved medication for the treatment of stroke within 3 hours of symptom onset.

## Signs of Cardiac Arrest

Cardiac arrest strikes immediately and without warning. Here are the signs:

- Sudden loss of responsiveness.

- No response to tapping on shoulders.

- No normal breathing.

- The victim does not take a normal breath for at least 5 seconds when you tilt the head up and check.

If these signs of cardiac arrest are present, tell someone else to call 9-1-1 and to get an AED if one is available before you begin cardiopulmonary resuscitation (CPR). Use the AED as soon as it arrives.

**SOURCE:** American Heart Association, 2010. *Heart Attack, Stroke, and Cardiac Arrest Warning Signs.* Reprinted with permission. www.american heart.org. Copyright © 2010 American Heart Association.

---

platelets in the blood from sticking to arterial plaques and forming clots; it also reduces inflammation. Low-dose aspirin therapy appears to help prevent first heart attacks in men, second heart attacks in men and women, and strokes in women over age 65. In addition to aspirin, prescription drugs can also help reduce the strain on the heart.

Several surgical treatments are available to treat certain forms of heart disease. *Balloon angioplasty* involves threading a catheter with an inflatable balloon tip through a coronary artery until it reaches the area of blockage; the balloon is then inflated, flattening the plaque and widening the arterial opening. Many surgeons permanently implant coronary *stents*—flexible stainless steel tubes—to prop the artery open and prevent reclogging after angioplasty. In coronary bypass surgery, healthy blood vessels are grafted to coronary arteries to bypass blockages.

## Stroke

A **stroke**, also called a *cerebrovascular accident* (CVA), occurs when the blood supply to the brain is cut off. If brain cells are deprived of blood for more than a few minutes, they die. Once brain cells begin dying, about 2 million cells are lost every minute that blood flow is not restored. Prompt treatment of stroke can greatly decrease the risk of permanent disability. The American Heart Association estimates that 795,000 Americans suffer a stroke each year.

A stroke may be caused by a blood clot that blocks an artery (*ischemic stroke*) or by a ruptured blood vessel (*hemorrhagic stroke*). Ischemic strokes, which account for 87% of all strokes, are often caused by atherosclerosis or certain types of arrhythmia. Hemorrhagic strokes may occur if there is a weak spot in an artery wall or following a head injury. The interruption of the blood supply to any area of the brain prevents the nerve cells there from functioning, in some cases causing death. Nerve cells control sensation and most body movements; depending on the area of the brain affected, a stroke may cause paralysis, walking disability, speech impairment, memory loss, and changes in behavior.

Effective treatment requires the prompt recognition of symptoms and correct diagnosis of the type of stroke that has occurred. Treatment may involve the use of clot-dissolving and antihypertensive drugs. Even if brain tissue has been damaged or destroyed, nerve cells in the brain can make new pathways, and some functions can be taken over by other parts of the brain.

Many people have strokes without knowing it, so they do not realize they may need treatment or evaluation for the risk of a full-blown stroke in the future. These silent strokes do not cause any noticeable symptoms while they are occuring. Although they may be mild, silent strokes leave their victims at a higher risk for subsequent and more serious strokes later in life. They also contribute to loss of mental and cognitive skills. In 2008, a study of MRI scans of 2000 elderly people revealed that 11% of the subjects had brain damage from one or more strokes but did not realize they had ever had a stroke. A 2009 study suggested that silent strokes may be five times more prevalent than full-blown strokes in people under age 65.

## Congestive Heart Failure

The heart's pumping mechanism can be damaged by a number of conditions, including high blood pressure, heart attack, atherosclerosis, viral infections, rheumatic fever, and birth defects. When the heart cannot maintain its regular pumping rate and force, fluids begin to back up. When extra fluid seeps through capillary walls, edema (swelling) results, usually in the legs and ankles, but sometimes in other parts of the body as well. Fluid

can collect in the lungs and interfere with breathing, particularly when a person is lying down. This condition is called *pulmonary edema,* and the entire process is known as **congestive heart failure.** Treatment includes reducing the workload on the heart, modifying salt intake, and using drugs that help the body eliminate excess fluid.

# PROTECTING YOURSELF AGAINST CARDIOVASCULAR DISEASE

You can take several important steps right now to lower your risk of developing CVD (Figure 11.4). Reducing CVD risk factors when you are young can pay off with many extra years of life and health.

## Eat a Heart-Healthy Diet

For most Americans, changing to a heart-healthy diet involves cutting total fat intake, substituting unsaturated fats for saturated and trans fats, and increasing intake of whole grains and fiber. The following aspects of nutrition apply directly to heart health:

- *Decreased fat and cholesterol.* The National Cholesterol Education Program (NCEP) recommends that all Americans over age 2 adopt a diet in which fats account for no more than 30% of total daily calories, with no more than one-third of total fat calories (10% of total daily calories) coming from saturated fat. The American Heart Association and the 2010 Dietary Guidelines Advisory Committee recommend that no more than 7% of daily calories come from saturated fats. The NCEP recommends that most Americans limit dietary cholesterol intake to no more than 300 milligrams per day; for people with heart disease or high LDL levels, the suggested daily limit is 200 milligrams.

- *Fiber.* Studies have shown that a high-fiber diet is associated with a 40–50% reduction in the risk of heart attack and stroke. To get the recommended 25–38 grams of dietary fiber a day, eat whole grains, fruits, and vegetables. Good sources of fiber include oatmeal, some breakfast cereals, barley, legumes, and most fruits and vegetables.

- *Sodium and potassium.* Reducing sodium intake to recommended levels, while also increasing potassium intake, can help reduce blood pressure for many people. The American Heart Association and the 2010 Dietary Guidelines Advisory Committee recommend that sodium intake be reduced to no more than 1500 mg per day for all Americans.

- *Alcohol.* Moderate alcohol use may increase HDL cholesterol; it may also reduce stroke risk, possibly by dampening the inflammatory response or by affecting blood clotting. For most people under age 45, however, the risks of alcohol use probably outweigh any health

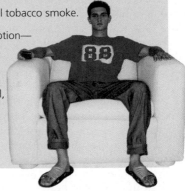

**Do More**

- Eat a diet rich in fruits, vegetables, whole grains, and low-fat or fat-free dairy products. Eat five to nine servings of fruits and vegetables each day.

- Eat several servings of high-fiber foods each day.

- Eat two or more servings of fish per week; try a few servings of nuts and soy foods each week.

- Choose unsaturated fats rather than saturated and trans fats.

  - Be physically active; do both aerobic exercise and strength training on a regular basis.

  - Achieve and maintain a healthy weight.

- Develop effective strategies for handling stress and anger. Nurture old friendships and family ties, and make new friends; pay attention to your spiritual side.

- Obtain recommended screening tests and follow your physician's recommendations.

**Do Less**

- Don't use tobacco in any form: cigarettes, spit tobacco, cigars and pipes, bidis and clove cigarettes.

- Limit consumption of fats, especially trans fats and saturated fats.

- Limit consumption of salt to no more than 2300 mg of sodium per day (1500 mg if you have or are at high risk for hypertension).

- Avoid exposure to environmental tobacco smoke.

- Avoid excessive alcohol consumption—no more than one drink per day for women and two drinks per day for men.

- Limit consumption of cholesterol, added sugars, and refined carbohydrates.

- Avoid excess stress, anger, and hostility.

**FIGURE 11.4 Strategies for reducing your risk of cardiovascular disease.**

## Wellness Tip

Oatmeal can actually lower your level of LDL cholesterol. Oatmeal contains soluble fiber, which prevents LDL particles from entering the bloodstream.

## Ask Yourself

**QUESTIONS FOR CRITICAL THINKING AND REFLECTION**

Has anyone you know ever had a heart attack? If so, was the onset gradual or sudden? Were appropriate steps taken to help the person (for example, call 9-1-1, give CPR, or use an AED)? Do you feel comfortable dealing with a cardiac emergency? If not, what can you do to improve your readiness?

benefit. Excessive alcohol consumption increases the risk of a variety of serious health problems, including hypertension, stroke, some cancers, liver disease, alcohol dependence, and injuries.

## Exercise Regularly

You can significantly reduce your risk of CVD with a moderate amount of physical activity (see the box "How Does Exercise Affect CVD Risk?"). A formal exercise program can provide even greater benefits. The information in Chapters 2–7 can help you create and implement a complete exercise program that meets your needs for fitness and prevention of chronic disease.

## Avoid Tobacco

The number-one risk factor for CVD that you can control is smoking. If you smoke, quit. If you don't, don't start. If you live or work with people who smoke, encourage them to quit—for their sake and yours. If you find yourself breathing in smoke, take steps to prevent or stop this exposure.

## Know and Manage Your Blood Pressure

If you have no CVD risk factors, have your blood pressure measured at least once every 2 years; yearly tests are recommended if you have other risk factors. If your blood pressure is high, follow your physician's advice on lowering it.

## Ask Yourself

**QUESTIONS FOR CRITICAL THINKING AND REFLECTION**

Do you know what your blood pressure and cholesterol levels are? If not, is there a reason you don't know? Is there something preventing you from getting this information about yourself? How can you motivate yourself to have these easy but important health checks?

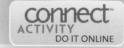

# How Does Exercise Affect CVD Risk?

Regular exercise directly and indirectly benefits your cardiovascular health and can actually help you avoid having a heart attack or stroke. The evidence comes from dozens of large-scale, population-based studies conducted over the past several decades. There is so much evidence about the cardiovascular health benefits of exercise, in fact, that physicians regard physical activity as a magic bullet against heart disease.

Physical activity has an inverse relationship with cardiovascular disease, meaning that the more exercise you get, the less likely you are to develop or die from CVD. Compared to sedentary individuals, people who engage in regular, moderate physical activity lower their risk of CVD by 20% or more. People who get regular, vigorous exercise reduce their risk of CVD by 30% or more. This positive benefit applies regardless of gender, age, race, or ethnicity.

Most studies focus on various aerobic endurance exercises, such as walking, running on a treadmill, or biking. As noted in Chapter 1, the type of exercise performed is less important than the amount of energy expended during the activity. The greater the energy expenditure, the greater the health benefits. In three different studies conducted between 1999 and 2002, for example, researchers focused on women of various ages who walked for exercise. All three studies showed that the women's relative risk of CVD dropped as they expended more and more energy by walking.

Exercise affects heart health via many mechanisms, all of which are being studied. For example, exercise helps people lose weight and improve body composition. Weight loss can improve heart health by reducing the amount of stress on the heart. Changing body composition to a more positive ratio of fat to fat-free mass boosts resting metabolic rate. Exercise directly strengthens the heart muscle itself, and it improves the balance of fats in the blood by boosting HDL and reducing LDL and triglyceride levels.

Exercise can also prevent metabolic syndrome and reverse many of its negative effects on the body. For example, exercise improves the health and function of the endothelial cells—the inner lining of the arteries. These cells secrete nitric oxide, which regulates blood flow, improves nerve function, strengthens the immune system, enhances reproductive health, and suppresses inflammation. Exercise training also improves the function of cell sodium-potassium pumps, which regulate fluid and electrolyte balance and cellular communication throughout the body.

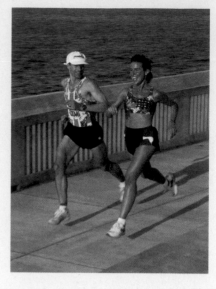

One of the clearest positive effects of exercise is on hypertension. Many studies, involving thousands of people, have shown that physical activity reduces both systolic and diastolic blood pressure. These studies showed that people who engaged in regular aerobic exercise lowered their resting blood pressure by 2–4%, on average. Lowered blood pressure itself reduces the risk of other kinds of cardiovascular disease.

Fewer studies have been conducted on exercise and risk of stroke. Even with limited evidence, however, there appears to be a similar inverse relationship between physical activity and stroke. According to a handful of studies, the most physically active people reduced their risk of both ischemic and hemorrhagic strokes by up to 30%. Although this benefit appears to apply equally to men and women, there is not sufficient evidence that it applies equally across races or ethnicities.

Of course, exercise isn't possible for everyone and may actually be dangerous for some people. People with CVD or serious risk factors for heart disease should work with their physician to determine whether or how to exercise.

SOURCES: Cornelissen, V. A., and R. H. Fagard. 2005. Effect of resistance training on resting blood pressure: A meta-analysis of randomized controlled trials. *Journal of Hypertension* 23(2): 251–259; Physical Activity Guidelines Advisory Committee. 2008. *Physical Activity Guidelines Advisory Committee Report, 2008.* Washington, D.C.: U.S. Department of Health and Human Services; Schnohr, P., et al. 2006. Long-term physical activity in leisure time and mortality from coronary heart disease, stroke, respiratory diseases, and cancer. The Copenhagen City Heart Study. *European Journal of Cardiovascular Prevention and Rehabilitation* 13(2): 173–179; Williams, M. A., et al. 2007. Resistance exercise in individuals with and without cardiovascular disease: 2007 update: A scientific statement from the American Heart Association Council on Clinical Cardiology and Council on Nutrition, Physical Activity, and Metabolism. *Circulation* 116(5): 572–584.

## Know and Manage Your Cholesterol Levels

All people age 20 and over should have their cholesterol checked at least once every 5 years. The NCEP recommends a fasting lipoprotein profile that measures total cholesterol, HDL, LDL, and triglyceride levels. Once you know your baseline numbers, you and your physician can develop an LDL goal and lifestyle plan.

## Develop Ways to Handle Stress and Anger

To reduce the psychological and social risk factors for CVD, develop effective strategies for handling the stress in your life. Shore up your social support network, and try some of the techniques described in this chapter for managing stress and anger.

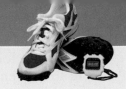

# Getting to Know Your Pulse Rate

Do you know what your resting pulse rate is? It's easy to find out, and it can be useful information for you and your doctor. Chapter 3 provides instructions for checking your own pulse. Practice a few times, and then check your resting pulse rate each day for 7 consecutive days. Write the results here:

| Day | Time | Pulse |
|-----|------|-------|
| 1. | _____ | _____ |
| 2. | _____ | _____ |
| 3. | _____ | _____ |
| 4. | _____ | _____ |
| 5. | _____ | _____ |
| 6. | _____ | _____ |
| 7. | _____ | _____ |

Be sure to rest for at least 10 minutes before checking your resting pulse rate, and don't check your pulse right after eating (some foods can increase your heart rate temporarily). For most people, a resting pulse rate between 60 and 100 beats per minute is considered normal. Very fit people may have a slower resting pulse rate.

## TIPS FOR TODAY AND THE FUTURE

Because cardiovascular disease is a long-term process that can begin when you're young, it's important to develop heart-healthy habits early in life.

### RIGHT NOW YOU CAN

- Make an appointment to have your blood pressure and cholesterol levels checked.
- List the key stressors in your life, and decide what to do about the ones that bother you most.
- Plan to replace one high-fat item in your diet with one that is high in fiber. For example, replace a doughnut with a bowl of whole-grain cereal.

### IN THE FUTURE YOU CAN

- Track your eating habits for one week, then compare them to the DASH eating plan. Make adjustments to bring your diet closer to the DASH recommendations.
- Sign up for a class in CPR. A CPR certification equips you with valuable lifesaving skills you can use to help someone who is choking, having a heart attack, or experiencing cardiac arrest.

## SUMMARY

- The major controllable risk factors for CVD are smoking, hypertension, unhealthy cholesterol levels, inactivity, overweight and obesity, and diabetes.

- Contributing factors for CVD that can be changed include high triglyceride levels, inadequate stress management, a hostile personality, depression, anxiety, lack of social support, poverty, and alcohol and drug use.

- Major risk factors for CVD that can't be changed are heredity, aging, being male, and ethnicity.

- Hypertension weakens the heart and scars and hardens arteries, causing resistance to blood flow. It is defined as blood pressure equal to or higher than 140 over 90.

- Atherosclerosis is a progressive hardening and narrowing of arteries that can lead to restricted blood flow and even complete blockage.

- Heart attacks, strokes, and congestive heart failure are the results of a long-term disease process; hypertension and atherosclerosis are usually involved.

- Reducing heart disease risk involves eating a heart-healthy diet, exercising regularly, avoiding tobacco, managing blood pressure and cholesterol levels, and handling stress and anger.

## FOR FURTHER EXPLORATION

### BOOKS

Heller, M. 2007. *The DASH Diet Action Plan, Based on the National Institutes of Health Research: Dietary Approaches to Stop Hypertension.* Northbrook, Ill.: Amidon Press. *Provides background information and guidelines for adopting the DASH diet; also includes meal plans to suit differing caloric needs and recipes.*

**Q** I know what foods to avoid to prevent CVD, but are there any foods I should eat to protect myself from CVD?

**A** The most important dietary change for CVD prevention is a negative one: cutting back on foods high in saturated and trans fat. However, certain foods can be helpful. The positive effects of unsaturated fats, soluble fiber, and alcohol on heart health were discussed earlier in the chapter. Other potentially beneficial foods include those rich in the following:

- *Omega-3 fatty acids.* Found in fish, shellfish, and some nuts and seeds, omega-3 fatty acids reduce clotting and inflammation and may lower the risk of fatal arrhythmia.
- *Folic acid, vitamin B-6, and vitamin B-12.* These vitamins may affect CVD risk by lowering homocysteine levels; see Table 8.4 for a list of food sources.
- *Plant stanols and sterols.* Plant stanols and sterols, found in some types of trans fat–free margarines and other products, reduce the absorption of cholesterol in the body and help lower LDL levels.
- *Soy protein.* Replacing some animal protein with soy protein can lower LDL cholesterol. Soy-based foods include tofu, tempeh, and soy-based beverages.
- *Calcium.* Diets rich in calcium may help prevent hypertension and possibly stroke by reducing insulin resistance and platelet aggregation. Low-fat and fat-free dairy products are rich in calcium; refer to Chapter 8 for other sources.

**Q** The advice I hear from the media about protecting myself from CVD seems to be changing all the time. What am I supposed to believe?

**A** Health-related research is now described in popular newspapers and magazines rather than just medical journals, meaning that more and more people have access to the information. Researchers do not deliberately set out to mislead or confuse people. However, news reports may oversimplify the results of research studies, leaving out some of the qualifications and questions the researchers present with their findings. In addition, news reports may not differentiate between a preliminary finding and a result that has been verified by a large number of long-term studies. And researchers themselves must strike a balance between reporting promising preliminary findings to the public, thereby allowing people to act on them, and waiting 10–20 years until long-term studies confirm (or disprove) a particular theory.

Although you cannot become an expert on all subjects, there are some strategies you can use to assess the health advice that appears in the media; see the box "Evaluating Health News."

**Q** What's a heart murmur, and is it dangerous?

**A** A heart murmur is an extra or altered heart sound heard during a routine medical exam. The source is often a problem with one of the heart valves that separate the chambers of the heart. Congenital defects and

Lipsky, M. S., et al. 2008. *American Medical Association Guide to Preventing and Treating Heart Disease.* New York: Wiley. *A team of doctors provides advice to consumers on heart health.*

Manger, W. M., and N. M. Kaplan. 2011. *101 Questions and Answers about Hypertension.* Alameda, Calif.: Hunter House. *A team of doctors answers questions about preventing, treating, and living with high blood pressure.*

Mostyn, B. 2007. *Pocket Guide to Low Sodium Foods,* 2nd ed. Olympia, Wash.: InData Publishing. *Lists thousands of low-sodium products that can be purchased in supermarkets, as well as low-sodium choices available in many restaurants.*

**ORGANIZATIONS AND WEB SITES**

*American Heart Association.* Provides information on hundreds of topics relating to the prevention and control of CVD.
    http://www.heart.org (general information)
*The Human Heart: An On-Line Exploration.* An online museum exhibit containing information on the structure and function of the heart, how to monitor your heart's health, and how to maintain a healthy heart.
    http://www.fi.edu/learn/heart/index.html
*MedlinePlus: Blood, Heart and Circulation Topics.* Provides links to reliable sources of information on cardiovascular health.
    http://www.nlm.nih.gov/medlineplus/bloodheartandcirculation.html

*National Cholesterol Education Program (NCEP): Cholesterol Counts for Everyone.* Provides information on cholesterol for people with heart disease and people who want to avoid it.
    http://rover.nhlbi.nih.gov/chd
*National Heart, Lung, and Blood Institute.* Provides information on a variety of topics relating to cardiovascular health and disease, including cholesterol, smoking, obesity, hypertension, and the DASH diet.
    http://www.nhlbi.nih.gov
*National Stroke Association.* Provides information and referrals for stroke victims and their families; the Web site has a stroke risk assessment.
    http://www.stroke.org
See also the listings for Chapters 9 and 10.

**SELECTED BIBLIOGRAPHY**

Albert, C. M., et al. 2008. Effect of folic acid and B vitamins on risk of cardiovascular events and total mortality among women at high risk for cardiovascular disease: A randomized trial. *Journal of the American Medical Association* 299(17): 2027–2036.
American Cancer Society. 2011. *Cancer Facts and Figures, 2011.* Atlanta, Ga.: American Cancer Society.
American Heart Association. 2011. *Heart Disease and Stroke Statistics—2011 Update.* Dallas, Texas: American Heart Association.

certain infections can cause abnormalities in the valves. The most common heart valve disorder is mitral valve prolapse (MVP), which occurs in about 4% of the population. MVP is characterized by a "billowing" of the mitral valve, which separates the left ventricle and left atrium, during ventricular contraction. In some cases, blood leaks from the ventricle into the atrium. Most people with MVP have no symptoms; they have the same ability to exercise and live as long as people without MVP.

MVP can be confirmed with echocardiography. Treatment is usually unnecessary, although surgery may be needed in the rare cases where leakage through the faulty valve is severe. Experts disagree over whether patients with MVP should take antibiotics prior to dental procedures, a precautionary step used to prevent bacteria, which may be dislodged into the bloodstream during some types of dental and surgical procedures, from infecting the defective valve. Most often, only those patients with significant blood leakage are advised to take antibiotics.

Although MVP usually requires no treatment, more severe heart valve disorders can impair blood flow through the heart. Treatment depends on the location and severity of the problem. More serious defects may be treated with surgery to repair or replace a valve.

## Q How does stress contribute to cardiovascular disease?

**A** With stress, the brain tells the adrenal glands to secrete cortisol and other hormones and neurotransmitters, which in turn activate the sympathetic nervous system—causing the fight-or-flight response. This response increases heart rate and blood pressure so that more blood is distributed to the heart and other muscles in anticipation of physical activity. Blood glucose concentrations and cholesterol also increase to provide a source of energy, and the platelets become activated so that they will be more likely to clot in case of injury. Such a response can be adaptive if you're being chased by a hungry lion but may be more detrimental than useful if you're sitting at a desk taking an exam or feeling frustrated by a task given to you by your boss.

If you are healthy, you can tolerate the cardiovascular responses that take place during stress, but if you already have CVD, stress can lead to adverse outcomes such as abnormal heart rhythms, heart attacks, and sudden cardiac death. It has long been known that an increase in heart rhythm problems and deaths is associated with acute mental stress. For example, the rate of potentially life-threatening arrhythmias in patients who already had underlying heart disease doubled during the month after the September 11 terrorist attacks; this increase was not limited to people in proximity to Manhattan.

Because avoiding all stress is impossible, having healthy mechanisms to cope with it is your best defense. Instead of adopting unhealthy habits such as smoking, drinking, or overeating to deal with stress, try healthier coping techniques such as exercising, getting enough sleep, and talking to family and friends.

*For more Common Questions Answered about heart health, visit the Online Learning Center at www.mhhe.com/fahey.*

Bibbins-Doming, K., et al. 2010. Projected effect of dietary salt reductions on future cardiovascular disease. *New England Journal of Medicine* 362(7): 590–599.

Berger, J. S., et al. 2006. Aspirin for the primary prevention of cardiovascular events in women and men: A sex-specific meta-analysis of randomized controlled trials. *Journal of the American Medical Association* 295(3): 306–313.

Bonaa, K. H., et al. 2006. Homocysteine lowering and cardiovascular events after acute myocardial infarction. *New England Journal of Medicine* 354(15): 1578–1588.

Centers for Disease Control and Prevention. 2008. Awareness of stroke warning symptoms—13 states and the District of Columbia, 2005. *Morbidity and Mortality Weekly Report* 57(18): 481–485.

Centers for Disease Control and Prevention. 2009. Application of lower sodium intake recommendations to adults—United States, 1999–2006. *Morbidity and Mortality Weekly Report* 58(11): 281–283.

de Torbal, A., et al. 2006. Incidence of recognized and unrecognized myocardial infarction in men and women aged 55 and older: The Rotterdam Study. *European Heart Journal* 27(6): 729–736.

Elliott, P., et al. 2006. Association between protein intake and blood pressure: The INTERMAP study. *Archives of Internal Medicine* 166(1): 79–87.

Giovannucci, E., et al. 2008. 25-hydroxyvitamin D and risk of myocardial infarction in men: A prospective study. *Archives of Internal Medicine* 168(11): 1174–1180.

Gommans, J., et al. 2009. Preventing strokes: The assessment and management of people with transient ischemic attack. *New Zealand Medical Journal* 122(1293): 50–60.

Gurfinkel, E. P., et al. 2007. Invasive vs. non-invasive treatment in acute coronary syndromes and prior bypass surgery. *International Journal of Cardiology* 119(1): 65–72.

Harvard Medical School. 2008. The status of statins. *Harvard Women's Health Watch* 15(6): 1–3.

Jenkins, D. J., et al. 2006. Assessment of the longer-term effects of a dietary portfolio of cholesterol-lowering foods in hypercholesterolemia. *American Journal of Clinical Nutrition* 83(3): 582–591.

Kidambi, S., et al. 2009. Hypertension, insulin resistance, and aldosterone: Sex-specific relationships. *Journal of Clinical Hypertension* 11(3): 130–137.

Marshall, D. A., et al. 2009. Achievement of heart health characteristics through participation in an intensive lifestyle change program (Coronary Artery Disease Reversal Study). *Journal of Cardiopulmonary Rehabilitation and Prevention* 29(2): 84–94.

Mirmiran, P., et al. 2009. Fruit and vegetable consumption and risk factors for cardiovascular disease. *Metabolism* 58(4): 460–468.

Muller, D., et al. 2006. How sudden is sudden cardiac death? *Circulation* 114(11): 1146–1150.

National Center for Health Statistics. 2011. Deaths: Preliminary data for 2009. *National Vital Statistics Reports* 59(4).

Nita, C., et al. 2008. Hypertensive waist: First step of the screening for metabolic syndrome. *Metabolic Syndrome and Related Disorders* 7(2): 105–110.

Ostrom, M. P., et al. 2008. Mortality incidence and the severity of coronary atherosclerosis assessed by computed tomography angiography. *Journal of the American College of Cardiology* 52(16): 1335–1343.

Pickering, T. G., et al. 2008. Call to action on use and reimbursement for home blood pressure monitoring: A joint scientific statement from the

## Evaluating Health News

Americans face an avalanche of health information from newspapers, magazines, books, and television programs. It's not always easy to decide what to believe. The following questions can help you evaluate health news:

- *Is the report based on research or on an anecdote?* Information or recommendations based on one or more carefully designed research studies have more validity than one person's experiences.

- *What is the source of the information?* A study in a respected publication has been reviewed by editors and other researchers in the field—people who are in a position to evaluate the merits of the study and its results. Information put forth by government agencies and national research organizations is also usually considered reliable.

- *How big was the study?* A study that involves many subjects is more likely to yield reliable results than a study involving only a few people. Another indication that a finding is meaningful is if several different studies yield the same results.

- *Who were the people involved in the study?* Research findings are more likely to apply to you if you share important characteristics with the subjects of the study. For example, the results of a study on men over age 50 who smoke may not be particularly meaningful for a 30-year-old nonsmoking woman. Even less applicable are studies done in test tubes or on animals.

- *What kind of study was it?* Epidemiological studies involve observation or interviews in order to trace the relationships among lifestyle, physical characteristics, and diseases. Although epidemiological studies can suggest links, they cannot establish cause-and-effect relationships. Clinical or interventional studies involve testing the effects of different treatments on groups of people who have similar lifestyles and characteristics. They are more likely to provide conclusive evidence of a cause-and-effect relationship. The best interventional studies share the following characteristics:

  - *Controlled.* A group of people who receive the treatment is compared with a matched group who do not receive the treatment.

  - *Randomized.* The treatment and control groups are selected randomly.

  - *Double-blind.* Researchers and participants are unaware of who is receiving the treatment.

  - *Multicenter.* The experiment is performed at more than one institution.

- *What do the statistics really say?* First, are the results described as statistically significant? If a study is large and well designed, its results can be deemed statistically significant, meaning there is less than a 5% chance that the findings resulted from chance. Second, are the results stated in terms of relative or absolute risk? Many findings are reported in terms of *relative risk*, how a particular treatment or condition affects a person's disease risk. Consider the following examples of relative risk:

  - According to some estimates, taking estrogen without progesterone can increase a postmenopausal woman's risk of dying from endometrial cancer by 233%.

  - Giving antiviral medication to HIV-infected pregnant women reduces prenatal transmission of HIV by 90%.

The first of these two findings seems far more dramatic than the second—until one also considers *absolute risk*, the actual risk of the illness in the population being considered. The absolute risk of endometrial cancer is 0.3%; a 233% increase based on the effects of estrogen raises it to 1%, a change of 0.7%. Without treatment, about 25% of infants born to HIV-infected women will be infected with HIV; with treatment, the absolute risk drops to about 2%, a change of 23%. Because the absolute risk of an HIV-infected mother's passing the virus to her infant is so much greater than a woman's risk of developing endometrial cancer (25% compared with 0.3%), a smaller change in relative risk translates into a much greater change in absolute risk.

- *Is new health advice being offered?* If the media report new guidelines for health behavior or medical treatment, examine the source. Government agencies and national research foundations usually consider a great deal of evidence before offering health advice. Above all, use common sense, and check with your physician before making a major change in your health habits based on news reports.

American Heart Association, American Society of Hypertension, and Preventive Cardiovascular Nurses Association. *Hypertension* 52(1): 10–29.

Raggi, P., et al. 2008. Coronary artery calcium to predict all-cause mortality in elderly men and women. *Journal of the American College of Cardiology* 52(1): 17–23.

Refsum, H., et al. 2006. The Hordaland Homocysteine Study: A community-based study of homocysteine, its determinants, and associations with disease. *Journal of Nutrition* 136(6 Suppl.): 1731S–1740S.

Rho, R. W., and R. L. Page. 2007. The automated external defibrillator. *Journal of Cardiovascular Electrophysiology* 18: 1–4.

Ridker, P. M., et al. 2008. Rosuvastatin to prevent vascular events in men and women with elevated C-reactive protein. *New England Journal of Medicine* 359(21): 2195–2207.

Sesso, H. D., et al. 2008. Vitamins E and C in the prevention of cardiovascular disease in men: Physician's Health Study II randomized controlled trial. *Journal of the American Medical Association* 300(18): 2123–2133.

Sui, X., et al. 2007. Cardiorespiratory fitness and the risk of nonfatal cardiovascular disease in women and men with hypertension. *American Journal of Hypertension* 20(6): 608–615.

Tufts University. 2006. Pendulum swings on estrogen and women's heart health risk. *Health & Nutrition Newsletter* 24(3): 1–2.

University of California, Berkeley. 2008. Heart tests: Low- to high-tech. University of California, Berkeley, *Wellness Letter*, August, 5.

Wang, X., et al. 2007. Efficacy of folic acid supplementation in stroke prevention: A meta-analysis. *Lancet* 369(9576): 1876–1882.

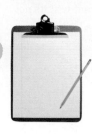

# LAB 11.1 Cardiovascular Health

## Part I  CVD Risk Assessment

Your chances of suffering a heart attack or stroke before age 55 depend on a variety of factors, many of which are under your control. To help identify your risk factors, circle the response for each risk category that best describes you.

1. Sex and Age

   0  Female age 55 or younger; male age 45 or younger

   2  Female over age 55; male over age 45

2. Heredity/Family History

   0  Neither parent suffered a heart attack or stroke before age 60.

   3  One parent suffered a heart attack or stroke before age 60.

   7  Both parents suffered a heart attack or stroke before age 60.

3. Smoking

   0  Never smoked

   3  Quit more than 2 years ago and lifetime smoking is less than 5 pack-years*

   6  Quit less than 2 years ago and/or lifetime smoking is greater than 5 pack-years*

   8  Smoke less than 1/2 pack per day

   13  Smoke more than 1/2 pack per day

   15  Smoke more than 1 pack per day

4. Environmental Tobacco Smoke

   0  Do not live or work with smokers

   2  Exposed to ETS at work

   3  Live with smoker

   4  Both live and work with smokers

5. Blood Pressure

   (If available, use the average of the last three readings.)

   0  120/80 or below

   1  121/81–130/85

   3  Don't know blood pressure

   5  131/86–150/90

   9  151/91–170/100

   13  Above 170/100

6. Total Cholesterol

   0 Lower than 19 0

   1  190–210

   2  Don't know

   3  211–240

   4  241–270

   5  271–300

   6  Over 300

7. HDL Cholesterol

   0  Over 60 mg/dl

   1  55–60

   2  Don't know HDL

   3  45–54

   5  35–44

   7  25–34

   12  Lower than 25

8. Exercise

   0  Exercise three times a week

   1  Exercise once or twice a week

   2  Occasional exercise less than once a week

   7  Rarely exercise

9. Diabetes

   0  No personal or family history

   2  One parent with diabetes

   6  Two parents with diabetes

   9  Type 2 diabetes

   13  Type 1 diabetes

10. Body Mass Index (kg/m2)

   0  <23.0

   1  23.0–24.9

   2  25.0–28.9

   3  29.0–34.9

   5  35.0–39.9

   7  ≥40

11. Stress

   0  Relaxed most of the time

   1  Occasionally stressed and angry

   2  Frequently stressed and angry

   3  Usually stressed and angry

### Scoring

Total your risk factor points. Refer to the list below to get an approximate rating of your risk of suffering an early heart attack or stroke.

| Score | Estimated Risk |
| --- | --- |
| Less than 20 | Low risk |
| 20–29 | Moderate risk |
| 30–45 | High risk |
| Over 45 | Extremely high risk |

*Pack-years can be calculated by multiplying the number of packs you smoked per day by the number of years you smoked. For example, if you smoked a pack and a half a day for 5 years, you would have smoked the equivalent of 1.5 × 5 = 7.5 pack-years.

connect™  http://www.mcgrawhillconnect.com/
FITNESS AND WELLNESS

## Part II   Hostility Assessment

Are you too hostile? To help answer that question, Duke University researcher Redford Williams, M.D., has devised a short self test. It's not a scientific evaluation, but it does offer a rough measure of hostility. Are the following statements true or false for you?

1. I often get annoyed at checkout cashiers or the people in front of me when I'm waiting in line.
2. I usually keep an eye on the people I work or live with to make sure they do what they should.
3. I often wonder how homeless people can have so little respect for themselves.
4. I believe that most people will take advantage of you if you let them.
5. The habits of friends or family members often annoy me.
6. When I'm stuck in traffic, I often start breathing faster and my heart pounds.
7. When I'm annoyed with people, I really want to let them know it.
8. If someone does me wrong, I want to get even.
9. I'd like to have the last word in any argument.
10. At least once a week, I have the urge to yell at or even hit someone.

According to Williams, five or more "true" statements suggest that you're excessively hostile and should consider taking steps to mellow out.

## Using Your Results

*How did you score?* (1) What is your CVD risk assessment score? Are you surprised by your score?

Are you satisfied with your CVD risk rating? If not, set a specific goal:

(2) What is your hostility assessment score? Are you surprised by the result?

Are you satisfied with your hostility rating? If not, set a specific goal:

*What should you do next?* Enter the results of this lab in the Preprogram Assessment column in Appendix C. (1) If you've set a goal for the overall CVD risk assessment score, identify a risk area that you can change, such as smoking, exercise, or stress. Then list three steps or strategies for changing the risk area you've chosen.
Risk area:
Strategies for change:

(2) If you've set a goal for the hostility assessment score, begin by keeping a log of your hostile responses. Review the anger management strategies in Chapter 10, and select several that you will try to use to manage your angry responses. Strategies for anger management:

Next, begin to put your strategies into action. After several weeks of a program to reduce CVD risk or hostility, do this lab again and enter the results in the Postprogram Assessment column of Appendix C. How do the results compare?

**SOURCES:** Hostility quiz from *Life Skills* by Virginia Williams and Redford Williams. New York: Times Books. Reprinted by permission of the authors.

# CHAPTER 12

# Cancer

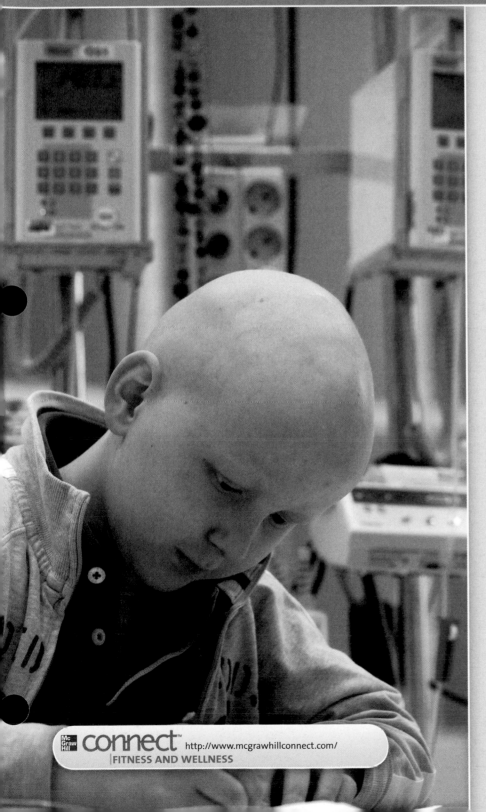

## LOOKING AHEAD...

After reading this chapter, you should be able to:

- Explain what cancer is and how it spreads
- List and describe common cancers, their risk factors, signs and symptoms, treatments, and approaches to prevention
- Discuss some of the causes of cancer and how they can be avoided or minimized
- Describe how cancer can be detected, diagnosed, and treated
- List specific actions you can take to lower your risk of cancer

## TEST YOUR KNOWLEDGE

1. Eating which of these foods may help prevent cancer?
   a. chili peppers
   b. broccoli
   c. oranges
2. Testicular cancer is the most common cancer in men under age 30. True or false?
3. The use of condoms during sexual intercourse can prevent cancer in women. True or false?

**Answers**

1. **All three.** These and many other fruits and vegetables are rich in phytochemicals, naturally occurring substances that may have anti-cancer effects.
2. **True.** Although rare, testicular cancer is the most common cancer in men under age 30. Regular self-exams may aid in its detection.
3. **True.** The primary cause of cervical cancer is infection with the human papillomavirus (HPV), a sexually transmitted pathogen. The use of condoms helps prevent HPV infection.

Cancer is the second leading cause of death, after heart disease. In the United States, cancer is responsible for 1 in 4 deaths, claiming 1500 lives every day. Evidence indicates that most cancers in the United States could be prevented by simple changes in lifestyle. Tobacco use is responsible for about 30% of all cancer deaths (Figure 12.1). Diet and exercise, including their relationship with obesity, account for another 30% of cancer deaths.

## WHAT IS CANCER?

**Cancer** is the abnormal, uncontrolled multiplication of cells, which can ultimately cause death if left untreated.

### Tumors

Most cancers take the form of tumors, although not all tumors are cancerous. A **tumor** (or *neoplasm*) is a mass of tissue that serves no physiological purpose. It can be benign, like a wart, or malignant, like most lung cancers.

**Benign** (noncancerous) **tumors** are made up of cells similar to the surrounding normal cells and are enclosed in a membrane that prevents them from penetrating neighboring tissues. They are dangerous only if their physical presence interferes with body functions.

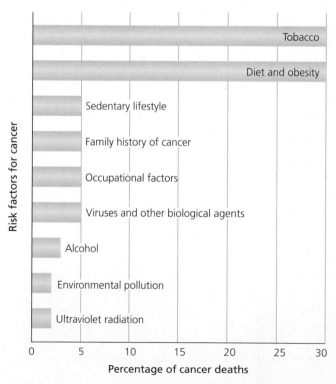

**FIGURE 12.1  Percentage of all cancer deaths linked to risk factors.**
**SOURCE:** Harvard Center for Cancer Prevention. 1996. Harvard reports on cancer prevention. Vol. 1: Human causes of cancer. *Cancer Causes and Control 7(Suppl. 1).*

The term **malignant tumor** is synonymous with cancer. A malignant tumor can invade surrounding structures, including blood vessels, the **lymphatic system**, and nerves. It can also spread to distant sites via the blood and lymphatic circulation, producing invasive tumors in almost any part of the body. A few cancers, like leukemia (cancer of the blood) do not produce a mass but still have the fundamental property of rapid, uncontrolled cell proliferation.

Every case of cancer begins as a change in a cell that allows it to grow and divide when it should not. A malignant cell divides into new cells without regard for normal control mechanisms and gradually produces a mass of abnormal cells, or a tumor. It takes about a billion cells to make a mass the size of a pea, so a single tumor cell must go through many divisions, often taking years, before the tumor grows to a noticeable size. Eventually, a tumor produces a sign or symptom that is detected. In an accessible location (such as a testicle), a tumor may be felt as a lump. In less accessible locations (such as the lungs), a tumor may be noticed only after considerable growth has taken place and may then be detected only by an indirect symptom such as a persistent cough or unexplained bleeding or pain.

### Metastasis

**Metastasis,** the spread of cancer cells, occurs because cancer cells do not stick to each other as strongly as normal cells do and therefore may not remain at the site of the *primary tumor,* the cancer's original location. They break away and can pass through the lining of lymph or blood vessels to invade nearby tissue. They can also drift to distant parts of the body and multiply, establishing new colonies of cancer cells. This traveling and seeding process is called *metastasizing,* and the new tumors are *secondary tumors,* or *metastases*.

The ability of cancer cells to metastasize makes early cancer detection critical. To control the cancer, every cancerous cell must be removed. Once cancer cells enter either the lymphatic system or the bloodstream, it is extremely difficult to stop their spread to other organs.

### COMMON CANCERS

Each year, more than 1.5 million Americans are diagnosed with cancer, and nearly 570,000 die (Figure 12.2). These statistics exclude the more than 1 million cases of the curable types of skin cancer. At current U.S. rates, nearly 1 in 2 men and more than 1 in 3 women will develop cancer at some point in their lives. Nearly 12 million living Americans have a history of cancer.

Until 1991, the number of cancer deaths increased fairly steadily in the United States, largely due to a wave of

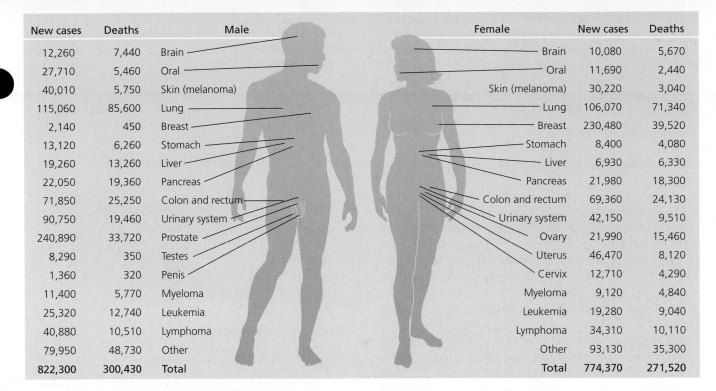

| New cases | Deaths | Male | Female | New cases | Deaths |
|---|---|---|---|---|---|
| 12,260 | 7,440 | Brain | Brain | 10,080 | 5,670 |
| 27,710 | 5,460 | Oral | Oral | 11,690 | 2,440 |
| 40,010 | 5,750 | Skin (melanoma) | Skin (melanoma) | 30,220 | 3,040 |
| 115,060 | 85,600 | Lung | Lung | 106,070 | 71,340 |
| 2,140 | 450 | Breast | Breast | 230,480 | 39,520 |
| 13,120 | 6,260 | Stomach | Stomach | 8,400 | 4,080 |
| 19,260 | 13,260 | Liver | Liver | 6,930 | 6,330 |
| 22,050 | 19,360 | Pancreas | Pancreas | 21,980 | 18,300 |
| 71,850 | 25,250 | Colon and rectum | Colon and rectum | 69,360 | 24,130 |
| 90,750 | 19,460 | Urinary system | Urinary system | 42,150 | 9,510 |
| 240,890 | 33,720 | Prostate | Ovary | 21,990 | 15,460 |
| 8,290 | 350 | Testes | Uterus | 46,470 | 8,120 |
| 1,360 | 320 | Penis | Cervix | 12,710 | 4,290 |
| 11,400 | 5,770 | Myeloma | Myeloma | 9,120 | 4,840 |
| 25,320 | 12,740 | Leukemia | Leukemia | 19,280 | 9,040 |
| 40,880 | 10,510 | Lymphoma | Lymphoma | 34,310 | 10,110 |
| 79,950 | 48,730 | Other | Other | 93,130 | 35,300 |
| 822,300 | 300,430 | Total | Total | 774,370 | 271,520 |

**FIGURE 12.2  Cancer cases and deaths by site and sex.**
**SOURCE:**  American Cancer Society. 2011. *Cancer Facts and Figures, 2011*. Atlanta, Ga.: American Cancer Society.

smoking-related lung cancers in men. In 1991, the death rate began to fall slowly; since then it has dropped more than 19% in men and 11% in women. Still, many more people could be saved from cancer. The American Cancer Society (ACS) estimates that 90% of skin cancer could be prevented by protecting the skin from the rays of the sun and 87% of lung cancer could be prevented by avoiding exposure to tobacco smoke.

A discussion of all types of cancer is beyond the scope of this book. This section looks at the most common cancers and their causes, prevention, and treatment.

## Lung Cancer

Lung cancer is the most common cause of cancer death in the United States; it is responsible for about 157,000 deaths each year. Since 1987, lung cancer has surpassed breast cancer as the leading cause of cancer death in women.

The chief risk factor for lung cancer is tobacco smoke, which currently accounts for 30% of all cancer deaths and 90% of lung cancer deaths. When smoking is combined with exposure to other **carcinogens**, such as asbestos particles, the risk of cancer can be multiplied by a factor of 10 or more. Quitting substantially reduces risk, but ex-smokers remain at higher risk than those who never smoked. And the smoker is not the only one at risk. Long-term exposure to environmental tobacco smoke (ETS), or secondhand smoke, also increases risk for lung cancer. ETS causes about 3400 lung cancer deaths in nonsmoking adults each year.

**Wellness Tip**

If you smoke, find a way to stop. There are many options for quitting smoking. See Chapter 13 for advice on giving up tobacco.

Symptoms of lung cancer usually do not appear until the disease has advanced to the invasive stage. Signals such as a persistent cough, chest pain, or recurring bronchitis may be the first indication of a tumor's presence. Lung cancer is most often treated by some combination of surgery, radiation, and **chemotherapy**; if all the

**KEY TERMS**

**cancer**  Abnormal, uncontrolled multiplication of cells.

**tumor**  A mass of tissue that serves no physiological purpose; also called a *neoplasm*.

**benign tumor**  A tumor that is not cancerous.

**malignant tumor**  A tumor that is cancerous and capable of spreading.

**lymphatic system**  A system of vessels that returns proteins, lipids, and other substances from fluid in the tissues to the circulatory system.

**metastasis**  The spread of cancer cells from one part of the body to another.

**carcinogen**  Any substance that causes cancer.

**chemotherapy**  The treatment of cancer with chemicals that selectively destroy cancerous cells.

tumor cells can be removed or killed, a cure is possible. Lung cancer is usually detected only after it has begun to spread, however, and only about 15% of lung cancer patients are alive 5 years after diagnosis.

## Colon and Rectal Cancer

Another common cancer in the United States is colon and rectal cancer (also called *colorectal cancer*). Colorectal cancer is the third most common type of cancer in both men and women. Age is a key risk factor, with 90% of cases diagnosed in people age 50 and older. Many cancers arise from preexisting polyps, small growths on the wall of the colon that may gradually develop into malignancies. Many colon cancers may be due to inherited gene mutations.

Lifestyle also affects colon cancer risk. Regular physical activity reduces risk; obesity increases risk. Although the mechanisms are unclear, high intake of red meat, smoked meat and fish, refined carbohydrates, and simple sugars appears to increase risk, as do excessive alcohol consumption and smoking. Protective lifestyle factors may include a diet rich in fruits, vegetables, and whole grains; adequate intake of folic acid, calcium, magnesium, and vitamin D; regular use of nonsteroidal anti-inflammatory drugs such as aspirin and ibuprofen; and, in women, use of oral contraceptives.

Young polyps and early-stage cancers can be removed before they spread. Because polyps may bleed, the standard warning signs of colon cancer are bleeding from the rectum and a change in bowel habits. The American Cancer Society recommends that regular screening be started at age 50. A yearly stool blood test can detect traces of blood in the stool long before obvious bleeding can be noticed. Another test is the *colonoscopy*, in which a flexible fiber-optic device is inserted through the rectum, allowing the colon to be examined and polyps to be removed (Figure 12.3). Studies show that screening could reduce the occurrence of colorectal cancer by up to 90%, but only about one-half of adults undergo these tests.

Surgery is the primary method of treatment for colon and rectal cancer. The 5-year survival rate is 90% for colon and rectal cancers detected early and 65% overall.

## Breast Cancer

Breast cancer is the most common cancer in women and causes almost as many deaths in women as lung cancer. In the United States, about 1 in 8 women will get breast cancer, and 1 woman in 30 will die from the disease. Breast cancer occurs only rarely in men.

**Risk Factors** There is a strong genetic factor in breast cancer. A woman who has two close relatives with breast cancer is more than four times more likely to develop the disease than a woman who has no relatives with it. However, only about 15% of breast cancers occur in women with a family history of the disease.

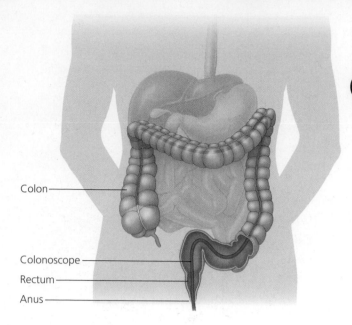

Colon

Colonoscope

Rectum

Anus

**FIGURE 12.3  Colonoscopy.**

Other risk factors include these:

- Early-onset menstruation or late-onset menopause
- Having no children or having a first child after age 30
- Current use of hormone replacement therapy
- Obesity
- Alcohol use

The female hormone estrogen may be a unifying element for some of these risk factors. Estrogen promotes cell growth in responsive tissues, such as the breast and uterus, so any factor that increases estrogen exposure may raise the risk of breast cancer. Fat cells produce estrogen, and estrogen levels are higher in obese women. Alcohol can increase estrogen in the blood as well.

**Prevention**  Although some risk factors cannot be changed, important lifestyle risk factors can be controlled. Eating a low-fat, vegetable-rich diet, exercising regularly, limiting alcohol intake, and maintaining a healthy body weight can minimize the chance of developing breast cancer, even for women at risk from family history or other factors.

**Detection**  The ACS stresses early detection of breast cancer through a three-part approach:

- *Mammography.* A **mammogram** is a low-dose breast X-ray that can spot breast abnormalities

### Fitness Tip

If you are a woman, staying physically active can reduce your risk of breast cancer. Strive to meet the recommended minimum of 150 minutes of moderate-intensity activity every week.

before physical symptoms arise. A newer type of mammography, called *digital mammography,* may provide more accurate results in some women, as may magnetic resonance imaging (MRI). The ACS recommends that women over 40 get a mammogram every year.

- *Clinical breast exams.* The ACS recommends that women between the ages of 20 and 39 have a clinical breast exam every 3 years and that women over 40 have one every year.

- *Breast self-exams.* By doing breast self-exams (BSEs), a woman can become familiar with her breasts and alert her physician to any changes (see the box "How to Perform a Breast Self-Exam"). Although the ACS encourages all women to perform regular breast self-exams, many women elect not to do them, fearing they may not perform them correctly. When women learn proper self-exam technique from a health care professional, however, they are much more likely to regularly examine their breasts. Women who choose to do self-exams should begin at age 20.

If any of these methods detects a lump in the breast, it can be **biopsied** or scanned by **ultrasonography** to determine whether it is cancerous. Most lumps are benign.

In 2009, the U.S. Preventive Services Task Force (U.S.P.S.T.F.) recommended against routine mammography before age 50, citing the anxiety and distress caused by false-positive results. The U.S.P.S.T.F. also recommended against teaching BSE. The debate about screening guidelines continues.

**Treatment** If a lump is cancerous, one of several surgical treatments may be used, ranging from a lumpectomy (removal of the lump and surrounding tissue) to a mastectomy (removal of the breast). Chemotherapy or radiation treatment may also be used to eradicate as many cancerous cells as possible.

Several drugs have been developed for preventing and treating breast cancer. These include selective estrogen-receptor modulators (SERMs), which act like estrogen in some tissues but block estrogen's effects in others. The two best-known SERMs are tamoxifen and raloxifene. Another category of drug, called trastuzumab, is a special type of antibody that binds to a specific cancer-related target in the body. Regardless of the treatments used, social support can also affect a patient's psychological and physical wellness.

If the tumor is discovered early, before it has spread to the adjacent lymph nodes, the patient with breast cancer has about a 98% chance of surviving more than 5 years. The survival rate for all stages is 90% at 5 years.

## Prostate Cancer

The prostate gland is situated at the base of the bladder in men; if enlarged, it can block the flow of urine. Prostate cancer is the most common cancer in men and the second

---

leading cause of cancer death in men. Nearly 241,000 new cases of prostate cancer are diagnosed and nearly 34,000 American men die from the disease each year.

Age is the strongest predictor of the risk of prostate cancer, with about 62% of cases diagnosed in men over age 65, and 97% of cases occurring in men over age 50. Inherited genetic predisposition may be responsible for 5–10% of cases; men with a family history of the disease should be vigilant about screening. Diets high in calories, dairy products, refined grains, and animal fats and low in plant foods have been implicated as possible culprits, as have obesity, inactivity, and a history of sexually transmitted diseases. Type 2 diabetes and insulin resistance are also associated with prostate cancer. Diet may be an important means of preventing prostate cancer. Soy foods, tomatoes, and cruciferous vegetables are being investigated for their possible protective effects.

Some cases are first detected by rectal examination during a routine physical exam. During this exam, a physician feels the prostate through the rectum to determine if the gland is enlarged or if lumps are present. Ultrasound and biopsy may also be used to detect and diagnose prostate cancer. A specialized test, called the **prostate-specific antigen (PSA) blood test**, is commonly used to detect prostate cancer and can be useful, but the test is controversial because it can yield false-positive results. The ACS recommends that men be given information about the benefits and limitations of the tests. Both the rectal exam and the PSA test should be offered annually, beginning at age 50 for men at average risk and at age 45 for men at high risk, including African Americans and those with a family history of the disease.

If the tumor is malignant, the prostate is usually removed surgically. However, a small, slow-growing tumor in an older man may be treated with watchful waiting because he is more likely to die from another cause before his cancer becomes life-threatening. A less invasive treatment involves radiation of the tumor by surgically implanting radioactive seeds in the prostate gland.

---

**KEY TERMS**

**mammogram**  A low-dose X-ray of the breasts used for the early detection of breast cancer.

**biopsy**  The removal and examination of a small piece of body tissue for the purpose of diagnosis.

**ultrasonography**  An imaging method in which inaudible high-pitched sound (ultrasound) is bounced off body structures to create an image on a monitor.

**prostate-specific antigen (PSA) blood test**  A diagnostic test for prostate cancer that measures blood levels of prostate-specific antigen (PSA).

---

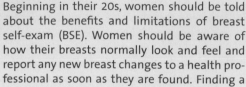

## Breast Awareness and Self-Exam

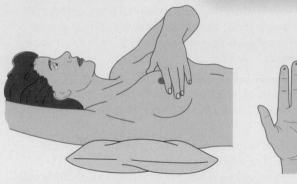

Beginning in their 20s, women should be told about the benefits and limitations of breast self-exam (BSE). Women should be aware of how their breasts normally look and feel and report any new breast changes to a health professional as soon as they are found. Finding a breast change does not necessarily mean there is a cancer.

A woman can notice changes by knowing how her breasts normally look and feel and feeling her breasts for changes (breast awareness), or by choosing to use a step-by-step approach and using a specific schedule to examine her breasts.

Women with breast implants can do BSE. It may be useful to have the surgeon help identify the edges of the implant so that you know what you are feeling. There is some thought that the implants push out the breast tissue and may make it easier to examine. Women who are pregnant or breast-feeding can also choose to examine their breasts regularly.

If you choose to do BSE, the following information provides a step-by-step approach for the exam. The best time for a woman to examine her breasts is when the breasts are not tender or swollen. Women who examine their breasts should have their technique reviewed during their periodic health exams by their health care professional.

It is acceptable for women to choose not to do BSE or to do BSE occasionally. Women who choose not to do BSE should still know how their breasts normally look and feel and report any changes to their doctor right away.

### How to examine your breasts

Lie down on your back and place your right arm behind your head. The exam is done while lying down, not standing up. This is because when lying down the breast tissue spreads evenly over the chest wall and is as thin as possible, making it much easier to feel all the breast tissue.

Use the finger pads of the 3 middle fingers on your left hand to feel for lumps in the right breast. Use overlapping dime-sized circular motions of the finger pads to feel the breast tissue.

Use 3 different levels of pressure to feel all the breast tissue. Light pressure is needed to feel the tissue closest to the skin; medium pressure to feel a little deeper; and firm pressure to feel the tissue closest to the chest and ribs. It is normal to feel a firm ridge in the lower curve of each breast, but you should tell your doctor if you feel anything else out of the ordinary. If you're not sure how hard to press, talk with your doctor or nurse. Use each pressure level to feel the breast tissue before moving on to the next spot.

Move around the breast in an up and down pattern starting at an imaginary line drawn straight down your side from the underarm and moving across the breast to the middle of the chest bone (sternum or breastbone). Be sure to check the entire breast

area going down until you feel only ribs and up to the neck or collar bone (clavicle).

There is some evidence to suggest that the up-and-down pattern (sometimes called the vertical pattern) is the most effective pattern for covering the entire breast without missing any breast tissue.

Repeat the exam on your left breast, putting your left arm behind your head and using the finger pads of your right hand to do the exam.

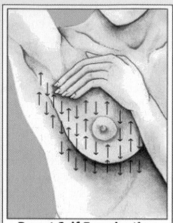

**Breast Self Examination**
Examine up to the collarbone, out to armpit, in to middle of chest, and down to bottom of rib cage

While standing in front of a mirror with your hands pressing firmly down on your hips, look at your breasts for any changes of size, shape, contour, or dimpling, or redness or scaliness of the nipple or breast skin. (The pressing down on the hips position contracts the chest wall muscles and enhances any breast changes.)

Examine each underarm while sitting up or standing and with your arm only slightly raised so you can easily feel in this area. Raising your arm straight up tightens the tissue in this area and makes it harder to examine.

This procedure for doing breast self-exam is different from previous recommendations. These changes represent an extensive review of the medical literature and input from an expert advisory group. There is evidence that this position (lying down), the area felt, pattern of coverage of the breast, and use of different amounts of pressure increase a woman's ability to find abnormal areas.

**SOURCE:** American Cancer Society's Web site www.cancer.org, 2011. Copyright © 2011 American Cancer Society, Inc. Reprinted with pemission.

---

Radiation from the seeds destroys the tumor and much of the normal prostate tissue but leaves surrounding tissue relatively untouched. Alternative or additional treatments include external radiation, hormones that shrink tumors, cryotherapy, and chemotherapy. The 5-year survival rate for all stages of prostate cancer is now nearly 100%.

## Cancers of the Female Reproductive Tract

Several types of cancer can affect the female reproductive tract, and a few of these cancers are relatively common.

**Cervical Cancer** Cancer of the cervix occurs frequently in women in their thirties and even twenties. In the United States, nearly 13,000 women are diagnosed with cervical cancer each year; the disease kills more than 4000 women annually.

Cervical cancer is at least in part a sexually transmitted disease (STD). Most cases of cervical cancer stem from infection by the human papillomavirus (HPV), which causes genital warts and is transmitted during unprotected sex. Smoking and prior infection with the STDs herpes and chlamydia may also be risk factors for cervical cancer.

Screening for the changes in cervical cells that precede cancer is done chiefly by means of the **Pap test.** During a pelvic exam, loose cells are scraped from the cervix and examined. If cells are abnormal but not yet cancerous—a condition referred to as *cervical dysplasia*—the Pap test is repeated at intervals. In about one-third of cases, the cellular changes progress toward malignancy. If this happens, the abnormal cells must be removed, either surgically or by destroying them with an ultracold (cryoscopic) probe or localized laser treatment. In more advanced cases, treatment may involve chemotherapy, radiation, or hysterectomy (surgical removal of the uterus).

Because the Pap test is highly effective, all sexually active women and women over the age of 18 should be tested. The recommended schedule for testing depends on risk factors, the type of Pap test performed, and whether the Pap test is combined with HPV testing.

Cervical cancer can be prevented by avoiding infection with HPV. Sexual abstinence, mutually monogamous sex with an uninfected partner, and regular use of condoms can reduce the risk of HPV infection (see Chapter 14 for more on HPV and other STDs).

Two HPV vaccines have been approved by the Food and Drug Administration (FDA) for the prevention of cervical cancer. Women who receive a vaccine should continue to receive routine Pap tests because the vaccines do not protect against all types of the virus.

**Uterine or Endometrial Cancer** Cancer of the lining of the uterus (the *endometrium*) most often occurs after age 55. Uterine cancer strikes more than 46,000 American women annually and kills more than 8000 women each year. The risk factors are similar to those for breast cancer. Endometrial cancer is usually detectable by pelvic examination. It is treated surgically, as well as by radiation, hormones, and chemotherapy.

**Ovarian Cancer** Although ovarian cancer is rare compared with cervical or uterine cancer, it causes more deaths than the other two combined. There are no screening tests to detect it, so it is often diagnosed late in its development. The risk factors are similar to those for breast and endometrial cancer. Anything that lowers a woman's lifetime number of ovulation cycles—pregnancy, breastfeeding, or use of oral contraceptives—reduces the risk of ovarian cancer.

In 2007, the Gynecologic Cancer Foundation announced that scientists had reached a consensus on symptoms of

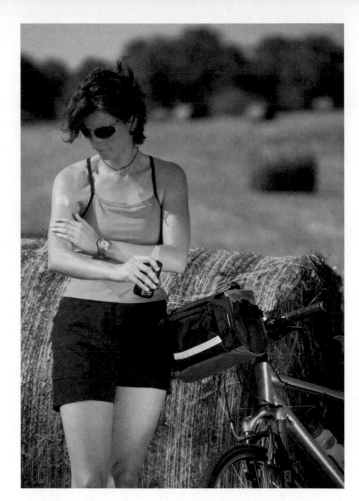

Sunscreen protects against skin cancer as well as sunburns.

ovarian cancer: bloating, pelvic or abdominal pain, difficulty eating or feeling full quickly, and urinary problems (urgency or frequency). Women who experience these symptoms almost daily for a few weeks should see their physician. Some ovarian cancers are also detected through regular pelvic exams. Ovarian cancer is treated by surgical removal of one or both ovaries, the fallopian tubes, and the uterus.

## Skin Cancer

Skin cancer is the most common cancer of all when cases of the highly curable forms are included in the count. Of the more than 1 million cases of skin cancer diagnosed each year, about 70,000 are of the most serious type, **melanoma.** Almost all cases of skin cancer can be traced to excessive exposure to **ultraviolet (UV) radiation** from the sun, including longer-wavelength ultraviolet A (UVA) and shorter-wavelength ultraviolet B (UVB) radiation. UVB radiation causes sunburns and can damage the eyes and immune system. UVA is less likely to cause an immediate sunburn, but it damages connective tissue and leads to premature aging of the skin. Tanning lamps and tanning salon beds emit mostly UVA radiation. Both solar and artificial sources of UVA and UVB radiation are human carcinogens that cause skin cancer.

Both severe, acute sun reactions (sunburns) and chronic low-level sun reactions (suntans) can lead to skin cancer. According to the American Academy of Dermatology, the risk of skin cancer doubles in people who have had five or more sunburns in their lifetime. People with fair skin have less natural protection against skin damage from the sun and a higher risk of skin cancer than people with naturally dark skin. Severe sunburns in childhood have been linked to a greatly increased risk of skin cancer in later life, so children in particular should be protected. Other risk factors include having many moles (particularly large ones), spending time at high altitudes, and having a family history of the disease.

There are three main types of skin cancer, named for the types of skin cell from which they develop. **Basal cell** and **squamous cell carcinomas** together account for about 95% of the skin cancers diagnosed each year. They are usually found in chronically sun-exposed areas, such as the face, neck, hands, and arms. They usually appear as pale, waxlike, pearly nodules, or red, scaly, sharply outlined patches. These cancers are often painless, although they may bleed, crust, and form an open sore.

Melanoma is by far the most dangerous skin cancer because it spreads so rapidly. It can occur anywhere on the body, but the most common sites are the back, chest, abdomen, and lower legs. A melanoma usually appears at the site of a preexisting mole. The mole may begin to enlarge, become mottled or varied in color (colors can include blue, pink, and white), or develop an irregular surface or irregular borders. Tissue invaded by melanoma may also itch, burn, or bleed easily.

To protect yourself against skin cancer, avoid overexposure to UV radiation. People of every age, including babies and children, need to be protected from the sun (see

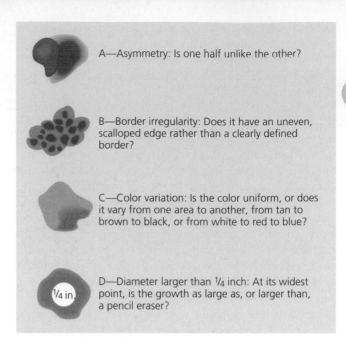

**FIGURE 12.4   The ABCD test for melanoma.**
To see a variety of photos of melanoma and benign moles, visit the National Cancer Institute's Visuals Online site (http://visualsonline.cancer.gov).

the box "Sunscreens and Sun-Protective Clothing"). You can help with early detection by examining your skin regularly. Most of the spots, freckles, moles, and blemishes on your body are normal, but if you notice an unusual growth, discoloration, or sore that does not heal, see your physician or a dermatologist immediately. The characteristics that may signal that a skin lesion is a melanoma are illustrated in Figure 12.4.

If you have an unusual skin lesion, your physician will examine it and possibly perform a biopsy. If the lesion is cancerous, it is usually removed surgically, a procedure that can almost always be performed in the physician's office using a local anesthetic. Treatment is usually simple and successful when the cancer is caught early. Even for melanoma, the outlook after removal in the early stages is good, with a 5-year survival rate of 98% if the tumor is localized but only 62% if the cancer has spread to adjacent lymph nodes. Most melanomas are detected in the early, localized stage.

## Head and Neck Cancers

Head and neck cancers—cancers of the oral cavity, pharynx, larynx, and nasal cavity—can be traced principally to cigarette, cigar, or pipe smoking, the use of spit tobacco, and the excessive consumption of alcohol. Additionally, 50% of cancers of the tonsils and tongue base are related to HPV infection. Head and neck cancer occurs twice as often in men as in women and most frequently in men over 40.

Chemotherapy, radiation, and surgery are the primary methods of treatment for head and neck cancers. Patients often endure intense mouth and throat inflammation and some require disfiguring surgeries, but many can be cured. The 5-year survival rate is about 61%.

## Wellness Tip

The Skin Cancer Foundation recommends that everyone see their physician at least once a year for a head-to-toe skin evaluation. Depending on individual risk factors, some people may need to have their skin checked more frequently.

**KEY TERMS**

**basal cell carcinoma**   Cancer of the deepest layers of the skin.

**squamous cell carcinoma**   Cancer of the surface layers of the skin.

# Sunscreens and Sun-Protective Clothing

With consistent use of the proper clothing, sunscreens, and common sense, you can lead an active outdoor life *and* protect your skin against most sun-induced damage.

## Clothing

• Wear long-sleeved shirts and long pants. Dark-colored, tightly woven fabrics provide reasonable protection from the sun. Another good choice is clothing made from special sun-protective fabrics; these garments have an ultraviolet protection factor (UPF) rating, similar to the SPF rating for sunscreens.

• Wear a hat. A good choice is a broad-brimmed hat or a legionnaire-style cap that covers the ears and neck. Wear sunscreen on your face even if you are wearing a hat.

• Wear sunglasses. Exposure to UV rays can damage the eyes and cause cataracts.

## Sunscreen

• Use a sunscreen and lip balm with a sun protection factor (SPF) of 15 or higher. An SPF rating refers to the amount of time you can stay out in the sun before you burn, compared with not using sunscreen. For example, a product with an SPF of 30 would allow you to remain in the sun without burning 30 times longer, on average, than if you didn't apply sunscreen. If you're fair-skinned, have a family history of skin cancer, are at high altitude, or will be outdoors for many hours, use a sunscreen with an even higher SPF.

• Choose a broad-spectrum sunscreen that protects against both UVA and UVB radiation. The SPF rating of a sunscreen currently applies only to UVB, but a number of ingredients, especially titanium dioxide and zinc oxide, are effective at blocking most UVA radiation. In 2011, the FDA announced that sunscreens would be required to pass a new broad-spectrum test to determine how effectively they protect against both UVA and UVB radiation. Starting in summer 2012, products that pass this test will be allowed to bear the "broad spectrum" label.

• Use a water-resistant sunscreen if you swim or sweat a great deal. Under the new FDA regulations, sunscreens cannot be labeled as "waterproof" or "sweatproof" because these claims overstate the products' actual effectivness. In order to be labeled as "water resistant," a product must remain effective for 40 minutes when the user is not swimming or sweating, or for 80 minutes if the user is swimming or sweating.

• If you have acne, look for a sunscreen that is labeled "non-comedogenic," which means that it will not cause pimples.

• Shake sunscreen before applying. Apply it 30 minutes before exposure to allow it time to bond to the skin. Reapply sunscreen frequently and generously to all sun-exposed areas (many people overlook their temples, ears, and sides and backs of their necks). Most people use less than half as much as they need to attain the full SPF rating. One ounce of sunscreen is enough to cover an average-size adult in a swimsuit. Reapply sunscreen every 2 hours. Also be sure to reapply sunscreen after activities, such as swimming, that could remove sunscreen.

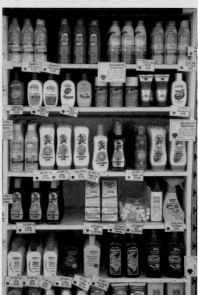

• If you're taking medications, ask your physician or pharmacist about possible reactions to sunlight or interactions with sunscreens. Medications for acne, allergies, and diabetes are just a few of the products that can trigger reactions. If you're using sunscreen and an insect repellent containing DEET, use extra sunscreen (DEET may decrease sunscreen effectiveness).

## Time of Day and Location

• Avoid sun exposure between 10:00 A.M. and 2:00 P.M., when the sun's rays are most intense. Clouds allow as much as 80% of UV rays to reach your skin. Stay in the shade when you can.

• Consult the day's UV Index, which predicts UV levels on a 0–10+ scale, to get a sense of the amount of sun protection you'll need. Take special care on days with a rating of 5 or above. UV Index ratings are available in local newspapers, from the weather bureau, or from certain Web sites.

• UV rays can penetrate at least 3 feet below the surface of water, so swimmers should wear water-resistant sunscreens. Snow, sand, water, concrete, and white-painted surfaces are also highly reflective of UV rays.

## Tanning Salons

• Stay away from tanning salons! Despite advertising claims to the contrary, the lights used in tanning parlors are damaging to your skin. Tanning beds and lamps emit mostly UVA radiation, increasing your risk of premature skin aging (such as wrinkles) and skin cancer.

# Testicular Cancer

Testicular cancer is relatively rare, accounting for only 1% of cancers in men (about 8300 cases per year), but it is the most common cancer in men age 20–35. Testicular cancer is much more common among white Americans than Latinos, Asian Americans, or African Americans. Men with undescended testicles are at increased risk for

## Testicle Self-Examination

The best time to perform a testicular self-exam is after a warm shower or bath, when the scrotum is relaxed.

First, stand in front of a mirror and look for any swelling of the scrotum. Then, examine each testicle with both hands. Place the index and middle fingers under the testicle and the thumbs on top. Roll each testicle gently between the fingers and thumbs. Don't worry if one testicle seems slightly larger than the other; that's common. Also, expect to feel the *epididymis*—the soft, sperm-carrying tube at the rear of each testicle.

Perform a self-exam each month. If you find a lump, swelling, or nodule, see your doctor right away. The abnormality may not be cancer, but only a physician can make a diagnosis.

Other possible signs of testicular cancer include a change in the way a testicle feels, a sudden collection of fluid in the scrotum, a dull ache in the lower abdomen or groin, a feeling of heaviness in the scrotum, or pain in a testicle or the scrotum.

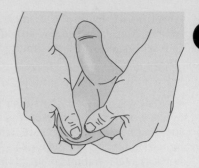

**SOURCES:** Testicular Cancer Resource Center. 2009. *How to Do a Testicular Self Examination* (http://tcrc.acor.org/tcexam.html; retrieved May 17, 2011); National Cancer Institute. 2010. *Testicular Cancer* (http://www.cancer.gov/cancertopics/types/testicular; retrieved May 17, 2011).

testicular cancer, and for this reason the condition should be corrected in early childhood. Self-examination may help in the early detection of testicular cancer (see the box "Testicle Self-Examination"). Tumors are treated by surgical removal of the testicle and, if the tumor has spread, by chemotherapy. The 5-year survival rate is 96%.

### Other Cancers

Several other cancers affect thousands of people each year. Some have identifiable risk factors (particularly smoking and obesity, which are controllable), but the causes of others are still under investigation.

- *Pancreatic cancer* causes nearly 38,000 deaths annually in the United States. The disease is usually well advanced before symptoms become noticeable, and no effective cure is available. About 3 out of 10 cases are linked to smoking. Other risk factors include being male, African American, or over age 60; having a family history of pancreatic cancer; having diabetes; being inactive and obese; and eating a diet high in fat and meat and low in vegetables.

- *Bladder cancer* is nearly four times as common in men as in women, and smoking is the key risk factor. The first symptoms are likely to be blood in the urine and/or increased frequency of urination. These

symptoms can also signal a urinary tract infection but should trigger a visit to a physician, who can evaluate the possibility of cancer. With early detection, 90% of bladder cancers are curable. There are about 69,000 new cases and nearly 15,000 deaths each year.

- *Kidney cancer* usually occurs in people over 50. Smoking and obesity are mild risk factors, as is a family history of the disease. Symptoms may include fatigue, pain in the side, and blood in the urine. There are about 61,000 new cases each year and about 13,000 deaths.

- *Brain cancer* commonly develops for no apparent reason and can arise from most of the cell types that are found in the brain. One of the few established risk factors for brain cancer is ionizing radiation, such as X-rays of the head. Symptoms are often nonspecific and include headaches, fatigue, behavioral changes, and sometimes seizures. Some brain tumors are curable by surgery or by radiation and chemotherapy, but most are not. There are about 22,000 new cases and 13,000 deaths each year.

- *Leukemia,* cancer of the white blood cells, starts in the bone marrow but can then spread to the lymph nodes, spleen, liver, other organs, and central nervous system. Some possible risk factors include smoking, radiation, certain chemicals, and infections. Most symptoms occur because leukemia cells crowd out the production of normal blood cells. The result can be fatigue, anemia, weight loss, and increased risk of infection. There are about 45,000 new cases and 22,000 deaths each year.

- *Lymphoma* is a form of cancer that begins in the lymph nodes and then may spread to almost any

**?** Ask Yourself

**QUESTIONS FOR CRITICAL THINKING AND REFLECTION**

Has anyone you know had cancer? If so, what type of cancer was it? What were its symptoms? Based on the information presented so far in this chapter, did the person have any of the known risk factors for the disease?

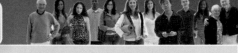

# Ethnicity, Poverty, and Cancer

Rates of cancer have declined among all U.S. ethnic groups in recent years, but significant disparities still exist.

- Among U.S. ethnic groups, African Americans have the highest incidence of and death rates from cancer.

- White women have a higher incidence of breast cancer, but African American women have the highest death rate. Black women are less likely to receive regular mammograms and more likely to experience delays in follow-up.

- African American men have a higher rate of prostate cancer than any other U.S. group and more than twice the death rate of other groups. However, black men are less likely than white men to undergo PSA testing for prostate cancer.

- Latinas have the highest incidence of cervical cancer, but African American women have the highest death rate. Language and cultural barriers and problems accessing screening services are thought to particularly affect Latinas, who have relatively low rates of Pap testing.

- Asian Americans and Pacific Islander Americans have the highest rates of liver and stomach cancers. Recent immigration helps explain these higher rates, as these cancers are usually caused by infections that are more prevalent in the recent immigrant's country of origin.

Some disparities in cancer risks and rates may be influenced by genetic or cultural factors. For example, certain genetic/molecular features of aggressive breast cancer are more common among African American women with the disease; they are more likely to be diagnosed at a later stage and with more aggressive tumors. Genetic factors may

also help explain the high rate of prostate cancer among black men. Women from cultures where early marriage and motherhood are common are likely to have a lower risk of breast cancer.

Most of the differences in cancer rates and deaths, however, are thought to be the result of socioeconomic inequities. People of low socioeconomic status are more likely to smoke, abuse alcohol, eat unhealthy foods, and be sedentary and overweight—all of which are associated with cancer. High levels of stress associated with poverty may impair the immune system, the body's first line of defense against cancer.

People with low incomes also are more likely to live in unhealthy environments. For example, Latinos and Asian and Pacific Islander Americans are more likely than other groups to live in areas that do not meet federal air quality standards. Low-income people may also have jobs that bring them into daily contact with carcinogenic chemicals. They may face similar risks in their homes and schools, where they may be exposed to asbestos or other carcinogens.

People with low incomes also have less exposure to information about cancer, are less aware of the early warning signs of cancer, and are less likely to seek medical care when they have such symptoms. Lack of health insurance is a key factor explaining higher death rates among people with low incomes. A study comparing low-income Americans and Canadians found that the Canadians were more likely to survive cancer, possibly due to Canada's system of universal health care, which ensures access to treatment regardless of income.

Public education campaigns that encourage healthy lifestyle habits, routine cancer screening, and participation in clinical trials may be one helpful strategy to reduce cancer disparities. But the

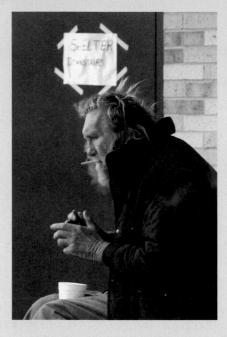

effects of poverty are more difficult to overcome. Some medical scientists look to policymakers for solutions and maintain that living and working conditions in the inner cities must be improved and that access to quality health care must be assured for all Americans. Then, even without new miracle drugs or medical breakthroughs, the United States could see a real decrease in cancer rates in low-income populations.

**SOURCES:** American Cancer Society. 2011. *Cancer Facts and Figures, 2011.* Atlanta, Ga.: American Cancer Society; Chlebowski, R. T., et al. 2005. Ethnicity and breast cancer: Factors influencing differences in incidence and outcome. *Journal of the National Cancer Institute* 97(6): 439–448; CDC Office of Minority Health and Health Disparities, 2009. *Eliminate Disparities in Cancer Screening and Management* (http://www.cdc.gov/omhd/AMH/factsheets/cancer.htm; retrieved May 17, 2011); National Cancer Institute. 2010. *Cancer Health Disparities* (http://www.cancer.gov/cancertopics/disparities; retrieved May 17, 2011).

**DIMENSIONS OF DIVERSITY**

part of the body. There are two types—Hodgkin's disease and non-Hodgkin's lymphoma (NHL). NHL is the more common and more deadly form of the disease. Risk factors for NHL are not well understood but may include genetic factors, radiation, and certain chemicals and infections.

## THE CAUSES OF CANCER

Although scientists do not know everything about what causes cancer, they have identified genetic, environmental, and lifestyle factors (see the box "Ethnicity, Poverty, and Cancer").

## The Role of DNA

Heredity and genetics are important factors in a person's risk of cancer. Certain genes may predispose some people to cancer, and specific gene mutations have been associated with cancer.

**DNA Basics**  The nucleus of each cell in your body contains 23 pairs of **chromosomes**, which are made up of tightly packed coils of **DNA** (deoxyribonucleic acid). Each chromosome contains hundreds or thousands of **genes**; you have about 25,000 genes in all. Each of your genes controls the production of a particular protein. By making different proteins at different times, genes can act as switches to alter the ways a cell works. Some genes are responsible for controlling the rate of cell division, and these genes often play a critical role in the development of cancer.

**DNA Mutations and Cancer**  A *mutation* is any change in the makeup of a gene. Some mutations are inherited; others are caused by environmental agents known as *mutagens*. Mutagens include radiation, certain viruses, and chemical substances in the air we breathe. (When a mutagen also causes cancer, it is called a *carcinogen*.) Some mutations are the result of copying errors that occur when DNA replicates itself as part of cell division.

A mutated gene no longer contains the proper code for producing its protein. It usually takes several mutational changes before a normal cell takes on the properties of a cancer cell. Genes that have mutations associated with the conversion of a normal cell into a cancer cell are known as **oncogenes.** In their undamaged form, many oncogenes play a role in controlling or restricting cell growth; they are called *tumor suppressor genes*. Mutational damage to suppressor genes releases the brake on growth and leads to rapid and uncontrolled cell division—a precondition for the development of cancer.

An example of an inherited mutated oncogene is BRCA1 (breast cancer gene 1). Women who inherit a damaged copy of this suppressor gene face a significantly increased risk of breast and ovarian cancer.

In most cases, however, mutational damage occurs after birth. For example, only about 5–10% of breast cancer cases can be traced to inherited copies of a damaged BRCA1 gene. In addition, lifestyle factors are important even for those who have inherited a damaged suppressor gene. Testing and identification of hereditary cancer risks can be helpful for some people, especially if it leads to increased attention to controllable risk factors and better medical screening.

**Cancer Promoters**  Substances known as *cancer promoters* make up another important piece of the cancer puzzle. These substances don't directly produce DNA mutations, but they accelerate the growth of cells, which means less time for a cell to repair DNA damage caused by other factors. Estrogen, which stimulates cellular growth in the female reproductive organs, is an example of a cancer promoter.

## Tobacco Use

Smoking is responsible for up to 90% of lung cancers and for about 30% of all cancer deaths. Overall, tobacco use is responsible for nearly 1 in 5 American deaths—nearly 444,000 premature deaths each year. The U.S. Surgeon General has reported that tobacco use is a direct cause of several types of cancer. In addition to lung and bronchial cancer, tobacco use is linked to cancer of the larynx, mouth, pharynx, esophagus, stomach, pancreas, kidneys, bladder, and cervix.

## Dietary Factors

Diet is one of the most important factors in cancer prevention, but it is also one of the most complex and controversial. Your food choices affect your cancer risk by both exposing you to potentially dangerous compounds and depriving you of potentially protective ones. The following dietary factors may affect cancer risk:

• *Dietary fat and meat:* Diets high in fat and meat may contribute to certain cancers, including colon, stomach, and prostate cancer. Certain types of fat may be riskier than others. Omega-6 polyunsaturated fats are associated with a higher risk of certain cancers; omega-3 fats are not. (See Chapter 8 for more information on types of fatty acids.)

• *Alcohol:* Alcohol is associated with an increased incidence of several cancers. For example, women who have 2 to 5 drinks daily have about 1.5 times the risk of women who drink no alcohol. Alcohol and tobacco interact as risk factors for oral cancer. Heavy users of both alcohol and tobacco have a risk for oral cancer many times greater than that of people who don't drink or use tobacco.

• *Fried foods:* Scientists have found high levels of the chemical acrylamide (a probable human carcinogen) in starch-based foods that have been fried or baked at high temperatures, especially french fries and certain types of snack chips and crackers. Acrylamide is also found in high concentrations in tobacco.

• *Fiber:* Various potential cancer-fighting actions have been proposed for fiber, but none has been firmly established. Further study is needed to clarify the relationship between fiber intake and cancer risk, but experts

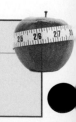

## Wellness Tip

Currently, the American Cancer Society does not recommend taking any type of dietary supplement, including vitamins or minerals, to prevent cancer.

## Table 12.1   Foods with Phytochemicals

| FOOD | PHYTOCHEMICAL | POTENTIAL ANTICANCER EFFECTS |
|---|---|---|
| Chili peppers (*Note:* Hotter peppers contain more capsaicin.) | Capsaicin | Neutralizes effect of nitrosamines; may block carcinogens in cigarette smoke from acting on cells |
| Oranges, lemons, limes, onions, apples, berries, eggplant | Flavonoids | Act as antioxidants; block access of carcinogens to cells; suppress malignant changes in cells; prevent cancer cells from multiplying |
| Citrus fruits, cherries | Monoterpenes | Help detoxify carcinogens; inhibit spread of cancer cells |
| Cruciferous vegetables (broccoli, cabbage, bok choy, cauliflower, kale, brussels sprouts, collards) | Isothiocyanates | Boost production of cancer-fighting enzymes; suppress growth; block effects of estrogen on cell growth |
| Garlic, onions, leeks, shallots, chives | Allyl sulfides | Increase levels of enzymes that break down potential carcinogens; boost activity of cancer-fighting immune cells |
| Grapes, red wine, peanuts | Resveratrol | Act as antioxidants; suppress tumor growth |
| Green, oolong, and black teas (*Note:* Drinking burning hot tea may *increase* cancer risk.) | Polyphenols | Increase antioxidant activity; prevent cancer cells from multiplying; help speed excretion of carcinogens from the body |
| Orange, deep yellow, red, pink, and dark green vegetables; some fruits | Carotenoids | Act as antioxidants; reduce levels of cancer-promoting enzymes; inhibit spread of cancer cells |
| Soy foods, whole grains, flax seeds, nuts | Phytoestrogens | Block effects of estrogen on cell growth; lower blood levels of estrogen |
| Whole grains, legumes | Phytic acid | Bind iron, which may prevent it from creating cell-damaging free radicals |

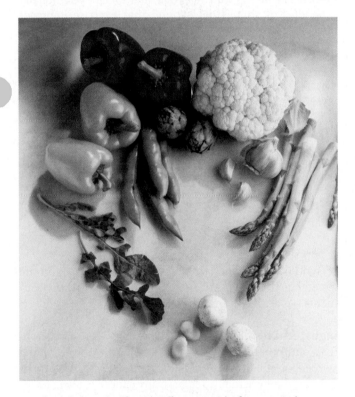

Your food choices significantly affect your risk of cancer. Red bell peppers, chili peppers, and garlic are just a few of the foods containing cancer-fighting phytochemicals.

against cancer. Some may prevent carcinogens from forming in the first place or block them from reaching or acting on target cells. Others boost enzymes that detoxify carcinogens and render them harmless. Some essential nutrients act as anticarcinogens. For example, vitamin C, vitamin E, selenium, and the **carotenoids** (vitamin A precursors) may help block cancer by acting as antioxidants.

Many other anti-cancer agents in the diet fall under the broader heading of **phytochemicals,** substances in plants that help protect against chronic diseases (Table 12.1). One of the first to be identified was sulforaphane, a potent anticarcinogen found in broccoli.

still recommend a high-fiber diet for its overall positive effect on health.

• *Fruits and vegetables:* Researchers have identified many mechanisms by which food components may act

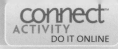

## THE EVIDENCE FOR EXERCISE

# How Does Exercise Affect Cancer Risk?

According to statistics from the International Agency for Research on Cancer (IARC), as many as 25% of cancers are due to overweight, obesity, and physical inactivity. Increasing levels of physical activity can potentially ward off several types of cancer.

The links between exercise and cancer prevention are not entirely clear. However, experts have associated increased physical activity and a reduced risk of several specific types of cancer. Studies show, for example, that people who do moderate aerobic exercise for 3–4 hours per week reduce their risk of colon cancer by 30%. Women who do the same amount of exercise can reduce their risk of breast cancer by as much as 40%. (Some studies suggest that women who meet certain criteria can reduce their breast cancer risk up to 80%.) Evidence also shows that, when compared with sedentary people, active people can reduce their risk of lung cancer (20%), endometrial cancer (30%), and ovarian cancer (20%). Researchers are continually trying to establish similar connections between exercise and other types of cancer.

As with all-cause mortality and cardiovascular disease, physical activity appears to have an inverse relationship with the types of cancer just listed. That is, the more you exercise, the lower your risk of developing these kinds of cancer. Energy balance also seems to be a factor, at least in relation to a few types of cancer, meaning that people who burn at least as many calories as they take in may further reduce their risk of some cancers. This positive effect may be due to the fact that reducing body fat (through exercise and a healthy diet) lowers the chemical and hormonal activities of adipose (fat) tissue—activities that may encourage some cancers to develop.

In addition to reducing the biological influences of adipose tissue, physical activity is known to reduce the inflammatory response and to boost immune function. Chronic inflammation, which can have many causes, leaves body tissues more vulnerable to infection. The immune system is the body's first line of defense against cancer, so supporting immune function through exercise may help prevent some cancers.

Emerging data also indicate that physical activity can help improve health outcomes in people who have cancer or are cancer survivors. For example, physical activity appears to restore cardiorespiratory fitness at least to some degree in patients whose heart muscles have been weakened by cancer treatments. This positive outcome was found in 13 separate studies, many of which found significant improvements in heart function among cancer survivors who performed moderate-intensity exercise for 20–40 minutes three times per week. The

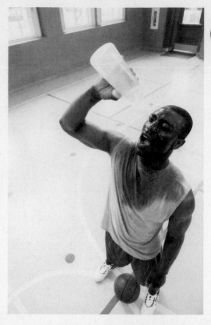

benefits were similar across several forms of aerobic exercise, including walking, yoga, and tai chi. Additionally, a handful of studies have found that exercise improves muscular strength and endurance and flexibility in patients whose muscles and joints have been weakened by cancer treatments.

SOURCES: Doyle, C., et al. 2006. Nutrition and physical activity during and after cancer treatment: An American Cancer Society guide for informed choices. *CA: A Cancer Journal for Clinicians* 56(6): 323–353. Irwin, M. L., and S. T. Mayne. 2008. Impact of nutrition and exercise on cancer survival. *Cancer Journal* 14(6): 435–441. Morris, G. S., et al. 2009. Pulmonary rehabilitation improves functional status in oncology patients. *Archives of Physical Medicine and Rehabilitation* 90(5): 837–841. Physical Activity Guidelines Advisory Committee. 2008. *Physical Activity Guidelines Advisory Committee Report, 2008.* Washington, D.C.: U.S. Department of Health and Human Services.

## Obesity and Inactivity

The ACS recommends maintaining a healthy weight throughout life by balancing caloric intake with physical activity, and by achieving and maintaining a healthy weight if you are currently overweight or obese. Being overweight or obese is linked with increased risk of several kinds of cancer, including breast and colon cancer (Figure 12.5). The ACS guidelines encourage everyone to adopt a physically active lifestyle (see the box "How Does Exercise Affect Cancer Risk?").

## Carcinogens in the Environment

Some carcinogens occur naturally in the environment, like viruses and the sun's UV rays. Others are manufactured or synthetic substances that show up occasionally in the general environment but more often in the work environments of specific industries.

**Ingested Chemicals** The food industry uses preservatives and other additives to prevent food from becoming spoiled or stale. Some of these compounds are antioxidants and may actually decrease any cancer-causing properties in the food.

Other compounds, like the nitrates and nitrites found in processed meats, are potentially more dangerous. Although nitrates and nitrites are not themselves carcinogenic, they can combine with dietary substances in the stomach and be converted to nitrosamines, which are highly potent carcinogens. Foods cured with nitrites, as well as those cured by salt or smoke, have been linked to

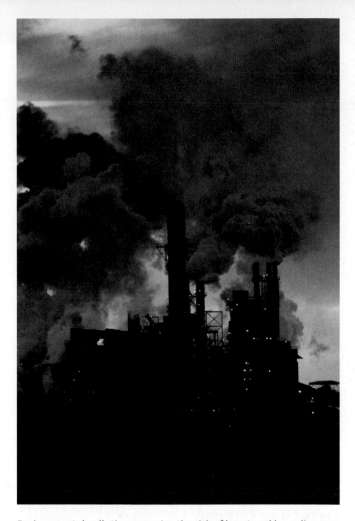

Relative risk of death from cancer

1.6 — Women
1.5
1.4
1.3 — Men
1.2
1.1
1.0

Normal weight → Obesity

**FIGURE 12.5  Body weight and cancer mortality.**
**SOURCE:** Calle, E. E., et al. 2003. Overweight, obesity, and mortality from cancer in a prospectively studied cohort of U.S. adults. *New England Journal of Medicine* 348(17): 1625–1638.

esophageal and stomach cancer, and they should be eaten only in modest amounts.

**Environmental and Industrial Pollution** The best available data indicate that less than 2% of cancer deaths are caused by general environmental pollution, such as substances in our air and water. Exposure to carcinogenic materials in the workplace is a more serious problem. Occupational exposure to specific carcinogens may account for about 4% of cancer deaths. With increasing industry and government regulations, industrial sources of cancer risk should continue to diminish.

**Radiation** All sources of radiation are potentially carcinogenic, including medical X-rays, radioactive substances (radioisotopes), and UV rays from the sun. Most physicians and dentists are quite aware of the risk of radiation, and successful efforts have been made to reduce the amount of radiation needed for mammography, dental X-rays, and other necessary medical X-rays.

**Microbes** About 15–20% of the world's cancers are caused by microbes, including viruses, bacteria, and parasites, although the percentage is much lower in developed countries like the United States. Certain types of human

Environmental pollution can raise the risk of heart and lung diseases, but it appears to account for only 2% of cancer deaths.

papillomavirus (HPV) are known to cause oropharyngeal cancer, cervical cancer, and other cancers, and the *Helicobacter pylori* bacterium has been definitely linked to stomach cancer.

The Epstein-Barr virus, best known for causing mononucleosis, is also suspected of contributing to Hodgkin's disease, cancer of the nasopharynx, and some stomach cancers. Human herpesvirus 8 has been linked to Kaposi's sarcoma and certain types of lymphoma. Hepatitis viruses B and C together cause as many as 80% of the world's liver cancers.

## Wellness Tip

Regular exposure to charred foods, particularly charred meats, may increase the risk of certain kinds of cancer. If you regularly eat grilled foods, avoid eating charred parts. In general, it's a good idea to avoid eating burned foods.

## Ask Yourself

**QUESTIONS FOR CRITICAL THINKING AND REFLECTION**

What do you think your risks for cancer are? Do you have a family history of cancer, or have you been exposed to carcinogens? How about your diet and exercise patterns? What can you do to reduce your risks?

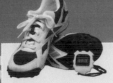

**PERSONAL CHALLENGE**

Based on the information in this chapter, how many cancer risks can you identify in your life? For example, do you smoke? Are you sedentary? Do you eat a lot of processed foods? Remember that risk factors can be hereditary or environmental, and environmental risk factors can include behaviors like smoking or working in a toxic environment. Consider the risk factors identified in the text, and list three risk factors that you are exposed to regularly or daily.

1. _____
2. _____
3. _____

Next, list steps you can take to reduce each of these risk factors. Target your steps to each specific risk factor.

1. _____
2. _____
3. _____

Finally, expand your thinking. Can you identify any cancer risk factors that exist in your community? If so, identify one such risk factor and think of ways people in your community can work together to reduce or eliminate that risk.

## DETECTING AND TREATING CANCER

Early cancer detection often depends on our willingness to be aware of changes in our own body and making sure we keep up with recommended diagnostic tests.

### Detecting Cancer

Unlike those of some other diseases, early signs of cancer are usually not apparent to anyone but the person who has them. Even pain is not a reliable guide to early detection, because the initial stages of cancer may be painless. Self-monitoring is the first line of defense. By being aware of the risk factors in your own life, your immediate family's cancer history, and your own history, you may bring a problem to the attention of a doctor long before it would be detected at a routine physical. In addition to self-monitoring, the ACS recommends routine cancer checkups, as well as specific screening tests for certain cancers (Table 12.2).

Physicians need to know the exact size and location of a tumor if they are to treat it effectively. A biopsy may be performed to confirm the tumor's type. Imaging studies or exploratory surgery may be required to identify a cancer's stage—that is, to determine the tumor's size and see if the cancer has spread to other sites. Several diagnostic imaging techniques are available, including MRI, computed tomography (CT) scanning, and ultrasonography.

### Treating Cancer

The ideal cancer therapy would kill or remove all cancerous cells while leaving normal tissue untouched.

Sometimes this is almost possible, as when a surgeon removes a small superficial tumor of the skin. Typically, however, the tumor is less accessible, so some combination of surgery, radiation therapy, and chemotherapy must be used.

**Surgery** For most cancers, surgery is the most useful treatment. In many cases, the organ containing the tumor is not essential for life and can be partially or completely removed. Surgery is less effective when the tumor involves cells of the immune system, which are widely distributed throughout the body, or when the cancer has already metastasized.

**Chemotherapy** Chemotherapy is the use of targeted drugs that destroy rapidly growing cancer cells. Many chemotherapy drugs work by interfering with DNA synthesis and replication in rapidly dividing cells. Normal cells, which usually grow slowly, are not destroyed by these drugs. However, some normal tissues such as intestinal, hair, and blood-forming cells are always growing, and damage to these tissues produces the unpleasant side effects of chemotherapy, including nausea, vomiting, diarrhea, and hair loss.

**Radiation** In cancer radiation therapy, a beam of X-rays or gamma rays is directed at the tumor, killing the tumor cells. Occasionally, when an organ is small enough, radioactive seeds are surgically placed inside the cancerous organ to destroy the tumor and then removed later if necessary. Radiation destroys both normal and cancerous cells, but because it can be precisely directed at the tumor it is usually less toxic for the patient than either surgery or

## Table 12.2 Screening Guidelines for the Early Detection of Cancer in Average-Risk Asymptomatic People

| CANCER SITE | POPULATION | TEST OR PROCEDURE | FREQUENCY |
|---|---|---|---|
| Breast | Women, age 20+ | Breast self-examination | Beginning in their early 20s, women should be told about the benefits and limitations of breast self-examination (BSE). The importance of prompt reporting of any new breast symptoms to a health professional should be emphasized. Women who choose to do BSE should receive instruction and have their technique reviewed on the occasion of a periodic health examination. It is acceptable for women to choose not to do BSE or to do BSE irregularly. |
| | | Clinical breast examination | For women in their 20s and 30s, it is recommended that clinical breast examination (CBE) be part of a periodic health examination, preferably at least every 3 years. Asymptomatic women aged 40 and over should continue to receive a clinical breast examination as part of a periodic health examination, preferably annually. |
| | | Mammography | Begin annual mammography at age 40*. |
| Colorectal[†] | Men and women, age 50+ | *Tests that find polyps and cancer:* Flexible sigmoidoscopy[†], or Colonoscopy, or Double-contrast barium enema (DCBE)[‡], or CT colonography (virtual colonoscopy)[‡] | Every 5 years, starting at age 50 Every 10 years, starting at age 50 Every 5 years, starting at age 50 Every 5 years, starting at age 50 |
| | | *Tests that mainly find cancer:* Fecal occult blood test (FOBT) with at least 50% test sensitivity for cancer, or Fecal immunochemical test (FIT) with at least 50% test sensitivity for cancer[‡§], or Stool DNA test (sDNA)[‡] | Annual, starting at age 50 Interval uncertain, starting at age 50 |
| Prostate | Men, age 50+ | Prostate-specific antigen (PSA) test with or without digital rectal examination (DRE) | Asymptomatic men who have at least a 10-year life expectancy should have an opportunity to make an informed decision with their health care provider about screening for prostate cancer after receiving information about the uncertainties, risks, and potential benefits associated with screening. Prostate cancer screening should not occur without an informed decision-making process.[¶] |
| Cervix | Women, age 18+ | Pap test | Cervical cancer screening should begin approximately 3 years after a woman begins having vaginal intercourse, but no later than 21 years of age. Screening should be done every year with conventional Pap tests or every 2 years using liquid-based Pap tests. At or after age 30, women who have had three normal test results in a row may get screened every 2–3 years with cervical cytology (either conventional or liquid-based Pap test) alone, or every 3 years with an HPV DNA test plus cervical cytology. Women 70 years of age and older who have had three or more normal Pap tests and no abnormal Pap tests in the past 10 years and women who have had a total hysterectomy may choose to stop cervical cancer screening. |
| Endometrial | Women, at menopause | At the time of menopause, women at average risk should be informed about risks and symptoms of endometrial cancer and strongly encouraged to report any unexpected bleeding or spotting to their physicians. | |

*(continued)*

| CANCER SITE | POPULATION | TEST OR PROCEDURE | FREQUENCY |
|---|---|---|---|
| Cancer-related checkup | Men and women, age 20+ | On the occasion of a periodic health examination, the cancer-related checkup should include examination for cancers of the thyroid, testicles, ovaries, lymph nodes, oral cavity, and skin, as well as health counseling about tobacco, sun exposure, diet and nutrition, risk factors, sexual practices, and environmental and occupational exposures. | |

*Beginning at age 40, annual clinical breast examination should be performed prior to mammography.

†Individuals with a personal or family history of colorectal cancer or adenomas, inflammatory bowel disease, or high-risk genetic syndromes should continue to follow the most recent recommendations for individuals at increased or high risk.

‡ Colonoscopy should be done if test results are positive.

§For FOBT or FIT used as a screening test, the take-home multiple sample method should be used. A FOBT or FIT done during a digital rectal exam in the doctor's office is not adequate for screening.

¶Information should be provided to men about the benefits and limitations of testing so that an informed decision can be made with the clinician's assistance.

**SOURCE:** American Cancer Society. *Cancer Facts and Figures, 2011.* Copyright © 2011 American Cancer Society, Inc. www.cancer.org. Reprinted with permission.

chemotherapy, and it can often be performed on an outpatient basis. Radiation may be used as an exclusive treatment or in combination with surgery and/or chemotherapy.

## TIPS FOR TODAY AND THE FUTURE

A growing body of research suggests that we can take an active role in preventing many cancers by adopting a wellness lifestyle.

### RIGHT NOW YOU CAN

- If you are a woman, do a breast self-exam; if you are a man, do a testicular self-exam.
- Buy multiple bottles of sunscreen and put them in places where you will most likely need them, such as your backpack, gym bag, or car.
- Check the cancer screening guidelines in this chapter, and make sure you are up-to-date on your screenings.

### IN THE FUTURE YOU CAN

- Learn where to find information about daily UV radiation levels in your area, and learn how to interpret the information. Many local newspapers and television stations (and their Web sites) report current UV levels every day.
- Gradually add foods with abundant phytochemicals to your diet, choosing from the list shown in Table 12.1.

## SUMMARY

- Cancer is an abnormal and uncontrolled multiplication of cells; cancer cells can metastasize (spread to other parts of the body).

- Lung cancer kills more people than any other type of cancer; tobacco smoke is the primary cause.

- Colon and rectal cancer are linked to age, heredity, obesity, and a diet rich in red meat and low in fruits and vegetables.

- Breast cancer has a genetic component, but lifestyle and hormones are also factors. Prostate cancer is chiefly a disease of aging; diet, heredity, and ethnicity are other risk factors.

- Cancers of the female reproductive tract include cervical, uterine, and ovarian cancer. Cervical cancer is linked to HPV infection; the Pap test is an effective screening test. Vaccination is recommended for girls and young women.

- Melanoma is the most serious form of skin cancer; excessive exposure to UV radiation in sunlight is the primary cause.

- Oral cancer is caused primarily by smoking, excess alcohol consumption, and use of spit tobacco.

- Testicular cancer can be detected early through self-examination.

- The genetic basis of some cancers appears to be mutational damage to suppressor genes, which normally limit cell division.

- Cancer-promoting dietary factors include meat, certain types of fat, and alcohol. Dietary elements that may protect against cancer include antioxidants and phytochemicals. An inactive lifestyle is associated with some cancers.

- Some carcinogens occur naturally in the environment; others are manufactured substances. Occupational exposure is a risk for some workers.

- All sources of radiation are potentially carcinogenic, including X-rays and UV rays from the sun.

- Self-monitoring and regular screening tests are essential to early cancer detection.

## Q What is a biopsy?

**A** A *biopsy* is the removal and examination of a small piece of body tissue. Biopsies enable cancer specialists to carefully examine cells that are suspected of having turned cancerous. Some biopsies are fairly simple to perform, such as those on tissue from moles or skin sores. Other biopsies may require the use of a needle or probe to remove tissue from inside the body, such as in the breast or stomach.

## Q Are other cancer treatments available beyond surgery, chemotherapy, and radiation?

**A** Some experimental techniques that show promise for some particular types of cancer include the following:

- **Bone marrow transplants.** Healthy bone marrow cells from a compatible donor are transplanted following the elimination of the patient's bone marrow by radiation or chemotherapy. Transplants of stem cells may provide a solution to the problem of donor incompatibility. These unspecialized cells can divide and produce many specialized cell types, including bone marrow cells. Stem cells can be grown outside the body and then transplanted back into the cancer patient, allowing safe repopulation of bone marrow.

- **Vaccines and genetically modified immune cells.** These enhance the reaction of a patient's own immune system.

- **Anti-angiogenesis agents.** These starve tumors by blocking their blood supply.

- **Proteasome inhibitors.** Proteasomes help control the cell cycle—the process through which cells divide. If proteasomes malfunction, as is often the case in cancer cells, then cells may begin multiplying out of control. Proteasome inhibitors block the action of proteasomes, halting cell division and killing the cells. One proteasome inhibitor is now being used against certain cancers, and other such drugs are in development.

- **Enzyme activators/blockers.** Normal cells die after dividing a given number of times. Scientists believe that the enzyme caspase triggers the death of normally functioning cells. In cancer cells, caspase activity may be blocked. Conversely, if the enzyme telomerase becomes active in cancer cells, the life/death cycle stops and the cells duplicate indefinitely. In effect, inactive caspase or active telomerase may make cancer cells "immortal." Researchers are studying compounds that can either activate caspase or deactivate telomerase; either type of drug might lead cancer cells to self-destruct. No such drugs are now in clinical use.

In the future, gene sequencing techniques may allow treatments to be targeted at specific cancer subtypes, much as specific antibiotics are now used to treat specific bacterial diseases.

*For more Common Questions Answered about cancer, visit the Online Learning Center at www.mhhe.com/fahey.*

---

- Methods of cancer diagnosis include MRI, CT scanning, and ultrasound.

- Cancer treatment usually consists of some combination of surgery, chemotherapy, and radiation.

## FOR FURTHER EXPLORATION

### BOOKS

American Cancer Society. 2009. *The American Cancer Society Complete Guide to Complementary & Alternative Cancer Therapies.* Atlanta, Ga.: American Cancer Society. *Provides in-depth information about cancer therapies being used alongside traditional Western medicine in treating cancer.*

American Institute for Cancer Research. 2005. *The New American Plate Cookbook.* Berkeley, Calif.: U.C. Berkeley Press. *Provides guidelines and recipes for healthy eating to prevent cancer and other chronic diseases.*

Hartmann, L. C., C. L. Loprinzi, and B. S. Gostout. 2005. *Mayo Clinic: Guide to Women's Cancers.* New York: Kensington. *Provides information about a variety of women's cancers.*

McKinnell, R. G., et al. 2006. *The Biological Basis of Cancer,* 2nd ed. Boston: Cambridge University Press. *Examines the underlying causes of cancer and discusses actual cases of the disease and its impact on patients and families.*

Rosenbaum, E., et al. 2008. *Everyone's Guide to Cancer Therapy,* rev. 5th ed. Riverside, N.J.: Andrews McMeel. *Reviewed by a panel of more than 100 oncologists; provides articles on the known causes, diagnoses, and treatments for many types of cancer.*

Turkington, C., and W. LiPera. 2005. *The Encyclopedia of Cancer.* New York: Facts on File. *Includes entries on a variety of topics relating to cancer causes, prevention, diagnosis, and treatment.*

### ORGANIZATIONS, HOTLINES AND WEB SITES

*American Academy of Dermatology.* Provides information on skin cancer prevention.
http://www.aad.org

*American Cancer Society.* Provides a wide range of free materials on the prevention and treatment of cancer.
http://www.cancer.org

*American Institute for Cancer Research.* Provides information on lifestyle and cancer prevention, especially nutrition.
http://www.aicr.org

*CureSearch National Childhood Cancer Foundation.* Offers information on childhood cancers and initiatives to raise awareness and funds for research.
http://www.curesearch.org

*EPA/Sunwise.* Provides information about the UV Index and the effects of sun exposure, with links to sites with daily UV Index ratings for U.S. and international cities.
http://www.epa.gov/sunwise/uvindex.html

*LiveStrong (The Lance Armstrong Foundation).* Provides resources on cancer and cancer support.
http://www.livestrong.org

*MedlinePlus: Cancers.* Provides links to reliable cancer information.
http://www.nlm.nih.gov/medlineplus/cancers.html

*National Cancer Institute.* Provides information on treatment options, screening, clinical trials, and newly approved drugs.
http://www.cancer.gov

*Skin Cancer Foundation.* Provides information on all types of skin cancers, their prevention, and treatment.
http://www.skincancer.org

*Susan G. Komen for the Cure.* Provides information and resources on breast cancer.
http://www.komen.org

*Washington University School of Medicine: Your Disease Risk.* Includes interactive risk assessments as well as tips for preventing common cancers.
http://www.yourdiseaserisk.wustl.edu

*World Health Organization: Cancer.* Home page of WHO's worldwide anti-cancer initiative.
http://www.who.int/cancer/en

## SELECTED BIBLIOGRAPHY

American Cancer Society. 2009. *Cancer Prevention and Early Detection Facts & Figures.* Atlanta, Ga.: American Cancer Society.

American Cancer Society. 2010. *Breast Cancer Facts & Figures, 2010.* Atlanta, Ga.: American Cancer Society.

American Cancer Society. 2010. *Colorectal Cancer Facts & Figures 2008–2010.* Atlanta, Ga.: American Cancer Society.

American Cancer Society. *Cancer Facts and Figures, 2011.* Atlanta, Ga.: American Cancer Society.

Chao, A., et al. 2005. Meat consumption and risk of colorectal cancer. *Journal of the American Medical Association* 293(2): 172–182.

Danaei, G., et al. 2005. Causes of cancer in the world: Comparative risk assessment of nine behavioral and environmental risk factors. *Lancet* 2005(366): 1784–1793.

Elmore, J. G., et al. 2005. Screening for breast cancer. *Journal of the American Medical Association* 293(10): 1245–1256.

Finn, O. J., 2008. Cancer immunology. *New England Journal of Medicine* 358(25): 2704–15.

Hu, J. C., et al. 2008. Patterns of care for radical prostatectomy in the United States from 2003 to 2005. *Journal of Urology* 180(5): 1969–1974.

Jones, K. L., et al. 2009. Evolving novel anti-HER2 strategies. *Lancet Oncology* 10(12): 1179–1187.

Kauff, N. D., et al. 2008. Risk-reducing salpingo-oophorectomy for the prevention of BRCA1- and BRCA2-associated breast and gynecologic cancer: A multicenter, prospective study. *Journal of Clinical Oncology* 26(8): 1331–1337.

Kavalerchik, E., et al. 2009. Chronic myeloid leukemia stem cells. *Journal of Clinical Oncology* 26(17): 2911–2915.

Kerbel, R. S., 2008. Tumor angiogenesis. *New England Journal of Medicine* 358(19): 2039–2049.

Kroenke, C. H., et al. 2005. Weight, weight gain, and survival after breast cancer diagnosis. *Journal of Clinical Oncology* 23(7): 1370–1378.

Ma, X., et al. 2010. Diet, lifestyle, and acute myeloid leukemia in the NIH-AARP cohort. *American Journal of Epidemiology* 171(3): 312–322.

Park, Y., et al. 2009. Dairy food, calcium, and risk of cancer in the NIH-AARP Diet and Health Study. *Archives of Internal Medicine* 169(4): 391–401.

Samet, J., et al. 2009. Lung cancer in never smokers: Clinical epidemiology and environmental risk factors. *Clinical Cancer Research* 15(18): 5626–5645.

Trimble, C. L., et al. 2005. Active and passive cigarette smoking and the risk of cervical neoplasia. *Obstetrics and Gynecology* 105(1): 174–181.

U.S. Preventive Services Task Force. 2008. Screening for prostate cancer: U.S. Preventive Services Task Force recommendation statement. *Annals of Internal Medicine* 149(3): 185–191.

Van Gils, C. H., et al. 2005. Consumption of vegetables and fruits and risk of breast cancer. *Journal of the American Medical Association* 293(3): 183–193.

Vogel, V. G., et al. 2006. Effects of tamoxifen vs raloxifene on the risk of developing invasive breast cancer and other disease outcomes: The NSABP Study of Tamoxifen and Raloxifene (STAR) P-2 trial. *Journal of the American Medical Association* 295(23): 2727–2741.

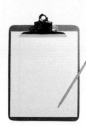

## LAB 12.1 Cancer Prevention

This lab looks at two areas of cancer prevention over which you have a great deal of individual control—diet and sun exposure. For a detailed personal risk profile for many specific types of cancer, complete the assessments at the Washington University School of Medicine's "Your Disease Risk" site (http://www.yourdiseaserisk.wustl.edu).

### Part I   Diet and Cancer

Track your diet for 3 days, recording the number of servings from each of the following groups that you consume.

| Day 1 | Day 2 | Day 3 | Potential Cancer Fighters |
|---|---|---|---|
| _____ | _____ | _____ | Orange, deep yellow, pink, and red vegetables and some fruits (for example, apricots, cantaloupe, carrots, corn, grapefruit, mangoes, nectarines, papayas, red and yellow bell peppers, sweet potatoes, pumpkin, tomatoes and tomato sauce, watermelon, winter squash such as acorn or butternut) |
| _____ | _____ | _____ | Dark green leafy vegetables (for example, broccoli rabe, chard, kale, romaine and other dark lettuces, spinach; beet, collard, dandelion, mustard, and turnip greens) |
| _____ | _____ | _____ | Cruciferous vegetables (bok choy, broccoli, brussels sprouts, cabbage, cauliflower, kohlrabi, turnips) |
| _____ | _____ | _____ | Citrus fruits (for example, grapefruit, lemons, limes, oranges, tangerines) |
| _____ | _____ | _____ | Whole grains (for example, whole-grain bread, cereal, and pasta; brown rice; oatmeal; whole-grain corn; barley; popcorn; bulgur) |
| _____ | _____ | _____ | Legumes (peas, lentils, and beans, including fava, navy, kidney, pinto, black, and lima beans) |
| _____ | _____ | _____ | Berries (for example, strawberries, raspberries, blackberries, blueberries) |
| _____ | _____ | _____ | Garlic and other allium vegetables (onions, leeks, chives, scallions, shallots) |
| _____ | _____ | _____ | Soy products (for example, tofu, tempeh, soy milk, miso, soybeans) |
| _____ | _____ | _____ | Other cancer-fighting fruits (apples, cherries, cranberries or juice, grapes, kiwifruit, pears, plums, prunes, raisins) |
| _____ | _____ | _____ | Other cancer-fighting vegetables (asparagus, beets, chili peppers, eggplant, green peppers, radishes) |
| _____ | _____ | _____ | **Daily totals (average for three days: _____)** |

The goal is to eat at least 7 (women) or 9 (men) servings of cancer-fighting fruits and vegetables each day; the more servings, the better. (Research is ongoing, and this list of cancer fighters is not comprehensive. Remember, nearly all fruits, vegetables, and grains are healthy choices.)

### Part II   Skin Cancer Risk Assessment

Your risk of skin cancer from the ultraviolet radiation in sunlight depends on several factors. Take the following quiz to see how sensitive you are. The higher your UV-risk score, the greater your risk of skin cancer—and the greater your need to take precautions against too much sun. Score 1 point for each true statement:

_____ 1. I have blond or red hair.

_____ 2. I have light-colored eyes (blue, gray, green).

_____ 3. I freckle easily.

_____ 4. I have many moles.

_____ 5. I had two or more blistering sunburns as a child.

_____ 6. I spent lots of time in a tropical climate as a child.

_____ 7. I have a family history of skin cancer.

_____ 8. I work outdoors.

_____ 9. I spend a lot of time in outdoor activities.

_____ 10. I like to spend as much time in the sun as I can.

_____ 11. I sometimes go to a tanning parlor or use a sunlamp.

_____ **Total score**

Mc Graw Hill **connect** http://www.mcgrawhillconnect.com/ |FITNESS AND WELLNESS

| Score | Risk of skin cancer from UV radiation |
|-------|---------------------------------------|
| 0 | Low |
| 1–3 | Moderate |
| 4–7 | High |
| 8–11 | Very high |

## Using Your Results

*How did you score?* (1) How close did you come to the goal of eating 7–9 or more servings of cancer fighters each day?

Are you satisfied with your diet in terms of cancer prevention? If not, set a specific goal for a target number of servings of cancer-fighting fruits and vegetables:

(2) What is your skin cancer risk assessment score? Does it indicate that you are at high or very high risk? Do you feel you need to take action because of your risk level?

*What should you do next?* Enter the results of this lab in the Preprogram Assessment column in Appendix C. (1) If you've set a goal for the diet and cancer portion of the lab, select a target number of additional cancer fighters from the list to try over the next few days; list the foods below, along with your plan for incorporating them into your diet (as a side dish, as a snack, on a salad, as a substitute for another food, etc.).

Cancer fighter to try:

Plan for trying:

(2) You cannot control all of your risk factors for skin cancer, but you can control your behavior with regard to sun exposure. Keep a journal to track your behavior on days when you are outdoors in the sun for a significant period of time. Compare your behavior with the recommendations for skin cancer prevention described in the chapter. Record information such as time of day, total duration of exposure, UV index for the day, clothing worn, type and amount of sunscreen used, frequency of sunscreen applications, and so on. From this record, identify ways to improve your behavior to lower your risk of skin cancer. Put together a behavior change plan.

Next, begin to put your strategies into action. After several weeks of a program to improve your diet or reduce your UV exposure, do this lab again and enter the results in the Postprogram Assessment column of Appendix C. How do the results compare?

SOURCE: Part II: Skin Cancer Risk Assessment, adapted from Shear, N. 1996. "What's Your UV-risk Score?" Copyright © 1996 by the Consumers Union of the United States, Inc., Yonkers, NY 10703-1057, a nonprofit organization. Reprinted with permission from the author.

# CHAPTER 13

# Substance Use and Abuse

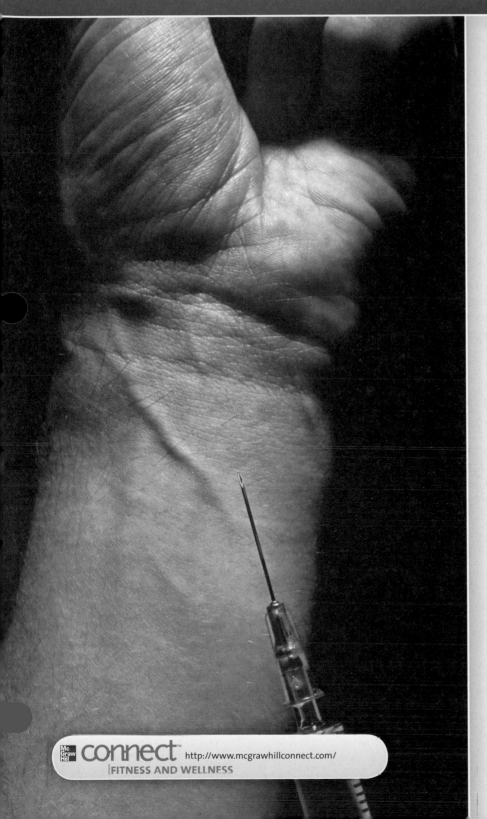

## LOOKING AHEAD...

After reading this chapter, you should be able to:

- Define and discuss the concepts of addictive behavior, substance abuse, and substance dependence

- List the major categories of psychoactive drugs and discuss how drug abuse can be prevented and treated

- Describe the short-term and long-term effects of alcohol use

- Identify strategies for drinking alcohol responsibly

- List the health hazards associated with tobacco use and exposure to environmental tobacco smoke

- Describe strategies that can help someone stop smoking

## TEST YOUR KNOWLEDGE

1. Which of the following is the most widely used illegal drug among college students?
   a. cocaine
   b. hallucinogens
   c. marijuana
   d. heroin

2. If a man and a woman of the same weight drink the same amount of alcohol, the woman will become intoxicated more quickly than the man. True or false?

3. Every day in the United States, about 1000 teens start smoking. True or false?

**Answers**

1. **c.** Marijuana ranks first, followed (in order) by hallucinogens, cocaine, and heroin. Alcohol, however, remains by far the most popular drug among college students.

2. **True.** Women usually have a higher percentage of body fat than men and a less active form of a stomach enzyme that breaks down alcohol. Both factors cause them to become intoxicated more quickly and to a greater degree.

3. **True.** Roughly 1000 Americans under 18 and 1800 over 18 start smoking every day.

The use of **drugs** for both medical and social purposes is widespread in America (Table 13.1). Many people believe that every problem has or should have a chemical solution. Advertisements, social pressures, and the human desire for quick solutions to life's difficult problems all contribute to the prevailing attitude that drugs can ease all pain. Unfortunately, using drugs can—and often does—have negative consequences.

The most serious consequences are abuse and addiction. The drugs most often associated with abuse are **psychoactive drugs**—those that alter a person's experiences or consciousness. In the short term, psychoactive drugs can cause **intoxication**, a state in which sometimes unpredictable physical and emotional changes occur. In the long term, recurrent drug use can have profound physical, emotional, and social effects.

This chapter examines the use of psychoactive drugs, including alcohol and tobacco, and explains their short- and long-term effects and their potential for abuse and addiction. The information provided is designed to help you make healthy, informed decisions about the role of drugs in your life. Before turning to the specific types of drugs, the following section examines addictive behavior in general.

## ADDICTIVE BEHAVIOR

Although addiction is most often associated with drug use, many experts now extend the concept of addiction to other areas. **Addictive behaviors** are habits that have gotten out of control, with resulting negative effects on a person's health.

## What Is Addiction?

Today, scientists view **addiction** as a psychological or physical dependence on a substance or behavior. Historically, the term was applied only when the habitual use of a drug produced chemical changes in the user's body. One such change is physical tolerance, in which the body adapts to a drug so that the initial dose no longer produces the same emotional or psychological effects. This process, caused by chemical

### VITAL STATISTICS

| Table 13.1 | Nonmedical Drug Use Among Americans, 2009 | |
|---|---|---|
| | **PERCENTAGE USING SUBSTANCE IN THE PAST 30 DAYS** | |
| | COLLEGE STUDENTS (AGE 18–25) | ALL AMERICANS (AGE 12 AND OLDER) |
| Illicit Drugs | 21.2 | 8.7 |
| Marijuana and hashish | 18.1 | 6.6 |
| Cocaine | 1.4 | 0.7 |
| Crack | 0.1 | 0.2 |
| Heroin | 0.2 | 0.1 |
| Methamphetamine | 0.2 | 0.2 |
| Hallucinogens | 1.8 | 0.5 |
|   LSD | 0.3 | 0.1 |
|   PCP | 0.0 | 0.0 |
|   Ecstasy | 0.9 | 0.3 |
| Inhalants | 0.4 | 0.2 |
| Nonmedical use of psychotherapeutics | 6.3 | 2.8 |
|   Pain relievers | 4.8 | 2.1 |
|     OxyContin | 0.5 | 0.2 |
| Tranquilizers | 1.8 | 0.8 |
| Stimulants | 1.3 | 0.5 |
| Sedatives | 0.2 | 0.1 |
| Tobacco (all forms) | 41.6 | 27.7 |
|   Cigarettes | 35.8 | 23.3 |
|   Smokeless tobacco | 6.1 | 3.4 |
|   Cigars | 11.4 | 5.3 |
|   Pipe tobacco | 1.7 | 0.8 |
| Alcohol | 61.8 | 51.9 |
|   Binge alcohol use | 41.7 | 23.7 |

**SOURCES:** Office of Applied Studies, Substance Abuse and Mental Health Services Administration. 2010. *Results from the 2009 National Survey on Drug Use and Health: Volume I. Summary of National Findings*. Rockville, Md.: Office of Applied Studies, NSDUH (Series H-38A, HHS Publication No. SMA 10-4856Findings); Office of Applied Studies, Substance Abuse and Mental Health Services Administration. 2010. *Results from the 2009 National Survey on Drug Use and Health: Volume II. Technical Appendices and Selected Prevalence Tables*. Rockville, Md.: Office of Applied Studies, NSDUH (Series H-38B, HHS Publication No. SMA 10-4856Appendices).

**KEY TERMS**

**drug** Any chemical other than food intended to affect the structure or function of the body.

**psychoactive drug** A drug that can alter a person's state of mind or consciousness.

**intoxication** The state of being mentally affected by a chemical (literally, a state of being poisoned).

**addictive behavior** Any habit that has gotten out of control, resulting in a negative effect on one's health.

**addiction** Psychological or physical dependence on a substance or behavior, characterized by a compulsive desire and increasing need for the substance or behavior and by harm to the individual or society.

changes in the brain, means the user has to take larger and larger doses of the drug to achieve the same high.

It is sometimes difficult to distinguish between a healthy habit and one that has become an addiction. Experts have identified some general characteristics typically associated with addictive behaviors.

- *Reinforcement.* The behavior produces pleasurable physical or emotional states or relieves negative ones.
- *Compulsion or craving.* The addict feels a compelling need to engage in the behavior.
- *Loss of control.* The addict loses control over the behavior and cannot block the impulse to do it.

- *Escalation.* More and more of the substance or activity is required to produce its desired effects.
- *Negative consequences.* The behavior continues despite serious negative consequences, such as problems with academic or job performance, difficulties with personal relationships, or health problems.

## The Development of Addiction

An addiction often starts when a person does something to bring pleasure or avoid pain. The activity may be drinking a beer, using the Internet, or going shopping. If it works, the person is likely to repeat it. He or she becomes increasingly dependent on the behavior, and tolerance may develop; over time, the person needs more of the behavior to feel the same effect. Eventually, the behavior becomes a central focus of the person's life, and there is a deterioration in other areas, such as school performance or relationships. The behavior no longer brings pleasure, but it is necessary to avoid the pain of going without it.

Although many common behaviors are potentially addictive, most people who engage in them don't develop problems. Risk for addiction depends on a combination of factors, including personality, lifestyle, heredity, the social and physical environment, and the nature of the substance or behavior in question. For example, nicotine (the psychoactive drug in tobacco) has a very high potential for physical addiction, but a person must try smoking—whether influenced by peer pressure, family factors, advertising, stress, or personality traits—to become addicted. Some studies have found that genetic factors play a role in risk for addiction, and some people may have a genetic predisposition for addiction to a particular drug.

## Examples of Addictive Behaviors

Some behaviors that are not related to drugs can become addictive for some people.

**Compulsive Gambling** Compulsive gamblers cannot resist the urge to gamble, even in the face of personal ruin. About 1% of adult Americans are compulsive (pathological) gamblers, and another 2% are "problem gamblers." Some 42% of students report having gambled at least once in the past year, and about 3% reported gambling at least once a week. The consequences of compulsive gambling are not just financial: The suicide rate among compulsive gamblers is 20 times higher than that of the general population. Many compulsive gamblers also have drug and alcohol abuse problems.

**Compulsive Buying** A compulsive buyer repeatedly gives in to the impulse to buy more than he or she needs or can afford. Compulsive spenders usually buy luxury items rather than daily necessities. Compulsive buyers are usually distressed by their behavior and its social,

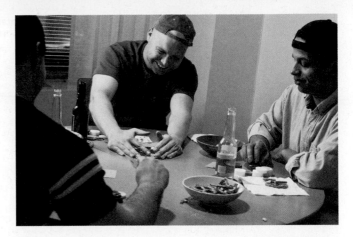
Many college students have gotten caught up in the poker craze.

personal, and financial consequences. Some experts link compulsive shopping with neglect or abuse during childhood; it also seems to be associated with eating disorders, depression, and bipolar disorder.

**Internet Addiction** Research indicates that surfing the Internet can also be addictive. To spend more time online, Internet addicts skip important school, social, or recreational activities. Despite negative financial, social, or academic consequences, they don't feel able to stop. As with other addictive behaviors, online addicts may be using their behavior to alleviate stress or avoid painful emotions. There is some concern that widespread access to the Internet may expose many more people to other potentially addictive behaviors, including gambling and shopping. By some estimates, millions of Americans have become compulsive Internet users—as much as 10% of the U.S. population. In one study of Internet addiction, addicts averaged 38 online hours per week.

Other behaviors that can become addictive include exercising, eating, watching TV, and working. Any substance or activity that becomes the focus of one's life at the expense of other needs can be damaging to health.

## PSYCHOACTIVE DRUGS

Psychoactive drugs include legal compounds such as caffeine, tobacco, and alcohol as well as illegal substances such as heroin, cocaine, and LSD (Figure 13.1). This

### Ask yourself

**QUESTIONS FOR CRITICAL THINKING AND REFLECTION**

Have you ever compulsively engaged in a behavior that had negative consequences? What was the behavior, and why did you continue? Were you able to bring the behavior under control? If so, how?

| Category | Representative drugs | Street names | Potential short-term effects | Potential long-term effects |
|---|---|---|---|---|
| **Opioids** | Heroin | Dope, H, junk, brown sugar, smack | Relief of anxiety and pain, euphoria, lethargy, apathy, drowsiness, confusion, inability to concentrate, nausea and vomiting, constipation, respiratory depression, lowered responsiveness to sexual stimulation, overdose and death | • Dependence, tolerance, and withdrawal; symptoms of withdrawal can include cramps, chills, nausea, tremors, feelings of panic<br>• Injection drug use can spread HIV and hepatitis and cause skin infections |
| | Opium | Big O, black stuff, hop | | |
| | Morphine | M, Miss Emma, monkey, white stuff | | |
| | Oxycodone, codeine, hydrocodone | Oxy, O.C., killer, Captain Cody, schoolboy, vike | | |
| **Central nervous system depressants** | Barbiturates | Barbs, reds, red birds, yellows, yellow jackets | Reduced anxiety, mood changes (irritability, abusiveness), lowered inhibitions, impaired muscle coordination, reduced pulse rate, drowsiness, loss of consciousness, respiratory depression, death | • Dependence, tolerance, and withdrawal; symptoms of withdrawal may include anxiety, weakness, convulsions, cardiovascular collapse, and death<br>• Brain damage, impaired ability to reason and make judgments<br>• Overdose, especially when combined with alcohol or another depressant<br>• Some are prescribed for insomnia and anxiety, to control seizures, and to calm patients before medical procedures; prescription depressants can also be abused |
| | Benzodiazepines (e.g., Valium, Xanax, Rohypnol) | Candy, downers, tranks, roofies, forget-me pill | | |
| | Methaqualone | Ludes, quad, quay | | |
| | Gamma hydroxy-butyrate (GHB) | G, Georgia home boy, grievous bodily harm | | |
| **Central nervous system stimulants** | Amphetamine, methamphet-amine | Bennies, speed, black beauties, uppers, chalk, crank, crystal, ice, meth | Increased heart rate, blood pressure, metabolism; increased mental alertness and energy; nervousness, insomnia, impulsive behavior, reduced appetite, disturbed sleep; high doses can cause death | • Dependence, tolerance, and withdrawal<br>• Severe behavioral disturbances, including delusions of persecution and unprovoked violence<br>• Brain damage, impaired judgment, and crashing (extreme sleepiness) when effects of a dose wear off<br>• Prenatal effects—miscarriage, premature labor, stillbirth, birth defects |
| | Cocaine, crack cocaine | Blow, C, candy, coke, flake, rock, toot | | |
| | Ritalin | JIF, MPH, R-ball, Skippy | | |
| **Marijuana and other cannabis products** | Marijuana | Dope, grass, joints, Mary Jane, reefer, skunk, weed | Euphoria, slowed thinking and reaction time, confusion, anxiety, impaired balance and coordination, increased heart rate, dilation of blood vessels in the eyes | • Throat and lung irritation, reduced lung function, precancerous changes in the lungs<br>• Decreased testosterone levels and sperm counts; increased sperm abnormalities<br>• Memory impairment, temporarily reduced IQ<br>• Prenatal effects—impaired growth and development of fetus |
| | Hashish | Hash, hemp, boom, gangster | | |
| **Hallucinogens** | LSD | Acid, boomers, blotter, yellow sunshines | Altered states of perception and feeling; nausea; increased heart rate, blood pressure; delirium; impaired motor function; numbness; weakness; panic; depersonalization | • Rapidly developing tolerance<br>• Unpredictable effects, including panic reactions and psychological disturbances |
| | Mescaline (peyote) | Buttons, cactus, mesc | | |
| | Psilocybin | Shrooms, magic mushrooms | | |
| | Ketamine | K, special K, cat Valium, vitamin K | | |
| | PCP | Angel dust, hog, love boat, peace pill | | |
| | MDMA (ecstasy) | X, peace, clarity, Adam | | |
| **Inhalants** | Solvents, aerosols, nitrites, anesthetics | Laughing gas, poppers, snappers, whippets | Stimulation, loss of inhibition, slurred speech, loss of motor coordination, loss of consciousness, death | • Damage to central nervous system, liver, kidneys, bone marrow, hearing<br>• Increased risk of cancer |

**FIGURE 13.1  Commonly abused drugs and their effects.**

SOURCES: The Partnership for a Drug-Free America. 2010. *Drug Guide by Name* (http://www.drugfree.org/portal/drug_guide; retrieved May 23, 2011); U.S. Drug Enforcement Agency. 2006. *Photo Library* (http://www.usdoj.gov/dea/photo_library.html; retrieved May 23, 2011); U.S. Drug Enforcement Agency. 2010. *Drug Information* (http://www.justice.gov/dea/concern/concern.htm; retrieved May 23, 2011); National Institute on Drug Abuse. 2010. *Commonly Abused Drugs* (http://www.drugabuse.gov/DrugPages/DrugsofAbuse.html; retrieved May 23, 2011)

section examines general issues that apply to the use of any psychoactive drug. Later sections discuss two commonly used and abused psychoactive drugs: alcohol and tobacco.

## Drug Use, Abuse, and Dependence

The American Psychiatric Association's (APA) *Diagnostic and Statistical Manual of Mental Disorders* is the authoritative reference for defining mental and behavioral disorders, including those related to drugs. The APA has chosen not to use the term *addiction*, in part because it is so broad and has so many connotations. Instead, the APA refers to two forms of substance (drug) disorders: substance abuse and substance dependence. Both are maladaptive patterns of substance use that lead to significant impairment or distress. Although the APA's definitions are more precise and more directly related to drug use, they clearly encompass the general characteristics of addictive behavior described in the preceding section.

**Abuse** As defined by the APA, **substance abuse** involves one or more of the following characteristics:

- Recurrent drug use, resulting in a failure to fulfill major responsibilities at work, school, or home
- Recurrent drug use in situations in which it is physically hazardous, such as before or while driving
- Recurrent drug-related legal problems
- Continued drug use despite persistent social or interpersonal problems caused by or worsened by the effects of the drug

The pattern of use may be constant or intermittent, and **physical dependence** may or may not be present. For example, a person who smokes marijuana once a week and cuts classes because he or she is high is abusing marijuana, even though he or she is not physically dependent.

**Dependence** **Substance dependence** is a more complex disorder and is what many people associate with the idea of addiction. The seven specific criteria the APA uses to diagnose substance dependence are listed below. The first two are associated with physical dependence; the final five are associated with compulsive use. To be considered dependent, a person must experience a cluster of three or more of these seven symptoms during a 12-month period.

1. *Developing tolerance to the substance.* When a person requires increased amounts of a substance to achieve the desired effect or notices a markedly diminished effect with continued use of the same amount, he or she has developed **tolerance** to the substance.

2. *Experiencing withdrawal.* In someone who has maintained prolonged, heavy use of a substance, a drop in its concentration within the body can result in unpleasant physical and cognitive **withdrawal** symptoms. Withdrawal symptoms are different for different drugs. For example, nausea, vomiting, and tremors are common withdrawal symptoms in people dependent on alcohol, opioids, or sedatives.

3. *Taking the substance in larger amounts or over a longer period than was originally intended.*

4. *Expressing a persistent desire to cut down on or regulate substance use.*

5. *Spending a great deal of time getting the substance, using the substance, or recovering from its effects.*

6. *Giving up or reducing important social, school, work, or recreational activities because of substance use.*

7. *Continuing to use the substance despite the knowledge that it is contributing to a psychological or physical problem.*

If a drug-dependent person experiences either tolerance or withdrawal, he or she is considered physically dependent. However, dependence can occur without a physical component, based solely on compulsive use.

## Who Uses Drugs?

Drug use and abuse occur at all income and education levels, among all ethnic groups, and across all age groups.

**KEY TERMS**

**substance abuse** A maladaptive pattern of using any substance that persists despite adverse social, psychological, or medical consequences; the pattern may be intermittent, with or without tolerance and physical dependence.

**physical dependence** The result of physiological adaptation that occurs in response to the frequent use of a drug; typically associated with tolerance and withdrawal.

**substance dependence** A cluster of cognitive, behavioral, and physiological symptoms that occur in someone who continues to use a substance despite suffering significant substance-related problems, leading to significant impairment or distress; also known as *addiction.*

**tolerance** Lower sensitivity to a drug so that a given dose no longer exerts the usual effect and larger doses are needed.

**withdrawal** Physical and psychological symptoms that follow the interrupted use of a drug on which a user is physically dependent; symptoms may be mild or life-threatening.

## Wellness Tip

Many over-the-counter medications contain drugs that can alter mood or reactions, including alcohol, caffeine, and dextromethrophan. Always use these medications with caution, and follow the label directions.

Society is concerned with the casual or recreational use of illegal drugs because it is not really possible to know when drug use will lead to abuse or dependence. Some casual users develop substance-related problems; others do not. Some psychoactive drugs, however, are more likely than others to lead to dependence (Table 13.2).

Characteristics that place people at higher-than-average risk for trying illegal drugs include being male, being young, being a troubled adolescent, being a thrill-seeker, being in a dysfunctional family, being in a peer group that accepts drug use, being poor, and beginning dating at a young age. Drug use is less common among young people who attend school regularly, get good grades, have strong personal identities, are religious, have a good relationship with their parents, and are independent thinkers whose actions are not controlled by peer pressure. Coming from a family that has a clear policy on drug use and deals with conflicts constructively is also associated with not using drugs.

Why do some people use psychoactive drugs without becoming dependent, while others aren't as lucky? The answer seems to be a combination of physical, psychological, and social factors. Some people may be born with a brain chemistry or metabolism that makes them more vulnerable to drug dependence. Psychological risk factors include having difficulty controlling impulses and having a strong need for excitement and immediate gratification. People may turn to drugs to numb emotional pain or to deal with difficult experiences or feelings such as rejection, hostility, or depression. Social factors that may increase the risk for dependence include exposure to drug-using family members or peers, poverty, and easy access to drugs (see the box "Club Drugs").

## Treatment for Drug Abuse and Dependence

Different types of programs are available to help people break their drug habits, but there is no single best method of treatment. The relapse rate is high for all types of treatment, but being treated is better than not being treated. Professional treatment programs usually take the form of drug substitution programs or treatment centers; nonprofessional self-help groups and peer counseling are also available. To be successful, a treatment program must deal with the reasons behind users' drug abuse and help them develop behaviors, attitudes, and a social support system that will help them remain drug free. See For Further Exploration at the end of the chapter for resources related to treatment.

Young people with drug problems are often unable to seek help on their own. In such cases, friends and family members may need to act on their behalf. The following signals suggest drug dependence:

- Sudden withdrawal or emotional distance
- Rebellious or unusually irritable behavior
- Loss of interest in usual activities or hobbies
- Decline in school performance
- Sudden change in group of friends
- Changes in sleeping or eating habits
- Frequent borrowing of money

## Preventing Drug Abuse and Dependence

The best solution to drug abuse is prevention. Government attempts at controlling the drug problem tend to focus on stopping the production, importation, and distribution of illegal drugs. Creative efforts are also being made to stop the demand for drugs. Approaches include building young people's self-esteem, improving their academic skills, increasing their recreational opportunities, providing them with honest information about the effects of drugs, and teaching them strategies for resisting peer pressure.

| Table 13.2 | Psychoactive Drugs and Their Potential for Producing Dependence | |
|---|---|---|
| | POTENTIAL FOR DEPENDENCE | |
| DRUG | PHYSICAL | PSYCHOLOGICAL |
| Heroin | High | High |
| Morphine | High | High |
| Hydrocodone | High | High |
| Oxycodone | High | High |
| Codeine | Moderate | Moderate |
| Gamma Hydroxybutric Acid | Moderate | Moderate |
| Bensodiazepines | Moderate | Moderate |
| Cocaine | Possible | High |
| Amphetamine/ Methamphetamine | Possible | High |
| Methylphenidate | Possible | High |
| MDMA (Ecstasy) | None | Moderate |
| LSD | None | Unknown |
| PCP | Possible | High |
| Marijuana | Unknown | Moderate |
| Hashish | Unknown | Moderate |
| Alcohol | High | High |

**SOURCE:** U.S. Department of Justice, Drug Enforcement Administration. 2005. *Drugs of Abuse.* Washington, D.C.: U.S. Department of Justice.

### Wellness Tip

Women should realize that date-rape drugs can be slipped into beverages. Never accept a drink unless you see it being poured, especially when you are at parties or socializing with strangers.

# Club Drugs

Some people refer to club drugs as soft drugs because they see them as recreational—for the casual, weekend user—rather than addictive. But club drugs have many negative effects and are particularly potent and unpredictable when mixed with alcohol. Substitute drugs are often sold in place of club drugs, putting users at risk for taking dangerous combinations of unknown substances.

**MDMA** Taken in pill form, MDMA (methylenedioxymethamphetamine) is a stimulant with mildly hallucinogenic and amphetamine-like effects. It can produce dangerously high body temperature and potentially fatal dehydration. Some users experience confusion, depression, anxiety, paranoia, muscle tension, involuntary teeth clenching, blurred vision, and seizures. Even low doses can affect concentration and driving ability. Use during pregnancy is linked to increased risk of birth defects.

Chronic use of MDMA may produce long-lasting, perhaps permanent, damage to the neurons that release serotonin. This may explain why heavy use is associated with persistent problems with learning and verbal and visual memory. MDMA users perform worse than nonusers on complex cognitive tasks of memory, attention, and general intelligence.

**Methamphetamine** A potent stimulant, methamphetamine is available in many forms and can be swallowed,

smoked, snorted, or injected. It causes the release of high levels of the neurotransmitter dopamine, which enhances mood and body movement. Other effects include insomnia, anxiety, irritability, paranoia, and aggressiveness. High doses can cause convulsions and death. Methamphetamine is highly addictive and may damage brain cells.

**LSD** A potent hallucinogen, LSD (lysergic acid diethylamide) is sold in tablets or capsules, in liquid form, or on small squares of paper called blotters. LSD increases heart rate and body temperature and may cause nausea, tremors, sweating, numbness, and weakness.

**Ketamine** A veterinary anesthetic that can be taken in powdered or liquid form, ketamine may cause hallucinations and impaired attention and memory. At higher doses, ketamine can cause delirium, amnesia, high blood pressure, and potentially fatal respiratory problems. Tolerance to ketamine develops rapidly.

**GHB** GHB (gamma hydroxybutyrate) can be produced in clear liquid, white powder, tablet, and capsule form. GHB is a central nervous system (CNS) depressant that in large doses or when taken with alcohol can cause sedation, loss of consciousness, respiratory arrest, and death. GHB may cause prolonged and potentially life-threatening withdrawal symptoms.

**Rohypnol** Taken in tablet form, Rohypnol (flunitrazepam) is a sedative ten times more potent than Valium. Its effects, which are magnified by alcohol, include reduced blood pressure, dizziness, confusion, gastrointestinal disturbances, and loss of consciousness. Users of Rohypnol may develop physical and psychological dependence on the drug.

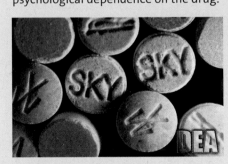

Rohypnol, GHB, and several other club drugs are sometimes used as "date-rape drugs." They can be surreptitiously added to beverages and unknowingly consumed by intended rape victims. In addition to depressant effects, some club drugs also cause *anterograde amnesia*, the loss of memory of events that occur while under the influence of the drug. Because of concern about such drugs, Congress passed the Drug-Induced Rape Prevention and Punishment Act, which increased penalties for use of any controlled substance to aid in sexual assault.

## The Role of Drugs in Your Life

Whatever your experience has been up to now, it is likely that you will encounter drugs at some point in your life. To make sure you'll have the inner resources to resist peer pressure and make your own decision, cultivate a variety of activities you enjoy doing, realize that you are entitled to have your own opinion, and keep your self-esteem high.

Before you try a psychoactive drug, consider the following questions:

- *What are the risks involved?* Many drugs carry an immediate risk of injury or death or legal consequences. Most carry long-term risk of abuse and dependence.
- *Is using the drug compatible with your goals?* Consider how drug use will affect your education

and career objectives, your relationships, your future happiness, and the happiness of those who love you.

- *What are your ethical beliefs about drug use?* Consider whether using a drug would cause you to go against your personal ethics, religious beliefs, social values, or family responsibilities.
- *What are the financial costs?* Many drugs are expensive, especially if you become dependent on them.
- *Are you trying to solve a deeper problem?* Drugs will not make emotional pain go away. In the long run, they will only make it worse. If you are feeling depressed or anxious, seek help from a mental health professional instead of self-medicating with drugs.

## Ask Yourself

Have you ever tried a psychoactive drug for fun? What were your reasons for trying it? Who was with you, and what were the circumstances? What was your experience like? What would you tell someone else who was thinking about trying the drug?

## ALCOHOL

You have probably noticed that alcohol seems to affect different people in different ways. One person seems to get drunk after just a drink or two, while another is able to tolerate a great deal of alcohol without apparent effect. These differences help explain why there are so many misconceptions about alcohol use. The following sections describe how alcohol works in the body, as well as the short- and long-term effects of alcohol use and abuse.

## Chemistry and Metabolism

**Ethyl alcohol** is the psychoactive ingredient in all alcoholic beverages. The concentration of alcohol varies with the type of beverage; it is indicated by the **proof value**, which is two times the percentage concentration. For example, if a beverage is 80 proof, it contains 40% alcohol. When alcohol consumption is discussed, **one drink** (a *standard drink)* refers to a 12-ounce bottle of beer, a 5-ounce glass of table wine, or a cocktail with 1.5 ounces of 80-proof liquor. Each of these drinks contains approximately 0.6 ounce of alcohol.

When consumed, alcohol is absorbed into the bloodstream from the stomach and small intestine. Once in the bloodstream, alcohol is distributed throughout the body's tissues, affecting nearly every body system (Figure 13.2). The main site of alcohol metabolism is the liver, which transforms alcohol into energy and other products.

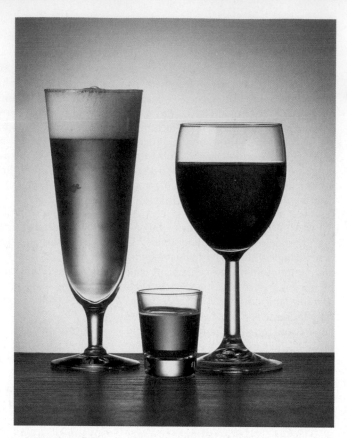

Ethyl alcohol is the common psychoactive drug in all alcoholic beverages. One drink—a 12-ounce beer, a 1.5-ounce cocktail, or a 5-ounce glass of wine—contains about 0.6 ounce of ethyl alcohol.

## Immediate Effects of Alcohol

**Blood alcohol concentration (BAC)**—the amount of alcohol in a person's blood—is a primary factor determining the effects of alcohol. BAC is determined by the amount of alcohol consumed and by individual factors such as heredity, body weight, and amount of body fat. Compared with a man who drinks the same amount of alcohol, a woman will typically have a higher BAC because of her smaller size, greater percentage of body fat, and less-active alcohol-metabolizing stomach enzymes.

Typically, the body can metabolize about half a drink in an hour. If a person drinks slightly less than that each hour, BAC remains low. People can drink large amounts of alcohol this way over a long period of time without becoming noticeably intoxicated; however, they still run the risk of significant long-term health problems. But if more alcohol is consumed than is metabolized, the BAC will increase steadily, as will the level of intoxication.

---

### KEY TERMS

**ethyl alcohol**   The intoxicating ingredient in fermented liquors; a colorless, pungent liquid.

**proof value**   Two times the percentage of alcohol in a beverage, measured by volume; a 100-proof beverage contains 50% alcohol.

**one drink**   The amount of a beverage that typically contains about 0.6 ounce of alcohol; also called a *standard drink.*

**blood alcohol concentration (BAC)**   The amount of alcohol in the blood in terms of weight per unit volume; used as a measure of intoxication.

---

### Wellness Tip

Beer contains 3–6% alcohol. Most wines are 9–14% alcohol. Hard liquor (gin, whiskey, rum, tequila, vodka, and liqueur) usually is 35–50% alcohol but can be stronger.

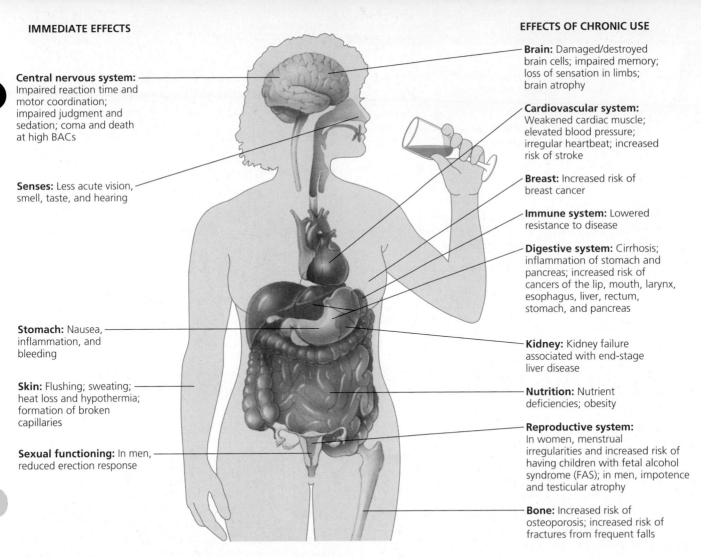

**Central nervous system:** Impaired reaction time and motor coordination; impaired judgment and sedation; coma and death at high BACs

**Senses:** Less acute vision, smell, taste, and hearing

**Stomach:** Nausea, inflammation, and bleeding

**Skin:** Flushing; sweating; heat loss and hypothermia; formation of broken capillaries

**Sexual functioning:** In men, reduced erection response

**Brain:** Damaged/destroyed brain cells; impaired memory; loss of sensation in limbs; brain atrophy

**Cardiovascular system:** Weakened cardiac muscle; elevated blood pressure; irregular heartbeat; increased risk of stroke

**Breast:** Increased risk of breast cancer

**Immune system:** Lowered resistance to disease

**Digestive system:** Cirrhosis; inflammation of stomach and pancreas; increased risk of cancers of the lip, mouth, larynx, esophagus, liver, rectum, stomach, and pancreas

**Kidney:** Kidney failure associated with end-stage liver disease

**Nutrition:** Nutrient deficiencies; obesity

**Reproductive system:** In women, menstrual irregularities and increased risk of having children with fetal alcohol syndrome (FAS); in men, impotence and testicular atrophy

**Bone:** Increased risk of osteoporosis; increased risk of fractures from frequent falls

**FIGURE 13.2** **The immediate and long-term effects of alcohol use.**

| Table 13.3 | Effects of Alcohol | |
|---|---|---|
| **BLOOD ALCOHOL CONCENTRATION (%)** | **COMMON BEHAVIORAL EFFECTS** | **HOURS REQUIRED TO METABOLIZE ALCOHOL** |
| 0.00–0.05 | Slight change in feelings, usually relaxation and euphoria; decreased alertness | 2–3 |
| 0.05–0.10 | Emotional instability with exaggerated feelings and behavior; reduced social inhibitions; impairment of reaction time and fine motor coordination; increasing impairment while driving. Legally drunk at 0.08% in all states. | 3–6 |
| 0.10–0.15 | Unsteadiness in standing and walking; loss of peripheral vision. Driving is extremely dangerous. | 6–10 |
| 0.15–0.30 | Staggering gait; slurred speech; impairment of pain perception and other sensory perceptions. | 10–24 |
| More than 0.30 | Stupor or unconsciousness; anesthesia. Death possible at 0.35% and above. Can result from rapid or binge drinking with few earlier effects. | More than 24 |

Low doses of alcohol induce relaxation and release inhibitions. Higher doses lead to less pleasant effects, including flushing and sweating; disturbed sleep; and hangover, characterized by headache, nausea, and generalized discomfort (Table 13.3). The combination of impaired judgment, weakened sensory perception, reduced inhibitions, impaired motor coordination, and, often, increased aggressiveness and hostility that characterizes alcohol intoxication can be dangerous or even deadly. Alcohol use contributes to over 50% of all

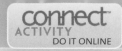

# Dealing with an Alcohol Emergency

**TAKE CHARGE**

Being very drunk is potentially life-threatening. Helping a drunken friend could save a life.

- Be firm but calm. Don't engage the person in an argument or discuss her drinking behavior while she is intoxicated.

- Get the person out of harm's way. Don't let him drive or wander outside. Don't let him drink anymore alcohol.

- If the person is unconscious, don't assume she is just "sleeping it off." Place her on her side with her knees up. This position helps prevent choking if she vomits.

- Stay with the person; you need to be ready to help if he vomits or stops breathing.

- Don't try to give the person anything to eat or drink, including coffee or other drugs. Don't give cold showers or try to make her walk around. None of these things help to sober up someone, and they can be dangerous.

Call 9-1-1 immediately in any of the following instances:

- You can't wake up the person even by shouting or shaking.

- The person is taking fewer than eight breaths per minute, or his breathing seems shallow or irregular.

- You think the person took other drugs in addition to alcohol.

- The person has had an injury, especially a blow to the head.

- The person drank a large amount of alcohol within a short time and then became unconscious. Death from alcohol poisoning most often occurs when the blood alcohol level rises very quickly due to rapid ingestion of alcohol.

If you aren't sure what to do, call 9-1-1. You may save a life.

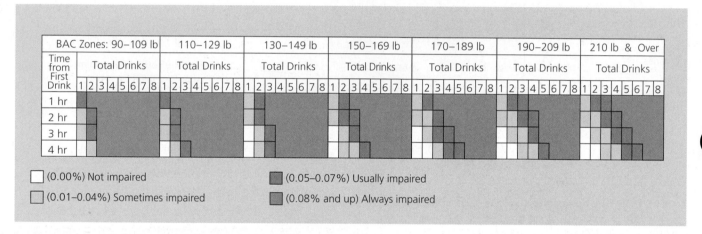

Legend:
- ☐ (0.00%) Not impaired
- ☐ (0.01–0.04%) Sometimes impaired
- ■ (0.05–0.07%) Usually impaired
- ■ (0.08% and up) Always impaired

**FIGURE 13.3 Approximate blood alcohol concentration and body weight.**
This chart shows the BAC an average person of a given weight would reach after drinking the specified number of drinks in the time shown. The legal limit for BAC is 0.08%. For drivers under 21 years of age, many states have zero-tolerance laws that set BAC limits of 0.01% or 0.02%.

murders, assaults, and rapes. Alcohol is frequently found in the bloodstreams of victims as well as perpetrators. In 2007, more than 2.6 million arrests were made for alcohol-related offenses. Through homicide, suicide, car crashes, and other incidents, alcohol use is linked to more than 75,000 American deaths a year. Alcohol poisoning is also a risk: Drinking large amounts of alcohol over a short time can rapidly raise the BAC into the lethal range (see the box "Dealing with an Alcohol Emergency").

## Drinking and Driving

People who drink and drive are unable to drive safely because their judgment is impaired, their reaction time is slower, and their coordination is reduced. In 2008, 11,773 Americans were killed in accidents involving drivers with a BAC of 0.08% or higher—about 32% of traffic fatalities

that year. Each year, more than 275,000 people are injured in alcohol-related car crashes. In the 2009 National Survey on Drug Use and Health, 16.6% of Americans age 18–20 admitted to using alcohol before driving.

In addition to increasing the risk of injury and death, driving while intoxicated can have serious legal consequences. The legal limit for BAC in all states is 0.08%; however, alcohol impairs the user even at much lower BACs (Figure 13.3). States now also have zero-tolerance laws regarding alcohol use by drivers under age 21. Under these laws, a young driver who has consumed any alcohol can have his or her license suspended. There are stiff penalties for drunk driving, including fines, loss of license, confiscation of vehicle, and jail time.

If you are out drinking, find an alternative means of transportation or follow the practice of having a designated driver—someone who refrains from drinking in order to provide safe transportation home for others in the group.

It's more difficult to protect yourself against a drunk driver. Learn to be alert to the erratic driving that signals an impaired driver. Warning signs include making wide, abrupt, and illegal turns; straddling the center line or lane marker; driving against traffic; driving on the shoulder; weaving, swerving, or nearly striking an object or another vehicle; following too closely; driving at erratic speeds; driving with headlights off at night; and driving with the window down in very cold weather.

## Effects of Chronic Alcohol Abuse

The average life span of alcohol abusers is 15 years shorter than that of nonabusers. **Cirrhosis**, a major cause of death in the United States, is one result of continued alcohol use. In this condition, liver cells are destroyed and replaced with fibrous scar tissue. Alcohol can also inflame the pancreas, causing nausea, vomiting, abnormal digestion, and severe abdominal pain. Although moderate doses of alcohol (one drink or less per day for women, and one to two drinks per day for men) may slightly reduce the chances of heart attack in some people, high doses are associated with cardiovascular problems, including high blood pressure and a weakening of the heart muscle. Alcohol is a known human carcinogen and is causally related to oral cancer; cancers of the esophagus, liver, stomach, and pancreas; and possibly breast cancer. Chronic alcohol abuse has also been linked to asthma, gout, diabetes, recurrent infections, nutritional deficiencies, and nervous system diseases. Psychiatric problems associated with excessive alcohol use include paranoia and memory gaps. Chronic drinking causes brain damage and impaired mental functioning in some people.

Maternal drinking during pregnancy can result in miscarriage, stillbirth, or **fetal alcohol syndrome (FAS).** Children with this syndrome are small at birth, are likely to have heart defects, and often have abnormal features such as small, wide-set eyes. Many are mentally impaired; others exhibit more subtle problems with learning and fine motor coordination. FAS is the most common preventable cause of mental retardation in the Western world. Full-blown FAS occurs in up to 15 out of every 10,000 live births in the United States. Many more babies are born with alcohol-related neurodevelopmental disorder (ARND). These children appear physically normal but often have learning and behavioral problems and are more likely as adults to develop substance abuse and legal problems. Getting drunk just one time during the final three months of pregnancy, when the fetus's brain cells are developing rapidly, can cause fetal brain damage. The safest course of action is to abstain from alcohol during pregnancy.

## Alcohol Abuse

**Alcohol abuse** is defined as recurrent alcohol use that has negative consequences, such as drinking in dangerous situations (such as before driving), or drinking patterns that result in academic, professional, interpersonal, or legal difficulties. **Alcohol dependence**, or **alcoholism**, involves more extensive problems with alcohol use, usually including physical tolerance and withdrawal. Various experts use different definitions to describe problems associated with drinking. The important point is that one does not have to be an alcoholic to have problems with alcohol. The person who drinks only once a month, perhaps after an exam, but then drives while intoxicated is an alcohol abuser. (Lab 13.1 includes an assessment to help you determine if alcohol is a problem in your life.)

How can you tell if you or someone you know is becoming alcohol-dependent? Look for the following warning signs:

- Drinking alone or secretively
- Using alcohol deliberately and repeatedly to perform or get through difficult situations
- Using alcohol as a way to "self-medicate" in order to dull strong emotions or negative feelings
- Feeling uncomfortable on certain occasions when alcohol is not available
- Escalating alcohol consumption beyond an already established drinking pattern
- Consuming alcohol heavily in risky situations, such as before driving
- Getting drunk regularly or more frequently than in the past
- Drinking in the morning or at other unusual times

## Binge Drinking

The National Institute on Alcohol Abuse and Alcoholism (NIAAA) defines **binge drinking** as a pattern of alcohol use that brings a person's BAC up to 0.08% or above (typically four drinks for men or three drinks for women), consumed within about 2 hours. The National Survey on

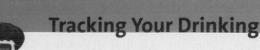

## Tracking Your Drinking

Many college students drink too much, but the best way to decide whether you do is to actually track your drinking habits over the course of time. Every time you drink over the next 2 weeks, log it in the following table, and make a note about the circumstances under which you drank. Remember to use the definition of "standard" drinks as you track your drinking; this will help you accurately determine how much alcohol you are actually consuming.

| WEEK 1 | | | | WEEK 2 | | |
|---|---|---|---|---|---|---|
| DAY | NO. OF DRINKS | CIRCUMSTANCES | | DAY | NO. OF DRINKS | CIRCUMSTANCES |
| Mon. | | | | Mon. | | |
| Tues. | | | | Tues. | | |
| Weds. | | | | Weds. | | |
| Thur. | | | | Thur. | | |
| Fri. | | | | Fri. | | |
| Sat. | | | | Sat. | | |
| Sun. | | | | Sun. | | |

Completing this log will also help you complete the log in Lab 13.1.

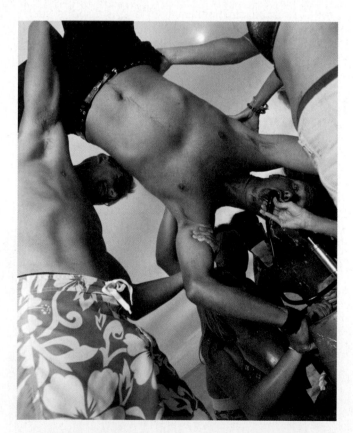

Binge drinking is very common among American college students.

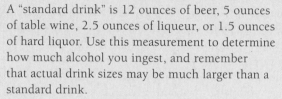

### Wellness Tip

A "standard drink" is 12 ounces of beer, 5 ounces of table wine, 2.5 ounces of liqueur, or 1.5 ounces of hard liquor. Use this measurement to determine how much alcohol you ingest, and remember that actual drink sizes may be much larger than a standard drink.

Drug Use and Health defines binge drinking as having five or more drinks within about 2 hours at least once within 30 days. The 2009 survey estimated that nearly 24% of Americans over the age of 12 were binge drinkers. Almost 7% were heavy drinkers, defined as having five or more drinks on the same occasion on each of 5 or more days in the past 30 days.

According to the NIAAA, 80% of all college students drink, including 60% of students age 18–20. More than 40% of college students binge drink. Binge drinking is a common form of alcohol abuse on college campuses, and it has a profound effect on students' lives. Frequent binge drinkers were found to be three to seven times more likely than nonbinge drinkers to engage in unplanned or unprotected sex, to drive after drinking, and to get hurt or injured. Binge drinkers were also more likely to miss classes, get behind in schoolwork, and argue with their friends. The more frequent the binges, the more problems the students encountered. Despite their experiences, fewer than 1% of the binge drinkers identify themselves as problem drinkers.

# Drinking Behavior and Responsibility

The responsible use of alcohol includes understanding your own attitudes and behaviors, managing your behavior, and encouraging responsible behavior in others.

## Examine Your Attitudes and Behavior

• **Consider your feelings about alcohol and drinking.** Do you care if alcohol is available at social activities? Do you consider it essential, or are you indifferent to its presence or absence? How do you feel about people who don't drink?

• **Consider where your attitudes toward drinking and alcohol come from.** How was alcohol used in your family when you were growing up? How is it used—or how do you think it is used—on your campus? How is it portrayed in ads? In other words, what influences might be shaping your alcohol use?

• **Consider your own drinking behavior.** If you drink, what are your reasons? Is your drinking moderate and responsible? Or do you drink too much and experience negative consequences?

## Drink Moderately and Responsibly

• **Drink slowly and space your drinks.** Sip your drinks and alternate them with nonalcoholic choices. Don't drink alcoholic beverages to quench your thirst. Avoid drinks made with carbonated mixers. Watch your drinks being poured or mixed so that you can be sure of what you're drinking.

• **Eat before and while drinking.** Don't drink on an empty stomach. Food in your stomach will slow the rate at which alcohol is absorbed and thus often lower the peak BAC.

• **Know your limits and your drinks.** Learn how different BACs affect you and how to keep your BAC under control.

• **Be aware of the setting.** In dangerous situations, such as driving, abstinence is the only appropriate choice.

• **Use designated drivers.** Arrange carpools to and from parties or events where alcohol will be served. Rotate the responsibility for acting as a designated driver.

• **Learn to enjoy activities without alcohol.** If you can't have fun without drinking, you may have a problem with alcohol.

## Encourage Responsible Drinking in Others

• **Encourage responsible attitudes.** Learn to express disapproval about someone who has drunk too much. Don't treat the choice to abstain as strange. The majority of American adults drink moderately or not at all.

• **Be a responsible host.** Serve only enough alcohol for each guest to have a moderate number of drinks, and offer nonalcoholic choices. Always serve food along with alcohol. Stop serving alcohol an hour or more before people will leave. Insist that a guest who drank too much take a taxi, ride with someone else, or stay overnight rather than drive.

• **Hold drinkers fully responsible for their behavior.** Pardoning unacceptable behavior fosters the attitude that the behavior is due to the drug rather than the person.

• **Take community action.** Find out about prevention programs on your campus or in your community. Consider joining an action group such as Students Against Destructive Decisions (SADD) or Mothers Against Drunk Driving (MADD).

# Alcoholism

As described earlier, alcoholism is usually characterized by tolerance and withdrawal. Everyone who drinks—even nonalcoholics—develops tolerance to alcohol after repeated use. When alcoholics stop drinking or cut their intake significantly, they have withdrawal symptoms, which can range from unpleasant to serious and even life-threatening distress. Symptoms of alcohol withdrawal include trembling hands (shakes, or jitters), a rapid pulse and breathing rate, insomnia, nightmares, anxiety, and gastrointestinal upset. Less common are seizures and the severe reaction known as the **DTs (delirium tremens),** characterized by confusion and vivid, usually unpleasant, hallucinations.

Some alcoholics recover without professional help, but the majority do not. Treatment is difficult. However, many different kinds of programs exist, including those that emphasize group and buddy support, those

that stress lifestyle management, and those that use drugs and chemical substitutes as therapy. Although not all alcoholics can be treated successfully, considerable optimism has replaced the older view that nothing can be done.

# Drinking and Responsibility

The responsible use of alcohol means drinking in a way that keeps your BAC low and your behavior under control. See the box "Drinking Behavior and Responsibility" for specific suggestions.

---

**DTs (delirium tremens)** A state of confusion brought on by the reduction of alcohol intake in an alcohol-dependent person; other symptoms are sweating, trembling, anxiety, hallucinations, and seizures.

# TOBACCO

According to the U.S. Surgeon General, smoking is the leading preventable cause of illness and death in the United States. Each year, 440,000 Americans die prematurely from smoking-related causes; tobacco use accounts for nearly one of every five adult deaths. Millions of Americans suffer chronic illnesses (such as cancer and heart disease) as a result of smoking. Tobacco in any form—cigarettes, cigars, pipes, chewing tobacco, clove cigarettes, or snuff—is unsafe.

Despite its well-known hazards, tobacco use is still widespread in our society (Table 13.4). According to the 2009 National Survey on Drug Use and Health, about 69.7 million Americans are tobacco users, including nearly 42% of college-age Americans. Thousands more join their ranks every day—including an estimated 1000 people under age 18.

## Nicotine Addiction

Regular tobacco use, and especially cigarette smoking, is not just a habit but an addiction, involving physical dependence on the psychoactive drug **nicotine**. Addicted tobacco users must keep a steady amount of nicotine circulating in the blood and going to the brain, where the drug triggers the release of powerful chemical messengers and causes a wide range of physical and emotional changes. If that amount falls below a certain level, they experience withdrawal symptoms that can include cravings, insomnia, confusion, tremors, difficulty concentrating, fatigue, muscle pains, headache, nausea, irritability, anger, and depression.

## Health Hazards of Cigarette Smoking

Cigarette smoking has negative effects on nearly every part of the body and increases the risk of many

### VITAL STATISTICS

| Table 13.4 | Who Smokes? | | |
|---|---|---|---|

| | PERCENTAGE OF SMOKERS | | |
|---|---|---|---|
| | MEN | WOMEN | TOTAL |
| **ETHNIC GROUP (AGE ≥ 18)** | | | |
| White | 24.5 | 19.8 | 22.1 |
| Black | 23.9 | 19.2 | 21.3 |
| Asian | 16.9 | 7.5 | 12.0 |
| American Indian/ Alaska Native | 29.7 | N/A | 23.2 |
| Latino | 19.0 | 9.8 | 14.5 |
| **EDUCATION (AGE ≥ 25)** | | | |
| < 8 years | 22.2 | 11.9 | 17.1 |
| 9–11 years | 36.5 | 30.5 | 33.6 |
| 12 years (no diploma) | 34.1 | 23.3 | 28.5 |
| GED | 53.2 | 44.7 | 49.1 |
| High school graduate | 29.0 | 21.5 | 25.1 |
| Associate degree | 20.6 | 19.1 | 19.7 |
| Undergraduate degree | 12.4 | 9.9 | 11.1 |
| Graduate degree | 4.9 | 6.3 | 5.6 |
| TOTAL | **23.5** | **17.9** | **20.6** |

**SOURCE:** Centers for Disease Control and Prevention. 2010. Vital Signs: Current cigarette smoking among adults aged ≥ 18 years—United States, 2009. *Morbidity and Mortality Weekly Report* 59(35): 1135–1140.

life-threatening diseases. Some of the many damaging chemicals in tobacco are carcinogens and cocarcinogens (agents that can combine with other chemicals to promote cancer). Others irritate the tissues of the respiratory system. Carbon monoxide, the deadly gas in automobile exhaust, is present in cigarette smoke in concentrations 400 times greater than the safety threshold set in workplaces. Low-tar and low-nicotine cigarettes deliver just as dangerous a dose of these chemicals as regular cigarettes because smokers inhale more deeply and frequently.

The effects of nicotine on smokers vary, depending on the size of the dose and the smoker's past smoking behavior. Nicotine can either excite or tranquilize the nervous system, generally resulting in stimulation that gives way to tranquility and then depression. Figure 13.4 summarizes the immediate effects of smoking.

In the short term, smoking interferes with the functions of the respiratory system and often leads rapidly to

**KEY TERM**

**nicotine** A poisonous, addictive substance found in tobacco and responsible for many of the effects of tobacco.

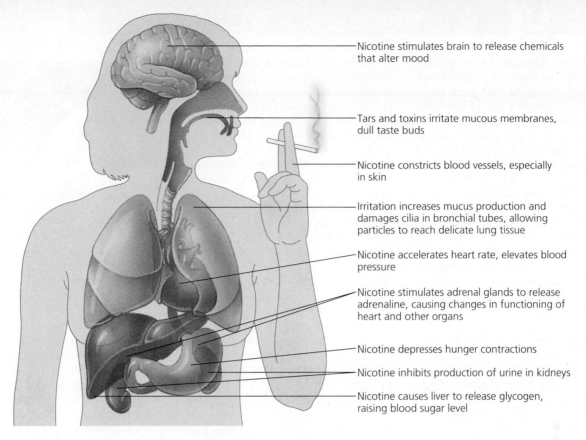

Nicotine stimulates brain to release chemicals that alter mood

Tars and toxins irritate mucous membranes, dull taste buds

Nicotine constricts blood vessels, especially in skin

Irritation increases mucus production and damages cilia in bronchial tubes, allowing particles to reach delicate lung tissue

Nicotine accelerates heart rate, elevates blood pressure

Nicotine stimulates adrenal glands to release adrenaline, causing changes in functioning of heart and other organs

Nicotine depresses hunger contractions

Nicotine inhibits production of urine in kidneys

Nicotine causes liver to release glycogen, raising blood sugar level

**FIGURE 13.4**   **The short-term effects of smoking a cigarette.**

shortness of breath and the conditions known as smoker's throat, smoker's cough, and smoker's bronchitis. Other common short-term complaints are loss of appetite, diarrhea, fatigue, hoarseness, weight loss, stomach pains, insomnia, and impaired visual acuity, especially at night.

Long-term effects fall into two general categories. The first is reduced life expectancy: On average, smokers lose about 14 years of life. The second category of long-term effects involves quality of life. Smokers have higher rates of acute and chronic diseases than those who have never smoked. The more people smoke, and the deeper and more often they inhale, the greater the risk of disease and other complications. Cigarette smoking increases the risk of all the following:

- Cardiovascular disease (coronary heart disease, heart attack, stroke, hypertension, high cholesterol levels), lung disease (emphysema, chronic bronchitis), osteoporosis, diabetes, and many types of cancer (lung, trachea, mouth, pharynx, esophagus, larynx, pancreas, bladder, kidney, breast, cervix, stomach, liver, colon)
- Tooth decay, gum disease, bad breath, colds, ulcers, hair loss, facial wrinkling, and discolored teeth and fingers

- Menstrual disorders, early menopause, impotence, infertility, stillbirth, and low birth weight (see the box "Gender and Tobacco Use")
- Motor vehicle crashes and fire-related injuries

When smokers quit, health improvements begin almost immediately. The younger people are when they stop smoking, the more pronounced are these improvements (see the box "Benefits of Quitting Smoking").

## Other Forms of Tobacco Use

Many smokers have switched from cigarettes to other forms of tobacco, such as cigars, pipes, clove cigarettes, and spit (smokeless) tobacco. However, these alternatives are far from safe.

**Cigars and Pipes**  Cigar and pipe smokers are at increased risk for many health problems, including cardiovascular and respiratory diseases and many types of cancer. Cigars contain more tobacco than cigarettes and so contain more nicotine and produce more tar when smoked. Cigar smokers who don't inhale have a six-times greater risk of throat cancer than nonsmokers; their risk of heart and lung disease approaches that of cigarette

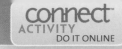

American men are currently more likely than women to smoke, but as the rate of smoking among women approaches that of men, so do rates of tobacco-related illness and death. Lung cancer, emphysema, and cardiovascular diseases sicken and kill both men and women who smoke, and more American women now die each year from lung cancer than from breast cancer.

Although overall risks for tobacco-related illness are similar for women and men, sex appears to make a difference in some diseases. Women, for example, are more at risk for smoking-related blood clots and strokes than are men, and the risk is even greater for women using oral contraceptives. Among men and women with the same smoking history, the odds of developing three major types of cancer, including lung cancer, are 1.2–1.7 times higher for women than men. Women may also have a greater biological vulnerability to lung cancer.

Tobacco use also is associated with sex-specific health problems. Men who smoke increase their risk of erectile dysfunction and infertility. Women who smoke have higher rates of osteoporosis (a bone-thinning disease that can lead to fractures), thyroid-related diseases, and depression.

Women who smoke also have risks associated with reproduction and the reproductive organs. Smoking is associated with greater menstrual bleeding, greater duration of painful menstrual cramps, and more variability in menstrual cycle length. Smokers have a more difficult time becoming pregnant, and they reach menopause on average a year or two earlier than nonsmokers. When women smokers become pregnant, they face increased chances of miscarriage, placental disorders, premature delivery, ectopic pregnancy, preeclampsia, and stillbirth. Smoking is a risk factor for cervical cancer, too.

Women are less successful than men in quitting. Women report more severe withdrawal symptoms when they stop

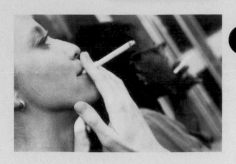

smoking and are more likely than men to report cravings in response to social and behavioral cues associated with smoking. For men, relapse to smoking is often associated with work or social pressure; women are more likely to relapse when sad or depressed or concerned about weight gain. Women and men also respond differently to medications: Nicotine replacement therapy appears to work better for men, whereas the non-nicotine medication bupropion appears to work better for women.

smokers. The risks are even higher for cigar smokers who inhale.

**Clove Cigarettes and Bidis** Clove cigarettes, imported from Indonesia and Pakistan, are made of tobacco mixed with chopped cloves. Also known as *kreteks*, they contain almost twice as much tar, nicotine, and carbon monoxide as conventional cigarettes. Some chemical constituents of cloves can be dangerous, and there have been a number of severe respiratory injuries and deaths from smoking clove cigarettes.

*Bidis*, or "beadies," are small cigarettes imported from India that contain a type of tobacco different from that used in U.S. cigarettes; they are rolled in ebony leaves and often flavored. Bidis contain up to four times more nicotine and twice as much tar as U.S. cigarettes.

**Spit (Smokeless) Tobacco** Spit tobacco comes in two main forms: snuff and chewing tobacco. Both forms have high levels of nicotine, and use can lead to nicotine addiction. Snuff is tobacco in the form of a coarse, moist powder, mixed with flavorings. The user places a pinch of tobacco between the lower lip or cheek and gum and sucks it. Long-term snuff use may increase the risk of cancer of the cheek and gums by as much as 50 times.

Chewing tobacco is in the form of shredded leaves, pressed into bricks or cakes or twisted into ropelike strands. The user places a wad of tobacco in the mouth and chews or sucks it, spitting out or swallowing the tobacco juice. Spit tobacco causes bad breath, tooth decay, and gum disease. One of the most serious effects of chewing tobacco is the increased risk of oral cancer—cancers of the lip, tongue, cheek, throat, gums, roof and floor of the mouth, and larynx.

**E-Cigarettes** The latest trend in smoking is the electronic cigarette, or *e-cig*. The e-cig is a battery-powered device that resembles a real cigarette. Instead of containing tobacco, the device uses a changeable filter that contains one or more chemicals, such as nicotine, flavorings, and other compounds. The user "smokes" an e-cig by sucking the filtered end; the device's battery heats the chemicals to create an inhalable vapor. During use, the device's tip even glows like the burning end of a real cigarette.

Marketers of e-cigs have claimed that the devices deliver only nicotine, making them a safe cigarette that does not cause cancer, and which can serve as an alternative to other nicotine replacement products such as gum and patches. According to the U.S. Food and Drug Administration (FDA), however, not all e-cigs actually contain nicotine.

# Benefits of Quitting Smoking

**Within 20 minutes of your last cigarette:**

- You stop polluting the air
- Blood pressure drops to normal
- Pulse rate drops to normal
- Temperature of hands and feet increases to normal

**8 hours:**

- Carbon monoxide level in blood drops to normal
- Oxygen level in blood increases to normal

**24 hours:**

- Chance of heart attack decreases

**48 hours:**

- Nerve endings start regrowing
- Ability to smell and taste is enhanced

**2 weeks–3 months:**

- Circulation improves
- Walking becomes easier
- Lung function increases up to 30%

**1–9 months:**

- Coughing, sinus congestion, fatigue, and shortness of breath all decrease

**1 year:**

- Heart disease risk declines to half that of a smoker

**5 years:**

- Stroke risk drops nearly to the risk for nonsmokers

**10 years:**

- Lung cancer death rate drops to 50% of that of continuing smokers
- Incidence of other cancers (mouth, throat, larynx, esophagus, bladder, kidney, and pancreas) decreases
- Risk of ulcer decreases

**15 years:**

- Risk of lung cancer is about 25% of that of continuing smokers
- Risks of heart disease and death are close to those of nonsmokers

## Wellness Tip

The Department of Health and Human Services classifies ETS as a "known human carcinogen," and the U.S. Surgeon General warns that there is no safe level of exposure to secondhand smoke.

Further, the FDA has warned consumers not to purchase or use e-cigs, after analysis of nearly 20 e-cig cartridges revealed they contained carcinogens, including at least one of the same carcinogens found in real cigarettes. Several samples contained a toxic chemical used in antifreeze.

## Environmental Tobacco Smoke

**Environmental tobacco smoke (ETS),** commonly called *secondhand smoke,* consists of **mainstream smoke,** the smoke exhaled by smokers, and **sidestream smoke,** the smoke that enters the atmosphere from the burning end of the cigarette, cigar, or pipe. Undiluted sidestream smoke is unfiltered by a cigarette filter or a smoker's lungs, so it contains significantly higher concentrations of toxic and carcinogenic compounds than mainstream smoke.

Nearly 85% of the smoke in a room where someone is smoking is sidestream smoke. Even though such smoke is diffuse, the concentrations can be considerable. In rooms where people are smoking, levels of carbon monoxide, for instance, can exceed those permitted by Federal Air Quality Standards for outside air.

**Effects of ETS** ETS is a known human carcinogen. ETS causes 3400 lung cancer deaths and about 46,000 deaths from heart disease each year in people who do not smoke. ETS also contributes to heart disease and aggravates respiratory conditions such as allergies and asthma.

Scientists have been able to measure changes capable of contributing to lung tissue damage and potential tumor promotion in the bloodstreams of healthy young test subjects who spent 3 hours in a smoke-filled room. After just 30 minutes of exposure to ETS, the function in the coronary arteries of healthy nonsmokers is reduced to the same level as that of smokers. And nonsmokers can still be affected by the harmful effects of ETS hours after they have left a smoky environment. Carbon monoxide, for example, lingers in the bloodstream for 5 hours.

**environmental tobacco smoke (ETS)** Smoke that enters the atmosphere from the burning end of a cigarette, cigar, or pipe, as well as smoke that is exhaled by smokers; also called *secondhand smoke.*

**mainstream smoke** Smoke that is inhaled by a smoker and then exhaled into the atmosphere.

**sidestream smoke** Smoke that enters the atmosphere from the burning end of a cigarette, cigar, or pipe.

**Children and ETS** Infants and children are particularly vulnerable to the harmful effects of ETS. Because they breathe faster than adults, they inhale more air and more of the pollutants it contains. Because they weigh less than adults, children inhale proportionately more pollutants per unit of body weight.

ETS triggers bronchitis, pneumonia, and other respiratory infections in infants and toddlers up to 18 months old, resulting in as many as 15,000 hospitalizations each year. Older children suffer, too. ETS can induce asthma in children and exacerbate symptoms in children who already have asthma.

**Avoiding ETS** If you are a nonsmoker, you have the right to breathe clean air, free from tobacco smoke. Try these strategies to keep the air around you safe:

- *Speak up tactfully.* Try something like, "Would you mind putting your cigarette out or moving to another spot? The smoke is bothering me."
- *Don't allow smoking in your home or room.* Get rid of ashtrays and ask smokers to light up outside.
- *Open a window.* If you cannot avoid being in a room with smokers, try to provide some ventilation.
- *Sit in the nonsmoking section in restaurants and other public areas.* Complain to the manager if none exists.
- *Fight for a smoke-free work environment.* For your sake and that of your coworkers, join with others either to eliminate all smoking indoors or to confine it to certain areas.
- *Discuss quitting strategies.* Social pressure is a major factor in many former smokers' decision to quit.

## Smoking and Pregnancy

Smoking almost doubles a pregnant woman's chance of having a miscarriage, and women who smoke also face an increased risk of **ectopic pregnancy.** Maternal smoking causes an estimated 4600 infant deaths in the United States each year, primarily due to premature delivery and smoking-related problems with the placenta, the organ that delivers blood, oxygen, and nutrients to the fetus. Infants whose mothers smoked during pregnancy are also more likely to die from sudden infant death syndrome (SIDS). Maternal smoking

> **ectopic pregnancy** A pregnancy in which the fertilized egg implants itself in an oviduct rather than in the uterus; the embryo must be surgically removed.

is a major factor in low birth weight, which puts newborns at high risk for infections and other potentially fatal problems.

Babies born to mothers who smoke more than two packs a day perform poorly on developmental tests in the first hours after birth when compared with babies of nonsmoking mothers. Later in life, obesity, hyperactivity, short attention span, and lower scores on spelling and reading tests all occur more frequently in children whose mothers smoked throughout pregnancy than in those born to nonsmoking mothers. Nevertheless, about 16% of pregnant women smoke throughout pregnancy.

## Action Against Tobacco

Individuals and communities have taken action against this major health threat. Thousands of local ordinances have been passed across the United States banning or restricting smoking in restaurants, stores, and other public places. Communities are also restricting many forms of tobacco advertising, such as billboards.

Action at the state level can have a significant effect. For example, California has one of the nation's most aggressive tobacco control programs, combining taxes on cigarettes, graphic ads, and bans on smoking in bars and restaurants. In the past decade, per-capita cigarette consumption fell by 50% in California, which now has the second lowest rate of smoking in the United States (Utah has the lowest rate). Both lung cancer cases and heart disease deaths have also declined in California.

Many states, as well as the federal government, have filed lawsuits against the tobacco industry to reclaim money spent on tobacco-related health care. A 1998 agreement requires the tobacco companies to pay states $206 billion over 25 years. For these and other reasons, tobacco consumption in the United States is declining among some groups. In response, the U.S. tobacco industry has increased its efforts to sell in foreign markets, especially in developing nations with few restrictions on tobacco advertising.

In 2009, Congress passed legislation granting the FDA regulatory powers over the packaging, marketing, and manufacturing of tobacco products, something the tobacco industry had fought for years. The Family Smoking Prevention and Tobacco Control Act cracks down on tobacco marketing to children and adolescents and prohibits the use of terms such as *light* and *low-tar* to describe products. Under the bill, manufacturers are required to use larger warning labels on cigarette packages, list cigarette ingredients on packages, and disclose changes in products as well as research findings. In addition, the FDA has the authority to require changes such as the removal of harmful ingredients.

# Smoking Cessation Products

Each year, millions of Americans visit their doctors in the hope of finding a drug that will help them stop smoking. Although pharmacological options are limited, the few available drugs have proved successful.

## Chantix (Varinicline)

The newest smoking cessation drug, marketed under the name Chantix, works in two ways: It reduces nicotine cravings, easing the withdrawal process, and it blocks the pleasant effects of nicotine. The drug acts on neurotransmitter receptors in the brain.

Unlike most smoking cessation products currently on the market, Chantix is not a nicotine replacement. For this reason, smokers may be advised to continue smoking for the first few days of treatment, to avoid withdrawal and to allow the drug to build up in their system. The approved course of treatment is 12 weeks, but the duration and recommended dosage depend on several factors, including the smoker's general health and the length and severity of his or her nicotine addiction.

Side effects reported with Chantix include nausea, headache, vomiting, sleep disruptions, and changes in taste perception. People with kidney problems or who take certain medications should not take Chantix, and it is not recommended for women who are pregnant or nursing. In 2008, the FDA issued a public health advisory warning that some Chantix users suffered adverse reactions, such as behavioral changes, agitation, depression, suicidal thoughts, and attempted suicide. Anyone taking Chantix should notify his or her doctor immediately of any sudden change in mood or behavior.

## Zyban (Bupropion)

Bupropion is an antidepressant (prescribed under the name Wellbutrin) as well as a smoking cessation aid (prescribed under the name Zyban). As a smoking cessation aid, bupropion eases the symptoms of nicotine withdrawal and reduces the urge to smoke. Like Chantix, it acts on neurotransmitter receptors in the brain.

Because the drug is not a nicotine replacement, the user may need to continue smoking for the first few days of treatment. A nicotine replacement product, such as a patch or gum, may be recommended to further ease withdrawal symptoms after the user stops smoking.

Bupropion users have reported an array of side effects, but they are rare. Side effects may be reduced by changing the dosage, taking the medicine at a different time of day, or taking it with or without food. Bupropion is not recommended for people with specific physical conditions or who take certain drugs. Zyban and Wellbutrin should not be taken together.

## Nicotine Replacement Products

The most widely used smoking cessation products replace the nicotine that the user would normally get from tobacco. The user continues to get nicotine, so withdrawal symptoms and cravings are reduced. Although still harmful, nicotine replacement products provide a cleaner form of nicotine, without the poisons and tars produced by burning tobacco. Less of the product is used over time, as the need for nicotine decreases.

Nicotine replacement products come in several forms, including patches, gum, lozenges, nasal sprays, and inhalers. They are available in a variety of strengths and can be worked into many different smoking cessation strategies. Most are available without a prescription.

# Giving Up Tobacco

Giving up tobacco is a long-term, difficult process, usually accompanied by psychological craving and physical withdrawal. Research shows that most tobacco users move through predictable stages—from being uninterested in stopping, to thinking about change, to making a concerted effort to stop, to finally maintaining abstinence. Most users attempt to quit several times before they finally succeed. Relapse is a normal part of the process, as with most behavior change plans. Quitting is an ongoing process, not a single event.

Quitting requires a strategy for success. Some people quit cold turkey, while others taper off slowly. There are over-the-counter and prescription products that help many people (see the box "Smoking Cessation Products"). Behavioral factors that have been shown to increase the chances of a smoker's permanent smoking cessation are support from others and regular exercise (see the box "How Does Exercise Help a Smoker Quit?"). Support can come from friends and family, Web sites, and/or formal group programs sponsored by organizations such as the American Cancer Society and the American Lung Association or by a college health center or community hospital.

If you are trying to quit, keeping track of cravings and urges in a health journal can help you deal with them. (Lab 13.2 can help identify your smoking triggers.) When you have an urge to use tobacco, use a relaxation technique, take a brisk walk, chew gum, or substitute some other activity. Practice stress management and time management so you don't get overwhelmed at school or work. Eat sensibly and get enough sleep. Quitting can be hard, but the benefits are lifelong.

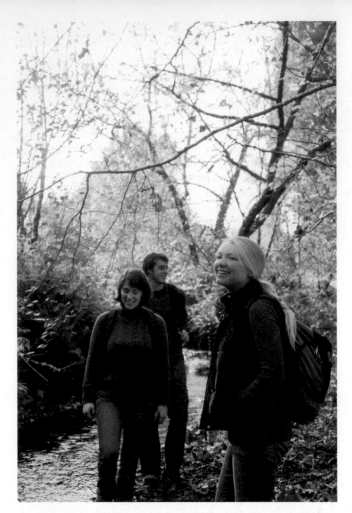

Regular physical activity and social support can make it easier to stop smoking.

## TIPS FOR TODAY AND THE FUTURE

The best treatment for dependence is prevention—not starting in the first place—but it's never too late to regain control of your life.

### RIGHT NOW YOU CAN

- Carefully consider your use of drugs, alcohol, or tobacco —if any—and decide whether this is the time for you to stop. If it is, throw away the offending products.
- List five things you can do instead of giving in to the temptation to use a drug, alcohol, or tobacco.

### IN THE FUTURE YOU CAN

- Look for local resources that can help you stop using drugs, alcohol, or tobacco. Your school may offer counseling or support services, such as a smoking cessation program. It can also be informative and inspiring to attend an Alcoholics Anonymous (AA) meeting.
- Track your progress toward quitting for good. Use a journal to record your cravings or urges and to describe the tactics you use to overcome them.

## Ask Yourself

### QUESTIONS FOR CRITICAL THINKING AND REFLECTION

Despite all the information available about the dangers of tobacco use, one-fifth of Americans still smoke. Why do you think this is the case? In your experience, what influences a person's decision to start smoking?

## SUMMARY

- Addictive behaviors are habits that have gotten out of control and have a negative impact on a person's health. Characteristics of addictive behaviors include reinforcement, craving, loss of control, escalation, and negative consequences.

- Drug abuse is a maladaptive pattern of drug use that persists despite adverse social, psychological, or medical consequences. Drug dependence involves taking a drug compulsively; tolerance and withdrawal symptoms are often present.

- Factors to consider when deciding whether to try a psychoactive drug include short- and long-term risks of drug use, your future goals and ethical beliefs, the financial cost of the drug, and your reasons for drug use.

- At low doses, alcohol causes relaxation; at higher doses, it interferes with motor and mental functioning and is associated with injuries; at very high doses, alcohol poisoning, coma, and death can occur.

- Continued alcohol use has negative effects on the digestive and cardiovascular systems and increases cancer risk and overall mortality. Women who drink while pregnant risk giving birth to children with fetal alcohol syndrome.

- Alcohol abuse involves drinking in dangerous situations or drinking to a degree that causes academic, professional, interpersonal, or legal difficulties.

- Alcohol dependence, or alcoholism, is characterized by more extensive problems with alcohol, usually involving tolerance and withdrawal.

- Binge drinking is a common form of alcohol abuse on college campuses that has negative effects on both drinking and nondrinking students.

- Nicotine is the addictive psychoactive drug in tobacco products.

- In the short term, smoking can either excite or tranquilize the nervous system; it also interferes with the functions of the respiratory system. Long-term effects of smoking include higher rates of acute and chronic diseases and reduced life expectancy.

- Other forms of tobacco use—cigars, pipes, clove cigarettes, and spit tobacco—also have serious associated health risks.

# How Does Exercise Help a Smoker Quit?

Most smokers trying to quit experience hard-to-manage cravings for tobacco that make it difficult to stay with their plan. A growing body of evidence shows that exercise can help people handle these cravings and resist relapse.

For example, a 2009 study looked at how exercise affects self-reported cravings in smokers following 15 hours of nicotine abstinence. The study also used MRI scanning to assess activation in various parts of the brain associated with reward, motivation, and attention. The researchers found that after only 10 minutes of moderate-intensity exercise, smokers reported lower cravings in response to smoking images, and MRI scans showed less activation in associated parts of the brain. Although the study was small, it confirmed previous evidence that a single session of exercise can reduce cigarette cravings. The study also provided the first evidence of a shift in regional brain activation in response to smoking cues following exercise.

Another study, from 2007, showed that smokers' withdrawal symptoms and nicotine cravings decreased significantly during a single bout of aerobic exercise and remained measurably lower for nearly an hour after exercising. The positive effects were seen whether participants exercised vigorously or at a low level of exertion. An earlier study conducted by the American College of Sports Medicine showed that moderate-intensity physical activity can be a useful adjunct to standard smoking cessation treatment. This study revealed that the more smokers exercised, the less likely they were to resume smoking.

Not all research has provided similar results. In fact, numerous studies have shown no difference in quit rates between smokers who exercise and those who don't. Even so, many experts believe that physicians and therapists should prescribe an appropriate level of physical activity to their patients who want to quit smoking.

As described in the chapter, the physical benefits of quitting smoking are tremendous. Regular physical activity enhances some of these benefits, such as improved lung function, blood pressure, and overall fitness. The jury is still out, however, on whether exercise further decreases the risk of certain diseases (including heart disease and cancer) among current and former smokers, beyond the risk reduction achieved simply by quitting smoking. A great deal of research is being done on this question.

Many smokers worry about weight gain associated with quitting. Although most ex-smokers gain a few pounds, at least temporarily, incorporating exercise into a new, tobacco-free lifestyle lays the foundation for healthy weight management. Research findings vary on the effect of exercise on weight gain after quitting smoking, but at least one new study shows that while exercise might not reduce short-term weight gain among new ex-smokers, physical activity does produce weight loss over the long term. Regardless, the health risks of adding a few pounds are far outweighed by the risks of continued smoking. According to one estimate, an ex-smoker would have to gain 75–100 pounds to equal the health risks of smoking a pack of cigarettes a day.

SOURCES: Parsons, A. C., et al. 2009. Interventions for preventing weight gain after smoking cessation. *Cochrane Database of Systematic Reviews* (Online) (1): CD006219; Taylor, A. H., et al. 2007. The acute effects of exercise on cigarette cravings, withdrawal symptoms, affect and smoking behavior: A systematic review. *Addiction* 102(4): 534–543; Van Rensburg, J. K., et al. 2009. Acute exercise modulates cigarette cravings and brain activation in response to smoking-related images: An fMRI study. *Psycho-pharmacology* 203(3): 589–598; Williams, D. M., et al. 2005. The effect of moderate intensity exercise on smoking cessation. *Medicine and Science in Sports and Exercise* 35(7) Supplement May 2005: S175.

THE EVIDENCE FOR EXERCISE

- Environmental tobacco smoke contains toxic and carcinogenic compounds in high concentrations. It causes health problems, including cancer and heart disease, in nonsmokers exposed to it; infants and children are especially at risk.

- Many approaches and products are available to aid people in quitting smoking.

## FOR FURTHER EXPLORATION

### BOOKS

Brandt, A. M. 2009. *The Cigarette Century: The Rise, Fall, and Deadly Persistence of the Product That Defined America, First Reprint ed.* New York: Basic Books. *A detailed study of the cigarette's impact on American history and Americans' efforts to overcome the addictive power of smoking.*

Carr, A. 2010. *The Easy Way to Stop Smoking.* New York: Sterling. *A best-selling self-help book for smokers who want to stop.*

Herrick, C. 2007. *100 Questions & Answers About Alcoholism & Drug Addiction.* Boston: Jones and Bartlett. *Answers a range of specific questions about alcohol abuse, dependence, and treatment options.*

Karch, S. B. 2006. *Drug Abuse Handbook,* 2nd ed. London: CRC Press. *Explores drug abuse from a variety of perspectives, including clinical and criminological.*

Kinney, J. 2009. *Loosening the Grip: A Handbook of Alcohol Information,* 9th ed. New York: McGraw-Hill. *A fascinating book about alcohol, including information on physical effects, abuse, alcoholism, and cultural aspects of alcohol use.*

Ksir, C., C. L. Hart, and O. S. Ray. 2008. *Drugs, Society, and Human Behavior,* 12th ed. New York: McGraw-Hill. *Examines drugs from the behavioral, pharmacological, historical, social, legal, and clinical perspectives.*

U.S. Institute of Medicine. 2007. *Ending the Tobacco Problem: A Blueprint for the Nation.* Washington, D.C.: National Academies Press. *Reviews tobacco policy and public approaches to stopping smoking.*

## Q Is there anything I can do for someone I know who has a drug problem?

**A** If you believe a friend or family member has a drug problem, obtain information about resources for drug treatment available on your campus or in your community. Communicate your concern, provide information about treatment options, and offer your support during treatment.

If the person denies having a problem, you may want to talk with an experienced counselor about setting up an intervention—a formal, structured confrontation designed to end denial by having family, friends, and other caring individuals present their concerns to the drug user. Participants in an intervention point out the ways in which the abuser is hurting others as well as him- or herself. If your friend or family member agrees to treatment, encourage him or her to attend a support group such as Narcotics Anonymous or Alcoholics Anonymous.

In addition, examine your relationship with the abuser for signs of codependency. A *codependent* is someone whose actions help or enable a person to remain dependent on a drug by removing or softening the effects of the drug use on the user. Common actions by codependents include making excuses or lying for someone, loaning money to someone to continue drug use, and not confronting someone who is obviously intoxicated or high on a drug.

The habit of enabling can prevent a person from experiencing the consequences of her or his behavior and so delay recovery. If you see yourself developing a codependent relationship, get help for yourself. Al-Anon and Alateen are organizations dedicated to helping people who are affected by someone else's drinking.

## Q Does drinking coffee help an intoxicated person sober up more quickly?

**A** No. Once alcohol is absorbed into the body, there are no ways to accelerate its breakdown. The rate of alcohol metabolism varies among individuals, largely as a result of heredity, but it is not affected by caffeine, exercise, fresh air, or other stimulants. To sober up, you simply have to wait until your body has had sufficient time to metabolize all the alcohol you have consumed.

## Q Is it true that marijuana can be used medically?

**A** Yes, although its use is restricted. Even though marijuana is considered an illegal drug in the United States and some other countries, there is a growing movement to make it legally available to treat certain illnesses and medical conditions. A report issued in 1999 by the National Academy of Sciences' Institute of Medicine found that marijuana appears to be helpful in treating pain, nausea, AIDS-related weight loss, muscle spasms in multiple sclerosis, and other problems. Many cancer patients and people with AIDS use marijuana because they find it effective in relieving nausea and restoring appetite. Research is under way to find methods of administering the drug that don't subject the user to the hazards of cancer, lung damage, and emphysema.

*For more Common Questions Answered about tobacco, alcohol, and other drugs, visit the Online Learning Center at www.mhhe.com/fahey.*

## ORGANIZATIONS, HOTLINES, AND WEB SITES

*Action on Smoking and Health (ASH).* Provides statistics, news briefs, and other information about smoking.
http://www.ash.org

*Al-Anon Family Group Headquarters.* Provides information and referrals to local Al-Anon and Alateen groups.
http://www.al-anon.org

*Alcoholics Anonymous (AA) World Services.* Provides information on AA, literature on alcoholism, and information about AA meetings.
http://www.aa.org

*American Cancer Society (ACS).* Sponsor of the annual Great American Smokeout; provides information on the dangers of tobacco, as well as tools for preventing and stopping the use of tobacco products.
http://www.cancer.org

*American Lung Association.* Provides information on lung diseases, tobacco control, and environmental health.
http://www.lungusa.org

*American Psychiatric Association: College Age Students.* Covers a variety of mental health issues affecting college students, including alcohol abuse and treatment.
http://www.healthyminds.org/More-Info-For/College-Age-Students.aspx

*CDC: Smoking and Tobacco Use.* Provides educational materials and tips on how to quit smoking.
http://www.cdc.gov/tobacco

*Facts on Tap.* Provides information about alcohol and college life, and sex and alcohol, as well as tips for students who have been negatively affected by other students' alcohol use.
http://www.factsontap.org

*Higher Education Center for Alcohol and Other Drug Abuse and Violence Prevention.* Provides information about alcohol and drug abuse on campus and links to related sites.
http://www.higheredcenter.org

*National Clearinghouse for Alcohol and Drug Information.* Provides statistics, information, and publications on substance abuse, including resources for people who want to help friends and family members overcome substance-abuse problems.

http://ncadi.samhsa.gov

*National Institute on Alcohol Abuse and Alcoholism (NIAAA)*. Provides booklets and other publications on a variety of alcohol-related topics, including fetal alcohol syndrome, alcoholism treatment, and alcohol use and minorities.

http://www.niaaa.nih.gov

*National Institute on Drug Abuse*. Develops and supports research on drug abuse prevention programs; fact sheets on drugs of abuse are available on the Web site.

http://www.drugabuse.gov

*Quitnet*. Provides interactive tools and questionnaires, support groups, a library, and the latest news on tobacco issues.

http://www.quitnet.org

*Smokefree.gov*. Provides step-by-step strategies for quitting as well as expert support via telephone or instant messaging.

http://www.smokefree.gov

The following hotlines provide support and referrals:

800-ALCOHOL

800-662-HELP

## SELECTED BIBLIOGRAPHY

Addolorato, G., et al. 2006. Baclofen: A new drug for the treatment of alcohol dependence. *International Journal of Clinical Practice* 60(8): 1003–1008.

American Cancer Society. 2011. *Cancer Facts and Figures, 2011*. Atlanta, Ga.: American Cancer Society.

American Lung Association. 2010. Trends in Tobacco Use (www.lungusa.org/finding-cures/our-research/trend-reports/Tobacco-Trend-Report.pdf; retrieved May 23, 2011).

American Lung Association. 2010. State of Tobacco Control 2009. New York: American Lung Association.

American Psychiatric Association. 2000. *Diagnostic and Statistical Manual of Mental Disorders*, 4th ed., text revision. (DSM-IV-TR). Washington, D.C.: American Psychiatric Association.

Anton, R. F., et al. 2006. Combined pharmacotherapies and behavioral interventions for alcohol dependence: The COMBINE study: A randomized controlled trial. *Journal of the American Medical Association* 295(17): 2003–2017.

Beers, M. H., et. al. 2006. *The Merck Manual of Diagnosis and Therapy*, 18th ed. New York: Wiley.

Centers for Disease Control and Prevention. 2008. Surveillance for cancers associated with tobacco use—United States, 1999–2004. *Morbidity and Mortality Weekly Report* 57(SS-08): 1–33.

Centers for Disease Control and Prevention. 2009. Alcohol Use Among Pregnant and Nonpregnant Women of Childbearing Age: United States, 1991–2005. *Morbidity and Mortality Weekly Report* 58(19): 529–532.

Centers for Disease Control and Prevention. 2009. Cigarette smoking among adults and trends in smoking cessation—United States, 2008. *Morbidity and Mortality Weekly Report* 58(44): 1227–1232.

Centers for Disease Control and Prevention. 2010. Alcohol and Public Health (http://www.cdc.gov/alcohol/index.htm; retrieved May 23, 2011).

Centers for Disease Control and Prevention. 2010. Vital Signs: Current cigarette smoking among adults aged ≥ 18 years—United States, 2009. *Morbidity and Mortality Weekly Report* 59(35): 1135–1140.

Centers for Disease Control and Prevention. 2010. Vital Signs: Nonsmokers' exposure to secondand smoke—United States, 1999–2009. *Morbidity and Mortality Weekly Report* 59(35): 1141–1146.

Centers for Disease Control and Prevention. 2010. Youth risk behavior surveillance—United States, 2009. *Morbidity and Mortality Weekly Report* 59(SS-05): 1–148.

Centers for Disease Control and Prevention. 2010. Smoking and Tobacco Use Fact Sheet: Tobacco-Related Mortality (http://www.cdc.gov/tobacco/data_statistics/fact_sheets/health_effects/tobacco_related_mortality; retrieved May 23, 2011).

Clifasefi, S. L., et al. 2006. Blind drunk: The effects of alcohol on inattentional blindness. *Applied Cognitive Psychology* 20(5): 697–704.

College Drinking Prevention. 2010. A Snapshot of Annual High-Risk College Drinking Consequences (http://www.collegedrinkingprevention.gov/StatsSummaries/snapshot.aspx; retrieved May 23, 2011).

Collins, G. B., et al. 2006. Drug adjuncts for treating alcohol dependence. *Cleveland Clinic Journal of Medicine* 73(7): 641–644.

Costello, R. M. 2006. Long-term mortality from alcoholism: A descriptive analysis. *Journal of Studies on Alcohol* 67(5): 694–699.

Department of Health and Human Services. 2007. *The Surgeon General's Call to Action to Prevent and Reduce Underage Drinking*. Washington, D.C.: Department of Health and Human Services, Office of the Surgeon General.

Fiore, M. C., et al. 2008. *Treating Tobacco Use and Dependence: 2008 Update. Clinical Practice Guideline*. Rockville, Md.: U.S. Department of Health and Human Services, Public Health Service.

Food and Drug Administration. 2008. Consumer Update: New Safety Warnings for Chantix (http://www.fds.gov/consumer/updates/chantix020508.html; retrieved May 23, 2011).

Grant, J. E., et al. 2006. Multicenter investigation of the opioid antagonist nalmefene in the treatment of pathological gambling. *American Journal of Psychiatry* 163(2): 303–312.

Gruenewald, P. J., and L. Remer. 2006. Changes in outlet densities affect violence rates. *Alcoholism: Clinical and Experimental Research* 30(7): 1184–1193.

Heilig, M., and M. Egli. 2006. Pharmacological treatment of alcohol dependence: Target symptoms and target mechanisms. *Pharmacology and Therapeutics* 111(3): 855–876.

Hingson, R. W., et al. 2006. Age at drinking onset and alcohol dependence: Age at onset, duration, and severity. *Archives of Pediatrics and Adolescent Medicine* 160(7): 739–746.

Iannone, M., et al. 2006. Electrocortical effects of MDMA are potentiated by acoustic stimulation in rats. *BMC Neuroscience* 7: 13.

Kim, S. W., et al. 2006. Pathological gambling and mood disorders: Clinical associations and treatment implications. *Journal of Affective Disorders* 92(1): 109–116.

Krampe, H., et al. 2006. Follow-up of 180 alcoholic patients for up to 7 years after outpatient treatment: Impact of alcohol deterrents on outcome. *Alcohol: Clinical and Experimental Research* 30(1): 86–95.

Mannino, D. M., and A. S. Buist. 2007. Global burden of COPD: Risk factors, prevalence, and future trends. *Lancet* 370(9589): 765–773.

Mayo Clinic. 2006. Pain relievers and alcohol: A potentially risky combination. *Mayo Clinic Health Letter*, May.

Messinis, L., et al. 2006. Neuropsychological deficits in long-term frequent cannabis users. *Neurology* 66(5): 737–739.

Miller, T. R., et al. 2006. Societal costs of underage drinking. *Journal of Studies on Alcohol* 67(4): 519–528.

National Council on Problem Gambling. 2010. What Is Problem Gambling? (http://www.ncpgambling.org/i4a/pages/index.cfm?pageid=1; retrieved May 23, 2011).

National Institute on Drug Abuse. 2008. *Comorbidity: Addiction and Other Mental Illnesses*. Bethesda, Md.: National Institute on Drug Abuse, NIH Publication No. 08-5771.

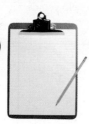

### LAB 13.1   Is Alcohol a Problem in Your Life?

## Part I   Do You Have a Problem with Alcohol?

For each question, choose the answer that best describes your behavior. Then total your scores.

| Questions | Points | | | | | Your Score |
|---|---|---|---|---|---|---|
| | **0** | **1** | **2** | **3** | **4** | |
| 1. How often do you have a drink containing alcohol? | Never | Monthly or less | 2 to 4 times a month | 2 to 3 times a week | 4 or more times a week | _____ |
| 2. How many drinks containing alcohol do you have on a typical day when you are drinking? | 1 or 2 | 3 or 4 | 5 or 6 | 7 to 9 | 10 or more | _____ |
| 3. How often do you have six or more drinks on one occasion? | Never | Less than monthly | Monthly | Weekly | Daily or almost daily | _____ |
| 4. How often during the past year have you found that you were not able to stop drinking once you had started? | Never | Less than monthly | Monthly | Weekly | Daily or almost daily | _____ |
| 5. How often during the past year have you failed to do what was normally expected from you because of drinking? | Never | Less than monthly | Monthly | Weekly | Daily or almost daily | _____ |
| 6. How often during the past year have you needed a first drink in the morning to get yourself going after a heavy drinking session? | Never | Less than monthly | Monthly | Weekly | Daily or almost daily | _____ |
| 7. How often during the past year have you had a feeling of guilt or remorse after drinking? | Never | Less than monthly | Monthly | Weekly | Daily or almost daily | _____ |
| 8. How often during the past year have you been unable to remember what happened the night before because you had been drinking? | Never | Less than monthly | Monthly | Weekly | Daily or almost daily | _____ |
| 9. Have you or has someone else been injured as a result of your drinking? | No | Yes, but not in the past year (2 points) | | Yes, during the past year (4 points) | | _____ |
| 10. Has a relative or friend or a doctor or other health worker been concerned about your drinking or suggested you cut down? | No | Yes, but not in the past year (2 points) | | Yes, during the past year (4 points) | | _____ |

**Total** _____

A total score of 8 or more indicates a strong likelihood of hazardous or harmful alcohol consumption.

connect™  http://www.mcgrawhillconnect.com/
FITNESS AND WELLNESS

## Part II   Are You Troubled by Someone's Drinking?

Millions of people are affected by the excessive drinking of someone close to them. The following questions are designed to help you decide whether you need Al-Anon. If you answer yes to any question, put a check next to it.

_____ 1. Do you worry about how much someone else drinks?

_____ 2. Do you have money problems because of someone else's drinking?

_____ 3. Do you tell lies to cover up for someone else's drinking?

_____ 4. Do you feel that if the drinker cared about you, he or she would stop drinking to please you?

_____ 5. Do you blame the drinker's behavior on his or her companions?

_____ 6. Are plans frequently upset or canceled or meals delayed because of the drinker?

_____ 7. Do you make threats, such as, "If you don't stop drinking, I'll leave you"?

_____ 8. Do you secretly try to smell the drinker's breath?

_____ 9. Are you afraid to upset someone for fear it will set off a drinking bout?

_____ 10. Have you been hurt or embarrassed by a drinker's behavior?

_____ 11. Are holidays and gatherings spoiled because of drinking?

_____ 12. Have you considered calling the police for help because of fear of abuse?

_____ 13. Do you search for hidden alcohol?

_____ 14. Do you often ride in a car with a driver who has been drinking?

_____ 15. Have you refused social invitations out of fear or anxiety?

_____ 16. Do you feel like a failure because you can't control the drinker?

_____ 17. Do you think that if the drinker stopped drinking, your other problems would be solved?

_____ 18. Do you ever threaten to hurt yourself to scare the drinker?

_____ 19. Do you feel angry, confused, or depressed most of the time?

_____ 20. Do you feel there is no one who understands your problems?

If you answered yes to three or more of these questions, Al-Anon or Alateen may be able to help.

## Using Your Results

*How did you score?* (1) What is your alcohol use assessment score from Part I? Are you surprised by your score? Does your score indicate a problem?

(2) Did the Al-Anon quiz indicate that you are affected by someone else's excessive drinking? Are you surprised by the result?

*What should you do next?* If your alcohol use assessment score indicates hazardous or harmful alcohol consumption, or if you are encountering drinking-related problems with your academic performance, job, relationships, or health, or with the law, you should consider seeking help. Check for campus or community resources, including counseling, self-help groups, AA, and formal treatment programs.

If you are troubled by someone else's drinking, you can contact Al-Anon or Alateen by looking in your local telephone directory or contacting Al-Anon's main office (1600 Corporate Landing Parkway, Virginia Beach, VA 23454; 800-344-2666; http://www.al-anon.org).

SOURCES: Part I from Saunders, J. B., et al. 1993. Development of the Alcohol Use Disorders Identification Test (AUDIT): WHO Collaborative Project on Early Detection of Persons with Harmful Alcohol Consumption—II. *Addiction* 88: 791–804, June. Carfax Publishing Ltd. Reprinted with permission from Blackwell Publishing. Part II from Are You Troubled by Someone's Drinking? (http://www.al-anon.alateen.org/quiz.html). Copyright © 1980 Al-Anon Family Group Headquarters, Inc. Reprinted by permission of Al-Anon Family Group Headquarters, Inc.

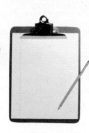

# LAB 13.2  For Smokers Only: Why Do You Smoke?

Although smoking cigarettes is physiologically addictive, people smoke for reasons other than nicotine craving. What kind of smoker are you? Knowing what your motivations and satisfactions are can ultimately help you quit. This test is designed to provide you with a score on each of six factors that describe many people's smoking. Read the statements and then circle the number that represents how often you feel this way when you smoke cigarettes. Be sure to answer each question.

| | | Always | Frequently | Occasionally | Seledom | Never |
|---|---|---|---|---|---|---|
| A. | I smoke cigarettes to keep myself from slowing down. | 5 | 4 | 3 | 2 | 1 |
| B. | Handling a cigarette is part of the enjoyment of smoking it. | 5 | 4 | 3 | 2 | 1 |
| C. | Smoking cigarettes is pleasant and relaxing. | 5 | 4 | 3 | 2 | 1 |
| D. | I light up a cigarette when I feel angry about something. | 5 | 4 | 3 | 2 | 1 |
| E. | When I have run out of cigarettes, I find it almost unbearable until I can get them. | 5 | 4 | 3 | 2 | 1 |
| F. | I smoke cigarettes automatically without even being aware of it. | 5 | 4 | 3 | 2 | 1 |
| G. | I smoke cigarettes for stimulation, to perk myself up. | 5 | 4 | 3 | 2 | 1 |
| H. | Part of the enjoyment of smoking a cigarette comes from the steps I take to light up. | 5 | 4 | 3 | 2 | 1 |
| I. | I find cigarettes pleasurable. | 5 | 4 | 3 | 2 | 1 |
| J. | When I feel uncomfortable or upset about something, I light up a cigarette. | 5 | 4 | 3 | 2 | 1 |
| K. | I am very much aware of the fact when I am not smoking a cigarette. | 5 | 4 | 3 | 2 | 1 |
| L. | I light up a cigarette without realizing I still have one burning in the ashtray. | 5 | 4 | 3 | 2 | 1 |
| M. | I smoke cigarettes to get a "lift." | 5 | 4 | 3 | 2 | 1 |
| N. | When I smoke a cigarette, part of the enjoyment is watching the smoke as I exhale it. | 5 | 4 | 3 | 2 | 1 |
| O. | I want a cigarette most when I am comfortable and relaxed. | 5 | 4 | 3 | 2 | 1 |
| P. | When I feel "blue" or want to take my mind off cares and worries, I smoke cigarettes. | 5 | 4 | 3 | 2 | 1 |
| Q. | I get a real gnawing hunger for a cigarette when I haven't smoked for a while. | 5 | 4 | 3 | 2 | 1 |
| R. | I've found a cigarette in my mouth and didn't remember putting it there. | 5 | 4 | 3 | 2 | 1 |

## How to Score

Enter the numbers you have circled in the spaces provided. Total the scores on each line. Total scores can range from 3 to 15. Any score of 11 or above is high; any score of 7 or below is low.

|  |  |  |  |  |  |  | Totals |
|---|---|---|---|---|---|---|---|
| _____ A | + | _____ G | + | _____ M | = | _____ | Stimulation |
| _____ B | + | _____ H | + | _____ N | = | _____ | Handling |
| _____ C | + | _____ I | + | _____ O | = | _____ | Pleasurable relaxation |
| _____ D | + | _____ J | + | _____ P | = | _____ | Crutch: tension reduction |
| _____ E | + | _____ K | + | _____ Q | = | _____ | Craving: strong physiological or psychological addition |
| _____ F | + | _____ L | + | _____ R | = | _____ | Habit |

## Using Your Results

*How did you score?* For which factors did you score the highest? Are you surprised by the results of the assessment?

*What should you do next?* Use the information from this assessment to help plan a successful approach for quitting. The six factors measured by this test describe ways of experiencing or managing certain kinds of feelings. The higher your score on a particular factor, the more important that factor is in your smoking, and the more useful the tips below will be in your attempt to quit. Highlight or make a list of the strategies that seem most helpful to you and post the list in a prominent place.

**Stimulation:** If you score high on this factor, it means you are stimulated by a cigarette—you feel that it helps wake you up, organize your energies, and keep you going. If you try to give up smoking, you may want a safe substitute—a brisk walk or moderate exercise, for example—whenever you feel the urge to smoke.

**Handling:** Handling things can be satisfying, but there are many ways to keep your hands busy without lighting up or playing with a cigarette. Try doodling or toying with a pen, pencil, or other small object.

**Pleasurable relaxation:** Those who do get real pleasure from smoking often find that an honest consideration of the harmful effects of their habit is enough to help them quit. They substitute social or physical activities and find they do not seriously miss their cigarettes.

**Crutch:** Many smokers use cigarettes as a kind of crutch in moments of stress or discomfort, and occasionally it may work; but heavy smokers are apt to discover that cigarettes do not help them deal with their problems effectively. When it comes to quitting, this kind of smoker may find it easy to stop when everything is going well but may be tempted to start again in a time of crisis. Physical exertion or social activity may serve as a useful substitute for cigarettes.

**Craving:** Quitting smoking is difficult for people who score high on this factor. It may be helpful for them to smoke more than usual for a day or two, so that the taste for cigarettes is spoiled, and then isolate themselves completely from cigarettes until the craving is gone.

**Habit:** These smokers light up frequently without even realizing it; they no longer get much satisfaction. They may find it easy to quit and stay off if they can break the habit patterns they have built up. The key to success is becoming aware of each cigarette when it's smoked. Ask, "Do I really want this cigarette?"

SOURCES: National Institutes of Health. 1990. *Why Do You Smoke?* NIH Pub. no. 90-1822. U.S. Department of Health and Human Services. Public Health Service.

# CHAPTER 14

# Sexually Transmitted Diseases

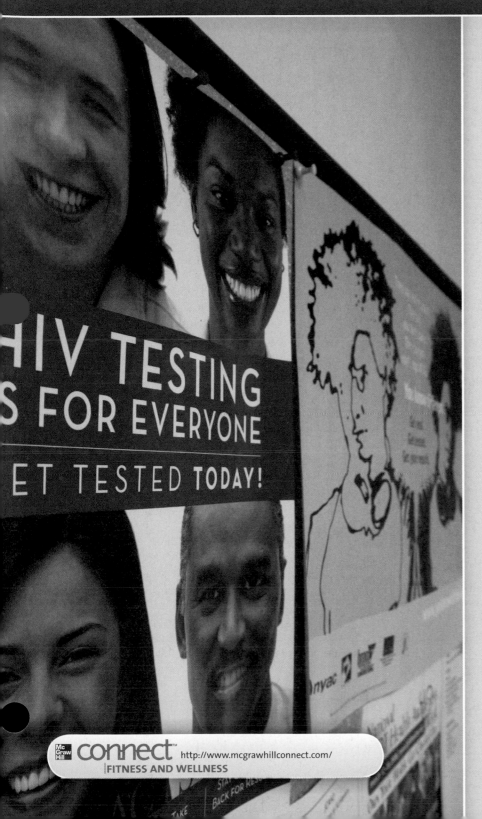

## LOOKING AHEAD...

After reading this chapter, you should be able to:

- Explain how HIV infection affects the body and how it is transmitted, diagnosed, and treated
- Discuss the symptoms, risks, and treatments of other major STDs
- List strategies for protecting yourself from STDs

## TEST YOUR KNOWLEDGE

1. Worldwide, HIV infection is spread primarily via which of the following?
   a. injection drug use
   b. sex between men
   c. mother-to-child transmission
   d. heterosexual sex

2. A man with an STD is more likely to transmit the infection to a female partner than vice versa. True or false?

3. After you have had an STD once, you become immune to that disease and cannot get it again. True or false?

**Answers**

1. **d.** The vast majority of HIV infection cases worldwide result from heterosexual contact, and the majority of new cases occur in teenage girls and young women.

2. **True.** For many STDs, infected men are at least twice as likely as infected women to transmit the disease to their partner.

3. **False.** Reinfection with STDs is very common. For example, if you are treated for and cured of chlamydia and then you have sex with your untreated partner, the chances are very good that you will be infected again.

**C**onsidering the intimate nature of sexual activity, it is not surprising that many diseases can be transmitted from one person to another through sexual contact. Of course, colds, influenza, and many other infections can spread from one sexual partner to another, but sexual contact is not the primary means of transmission for these illnesses. **Sexually transmitted diseases (STDs)**—also called **sexually transmitted infections (STIs)**—spread from person to person mainly through sexual activity. STDs are a particularly insidious group of illnesses because a person can be infected and able to transmit a disease, yet not look or feel sick; this is why the term *sexually transmitted infection (STI)* is coming into common use.

STDs can be prevented. Many STDs can also be cured if treated early and properly. This chapter introduces the major forms of STDs. It also provides information about healthy, safer sexual behavior to help you understand how to reduce the further spread of these diseases.

## THE MAJOR STDs

The following seven STDs pose a major health threat:

- HIV/AIDS
- Chlamydia
- Gonorrhea
- Human papillomavirus (HPV)
- Herpes
- Hepatitis
- Syphilis

These diseases are considered major threats because they are serious in themselves, cause serious complications if left untreated, and pose risks to a fetus or newborn. STDs often result in serious long-term consequences, including chronic pain, infertility, stillbirths, genital cancers, and death.

## Wellness Tip

STDs are caused by more than 30 different organisms, including viruses, bacteria, fungi, and protozoa.

**KEY TERMS**

**sexually transmitted disease (STD)** or **sexually transmitted infection (STI)**   A disease that can be transmitted by sexual contact; some can also be transmitted by other means.

**human immunodeficiency virus (HIV)**   The virus that causes HIV infection and AIDS.

**acquired immunodeficiency syndrome (AIDS)**   A generally fatal, incurable, sexually transmitted viral disease.

**HIV infection**   A chronic, progressive viral infection that damages the immune system.

| Table 14.1 | Annual New Cases of STDs in the United States |
| --- | --- |

| STD | NEW CASES |
| --- | --- |
| Trichomoniasis | 7,400,000 |
| HPV | 6,200,000 |
| Chlamydia | 1,211,000 |
| Genital herpes | 292,000 |
| Gonorrhea | 337,000 |
| HIV infection | 56,000 |
| Hepatitis B | 46,000 |
| Syphilis (all stages) | 41,000 |

**SOURCES:** Centers for Disease Control and Prevention, National Center for HIV/AIDS, Viral Hepatitis, STD, and TB Prevention. 2008. *2006 Disease Profile* (http://www.cdc.gov/nchhstp/Publications/docs/2006_Disease_Profile_508 _FINAL.pdf; retrieved October 4, 2010); Centers for Disease Control and Prevention. 2008. *Genital HPV Infection—CDC Fact Sheet* (http://www.cdc .gov/std/hpv/stdfact-hpv.htm; retrieved October 4, 2010); Centers for Disease Control and Prevention. 2009. *Sexually Transmitted Disease Surveillance, 2008.* Atlanta, Ga.: Centers for Disease Control and Prevention.

All of these diseases have a relatively high incidence among Americans (Table 14.1). In fact, the United States has the highest rate of STDs of any developed nation; at current rates, half of all young people will acquire an STD by age 25. The Centers for Disease Control and Prevention (CDC) reports that many of the most common STDs are on the rise in the United States. In 2008, the CDC estimated that 65 million Americans were infected with an STD. About 19 million Americans become newly infected with an STD each year.

## HIV Infection and AIDS

The **human immunodeficiency virus (HIV)** causes **acquired immunodeficiency syndrome (AIDS)**, a disease that without treatment ultimately kills most of its victims. On average, with the best treatment currently available, someone with HIV infection will live 20 to 30 years or more after diagnosis. For most people infected with HIV worldwide, however, adequate treatment is not available, and most infected persons die within 10 years.

An estimated total of 65 million people have been infected since the epidemic began in 1981—nearly 1% of the world's population—and tens of millions of those people have died. Currently, about 33 million people are infected with HIV/AIDS worldwide.

Worldwide, the number of people living with HIV infection has leveled off. Many experts believe that the global HIV epidemic peaked in the late 1990s, at about 3.5 million new infections per year, compared with an estimated 2.7 million new infections in 2008. Despite a slowing of the epidemic, however, AIDS remains a primary cause of death in Africa and continues to be a major cause of mortality around the world.

# Does Exercise Help or Harm the Immune System?

Like any infectious illness, STDs attract the attention of the body's immune system—an information network operating through billions of specialized white blood cells to protect the body from disease. When an infection is detected inside the body, these cellular defenders—including lymphocytes, macrophages ("big eaters"), and "natural killer" cells, among others—spring into action. They attack invading pathogens, destroy body cells that are already infected, and prime the immune system in case of future infections by the same agent. This is even the case in HIV infection. Although HIV targets specific types of immune system cells—primarily CD4 T cells and other kinds of T cells—other immune cells pick up the fight and attempt to rid the body of the virus.

A strong immune system can help defend your body against infections, including STDs, if only by keeping the infection at bay and minimizing damage until medical therapy (such as antibiotics) can be started. Many lifestyle factors, including nutrition, sleep, and stress management, are known to support immune function. The effects of physical activity and exercise on the immune system are more complex. It appears that effects vary depending on the intensity of the activity. Research has demonstrated that moderate-intensity exercise tends to improve immune function, whereas vigorous-intensity exercise tends to impair immunity temporarily.

On the positive side, a 2008 systematic review of 17 different research studies found that regular activity, particularly aerobic exercise, enhances immune system function in otherwise healthy adults. A 2009 study of sedentary women found that positive changes occurred in immune cell function following both moderate and intense exercise, but greater changes occurred following moderate exercise, and only moderate exercise improved inflammatory response. The study also found that moderate exercise reduced levels of cortisol and other stress hormones, another mechanism by which exercise may enhance immune function (since stress is known to impair immunity). Other studies have examined the effects of exercise on specific components of the immune system (such as natural killer cells, neutrophils, and dendritic cells) and found that the overall immune system response to physical activity is positive.

On the other hand, many studies have found that people who exercise vigorously, for prolonged periods, or without proper nutrition experience temporary declines in immune system function, although full function is typically recovered in a matter of hours or days. For example, a 2009 literature review looked at the relationship among exercise, physical activity, sports training, and susceptibility to upper respiratory tract infections. The study found that intense bouts of exercise temporarily impaired immune function and that, compared with less active people, athletes experienced more upper respiratory tract infections after training and competitions.

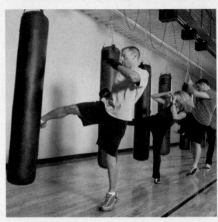

In less active people, more physical activity was associated with lower risk of upper respiratory tract infections.

These researchers point out that vulnerability to infection is influenced by many factors besides exercise, including heredity, nutrition, and general level of fitness. They also point out that the exact relationship between amount and intensity of exercise and suppression of the immune system (the dose-response relationship) is an area for further research. In other words, it isn't clear at exactly what level of exercise the immune system begins to be affected negatively. It also is not known exactly why this effect occurs.

Because of this greater susceptibility, athletes should avoid overtraining and be especially vigilant about supporting the immune system through nutrition, sleep, and other healthy lifestyle habits. For the average person, the evidence strongly indicates that regular moderate-intensity exercise promotes immune system function in many ways.

**SOURCES:** Giraldo, E., et al. 2009. Exercise intensity-dependent changes in the inflammatory response in sedentary women: Role of neuroendocrine parameters in the neutrophil phagocytic process and the pro-/anti-inflammatory cytokine balance. *Neuroimmunomodulation* 16(4): 237–244; Gavrieli, R., et al. 2008. The effect of aerobic exercise on neutrophil functions. *Medicine and Science in Sports and Exercise* 40(9): 1623–1628; Gleeson, M. 2007. Immune function in sport and exercise. *Journal of Applied Physiology* 103(2): 693–699; Haaland, D. A. 2008. Is regular exercise a friend or foe of the aging immune system? A systematic review. *Clinical Journal of Sport Medicine* 18(6): 539–548; Moreira, A., et al. 2009. Does exercise increase the risk of upper respiratory tract infections? *British Medical Bulletin* 90: 111–131.

---

In the United States, nearly 1.2 million people have been infected with HIV; about 50,000 new HIV infections are reported each year. Today, about 236,000 HIV-infected Americans are unaware of their infection. More than 576,000 Americans have died from AIDS since the start of the epidemic.

**What Is HIV Infection?** **HIV infection** is a chronic disease that progressively damages the body's immune system, making an otherwise healthy person less able to resist a variety of infections and disorders. Normally, when a virus or other pathogen enters the body, it is targeted and destroyed by the immune system. But HIV attacks the immune system itself, taking over immune system cells and forcing them to produce new copies of HIV. It also makes them incapable of performing their immune functions (see the box "Does Exercise Help or Harm the Immune System?").

The destruction of the immune system is signaled by the loss of **CD4 T cells.** As the number of CD4 T cells declines, an infected person may begin to experience mild to moderately severe symptoms. A person is diagnosed with AIDS when he or she develops one of the conditions defined as a marker for AIDS or when the number of CD4 T cells in the blood drops below a certain level (200/μl). People with AIDS are vulnerable to a number of serious—often fatal—secondary, or opportunistic, infections.

The asymptomatic period of HIV—the time between the initial viral infection and the onset of disease symptoms—may range from 2 to 20 years, with an average of 11 years in untreated adults. Most, but not all, infected people experience flulike symptoms shortly after the initial infection, but most remain generally healthy for years. During this time, however, the virus is progressively infecting and destroying the cells of the immune system. People infected with HIV can pass the virus to others—even if they have no symptoms and especially if they do not know they have been infected.

**Transmitting the Virus** HIV lives only within cells and body fluids, not outside the body. It is transmitted by blood and blood products, semen, vaginal and cervical secretions, and breast milk. It cannot live in air, in water, or on objects or surfaces such as toilet seats, eating utensils, or telephones. A person is not at risk of getting HIV infection by being in the same classroom, dining room, or even household with someone who is infected.

There are three main routes of HIV transmission:

- Specific kinds of sexual contact
- Direct exposure to infected blood
- Contact between an HIV-infected woman and her child during pregnancy, childbirth, or breastfeeding

These means of transmission are discussed in the following sections.

**SEXUAL CONTACT** HIV is more likely to be transmitted through unprotected vaginal or anal intercourse than by other sexual activities. During vaginal intercourse, male-to-female transmission is more likely to occur than female-to-male transmission. HIV has been found in preejaculatory fluid, so transmission can also occur before ejaculation. Any trauma or irritation of tissues, such as those that can occur through rough or unwanted intercourse or through the overuse of spermicides, increases the risk of HIV transmission. The presence of lesions or blisters from other STDs also makes it easier for the virus to be passed.

Oral-genital contact carries some risk of transmission, although less than vaginal or anal intercourse. The risk of HIV transmission during oral sex increases if a participant

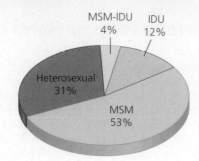

* MSM = Men who have sex with men
IDU = Injection drug users

**FIGURE 14.1  Routes of HIV transmission among Americans.**
**SOURCE:** Centers for Disease Control and Prevention. 2009. *HIV/AIDS in the United States* (http://www.cdc.gov/hiv/resources/factsheets/us.htm; retrieved August 15, 2011).

has oral sores, has poor oral hygiene practices, or brushes or flosses just before or after oral sex. Some evidence suggests that drinking alcohol before oral sex may make the cells that line the mouth more susceptible to infection with HIV.

Among Americans with AIDS, the most common means of HIV exposure is sexual activity between men; heterosexual contact and injection drug use (IDU) are the next most common (Figure 14.1).

**CONTACT WITH INFECTED BLOOD** Direct contact with infected blood is another major route of HIV transmission. Needles used to inject drugs (including heroin, cocaine, and anabolic steroids) are usually contaminated with the user's blood. If needles are shared, small amounts of one person's blood are injected into another person's bloodstream. HIV can be transmitted through subcutaneous and intramuscular injection as well, from needles or blades used in acupuncture, tattooing, ritual scarring, and piercing of any body part. About 20–25% of all new U.S. cases of HIV are caused, directly or indirectly, through the sharing of drug injection equipment contaminated with HIV.

**CONTACT BETWEEN MOTHER AND CHILD** The final major route of HIV transmission is mother-to-child, also called *vertical,* or *perinatal, transmission,* which can occur during pregnancy, childbirth, or breastfeeding. The number of new cases of HIV/AIDS among American infants has declined more than 90% since 1992 because of testing and treatment of infected women with anti-HIV drugs. Treatment is expensive, however, and vertical transmission continues to be a major threat worldwide (see the box "HIV Infection Around the World"). Cesarean

*Wellness Tip*

The American Blood Bank Association estimates that fewer than 1 in 2 million units of blood products is capable of transmitting HIV. The risk of being infected with HIV through a blood transfusion is very low, and there is no risk of infection from donating blood.

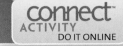
# HIV Infection Around the World

In 2011, the world marked the thirtieth year since AIDS was diagnosed in five young gay men in Los Angeles. HIV is now a worldwide scourge, with 65 million people infected and more than 25 million deaths since the epidemic began.

The vast majority of cases—95%—have occurred in developing countries, where heterosexual contact is the primary means of transmission, responsible for 85% of all adult infections. In the developed world, HIV is increasingly becoming a disease that disproportionately affects the poor and ethnic minorities. Worldwide, women are the fastest-growing group of newly infected people; half of adults living with HIV in 2008 were women. Some 2 million children now live with HIV infection, and about 15 million children are AIDS orphans.

The HIV epidemic seems to have stabilized in many parts of the world. Rates of new infections have remained steady or have even dropped in a few regions. Sub-Saharan Africa remains the hardest-hit area of the world, but even there the number of new infections dropped from 2.3 million in 2001 to 1.9 million in 2008. Despite gradual improvement, two-thirds of all HIV-infected people in the world live in Sub-Saharan Africa, and nearly three-quarters of all deaths due to AIDS in 2008 occurred there. However, treatment rates are up to 48% in eastern and southern Africa.

Eastern Europe and parts of Asia have also been hit hard by HIV. For example, former Soviet countries have seen a 50-fold increase in HIV infection in the last decade. In many of these areas, HIV infection was initially seen primarily in intravenous drug users, but in recent years sexual transmission has become much more common.

Efforts to combat AIDS are complicated by political, economic, and cultural barriers. Education and prevention programs are often hampered by resistance from social and religious institutions and by the taboo on openly discussing sexual issues. Condoms are not commonly used in many countries, and women in many societies do not have sufficient control over their lives to demand that men use condoms during sex. Successful prevention approaches include STD treatment and education, public education campaigns about safer sex, and syringe exchange programs for injection drug users.

In countries where there is a substantial imbalance in the social power of men and women, empowering women is a crucial priority in reducing the spread of HIV. In particular, reducing sexual violence against women, allowing women property and inheritance rights, and increasing women's access to education and employment are essential.

International efforts are under way to make condoms more available by lowering their price and to develop effective antiviral creams that women can use without the knowledge of their partners. Other potential strategies for fighting the spread of HIV include the widespread use of drugs to suppress genital herpes simplex, an extremely common STD that can dramatically increase transmission of HIV. Also, male circumcision might be useful in reducing the spread of HIV (and chlamydia, discussed later in this chapter). Recent research has shown a 60% reduction in HIV transmission among circumcised men compared with uncircumcised men, even when controlling for other factors.

In developed nations such as the United States, new drugs are easing AIDS symptoms and lowering viral levels dramatically for some patients. In the past few years, a small but growing number of people in poor countries have gained access to antiviral drugs because of the introduction of inexpensive generic drugs and increasing international funding for HIV treatment. Still, the vast majority of people with HIV remain untreated.

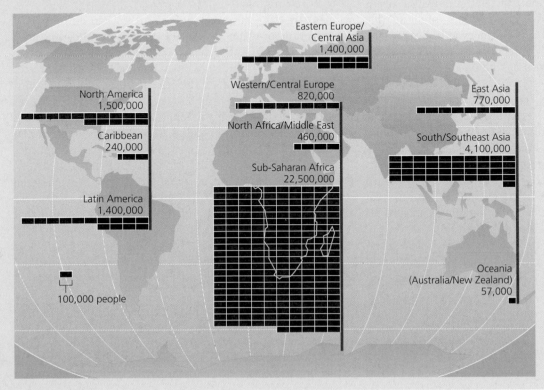

Approximate number of people living with HIV/AIDS in 2009.

**SOURCE:** Joint United Nations Programme on HIV/AIDS (UNAIDS). 2010. *Global Report: UNAIDS Report on the Global AIDS Epidemic, 2010.* Geneva: UNAIDS.

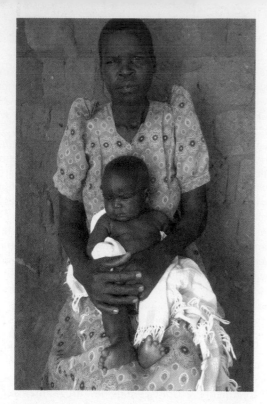

Currently available treatments can significantly increase the chance that this baby, born to an HIV-infected mother, will be free of the virus.

delivery further reduces the risk of HIV transmission in women with high blood levels of HIV.

**Symptoms** Within a few days or weeks of infection with HIV, some victims develop symptoms of *primary HIV infection*. These can include fever, fatigue, rashes, headache, swollen lymph nodes, body aches, night sweats, sore throat, nausea, and ulcers in the mouth. Because the symptoms of primary HIV infection are similar to those of many common viral illnesses, the condition often goes undiagnosed.

Because the immune system is weakened, people with HIV infection are highly susceptible to other infections, both common and uncommon. The infection most often seen among people with HIV is *Pneumocystis* pneumonia, a fungal infection. Kaposi's sarcoma, a once-rare form of cancer, is common in HIV-infected men. Women with HIV infection often have frequent and difficult-to-treat vaginal yeast infections. Cases of tuberculosis are also increasingly being reported in people with HIV.

**Diagnosis** The most commonly used screening blood test for HIV is the HIV antibody test. This procedure

consists of an initial screening called an ELISA test and a more specific confirmation test called the Western blot. These tests determine whether a person has antibodies to HIV circulating in the bloodstream, a sign that the virus is present in the body (see the box "Getting an HIV Test").

If a person is diagnosed as **HIV-positive,** the next step is to determine the current severity of the disease in order to plan appropriate treatment. The status of the immune system can be gauged by taking CD4 T cell measurements every few months. The infection itself can be monitored by tracking the amount of virus in the body (the viral load) through a test that measures the amount of HIV RNA in a blood sample.

A new diagnostic test that may help guide treatment decisions is called HIV Replication Capacity. This test shows how fast HIV from a patient's blood sample can reproduce itself. It is a measure of viral fitness and may be helpful when used in conjunction with CD4 and viral load tests in predicting how quickly a given person may progress to more serious disease.

Being tested once is not enough. Periodic routine testing is the best way for anyone to find out if he or she has HIV. The frequency of testing depends on multiple factors. For example, the CDC recommends that men who have sex with men should be tested at least once a year. People who engage in high-risk behavior (such as unprotected anal sex) should be tested more often. Rather than testing only at-risk individuals, the CDC also recommends universal HIV testing as part of routine medical care for everyone age 13–64. The CDC hopes that routine HIV testing will increase the odds that people with HIV are diagnosed earlier.

**Treatment** Although there is no known cure for HIV infection or AIDS, medications can significantly alter the course of the disease and extend life. The main types of antiviral drugs used against HIV/AIDS are reverse transcriptase inhibitors, protease inhibitors, integrase inhibitors, and entry inhibitors. These drugs either block HIV from replicating itself or prevent it from infecting other cells. Research has shown that using combinations of antiviral drugs can sometimes reduce HIV levels in the blood to undetectable levels. However, people on antiviral drugs can still pass the infection on, and concerns are growing that even these very aggressive treatments are starting to fail and that drug-resistant strains of HIV are developing rapidly. In addition to antiviral drugs, most patients with low CD4 T cell counts take a variety of antibiotics to help prevent opportunistic infections such as pneumonia and tuberculosis.

The best hope for stopping the spread of HIV worldwide rests with the development of a safe, effective, and inexpensive vaccine. Many different approaches to the development of an AIDS vaccine are currently under investigation, and human trials have begun on

# Getting an HIV Test

You should strongly consider being tested for HIV if any of the following apply to you or to any past or current sexual partner:

- You have had unprotected sex (vaginal, anal, or oral) with more than one partner or with a partner who was not in a mutually monogamous relationship with you

- You have used or shared needles, syringes, or other paraphernalia for injecting drugs (including steroids)

- You received a transfusion of blood or blood products between 1978 and 1985

- You have been diagnosed with an STD

If you decide to get an HIV test, you can either visit a physician or health clinic or take a home test.

## Physician or Clinic Testing

Your physician, student health clinic, Planned Parenthood, public health department, or local AIDS association can arrange your HIV test. Testing usually costs $50–$100, but public clinics often charge little or nothing. The standard test involves drawing a sample of blood that is sent to a lab, which checks for antibodies. If the first stage of testing is positive, a confirmatory test is done. This standard test takes 1–2 weeks, and you'll be asked to phone or come in personally to obtain your results, which should also include appropriate counseling.

Alternative tests are available at some clinics. The Orasure test uses oral fluid, which is collected by placing a treated cotton pad in the mouth; urine tests are also available. New rapid tests are also available at some locations. These tests involve the use of blood or oral fluid and can provide results in as little as 20 minutes. If a rapid test is positive for HIV infection, a confirmatory test will be performed.

Before getting tested, be sure you understand what will be done with the results. Results from confidential tests may still become part of your medical record and/or be reported to state and federal public health agencies. If you decide you want to be tested anonymously, ask your physician or counselor about an anonymous test, or use a home test.

## Home Testing

Home HIV test kits are available and cost about $40–$70. (Avoid test kits that are not FDA approved; unapproved kits are sold over the Internet. As of this printing, the only FDA-approved home test kit for HIV was manufactured by Home Access.) To use a home test, you prick a finger with a supplied lancet, blot a few drops of blood onto blotting paper, and mail it to the company's lab. In about a week (or within 3 business days for more expensive "express" tests), you call a toll-free number to learn your results. Anyone testing positive is routed to a trained counselor who can provide emotional and medical support. The results of home test kits are completely anonymous.

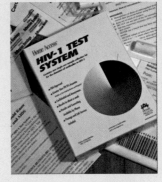

## Understanding the Results

A negative test result means that no antibodies were found in your sample. However, it usually takes at least a month (and possibly as long as 6 months in some people) after exposure to HIV for antibodies to appear. Therefore, an infected person may get a false-negative result. If you think you've been exposed to HIV, get a test immediately; if it's negative but your risk of infection is high, ask for an HIV RNA assay, which allows very early diagnosis.

A positive result means that you are infected. It is important to seek medical care and counseling immediately. Rapid progress is being made in treating HIV, and treatments are potentially much more successful when begun early. For more information on testing, visit the National HIV and STD Testing Resources Web site (http://www.hivtest.org).

---

several vaccines. However, no vaccine is likely to be ready for widespread use within the next decade. Researchers are making more rapid progress in producing a microbicide that could be used to prevent HIV and other STDs. A microbicide in the form of a cream, gel, sponge, or suppository could function as a kind of chemical condom.

**Prevention** Although AIDS is currently incurable, it is preventable. You can protect yourself by avoiding behaviors that may bring you into contact with HIV. This means making careful choices about sexual activity and not sharing needles if you inject drugs (Figure 14.2).

Anal and vaginal intercourse are the sexual activities associated with the highest risk of HIV infection. If you have intercourse, always use a condom (see the box

### Wellness Tip

All STDs, including HIV, are preventable. Follow the guidelines given throughout this chapter and make responsible sexual choices, and you can greatly reduce your risk of exposure to STDs.

**High Risk**

**Unprotected anal sex** is the riskiest sexual behavior, especially for the receptive partner.

**Unprotected vaginal intercourse** is the next riskiest, especially for women, who are much more likely to be infected by an infected male partner than vice versa.

**Oral sex** is probably considerably less risky than anal and vaginal intercourse but can still result in HIV transmission.

**Sharing of sex toys** can be risky because they can carry blood, semen, or vaginal fluid.

**Use of a condom** reduces risk considerably but not completely for any type of intercourse. Anal sex with a condom is riskier than vaginal sex with a condom; oral sex with a condom is less risky, especially if the man does not ejaculate.

**Hand-genital contact and deep kissing** are less risky but could still theoretically transmit HIV; the presence of cuts or sores increases risk.

**Sex with only one uninfected and totally faithful partner** is without risk but effective only if both partners are uninfected and completely monogamous.

**Activities that don't involve the exchange of body fluids** carry no risk: hugging, massage, closed-mouth kissing, masturbation, phone sex, and fantasy.

**Abstinence** is completely without risk. For many people, it can be an effective and reasonable method of avoiding HIV infection and other STDs during certain periods of life.

**No Risk**

**FIGURE 14.2** **What's risky and what's not: the approximate relative risk of HIV transmission of various sexual activities.**

"Using Male Condoms"). The use of a lubricated condom reduces the risk of transmitting HIV during all forms of intercourse. Condoms are not perfect, and they do not provide risk-free sex. When used properly, however, a condom provides a high level of protection against HIV and other STDs. Experts also suggest the use of latex squares and dental dams, devices that can be used as barriers during oral-genital or oral-anal sexual contact. Also, avoid using lubricants and lubricated condoms that contain the spermicide nonoxynol-9 (N-9). This spermicide has been shown to cause tissue irritation, which can make STD transmission more likely.

## Chlamydia

*Chlamydia trachomatis* causes **chlamydia,** the most prevalent bacterial STD in the United States. According to the CDC, more than 1.2 million new cases of chlamydia were officially reported in 2009, but because the disease is underreported, the CDC estimates that about 2.8 million actual new cases of chlamydia occur every year in the United States. The highest rates of infection occur in single people between ages 15 and 24. African American women experience chlamydia infections at nearly eight times the rate of white women.

Both men and women are susceptible to chlamydia, but women bear the greater burden because of possible complications from and consequences of the disease. If left untreated, chlamydia can lead to *pelvic inflammatory disease* (PID), a serious infection that can cause infertility. PID is discussed later in this chapter.

Chlamydia can also lead to infertility in men, although not as often as in women. In men under age 35, chlamydia is the most common cause of *epididymitis*—inflammation of the sperm-carrying ducts. (See Figure 14.3 and

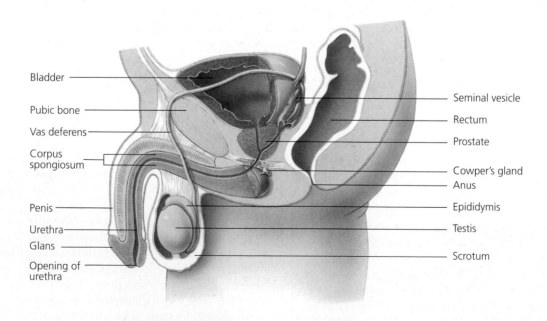

Bladder
Pubic bone
Vas deferens
Corpus spongiosum
Penis
Urethra
Glans
Opening of urethra

Seminal vesicle
Rectum
Prostate
Cowper's gland
Anus
Epididymis
Testis
Scrotum

**FIGURE 14.3** **Male sexual anatomy.**

# Using Male Condoms

Although they're not 100% effective as a contraceptive or as protection from STDs—only abstinence is—condoms improve your chances on both counts. Use them properly:

- **Buy latex condoms.** If you're allergic to latex, use a polyurethane condom or wear a lambskin condom under a latex one.

- **Buy and use condoms while they are fresh.** Packages have an expiration date or a manufacturing date. Don't use condoms beyond the expiration date or more than 5 years after the manufacturing date (2 years if they contain spermicide).

- **Try different styles and sizes.** Male condoms come in a variety of textures, colors, shapes, lubricants, and sizes. Shop around until you find a brand that's right for you. Condom widths and lengths vary by about 10–20%. A condom that is too tight may be uncomfortable and more likely to break; one that is too loose may slip off.

- **Don't remove the condom from its individual, sealed wrapper until you're ready to use it.** Open the packet carefully. Don't use a condom if it is gummy, dried out, or discolored.

- **Store condoms correctly.** Don't leave condoms in extreme heat or cold, and don't carry them in a pocket or wallet.

- **Use only water-based lubricants such as K-Y Jelly.** Never use oil-based lubricants like Vaseline or hand lotion; they may cause the condom to break. Avoid oil-based vaginal products.

- **Avoid condoms with lubricants containing the spermicide.** N-9 causes tissue irritation that increases the risk of STD transmission.

- **Use condoms correctly.** Roll the condom down over the penis as soon as it's erect. Squeeze the air out of the reservoir tip or the top quarter-inch of the condom as you unroll it to leave room for semen. Make sure there are no air bubbles. Remove it after ejaculation but before the penis becomes flaccid. Use a new condom every time you have intercourse.

- **Practice.** Condoms aren't hard to use, but practice helps. Take one out of the wrapper; examine it and stretch it to see how strong it is. Practice by yourself and with your partner.

Open the discussion of using condoms with your partner *before* you have sex. Despite the embarrassment most people feel at bringing up the subject at all, at least one study has shown that even if you have to *insist* on using condoms, your partner will like you more, respect you more, be more likely to want a long-term relationship with you, and feel that the sexual encounter was more intimate and meaningful.

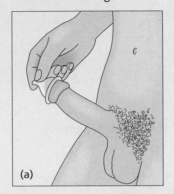
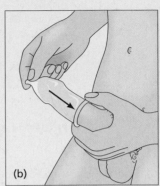
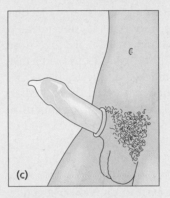
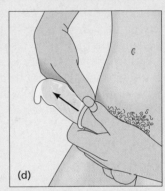

**USE OF THE MALE CONDOM.**
(a) Place the rolled-up condom over the head of the erect penis. Hold the top half-inch of the condom (with air squeezed out) to leave room for semen. (b) While holding the tip, unroll the condom onto the penis. Gently smooth out any air bubbles. (c) Unroll the condom down to the base of the penis. (d) To avoid spilling semen after ejaculation, hold the condom around the base of the penis as the penis is withdrawn. Remove the condom away from your partner, taking care not to spill any semen.

Figure 14.4 for basic information about human sexual anatomy.) In men, up to half of all cases of urethritis—inflammation of the urethra—are caused by chlamydia.

**Symptoms** Most people experience few or no symptoms from chlamydia infection, increasing the likelihood that they will inadvertently spread the infection to their partners. In men, symptoms can include painful urination, a slight watery discharge from the penis, and sometimes pain around the testicles.

Women may notice increased vaginal discharge, burning with urination, pain or bleeding with intercourse, and lower abdominal pain. Because infection rates are high and most women are asymptomatic, annual screening is recommended for sexually active young women.

**Diagnosis and Treatment** Chlamydia is diagnosed through a urine test or laboratory examination of fluid from the urethra or cervix. Once chlamydia has been

**chlamydia** An STD transmitted by the bacterium *Chlamydia trachomatis.*

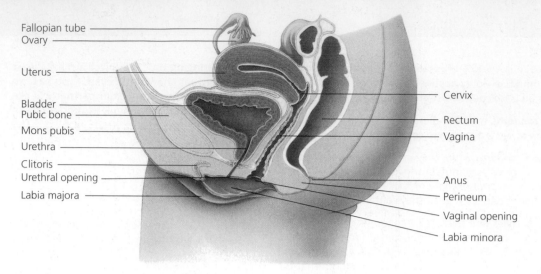

**FIGURE 14.4  Female sexual anatomy.**

diagnosed, the infected person and his or her partner(s) are given antibiotics—usually doxycycline, erythromycin, or a newer drug, azithromycin, which can cure chlamydia in a single dose. It is important for the infected person's partner to be tested and treated. If a one-dose treatment is used, couples should wait 7 days after taking their medication to resume sexual activity. The CDC now recommends that women who have been treated for chlamydia be retested 3 months after treatment is completed.

## Gonorrhea

**Gonorrhea** is caused by the bacterium *Neisseria gonorrhoeae*, which flourishes in mucous membranes. More than 300,000 new cases of gonorrhea were reported to the CDC in 2009, but because the infection often causes no symptoms, only about 50% of actual infections are reported. The highest incidence is among 15- to 24-year-olds. Like chlamydia, untreated gonorrhea can cause PID in women and urethritis and epididymitis in men. It can also cause arthritis and rashes, and it occasionally involves internal organs. An infant passing through the birth canal of an infected mother may contract *gonococcal conjunctivitis*, an infection in the eyes that can cause blindness if not treated.

**Symptoms**  In males, the incubation period for gonorrhea is brief, generally 2–7 days. The first symptoms are due to urethritis, which causes urinary discomfort and a thick, yellowish-white or yellowish-green discharge from the penis. The lips of the urethral opening may become inflamed and swollen. In some cases, the lymph glands in the groin become enlarged and swollen. Many males have very minor symptoms or none at all.

Most females with gonorrhea are asymptomatic. Those who have symptoms often experience urinary pain, increased vaginal discharge, and severe menstrual cramps. Women may also develop painful abscesses in the Bartholin's glands, a pair of glands located on either side of the opening of the vagina. Up to 40% of women with untreated gonorrhea develop PID.

Gonorrhea can also infect the throat or rectum of people who engage in oral or anal sex. Gonorrhea symptoms in the throat may be a sore throat or pus on the tonsils, and those in the rectum may be pus or blood in the feces or rectal pain and itching.

**Diagnosis and Treatment**  Several tests—gram stain, detection of bacterial genes or DNA, or culture—are available to detect gonorrhea. The physician may also collect samples of urine or cervical, urethral, throat, or rectal fluids.

Antibiotics can cure gonorrhea, but increasing drug resistance is a major concern. Today only one class of antibiotics, the cephalosporins, remains consistently effective against gonorrhea. People with gonorrhea often also have chlamydia, requiring additional antibiotics to treat chlamydia.

## Pelvic Inflammatory Disease

**Pelvic inflammatory disease (PID)** is a major complication in 10–40% of women who have been infected with either chlamydia or gonorrhea and have not

**Wellness Tip**

Like many other STDs, chlamydia and gonorrhea are often symptomless. For this reason alone, it's a good idea to talk to your doctor about your risks and the need for STD testing.

received treatment. PID occurs when the initial infection travels upward, often along with other bacteria, beyond the cervix into the uterus, oviducts, ovaries, and pelvic cavity. PID is often serious enough to require hospitalization and sometimes surgery. Even if the disease is treated successfully, about 25% of affected women will have long-term problems such as a continuing susceptibility to infection, ectopic pregnancy, infertility, and chronic pelvic pain. PID is the leading cause of infertility in young women.

**Symptoms** Symptoms of PID vary greatly. Some women, especially those with PID from chlamydia, may be asymptomatic; others may feel very ill with abdominal pain, fever, chills, nausea, and vomiting. Early symptoms are essentially the same as those described for chlamydia and gonorrhea. Symptoms often begin or worsen during or soon after a woman's menstrual period. Many women have abnormal vaginal bleeding—either bleeding between periods or heavy and painful menstrual bleeding.

**Diagnosis and Treatment** Diagnosis of PID is made on the basis of symptoms, physical examination, ultrasound, and laboratory tests. **Laparoscopy** may be used to confirm the diagnosis and obtain material for cultures.

Treatment should begin as quickly as possible to minimize damage to the reproductive organs. Antibiotics are usually started immediately; in severe cases, the woman may be hospitalized and antibiotics given intravenously. It is especially important that an infected woman's partners be treated. As many as 60% of the male contacts of women with PID are infected but asymptomatic.

# Human Papillomavirus (HPV)

**Human papillomavirus (HPV)** infection causes several human diseases, including common warts, **genital warts,** and genital cancers. HPV also causes virtually all cervical cancer, as well as penile cancer and some forms of anal and oropharyngeal cancer. Genital HPV is usually spread through sexual activity, including oral sex.

HPV is the most common STD in the United States; more than 80% of sexually active people will have been infected with HPV by age 50. HPV is especially common in young people, with some of the highest infection rates among college students.

Two HPV vaccines—Gardasil and Cervarix—have been approved by the FDA. Gardasil protects against four types of HPV virus that account for 90% of genital warts and 70% of cervical cancers; Gardasil has also been shown to prevent cancers of the vagina and vulva. Cervarix protects against two types of HPV, but not against the types that cause genital warts. Some studies show that Cervarix may be more effective and may provide longer-lasting protection against the viral strains that cause cervical cancer.

Vaccination with Gardasil is approved for girls and women age 9–26, and the CDC recommends the vaccine for all girls between the ages of 11 and 12. Cervarix is approved for girls and women age 10–25. Gardasil is also recommended for use in boys and men ages 9–26 to prevent anal cancer. Many experts believe that it makes sense to routinely vaccinate young males for HPV to protect them from HPV-related diseases and to protect their female partners.

**Symptoms** HPV-infected tissue often appears normal; it may also look like anything from a small bump on the skin to a large warty growth. Untreated warts can grow together to form a cauliflower-like mass. In males, they appear on the penis and often involve the urethra, appearing first at the opening and then spreading inside. The growths may cause irritation and bleeding, leading to painful urination and a urethral discharge. Warts may also appear around the anus or within the rectum.

In women, warts may appear on the labia or vulva and may spread to the *perineum,* the area between the vagina and the anus. If warts occur only on the cervix, the woman will generally have no symptoms or awareness that she has HPV.

The incubation period ranges from 1 month to 2 years from the time of contact. People can be infected with the virus and be capable of transmitting it to their sex partners without having any symptoms at all. The vast majority of people with HPV infection have no visible warts or symptoms of any kind.

**Diagnosis and Treatment** Genital warts are usually diagnosed based on the appearance of the lesions. Frequently, HPV infection of the cervix is detected on routine Pap tests.

Treatment of genital warts focuses on reducing the number and size of warts. The currently available treatments do not eradicate HPV infection. Warts may be removed by cryosurgery (freezing), electrocautery (burning), or laser surgery. Direct applications of a cytotoxic acid may be used, and there are treatments that patients can use at home.

Even after treatment and the disappearance of visible warts, the individual may continue to carry HPV in healthy-looking tissue and can probably still infect others. Anyone who has ever had HPV should inform all partners. Condoms should be used, even though they do not provide total protection. As with HIV, circumcision may provide some protection against HPV.

## Genital Herpes

**Genital herpes** affects about 1 in 6 adults in the United States. Two types of herpes simplex viruses, HSV 1 and HSV 2, cause genital herpes and oral-labial herpes (cold sores). Many people wrongly assume that they are unlikely to pick up an STD if they limit their sexual activity to oral sex, but this is not true, particularly in the case of genital herpes. HSV can also cause rectal lesions, usually transmitted through anal sex. Infection with HSV is generally lifelong; after infection, the virus lies dormant in nerve cells and can reactivate at any time.

HSV 1 infection is so common that 50–80% of adults have antibodies to HSV-1 (indicating previous exposure to the virus). Most people are exposed to HSV 1 during childhood. HSV 2 infection usually occurs during adolescence and early adulthood, most commonly between ages 18 and 25. About 16% of adults have antibodies to HSV 2.

HSV 2 is almost always sexually transmitted. The infection spreads readily whether people have active sores or are completely asymptomatic. If you have ever had an outbreak of genital herpes (that is, the appearance of genital sores), you should consider yourself always contagious and inform your partners. Avoid intimate contact when any sores are present, and use condoms during all sexual contact, including times when you have no symptoms. A recent study showed that using condoms for every act of intercourse results in a 30% decrease in the transmission of herpes compared with no condom use. Condoms are more effective in preventing the transmission of other STDs than for herpes, but this study shows that they can make a significant difference in preventing the spread of genital herpes.

Newborns can occasionally be infected with HSV, usually during passage through the birth canal of an infected mother. Without treatment, 65% of newborns with HSV will die, and most who survive will have some degree of brain damage. Pregnant women who have ever been exposed to genital herpes should inform their physician so that appropriate precautions can be taken to protect the baby from infection.

**Symptoms** Most people who are infected with HSV have no symptoms. Those who develop symptoms often first notice them within 2–20 days of having sex with an infected partner. The first episode of genital herpes frequently causes flulike symptoms in addition to genital lesions. The lesions usually heal within 3 weeks, but

the virus remains alive in an inactive state within nerve cells. A new outbreak of herpes can occur at any time. On average, newly diagnosed people will experience five to eight outbreaks a year, with a decrease in the frequency of outbreaks over time. Outbreaks can be triggered by stress, illness, fatigue, sun exposure, sexual intercourse, and menstruation.

**Diagnosis and Treatment** Genital herpes can be diagnosed on the basis of symptoms; a sample of fluid from the lesions may also be sent to a laboratory for evaluation. A new blood test that can determine if a person is infected with HSV 1 or HSV 2 is now available and may alert many asymptomatic people to the fact that they are infected.

There is no cure for herpes. Once infected, a person carries the virus for life. Antiviral drugs such as acyclovir can be taken at the beginning of an outbreak to shorten the severity and duration of symptoms. Support groups are available to help people learn to cope with herpes.

## Hepatitis B

**Hepatitis** (inflammation of the liver) can cause serious and sometimes permanent damage to the liver, which can result in death in severe cases. One of the many types of hepatitis is caused by hepatitis B virus (HBV). Hepatitis B virus is somewhat similar to HIV, but it is much more contagious than HIV, and it can also be spread through nonsexual close contact.

HBV is found in all body fluids, including blood and blood products, semen, saliva, urine, and vaginal secretions. It is easily transmitted through any sexual activity that involves the exchange of body fluids, the use of contaminated needles, and any blood-to-blood contact, including the use of contaminated razor blades, toothbrushes, and eating utensils. The primary risk factors for acquiring hepatitis B are sexual exposure and injection drug use; having multiple partners greatly increases risk.

**Symptoms** Many people infected with HBV never develop symptoms; they have what is known as a silent infection. The normal incubation period is 30–180 days. Mild cases of hepatitis cause flulike symptoms. As the illness progresses, there may be nausea, vomiting, dark-colored urine, abdominal pain, and jaundice.

People with hepatitis B sometimes recover completely, but they can also become chronic carriers of the virus, capable of infecting others for the rest of their lives. Some chronic carriers remain asymptomatic, while others develop chronic liver disease. Chronic hepatitis can cause cirrhosis, liver failure, and a deadly form of liver cancer. Hepatitis kills some 5000 Americans each year; worldwide, the annual death toll exceeds 600,000.

**Diagnosis and Treatment** Blood tests can diagnose hepatitis by analyzing liver function and detecting the infecting organism. There is no cure for HBV and no specific treatment for acute infections; antiviral drugs and immune system modulators may be used for chronic HBV infection. For people exposed to HBV, treatment with hepatitis B immunoglobulin can provide protection against the virus.

The vaccine for hepatitis B is safe and effective. Immunization is recommended for everyone under age 19 and for all adults at increased risk, including people who have more than one sex partner in 6 months, men who have sex with other men, those who inject illegal drugs, and health care workers who are exposed to blood and body fluids.

## Syphilis

**Syphilis,** a disease that once caused death and disability for millions, can now be treated effectively with antibiotics. In 2008, there were 13,500 new cases of early syphilis in the United States, and about 46,000 people were diagnosed at all stages of the disease.

Syphilis is caused by a corkscrew-shaped bacterium called *Treponema pallidum*. It requires warmth and moisture to survive and dies very quickly outside the human body. The bacterium passes through any break or opening in the skin or mucous membranes and can be transmitted by kissing, vaginal or anal intercourse, or oral-genital contact.

**Symptoms** Syphilis progresses through several stages. *Primary syphilis* is characterized by an ulcer called a **chancre** that appears within about 10–90 days after exposure. The chancre is usually found at the site where the organism entered the body, such as the genital area, but it may also appear in other sites such as the mouth, breasts, or fingers. Chancres contain large numbers of bacteria and make the disease highly contagious when present; they are often painless and typically heal on their own within a few weeks. If the disease is not treated during the primary stage, about a third of infected individuals progress to chronic stages of infection.

*Secondary syphilis* is usually marked by mild, flulike symptoms and a skin rash that appears 3–6 weeks after the chancre. The rash may cover the entire body or only a few areas, but the palms of the hands and soles of the feet are usually involved. Areas of skin affected by the rash are highly contagious but usually heal within several weeks or months. If the disease remains untreated, the symptoms of secondary syphilis may recur over a period of several years. Affected individuals may then lapse into an asymptomatic latent stage in which they experience no further consequences of infection. In about a third of cases of untreated secondary syphilis, however, the individual develops *late,* or *tertiary, syphilis*. Late syphilis can damage many organs of the body, possibly causing severe dementia, cardiovascular damage, blindness, and death.

In infected pregnant women, the syphilis bacterium can cross the placenta. If the mother is not treated, the probable result is stillbirth, prematurity, or congenital deformity. In some cases, the infant is born infected (*congenital syphilis*) and requires treatment.

**Diagnosis and Treatment** Syphilis is diagnosed by examination of infected tissues and with blood tests. All stages can be treated with antibiotics, but damage from late syphilis can be permanent.

## Other STDs

A few other diseases are transmitted sexually, but they can be avoided by observing responsible sexual behavior.

**Trichomoniasis,** often called *trich,* is a common STD. The single-celled organism that causes trich, *Trichomonas vaginalis,* thrives in warm, moist conditions, making women particularly susceptible to these infections in the vagina. Women who become symptomatic with trich develop a greenish, foul-smelling vaginal discharge and severe itching and pain in the vagina. Prompt treatment with metronidazole (Flagyl) is important because studies suggest that trich may increase the risk of HIV transmission and, in pregnant women, premature delivery.

**Bacterial vaginosis (BV)** is the most common cause of abnormal vaginal discharge in women of reproductive age. BV occurs when healthy bacteria that normally inhabit the vagina become displaced by unhealthy species. BV is clearly associated with sexual activity and often occurs after a change in partners. Symptoms of BV include vaginal discharge with a fishy odor and sometimes vaginal irritation. BV is treated with topical and oral antibiotics.

---

**KEY TERMS**

**genital herpes**   A sexually transmitted infection caused by the herpes simplex virus.

**hepatitis**   Inflammation of the liver, which can be caused by infection, drugs, or toxins; some forms of infectious hepatitis can be transmitted sexually.

**syphilis**   A sexually transmitted infection caused by the bacterium *Treponema pallidum*.

**chancre**   The sore produced by syphilis in its earliest stage.

**trichomoniasis**   A protozoal infection caused by *Trichomonas vaginalis,* transmitted sexually and externally.

**bacterial vaginosis (BV)**   A condition caused by an overgrowth of certain bacteria inhabiting the vagina.

## Protecting Yourself from STDs

**TAKE CHARGE**

- **Abstinence.** The only truly foolproof way to protect yourself from STDs is abstinence—abstaining from sexual relations with other people. Remember that it is OK to say no to sex.

- **Monogamy.** Next to abstinence, the most effective way to protect yourself is monogamy—having sex exclusively with one partner, who engages in sex with no one else but you, and who does not have an STD.

- **Communication.** If you choose to be sexually active, protect yourself by practicing open and honest communication and insisting on the same from your partner. Be truthful about your past, and ask your partner to do the same. Remember that you are indirectly exposing yourself to all of your partner's prior sexual contacts.

- **Safer sexual activities.** Know what sexual activities are risky (see Figure 14.2). Safer alternatives to intercourse include fantasy, hugging, massage, rubbing clothed bodies together, mutual masturbation, and closed-mouth kissing.

- **Condoms.** Always use latex condoms during every act of vaginal intercourse, anal intercourse, and oral sex. Multiple studies show that regular condom use can reduce the risk of several diseases, including HIV, chlamydia, and genital herpes.

- **Activities to avoid.** Don't drink or use drugs in sexual situations. Mood-altering drugs can affect your judgment and make you more likely to engage in risky behaviors. Limit the number of sexual partners; having multiple partners is associated with increased risk of STDs. Avoid sexual contact with partners who have an STD or have had unprotected sex in the past. Avoid sexual contact that could cause tears or cuts in the skin or tissue. Don't inject drugs; don't share needles, syringes, or anything that might have blood on it. Decontaminate needles and syringes with household bleach and water. If you are at risk for HIV infection, don't donate blood, sperm, or organs.

- **Other preventive measures.** Get tested for HIV during your next routine medical examination. Have periodic screenings for STDs if you are at risk. Make sure all your vaccinations are up-to-date. Girls and women age 9–26 should be vaccinated against HPV, unless there are medical reasons to avoid the vaccination. Ask your physician if it is appropriate for you to be vaccinated against hepatitis B.

---

**Pubic lice** (commonly known as *crabs*) and **scabies** are highly contagious parasitic infections. Treatment is generally easy, although lice infestation can require repeated applications of medications.

## WHAT YOU CAN DO ABOUT STDs

You can take responsibility for your health and help reduce the incidence of STDs.

## Education

Many schools have STD counseling and education programs. These programs allow students to practice communicating with potential sex partners and negotiating for safer sex, to engage in role-playing to build self-confidence, and to learn how to use condoms.

You can find free pamphlets and other literature about STDs at public health departments, health clinics, physicians' offices, student health centers, and Planned Parenthood; easy-to-understand books are available in libraries and bookstores. National hotlines provide free, confidential information and referral services to callers anywhere in the country (see For Further Exploration at the end of the chapter).

## Diagnosis and Treatment

Early diagnosis and treatment of STDs can help you avoid complications and can also help prevent the spread of infection. If you are sexually active, be alert and seek treatment for any sign or symptom of disease, such as a rash, a discharge, sores, or unusual pain. Many STDs can be asymptomatic, however, so a professional examination and testing are recommended following any risky sexual encounter—even in the absence of symptoms.

## Prevention

The only sure way to avoid exposure to STDs is to abstain from sexual activity. If you choose to be sexually active, think about prevention before you have a sexual

**KEY TERMS**

**pubic lice** Parasites that infest the hair of the pubic region; commonly called *crabs*.

**scabies** A contagious skin disease caused by burrowing parasitic mites.

### Ask yourself

**QUESTIONS FOR CRITICAL THINKING AND REFLECTION**

Have you ever engaged in sexual activities you regretted later? If so, what were the circumstances, and what influenced you to act the way you did? Were there any negative consequences? What preventive strategies can you use in the future to make sure it doesn't happen again?

encounter or find yourself in the "heat of the moment." Plan ahead for safer sex. For tips and strategies, see the box "Protecting Yourself from STDs." Remember that asking questions and being aware of signs and symptoms show that you care about yourself and your partner. Concern about STDs is an essential and mutually beneficial part of a sexual relationship.

If you are diagnosed as having an STD, begin treatment as quickly as possible. Inform your partner(s) and avoid any sexual activity until your treatment is complete.

## TIPS FOR TODAY AND THE FUTURE

Because STDs can have serious, long-term effects, it is important to be vigilant about exposure, treatment, and prevention.

### RIGHT NOW YOU CAN

- Make an appointment with your health care provider if you are worried about possible STD infection.
- Resolve to discuss condom use with your partner if you are sexually active and are not already using condoms.

### IN THE FUTURE YOU CAN

- Learn how to communicate effectively with a partner who resists safer sex practices or is reluctant to discuss his or her sexual history. Support groups and classes can help.
- Make sure all your vaccinations are up-to-date; ask your doctor if you should be vaccinated against any STDs. Follow instructions for treatment carefully and complete all the medication as prescribed.

## SUMMARY

- HIV damages the immune system and causes AIDS. People with AIDS are vulnerable to often-fatal opportunistic infections.

- HIV is carried in blood and blood products, semen, vaginal and cervical secretions, and breast milk; it is transmitted through the exchange of these fluids.

- Drugs have been developed to slow the course of HIV infection and to prevent or treat certain secondary infections, but there is no cure.

- Chlamydia is a bacterial infection that causes epididymitis and urethritis in men and can lead to PID in women.

- Untreated, gonorrhea can cause PID in women and epididymitis in men, leading to infertility. In infants, untreated gonorrhea can cause blindness.

- Pelvic inflammatory disease (PID), a complication of untreated chlamydia or gonorrhea, is an infection of the uterus and oviducts that may extend to the ovaries and pelvic cavity. It can lead to infertility, ectopic pregnancy, and chronic pelvic pain.

- Genital warts, caused by the human papillomavirus (HPV), are associated with cervical cancer. Treatment does not eradicate the virus, but vaccines are available, recommended for everyone age 9–26.

- Genital herpes is a common incurable viral infection characterized by outbreaks of lesions and periods of latency.

- Hepatitis B is a viral infection of the liver transmitted through sexual and nonsexual contact. Some people become chronic carriers of the virus and may develop serious, potentially fatal, complications.

- Syphilis is a highly contagious bacterial infection that can be treated with antibiotics. If left untreated, it can lead to deterioration of the central nervous system and death.

- Other common STDs include trichomoniasis, bacterial vaginosis, and pubic lice and scabies.

- Successful diagnosis and treatment of STDs involves being alert for symptoms, getting tested, informing partners, and following treatment instructions.

- All STDs are preventable; the key is practicing responsible sexual behaviors.

## FOR FURTHER EXPLORATION

### BOOKS

Engel, J. 2007. *The Epidemic: A Global History of AIDS*. New York: Collins. *A historical, social, and cultural perspective on the AIDS epidemic, from its beginning in 1981 to the present day, from a medical historian.*

Hyde, J. S., and J. D. DeLamater. 2010. *Understanding Human Sexuality*, 11th ed. New York: McGraw-Hill. *A comprehensive, multidisciplinary introduction to human sexuality; includes material on STDs.*

Klausner, J. D., and E. W. Hook. 2007. *Current Diagnosis and Treatment of Sexually Transmitted Diseases*. New York: McGraw-Hill. *Written for the clinician; provides an easy-to-use reference of the latest diagnostic and treatment information available on STDs.*

Marr, L. 2007. *Sexually Transmitted Diseases: A Physician Tells You What You Need to Know*. Baltimore, Md.: Johns Hopkins University Press. *Practical, up-to-date information on the diagnosis, treatment, and prevention of sexually transmitted diseases of all types.*

Moore, E. A. 2008. *Encyclopedia of Sexually Transmitted Diseases*, Illustrated ed. Jefferson, N. C.: McFarland. *Includes a variety of information on STDs in an easy-to-use format.*

### ORGANIZATIONS, HOTLINES, AND WEB SITES

*American College Health Association*. Offers free brochures on STDs, alcohol use, acquaintance rape, and other health issues.
http://www.acha.org

*American Social Health Association* (ASHA). Provides information and referrals on STDs; sponsors support groups for people with herpes and HPV.
http://www.ashastd.org

**Q** Why do young people, including college students, have high rates of STDs?

**A** Half of young Americans will have an STD by age 25. Contributing factors may include the following:

• *College students underestimate their risk of STDs and HIV.* Although students may know about STDs, they often feel the risks do not apply to them. One study of students with a history of STDs showed that more than half had unprotected sex while they were infected, and 25% of them continued to have sex without ever informing their partner(s).

• *Risky sexual behavior is common.* One study of college students found that fewer than half used condoms consistently and one-third had had ten or more sex partners. Another study found that 19% of male students and 33% of female students had consented to sexual intercourse simply because they felt awkward refusing. Nearly half of young adults are sexually active by age 18 (more than 95% by age 25), but they are not yet in long-term monogamous relationships; they are more likely to have more than one partner over time and to have a partner with an STD.

• *Alcohol and drug use play an important role.* Between one-third and one-half of college students report participating in sexual activity as a direct result of being intoxicated. Students who binge drink are more likely to have multiple partners, use condoms inconsistently, and delay seeking treatment for STDs than students who drink little or no alcohol. Sexual assaults occur more frequently when either the perpetrator or the victim has been drinking.

**Q** Does the success of the new AIDS drugs mean that I don't need to worry about HIV infection anymore?

**A** No. The new combination drug therapy has had dramatic effects for some people infected with HIV. In the United States, the number of HIV-infected people who progress to AIDS each year is declining, as is the death rate from AIDS. But the new drugs are expensive, can have serious side effects, and are not effective for everyone. Scientists do not yet know how long the drugs will keep HIV at bay, and no treatment has yet been shown to permanently eradicate HIV from the body. AIDS is still an incurable, fatal disease.

**Q** Which contraceptive methods protect best against STDs?

**A** Latex male condoms are the best known protection against HIV and other STDs. Condoms are not foolproof, however, and they do not protect against the transmission of diseases from sores that they do not cover.

Some other contraceptive methods may provide some protection against certain STDs. The diaphragm and cervical cap cover the cervix and may offer some protection against diseases that involve the infection of cervical cells. Combining these barrier methods with a condom can provide even greater protection.

Hormonal methods such as oral contraceptives do not protect against

---

*The Body: The Complete HIV/AIDS Resource.* Provides information about prevention, testing, and treatment, and includes an on-line risk assessment.
http://www.thebody.com

*CDC National Prevention Information Network.* Provides extensive information and links on AIDS and other STDs.
http://www.cdcnpin.org

*CDC National STD and AIDS Hotlines.* Callers can obtain information, counseling, and referrals for testing and treatment. The hotlines offer information on more than 20 STDs and include Spanish and TTY service.
800-342-AIDS or 800-227-8922; 800-344-SIDA (Spanish)
800-243-7889 (TTY, deaf access)

*HIV InSite: Gateway to AIDS Knowledge.* Provides information about prevention, education, treatment, statistics, clinical trials, and new developments.
http://hivinsite.ucsf.edu

*Joint United Nations Programme on HIV/AIDS (UNAIDS).* Provides statistics and information on the international HIV/AIDS situation.
http://www.unaids.org

*MedlinePlus: Sexually Transmitted Diseases.* Maintained by the CDC; a clearinghouse of links and information on STDs.
http://www.nlm.nih.gov/medlineplus/sexuallytransmitted diseases.html

*Planned Parenthood Federation of America.* Provides information on STDs, family planning, and contraception.
http://www.plannedparenthood.org

*Smarter Sex.* Designed for college students; provides tips and information on safer sex practices, relationships, STDs, and more.
http://www.smartersex.org

## SELECTED BIBLIOGRAPHY

American Association of Blood Banks. 2010. Blood FAQ (http://www.aabb.org/resources/bct/Pages/bloodfaq.aspx; retrieved October 4, 2010).

American College Health Association. 2009. American College Health Association–National College Health Assessment II: Reference Group Executive Summary Fall 2009. Linthicum, Md.: American College Health Association.

American Social Health Association. 2010. Frequently Asked Questions About Cervical Cancer/HPV Vaccines (http://www.ashastd.org/hpv/hpv_vaccines.cfm; retrieved October 4, 2010).

American Social Health Association. 2010. Herpes Testing Toolkit (http://www.ashastd.org/herpes/herpes_toolkit/; retrieved October 4, 2010).

Baeten, J. M., et al. 2005. Female-to-male infectivity of HIV-1 among circumcised and uncircumcised Kenyan men. *Journal of Infectious Diseases* 191(4): 546–553.

STDs in the lower reproductive tract but do provide some protection against PID. If vaginal irritation occurs from the use of spermicides, the risk of infection with HIV and other STDs may actually increase.

## Q Why are women hit harder by STDs than men?

A Sexually transmitted diseases cause suffering for all who are infected, but in many ways, women and girls are the hardest hit, for both biological and social reasons:

• *Male-to-female transmission of many infections is more likely to occur than female-to-male transmission.* This is particularly true of HIV.

• *Young women are even more vulnerable to STDs than older women because the less-mature cervix is more susceptible to injury and infection.* As a woman ages, the cells at the opening of the cervix gradually change so that the tissue becomes more resistant to infection.

Young women are also more vulnerable for social and emotional reasons: Lack of control in relationships, fear of discussing condom use, and having an older sex partner are all linked to increased STD risk.

• *Once infected, women tend to suffer more consequences of STDs than men.* For example, gonorrhea and chlamydia can cause PID and permanent damage to the oviducts in women, while these infections tend to have less serious effects in men. HPV infection causes nearly all cases of cervical cancer. HPV infection is also associated with penile cancer in men, but penile cancer is much less common than cervical cancer. Women also have the added concern of the potential effects of STDs during pregnancy.

• *Women with HIV infection often face greater challenges when they are ill.* Women may become sicker at lower viral loads compared to men. Women and men with HIV do about as well if they have similar access to treatment, but in many cases women are diagnosed later in the course of HIV infection, receive less treatment, and die sooner. In addition, they may be caring for family members who are also infected and ill. The proportion of new AIDS cases in women is increasing both in the United States and globally.

• *Worldwide, social and economic factors play a large role in the transmission and consequences of AIDS and other STDs for women.* Such practices as very early marriage for women, often to much older men who have had many sexual partners, places women at risk for infection. Cultural gender norms that promote premarital and extramarital relationships for men, combined with women's lack of power to negotiate safe sex, make infection a risk even for women who are married and monogamous. In some parts of the world, the stigma of AIDS hits women harder. In addition, lack of education and limited economic opportunities can force women into commercial sex work, placing them at high risk for all STDs. Solutions to the STD crisis in women include greater access to health care as well as empowerment in the social sphere.

*For more Common Questions Answered about STDs, visit the Online Learning Center at www.mhhe.com/fahey.*

Brown, D. R., et al. 2005. A longitudinal study of genital human papillomavirus infection in a cohort of closely followed adolescent women. *Journal of Infectious Diseases* 191(2): 182–192.

Buchbinder, Susan. 2010. HIV epidemiology, testing strategies and prevention interventions. *Topics in HIV Medicine* 18(2): 38–44.

Caskey, Rachel. 2009. Knowledge and early adoption of the HPV vaccine among girls and young women: Results of a national survey. *Journal of Adolescent Health* 45(5): 453–462.

Centers for Disease Control and Prevention. 2006. Revised recommendations for HIV testing of adults, adolescents, and pregnant women in health-care settings. *Morbidity and Mortality Weekly Report* 55(RR-14): 1–17.

Centers for Disease Control and Prevention. 2006. Trends in HIV-related risk behaviors among high school students—United States, 1991–2005. *Morbidity and Mortality Weekly Report* 55(31): 851–854.

Centers for Disease Control and Prevention. 2009. *Sexually Transmitted Disease Surveillance, 2008.* Atlanta: U.S. Department of Health and Human Services.

Centers for Disease Control and Prevention. 2010. *Genital HPV Infection—CDC Fact Sheet* (http://www.cdc.gov/std/hpv/stdfact-hpv.htm; retrieved October 4, 2010).

Centers for Disease Control and Prevention. 2010. *Chlamydia Fact Sheet* (http://www.cdc.gov/std/Chlamydia/STDFact-Chlamydia.htm; retrieved October 4, 2010).

Centers for Disease Control and Prevention. 2010. *Expedited Partner Therapy* (http://www.cdc.gov/std/ept/; retrieved October 4, 2010).

Centers for Disease Control and Prevention. 2010. *Hepatitis B Information for Health Professionals* (http://www.cdc.gov/hepatitis/HBV/HBVfaq.htm#overview; retrieved October 4, 2010).

Centers for Disease Control and Prevention. 2010. Seroprevalence of herpes simplex virus type 2 among persons aged 14 to 49 years–U.S. 2005–2008. *Morbidity and Mortality Weekly Report* 59(15): 456–459.

Erbelding, E. J., and J. M. Zenilman. 2005. Toward better control of sexually transmitted diseases. *New England Journal of Medicine* 352(7): 720–721.

Garland, S. 2010. Prevention strategies against human papillomavirus in males. *Gynecologic Oncology* 117(2010): S20–25.

Goetz, M. B., et al. 2010. HIV replication capacity is an independent predictor of disease progression in persons with untreated chronic HIV infection. *Journal of Acquired Immune Deficiency Syndrome* 53(4): 472–479.

Hampton, T. 2006. High prevalence of lesser-known STDs. *Journal of the American Medical Association* 295(21): 2467.

Hightow, L. B., et al. 2005. The unexpected movement of the HIV epidemic in the southeastern United States: Transmission among college students. *Journal of Acquired Immune Deficiency Syndrome* 38(5): 531–537.

Huppert, J. S. 2006. New detection methods for trichomoniasis may help curb more serious STIs. *Patient Care for the Nurse Practitioner* 40(5).

International AIDS Vaccine Initiative. 2010. *State of the Field* (http://www.iavi.org/research-development/Pages/state-of-field.aspx; retrieved October 4, 2010).

Kaiser Family Foundation. *2009 Survey of Americans on HIV/AIDS* (http://www.kff.org/kaiserpolls/7889.cfm; retrieved October 4, 2010).

Mathers, C. D., and D. Loncar. 2006. Projections of global mortality and burden of disease from 2002 to 2030. *Public Library of Science, Medicine* 3(11): 2011–2030.

National Institutes of Allergy and Infectious Diseases. 2009. *HIV Infection in Women* (http://www3.niaid.nih.gov/topics/HIVAIDS/Understanding /Population+Specific+Information/womenHiv.htm; retrieved October 4, 2010).

Ness, R. B., et al. 2005. Douching, pelvic inflammatory disease, and incident gonococcal and chlamydial genital infection in a cohort of high-risk women. *American Journal of Epidemiology* 61(2): 186–195.

Sanders, G. D., et al. 2005. Cost-effectiveness of screening for HIV in the era of highly active antiretroviral therapy. *New England Journal of Medicine* 352(6): 570–585.

Sepkowitz, K. 2006. One disease, two epidemics—AIDS at 25. *New England Journal of Medicine* 354(23): 2411–2414.

Voelker, Rebecca. 2010. Experts reconsider wisdom of limiting chlamydia screening only to women. *Journal of the American Medical Association* 303(9): 823–824.

Xu, F., et al. 2006. Trends in herpes simplex virus type 1 and type 2 sero prevalence in the United States. *Journal of the American Medical Association* 296(8): 964–973.

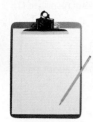

## LAB 14.1 Behaviors and Attitudes Related to STDs

### Part I   Risk Assessment

To identify your risk factors for STDs, read the following list of statements and mark whether they're true or false for you. *Note:* The statements in this assessment are worded in a way that assumes current sexual activity. If you have never been sexually active, you are not now at risk for STDs. Respond to the statements in the quiz based on how you realistically believe you would act. If you are currently in a mutually monogamous relationship with an uninfected partner or are not currently sexually active (but have been in the past), you are at low risk for STDs at this time. Respond to the statements in the quiz according to your attitudes and past behaviors. (For more on your risk factors for STDs, take the online assessment available at www.thebody.com.)

| True | False |  |
|------|-------|--|
| _____ | _____ | 1.  I have only one sex partner. |
| _____ | _____ | 2.  I always use a latex condom for each act of intercourse, even if I am fairly certain my partner has no infections. |
| _____ | _____ | 3.  I do not use oil-based lubricants with condoms. |
| _____ | _____ | 4.  I discuss STDs and prevention with new partners before having sex. |
| _____ | _____ | 5.  I do not use alcohol or another mood-altering drug in sexual situations. |
| _____ | _____ | 6.  I would tell my partner if I thought I had been exposed to an STD. |
| _____ | _____ | 7.  I am familiar with the signs and symptoms of STDs. |
| _____ | _____ | 8.  I regularly perform genital self-examination to check for signs and symptoms of STDs. |
| _____ | _____ | 9.  When I notice any sign or symptom of any STD, I consult my physician immediately. |
| _____ | _____ | 10.  I have been tested for HIV or plan to be tested at my next routine medical exam. |
| _____ | _____ | 11.  I obtain screenings for STDs regularly. In addition (if female), I obtain yearly pelvic exams and Pap tests. |
| _____ | _____ | 12.  I have been vaccinated for hepatitis B. In addition (if female), I have been vaccinated or plan to be vaccinated for HPV. |
| _____ | _____ | 13.  When diagnosed with an STD, I inform all recent partners. |
| _____ | _____ | 14.  When I have a sign or symptom of an STD that goes away on its own, I still consult my physician. |
| _____ | _____ | 15.  I do not use drugs prescribed for friends or partners or left over from other illnesses to treat STDs. |
| _____ | _____ | 16.  I do not share syringes or needles to inject drugs. |

## Using Your Results

*How did you score?* False responses indicate attitudes and behaviors that may put you at risk for contracting STDs or for suffering serious medical consequences from them. How many false responses did you give? Are you satisfied that you're doing everything you can to protect yourself from STDs?

*What should you do next?* Any false reponse indicates a factor that you could change to reduce your risk for STDs. Choose one as the focus of a behavior change program.

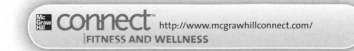

## Part II Communication

Good communication with sex partners or potential sex partners is a critical component of STD prevention. Regardless of your responses to the risk assessment, complete this communication exercise to help build your communication skills.

1. List three ways to bring up the subject of STDs with a new partner. How would you ask whether he or she has been exposed to any STDs or engaged in any risky behaviors? (Remember that because many STDs can be asymptomatic it is important to know about past behaviors even if no STD was diagnosed.)

   a. _____

   _____

   b. _____

   _____

   c. _____

   _____

2. List three ways to bring up the subject of condom use with your partner. How might you convince someone who does not want to use a condom?

   a. _____

   _____

   b. _____

   _____

   c. _____

   _____

3. If you have had an STD in the past that you might possibly still pass on (e.g., herpes, genital warts), how would you tell your partner(s)?

   _____

   _____

   _____

4. If you were diagnosed with an STD that you believe was given to you by your current partner, how would you begin a discussion of STDs with her or him?

   _____

   _____

   _____

# CHAPTER 15

# Environmental Health

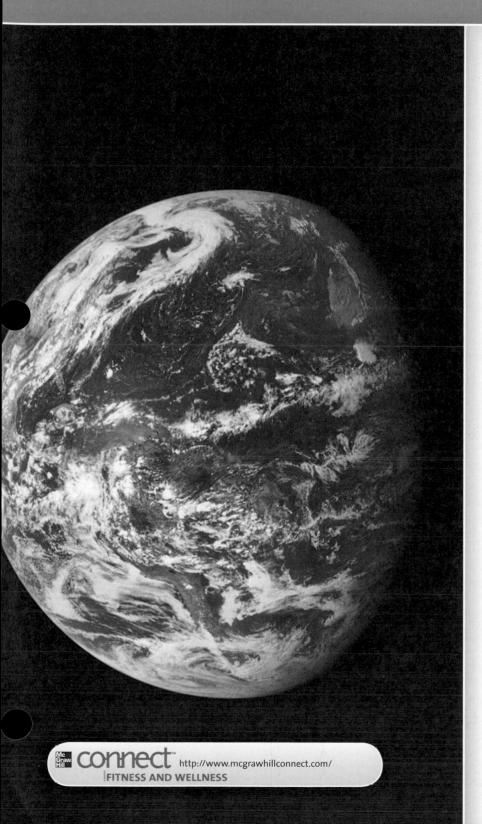

## LOOKING AHEAD...

After reading this chapter, you should be able to:

- Explain how population growth affects the earth's environment and contributes to pollution and climate change

- Discuss the causes and effects of air and water pollution, and describe strategies that people can take to protect these resources

- Discuss the issue of solid waste disposal and the impact it has on the environment and human health

- Identify some key sources of chemical and radiation pollution, and discuss methods for preventing such pollution

- Explain how energy use affects the environment, and describe steps everyone can take to use energy more efficiently

## TEST YOUR KNOWLEDGE

1. The world's current population is about what?
   a. .68 billion
   b. 6.8 billion
   c. 68 billion
   d. 680 billion

2. Air pollution can be naturally occurring, as well as human-made. True or false?

3. Compact fluorescent lightbulbs can last ten times longer than standard incandescent lightbulbs. True or false?

**Answers**

1. **b.** The world's current population is about 6.8 billion, and it is growing at a rate of about 75 million per year.
2. **True.** There are many types of naturally occurring air pollution, such as smoke from forest fires and dust from dust storms.
3. **True.** Compact fluorescent lightbulbs use 75% less energy and last up to ten times longer than regular lightbulbs.

We are constantly reminded of our intimate relationship with everything that surrounds us—our **environment.** Although the planet provides us with food, water, air, and everything else that sustains life, it also provides us with natural occurrences—earthquakes, tsunamis, hurricanes, drought, climate changes—that destroy life and disrupt society. In the past, humans frequently had to struggle against the environment to survive. Today, in addition to dealing with natural disasters, we also have to find ways to protect the environment from the by-products of our way of life.

This chapter introduces the concept of environmental health and explains how the environment affects us. The chapter also discusses the ways humans affect the planet and its resources, and it describes steps you can take to improve your personal environmental health while reducing your impact on the earth.

## ENVIRONMENTAL HEALTH DEFINED

The field of **environmental health** grew out of efforts to control communicable diseases. When certain insects and rodents were found to carry microorganisms that cause disease in humans, campaigns were undertaken to eradicate or control these animal vectors. It was also recognized that pathogens could be transmitted in sewage, drinking water, and food. These discoveries led to systematic garbage collection, sewage treatment, filtration and chlorination of drinking water, food inspection, and the establishment of public health enforcement agencies.

These efforts to control and prevent communicable diseases changed the health profile of the developed world. Americans rarely contract cholera, typhoid fever, plague, diphtheria, or other diseases that once killed large numbers of people, but these diseases have not been eradicated worldwide.

In the United States, a huge, complex public health system is constantly at work behind the scenes attending to the details of these critical health concerns. Every time the system is disrupted, danger recurs. After any disaster that damages a community's public health system—whether a natural disaster such as a hurricane or a human-made disaster such as a terrorist attack—prompt restoration of basic health services becomes crucial to human survival. Every time we venture beyond the boundaries of our everyday world, whether traveling to a

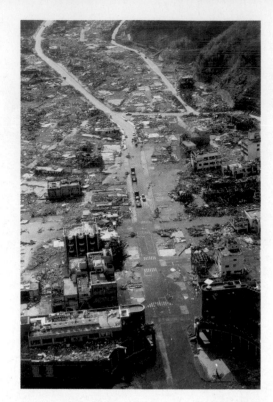

Natural disasters—such as the 2011 tsunami that struck several parts of Japan—can directly kill thousands of people while wiping out essential services, polluting water, and facilitating the spread of disease.

less-developed country or camping in a wilderness area, we are reminded of the importance of these basics: clean water, sanitary waste disposal, safe food, and insect and rodent control.

Over the last few decades, the focus of environmental health has expanded and become more complex, for several reasons. We now recognize that environmental pollutants contribute not only to infectious diseases but to many chronic diseases as well. In addition, technological advances have increased our ability to affect and damage the environment. Also, rapid population growth, which has resulted partly from past environmental improvements, means that far more people are consuming and competing for resources than ever before, magnifying the effect of humans on the environment.

Environmental health is therefore seen as encompassing all the interactions of humans with their environment

**KEY TERMS**

**environment**  The natural and human-made surroundings in which we spend our lives.

**environmental health**  The collective interactions of humans with the environment and the short-term and long-term health consequences of those interactions.

### Ask yourself

QUESTIONS FOR CRITICAL THINKING AND REFLECTION

How often do you think about the environment's impact on your personal health? In what ways do your immediate surroundings (your home, neighborhood, school, workplace) affect your well-being? In what ways do you influence the health of your personal environment?

and the health consequences of these interactions. Fundamental to this definition is a recognition that we hold the world in trust for future generations and for other forms of life. Our responsibility is to pass on a world no worse, and preferably better, than the one we live in today. Although many environmental problems are complex and seem beyond the control of the individual, there are ways that people can make a difference to the future of the planet.

## POPULATION GROWTH AND CONTROL

Throughout most of history, humans have been a minor pressure on the planet. About 300 million people were alive in the year 1 A.D.; by the time Europeans were settling in the United States 1600 years later, the world population had increased gradually to a little over 500 million. But then it began rising exponentially—zooming to 1 billion by about 1800, more than doubling by 1930, and then doubling again in just 40 years (Figure 15.1).

The world's population, currently about 6.8 billion, is increasing at a rate of about 75 million per year—approximately 150 people every minute. The United Nations projects that world population will reach 9.1 billion by 2050 and will continue to increase until it levels off above 10 billion in 2200.

Virtually all of this increase is taking place in less-developed regions. In 1950, the more-developed regions accounted for 32% of the world's population; their share dropped to 20% in 2000 and is expected to further decline to 13% in 2050. Changes are also projected for the world's age distribution: The proportion of people age 60 and over will increase from 10% in 2000 to 22% in 2050, and by 2050 there will be more older persons than children.

This rapid expansion of population, particularly in the past 50 years, is generally believed to be responsible for most of the stress humans put on the environment. A large and rapidly growing population makes it more difficult to provide the basic components of environmental health discussed earlier, including clean and disease-free food and water. It is also a driving force behind many of the relatively more recent environmental health concerns, including chemical pollution, global warming, and the thinning of the atmosphere's ozone layer.

### How Many People Can the World Hold?

No one knows how many people the world can support, but most scientists agree that there is a limit. A 2006 report from the United Nations' Convention on Biological Diversity states that the population's demand for resources already exceeds the earth's capacity by 20%. The primary factors that may eventually put a cap on human population are the following:

- *Food:* Enough food is currently produced to feed the world's entire population, but economic and sociopolitical factors have led to food shortages and famine. Food production can be expanded in the future, but better distribution of food will be needed to prevent even more widespread famine as the world's population keeps growing. For all people to receive adequate nutrition, the makeup of the world's diet may also need to change.

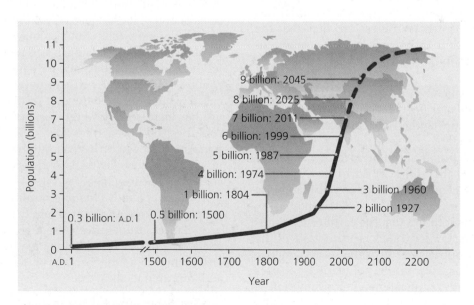

**FIGURE 15.1  World population growth.**
The United Nations estimates that the world's population will continue to increase dramatically until it stabilizes above 10 billion people in 2200.
**SOURCES:**  United Nations Population Division. 2009. *World Population Prospects: The 2009 Revision.* New York: United Nations; U.S. Census Bureau.

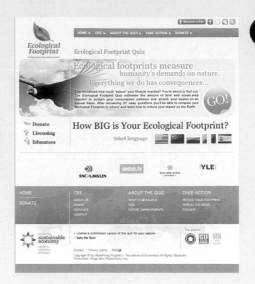

Environmental health may seem like a global challenge, but each person has a unique impact on our planet's health. In fact, there are ways to measure the environmental impact of your individual lifestyle.

For an estimate of how much land and water your lifestyle requires, take the Ecological Footprint quiz at www.myfootprint.org. You can also determine your "carbon footprint" at the Global Footprint Network Web site (www.footprintnetwork.org/en/index.php/GFN/page/calculators) or at the Nature Conservancy Web site (www.nature.org/initiatives/climatechange/calculator/?src=l12).

Go online and take one or all of these quizzes, and compare your results with the results of your classmates. Then identify ways you can reduce the size of your ecological and carbon footprints, both as an individual and as a class.

• *Available land and water:* Rural populations rely on trees, soil, and water for their direct sustenance, and a growing population puts a strain on these resources. Forests are cut for wood, soil is depleted, and water is withdrawn at ever-increasing rates. These trends contribute to local hardships and to many global environmental problems, including habitat destruction and species extinction.

• *Energy:* Currently, most of the world's energy comes from nonrenewable sources: oil, coal, natural gas, and nuclear power. As these sources are depleted, the world will have to shift to renewable (sustainable) energy sources, such as hydropower and solar, geothermal, wind, biomass, and ocean power. Supporting a growing population, maintaining economic productivity, and stemming environmental degradation will require both greater energy efficiency and an increased use of renewable energy sources.

• *Minimum acceptable standard of living:* The mass media have exposed the entire world to the American lifestyle and raised people's expectations of living at a comparable level. But such a lifestyle is supported by levels of energy consumption that the earth cannot support indefinitely. The United States has about 5% of the world's population but uses 25% of the world's energy. In contrast, India has 16% of the population but uses only 3% of the energy. China's energy consumption is rapidly increasing, and that nation accounts for 20% of the world's population. If all people are to enjoy a minimally acceptable standard of living, the population must be limited to a number that available resources can support.

## Factors That Contribute to Population Growth

Although it is apparent that population growth must be controlled, population trends are difficult to influence and manage. A variety of interconnecting factors fuel the current population explosion:

• *High fertility rates:* The combination of poverty, very high child mortality rates, and a lack of social provisions of every type is associated with high fertility rates in the developing world. Families may need to have more children to ensure that enough survive childhood to work for the household and to care for parents in old age. Most countries, both developed and developing, have experienced significant reductions in fertility as contraceptive use has increased. However, the majority of developing countries still have fertility levels that ensure substantial population growth. In a small number of countries, most of which are classified as least developed, fertility levels continue to be very high.

• *Lack of family planning resources:* Half the world's couples don't use any form of family planning.

• *Lower death rates:* Although death rates remain relatively high in the developing world, they have decreased in recent years because of public health measures and improved medical care.

Changes in any of these factors can affect population growth, but the issues are complex. Increasing death rates through disease, famine, or war might slow population growth, but few people would argue in favor of these as methods of population control. Although the increased availability of family planning services is a crucial part of population management, cultural, political, and religious factors also need to be considered. To be successful, population management policies must change the condition of people's lives, especially poverty, to remove the pressures to have large families. Research indicates that the combination of improved health, better education, and increased literacy and employment opportunities for women works together with family planning to decrease fertility rates. Unfortunately, in the fastest-growing countries, the needs of a rapidly increasing population use up financial resources that might otherwise be used to improve lives and ultimately slow population growth.

## AIR QUALITY AND POLLUTION

Air pollution is not a human invention or even a new problem. The air is polluted naturally with every forest fire, pollen bloom, and dust storm, as well as with countless other natural pollutants. To these natural sources, humans have always contributed the by-products of our activities.

Air pollution is linked to a wide range of health problems, and the very young and the elderly are among the most susceptible to air pollution's effects. For people with chronic ailments such as diabetes or heart failure, even relatively brief exposure to particulate air pollution increases the risk of death by nearly 40%. Recent studies have linked exposure to air pollution to reduced birth weight in infants, reduced lung capacity in teens, and atherosclerosis (thickening of the arteries) in adults.

## Air Quality and Smog

The U.S. Environmental Protection Agency (EPA) uses a measure called the **Air Quality Index (AQI)** to indicate whether air pollution levels pose a health concern. The AQI is used for five major air pollutants:

- *Carbon monoxide (CO):* An odorless, colorless gas, CO forms when the carbon in **fossil fuels** does not completely burn. The primary sources of CO are vehicle exhaust and fuel combustion in industrial processes. CO deprives body cells of oxygen, causing headaches, fatigue, and impaired vision and judgment. It also aggravates cardiovascular diseases.
- *Sulfur dioxide ($SO_2$):* $SO_2$ is produced by the burning of sulfur-containing fuels such as coal and oil, during metal smelting, and by other industrial processes; power plants are a major source. In humans, $SO_2$ narrows the airways, which may cause wheezing, chest tightness, and shortness of breath, particularly in people with asthma. $SO_2$ may also aggravate symptoms of CVD.
- *Nitrogen dioxide ($NO_2$):* $NO_2$ is a reddish-brown, highly reactive gas formed when nitric oxide combines with oxygen in the atmosphere; major sources include motor vehicles and power plants. In people with respiratory diseases such as asthma, $NO_2$ affects lung function and causes symptoms such as wheezing and shortness of breath. $NO_2$ exposure may also increase the risk of respiratory infections.
- *Particulate matter (PM):* Particles of different sizes are released into the atmosphere from a variety of sources, including combustion of fossil fuels, crushing or grinding operations, industrial processes, and dust from roadways. PM can accumulate in the respiratory system, aggravate cardiovascular and lung diseases, and increase the risk of respiratory infections.
- *Ground-level ozone:* At ground level, ozone is a harmful pollutant. Where it occurs naturally in the upper atmosphere, it shields the earth from the sun's harmful ultraviolet rays. (The health hazards from the thinning of this protective ozone layer are discussed later in the chapter.) Ground-level ozone is formed when pollutants emitted by cars, power plants, industrial plants, and other sources react chemically in the presence of sunlight (photochemical reactions). Ozone can irritate the respiratory system, reduce lung function, aggravate asthma, increase susceptibility to respiratory infections, and damage the lining of the lungs. Short-term elevations of ozone levels have also been linked to increased death rates.

**Air Quality Index (AQI)**   A measure of local air quality and what it means for health.

**fossil fuels**   Buried deposits of decayed animals and plants that are converted into carbon-rich fuels by exposure to heat and pressure over millions of years; oil, coal, and natural gas are fossil fuels.

**KEY TERMS**

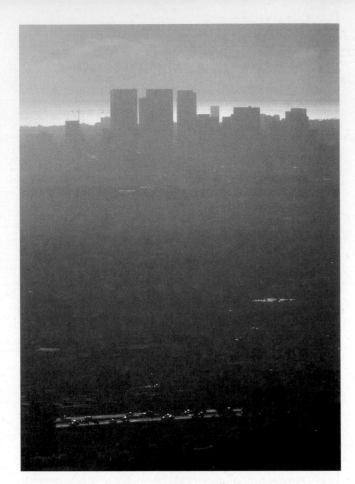

Smog tends to form over Los Angeles because of the natural geographical feaures of the area and because of the tremendous amount of motor vehicle exhaust in the air.

| Table 15.1 | Sources of Greenhouse Gases |
| --- | --- |
| GREENHOUSE GAS | SOURCES |
| Carbon dioxide | Fossil fuel and word burning, factory emissions, car exhaust, deforestation |
| Chlorofluorocarbons (CFCs) | Refrigeration and air conditioning, aerosols, foam products, solvents |
| Methane | Cattle, wetlands, rice paddies, land-fills, gas leaks, coal and gas industries |
| Nitrous oxide | Fertilizers, soil cultivation, deforesta-tion, animal feedlots and wastes |
| Ozone and other trace gases | Photochemical reactions, car exhaust, power plant emissions, solvents |

AQI values run from 0 to 500; the higher the AQI, the greater the level of pollution and associated health danger. When the AQI exceeds 100, air quality is considered unhealthy, at first for certain sensitive groups of people and then for everyone as AQI values get higher. For local areas, AQI values are calculated for each of the five pollutants listed above, and the highest value becomes the AQI rating for that day. Depending on the AQI value, local officials may issue precautionary health advice. Local AQI information is often available in newspapers, on television and radio, on the Internet, and from state and local telephone hotlines.

The term **smog** was first used in the early 1900s in London to describe the combination of smoke and fog. What we typically call smog today is a mixture of pollutants, with ground-level ozone being the key ingredient. Major smog occurrences are linked to the combination of several factors: Heavy motor vehicle traffic, high temperatures, and sunny weather can increase the production of ozone. Pollutants are also more likely to build up in areas with little wind and/or where a topographic feature such as a mountain range or valley prevents the wind from pushing out stagnant air.

## The Greenhouse Effect and Global Warming

The temperature of the earth's atmosphere depends on the balance between the amount of energy the planet absorbs from the sun (mainly as high-energy ultraviolet radiation) and the amount of energy radiated back into space as lower-energy infrared radiation. Key components of temperature regulation are carbon dioxide, water vapor, methane, and other **greenhouse gases**—so named because, like the glass panes in a greenhouse, they let through visible light from the sun but trap some of the resulting infrared radiation and reradiate it back to the earth's surface. This reradiation causes a buildup of heat that raises the temperature of the lower atmosphere, a natural process known as the **greenhouse effect.** Without it, the atmosphere would be far cooler and much more hostile to life.

There is growing consensus that human activity is causing **global warming,** or *climate change*. The concentration of greenhouse gases is increasing because of human activity, especially the combustion of fossil fuels (Table 15.1). Carbon dioxide levels in the atmosphere have increased rapidly in recent decades. The use of fossil fuels pumps more than 20 billion tons of carbon dioxide into the atmosphere every year. Experts believe carbon dioxide may account for about 60% of the greenhouse effect. Analysis of ice core samples shows that carbon dioxide levels are now about 25% higher than at any other time in

*Fitness Tip*

Exercising in polluted outdoor air can actually reduce lung function, at least temporarily. When the air quality outside is bad, exercise indoors.

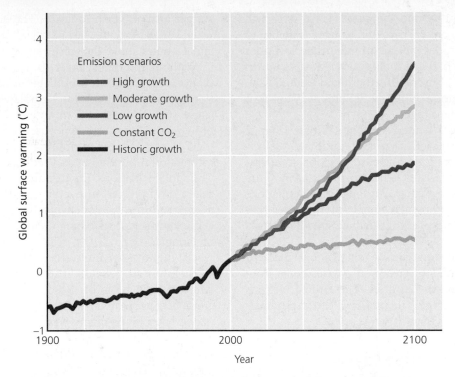

**FIGURE 15.2  Temperature projections to the year 2100, based on different greenhouse gas growth scenarios.**
The orange line shows that temperatures would change only slightly if greenhouse gas emissions stopped rising.
**SOURCE:** Environmental Protection Agency, 2007. *Future Temperature Changes* (http://www.epa.gov/climatechange/science/futuretc.html; retrieved June 15, 2011).

the last 650,000 years. The United States is responsible for one-third of the world's total emissions of carbon dioxide. Deforestation, often by burning, also sends carbon dioxide into the atmosphere and reduces the number of trees available to convert carbon dioxide into oxygen.

To date, 2005 was the warmest year on record since record keeping began in 1880, but 2010 may surpass it when data are analyzed. The global temperature has risen more than 1 degree Fahrenheit since 1900. There is growing agreement among scientists that temperatures will continue to rise, although estimates vary as to how much they will change. If global warming persists, experts say the impact may be devastating. Possible consequences include the following:

- Increased rainfall and flooding in some regions, increased drought in others. Coastal zones, where half the world's people live, would be severely affected.

- Increased mortality from heat stress, urban air pollution, and tropical diseases. Deaths from weather events such as hurricanes, tornadoes, droughts, and floods might also increase.

- A poleward shift of about 50–350 miles (150–550 km) in the location of vegetation zones, affecting crop yields, irrigation demands, and forest productivity.

- Increasingly rapid and drastic melting of the earth's polar ice caps. Arctic ice melts to some extent during

the summer each year, but during the 2007 melting season, arctic ice formations melted faster and farther than any other time since observations began. Experts predicted that as soon as 2030, the arctic sea ice could melt away completely during the summer, though it would return in the winter months. Such extensive melting could mean increased flooding in the Northern Hemisphere, further changes in weather patterns, and the elimination of habitat for species that live in the Arctic.

According to estimates from the Environmental Protection Agency (EPA), the earth's average surface temperature is likely to increase 2.0–11.5°F (1.1–6.4°C) by the end of the twenty-first century (Figure 15.2). Warming will not

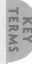

be evenly distributed around the globe. Land areas will warm more than oceans in part due to water's ability to store heat. High latitudes will warm more than low ones in part due to the effects of melting ice. Most of North America, all of Africa, Europe, Northern and Central Asia, and most of Central and South America are likely to warm more than the global average.

Parties at the 2009 United Nations Climate Change Conference in Copenhagen, Denmark, endorsed the scientific view that keeping the increase in global temperature below 2 degrees Celsius is necessary to stave off the worst effects of climate change. Although this conference did not end with a binding agreement among the world's nations, the parties did pledge to reduce greenhouse gas emissions.

Increasing research on climate change has revealed that significant amounts of greenhouse gases come from sources other than industrial ones. The United Nations has reported, for example, that raising cattle produces more greenhouse gases than driving cars.

## Thinning of the Ozone Layer

Another air pollution problem is the thinning of the **ozone layer** of the atmosphere, a fragile, invisible layer about 10–30 miles above the earth's surface that shields the planet from the sun's hazardous ultraviolet (UV) rays. Since the mid-1980s, scientists have observed the seasonal appearance and growth of a hole in the ozone layer over Antarctica. More recently, thinning over other areas has been noted.

The ozone layer is being destroyed primarily by **chlorofluorocarbons (CFCs),** industrial chemicals used as coolants in refrigerators and air conditioners, as foaming agents in some rigid foam products, as propellants in some kinds of aerosol sprays (most of which were banned in 1978), and as solvents. When CFCs rise into the atmosphere, winds carry them toward the polar regions. During winter, circular winds form a vortex that keeps the air over Antarctica from mixing with air from elsewhere. CFCs react with airborne ice crystals, releasing chlorine atoms, which destroy ozone. When the polar vortex weakens in the summer, winds richer in ozone from the north replenish the lost Antarctic ozone.

In the Northern Hemisphere, ozone levels have declined by about 10% since 1980, and certain areas may be temporarily depleted in late winter and early spring by as much as 40%. The largest and deepest ozone hole on record occurred in late September 2006, reaching 10.6 million square miles, considerably larger than the surface area of North America. The hole also had an unusual vertical extent, with nearly all the ozone between 8 and 13 miles above the earth's surface destroyed.

Without the ozone layer to absorb the sun's UV radiation, life on Earth would be impossible. (UV radiation levels under the Antarctic hole were high enough to cause sunburn within 7 minutes.) The potential effects of increased long-term exposure to UV light for humans include skin cancer, wrinkling and aging of the skin, cataracts and blindness, and reduced immune response. The United Nations Environment Programme predicts that a drop of 10% in overall ozone levels would cause a 26% rise in the incidence of nonmelanoma skin cancers. Some scientists blame ozone loss for many cases of melanoma.

UV light may interfere with photosynthesis and cause lower crop yields; it may also kill phytoplankton and krill, the basis of the ocean food chain. And because heat generated by the absorption of UV rays in the ozone layer helps create stratospheric winds, the driving force behind weather patterns, a drop in the concentration of ozone could potentially alter the earth's climate systems.

Worldwide production and use of CFCs have declined rapidly since the danger to the ozone layer was recognized. Industrialized nations agreed to eliminate CFC production as of the year 2000, and limits have also been placed on other agents that destroy ozone. Ozone-depleting substances have very long lifetimes in the atmosphere, however, so despite these efforts, the ozone hole is not expected to recover until 2070. The gradual recovery is masked by annual variations caused by weather fluctuations over Antarctica.

## Energy Use and Air Pollution

Americans are the biggest energy consumers in the world. We use energy to create electricity, transport us, power our industries, and run our homes. About 85% of the energy we use comes from fossil fuels—oil, coal, and natural gas. The remainder comes from nuclear power and renewable energy sources (such as hydroelectric, wind, and solar power).

Energy consumption is at the root of many environmental problems, especially those relating to air pollution. Automobile exhaust and the burning of oil and coal by industry and by electric power plants are primary causes of smog, acid precipitation, and the greenhouse effect. The mining of coal and the extraction and transportation of oil cause pollution on land and in the water; the 2010 oil spill in the Gulf of Mexico was the worst environmental disaster in American history and one of the largest oil spills ever to occur. Nuclear power generation creates hazardous wastes and carries the risk of dangerous releases of radiation.

Two key strategies for controlling energy use are conservation and the development of nonpolluting, renewable

**KEY TERMS**

**ozone layer**   A layer of ozone molecules ($O_3$) in the upper atmosphere that screens out UV rays from the sun.

**chlorofluorocarbons (CFCs)**   Chemicals used as spray-can propellants, refrigerants, and industrial solvents, implicated in the destruction of the ozone layer.

sources of energy. Although the use of renewable energy sources has increased in recent years, renewables still supply only a small proportion of our energy, in part because of their cost. Some countries have chosen to promote energy efficiency by removing subsidies or adding taxes on the use of fossil fuels. This strategy is reflected in the varying prices drivers pay for gasoline.

Despite increases in U.S. consumer gas prices, more than 70% of commuters drive alone to work, and low fuel-economy sport utility vehicles (SUVs) remain popular. Every gallon of gas burned puts about 20 pounds of carbon dioxide into the atmosphere; some SUVs average fewer than 10 miles per gallon, and the largest SUVs increase greenhouse gas emissions by 6 or more tons per year more than an average car.

**Alternative Fuels** The U.S. Department of Energy (DOE) is encouraging researchers and automobile manufacturers to produce vehicles that can handle alternative fuels such as ethanol. Ethanol, a form of alcohol, is a renewable and largely domestic transportation fuel produced from fermenting plant sugars such as corn, sugar cane, and other starchy agricultural products. Ethanol use reduces the amount of imported oil required to produce gasoline, reduces overall greenhouse gas emissions from automobiles, and supports the U.S. agricultural industry.

Another type of alternative fuel is E85, which is a mixture of 85% ethanol and 15% gasoline. E85 is becoming more popular in the Midwest region (the "corn belt") of the United States. E85 provides lower mileage than gasoline, though it typically costs the same as regular gasoline. Ethanol has been mixed with gasoline for years in the United States, but several other countries (such as Brazil) use ethanol much more extensively.

Ethanol, however, has its critics, who say the alternative fuel may do more harm than good. For one thing, some reports show that corn-based ethanol requires more energy to produce than it yields when burned as fuel. Other reports dispute this point, and improvements in manufacturing processes may reduce the amount of energy required to make the fuel. Regardless, ethanol made from sugar cane and other plant matter may be far more energy-efficient, say some experts.

One huge potential drawback of ethanol is the diversion of corn crops from the food supply to produce the fuel. In 2007 and 2008, this practice was blamed for skyrocketing food prices and food shortages around the world, which led to food riots in several countries. At the same time, the federal government gave billions of dollars in subsidies to corn farmers to raise the grain for ethanol production, even as grain prices soared. The food-related concerns prompted the United Nations to call for a moratorium on food-based ethanol production until nonfood sources of alternative fuels could be developed.

**Hybrid and Electric Vehicles** A more positive trend has been the introduction of hybrid electric vehicles (HEVs). Hybrid vehicles use two or more distinct power sources to propel the vehicle, such as an on-board energy storage system (batteries, for example) and an internal combustion engine and electric motor. The hybrid vehicle typically realizes greater fuel economy than a conventional car does and produces fewer polluting emissions. Hybrids also tend to run with less noise than conventional vehicles. Several hybrid models are currently available in the United States, but they typically cost several thousand dollars more than their conventional gas-powered counterparts. Still, hybrids are gaining popularity with consumers and are being more commonly used in both corporate and government vehicle fleets.

Researchers hope that hybrid technology can be extended to all classes of vehicles and that Americans can be convinced to use more fuel-efficient vehicles and to travel more frequently on public transportation, in carpools, or on foot.

Another type of alternative vehicle is all-electric. In these vehicles, electricity is stored in battery packs and then converted into mechanical power that runs the vehicle. After a given number of miles, the batteries must be recharged. These vehicles do not produce tailpipe emissions, but generators that produce the electricity for the batteries do emit pollutants.

Even when mass production begins, electric vehicles are expected to cost more than conventionally fueled ones. Even with lower "fuel" and maintenance costs (electric vehicles have fewer moving parts than gas-powered cars), the lead-acid battery packs must be replaced every few years, adding to the overall cost of electric vehicles.

## Indoor Air Pollution

Although most people associate air pollution with the outdoors, your home may also harbor potentially dangerous pollutants. Some of these compounds trigger allergic responses, and others have been linked to cancer. Common indoor pollutants include the following:

- *Environmental tobacco smoke* (*ETS*), a human carcinogen that also increases the risk of asthma, bronchitis, and cardiovascular disease (see Chapter 11). Several states and cities have passed legislation known as Clean Indoor Air Acts, which state that any enclosed, indoor areas used by the public shall be smoke-free except for certain designated areas.
- *Carbon monoxide and other combustion by-products,* which can cause chronic bronchitis, headaches, dizziness, nausea, fatigue, and even death. Common sources in the home are woodstoves, fireplaces, kerosene heaters and lamps, and gas ranges. In poverty-stricken areas, especially in Asia and Africa, people commonly burn solid fuels like coal for cooking and heating their homes. The World Health Organization (WHO) says the smoke and

by-products from these indoor fires kill about 1.5 million people annually—mostly children.

- *Formaldehyde gas,* which can cause eye, nose, and throat irritation; shortness of breath; headaches; nausea; lethargy; and, over the long term, cancer. This gas can seep from certain construction materials, paints, floor finishes, permanent press clothing, and nail polish.

- *Biological pollutants,* including bacteria, dust mites, mold, and animal dander, which can cause allergic reactions and other health problems. These allergens are typically found in bathrooms, damp or flooded basements, humidifiers, air conditioners, and even some carpets and furniture.

- *Indoor mold,* the fuzzy black substance growing on shower tiles and damp basement walls, is an indoor pollutant not to be taken lightly. More than 100 common indoor molds have been classified as potentially hazardous to people, but only a few are serious threats to human health. One of the most common of these is *Stachybotrys* mold, commonly known as "toxic black mold." It is greenish black in color and appears slimy when wet. Toxic mold spores permeate the air and can cause health problems when inhaled, especially for people with asthma and other respiratory conditions.

## Preventing Air Pollution

You can do a great deal to reduce air pollution. Here are a few ideas:

- Cut back on driving. Ride your bike, walk, use public transportation, or carpool in a fuel-efficient vehicle.

- Keep your car tuned and well maintained. Keep your tires inflated at recommended pressures. To save energy when driving, avoid quick starts, stay within the speed limit, limit the use of air conditioning, and don't let your car idle unless absolutely necessary. Have your car's air conditioner checked and serviced by a station that uses environmentally friendly refrigerants (automotive air conditioners made before 1994 are a major source of CFCs).

- Buy energy-efficient appliances and use them only when necessary. Run the washing machine, dryer, and dishwasher only when you have full loads, and do laundry in warm or cold water instead of hot; don't overdry your clothes. Clean refrigerator coils and clothes dryer lint screens frequently. Towel or air-dry your hair rather than using an electric dryer.

- Replace incandescent bulbs with compact fluorescent bulbs (not fluorescent tubes). For more information, see the box "Compact Fluorescent Lightbulbs."

- Make sure your home is well insulated with ozone-safe agents; use insulating shades and curtains to keep heat in during winter and out during summer.

- Plant and care for trees in your yard and neighborhood. They recycle carbon dioxide, so trees work against global warming. They also provide shade and cool the air, so less air conditioning is needed.

- Before discarding a refrigerator, air conditioner, or humidifier, check with the waste hauler or your local government to ensure that ozone-depleting refrigerants will be removed prior to disposal.

- Keep your house adequately ventilated, and buy some houseplants; they have a natural ability to rid the air of harmful pollutants.

- Keep paints, cleaning agents, and other chemical products tightly sealed in their original containers.

- Don't smoke, and don't allow others to smoke in your room, apartment, or home. If these rules are too strict for your situation, limit smoking to a single, well-ventilated room.

- Clean and inspect chimneys, furnaces, and other appliances regularly. Install carbon monoxide detectors.

## WATER QUALITY AND POLLUTION

Few parts of the world have enough safe, clean drinking water, and yet few things are as important to human health.

## Water Contamination and Treatment

Many cities rely at least in part on wells that tap local groundwater, but often it is necessary to tap lakes and rivers to supplement wells. Because such surface water is more likely to be contaminated with both organic matter and pathogenic microorganisms, it is purified in water treatment plants before being piped into the community. At treatment facilities, the water is subjected to various physical and chemical processes, including screening, filtration, and disinfection (often with chlorine), before it is introduced into the water supply system. **Fluoridation,** a water-treatment process that reduces tooth decay by 15–40%, has been used successfully in the United States for more than 60 years.

In most areas of the United States, water systems have adequate, dependable supplies, are able to control

Ask yourself
QUESTIONS FOR CRITICAL THINKING AND REFLECTION

What are your views on the issue of climate change? Do you believe it is a real problem, or that it has been overly hyped by the media and some politicians and activist groups? How do you support your views?

# Compact Fluorescent Lightbulbs

A good way to cut your home's energy use, lower your energy bills, and reduce your environmental footprint is by using energy-efficient lightbulbs, commonly called *compact fluorescent lightbulbs (CFLs)*.

According to the EPA, CFLs are cost-efficient because they use 75% less energy than traditional incandescent lightbulbs. Although CFLs initially cost more than regular lightbulbs, over the long term they save money for the user. This is because they use less energy by requiring less electricity to produce light. For example, a 15-watt CFL is equivalent to a 60-watt incandescent lightbulb. CFLs also last up to ten times longer than conventional lightbulbs.

The EPA says that if every American home replaced one incandescent bulb with a CFL, enough energy would be saved in one year to light 3 million homes. It would also reduce greenhouse gas emissions by an amount equal to the output of 800,000 cars.

In some countries, consumer reluctance to switch to CFLs has resulted in government action. Australia and Canada have instituted bans on incandescent bulbs. Many other countries are contemplating similar measures, and various organizations are lobbying for the use of CFLs.

In spite of their positive attributes, compact fluorescent bulbs have a downside: They contain a gas that includes low-pressure mercury and argon. Mercury vapor from broken bulbs can harm babies, children, and pregnant women, and the bulbs can pollute the environment if dumped in the trash. If all the CFLs currently in use were disposed of in landfills,

they could generate about 30,000 pounds of mercury that could eventually leech into the groundwater system. For this reason, it is best to take your burned-out CFLs (and all fluorescent bulbs) to a recycling center for proper disposal instead of tossing them in the trash.

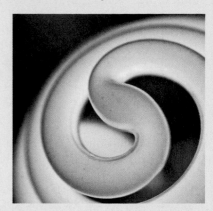

Even though the amount of mercury in a single CFL is very small, you should take extra precautions when cleaning up a broken bulb. If a CFL breaks, shut off the central heating/air conditioning system, open a window, and clear all people and animals out of the room for at least 15 minutes. Put on rubber or latex gloves, and carefully pick up the large pieces of glass. Put the pieces in a glass jar that can be closed with a lid or in a heavy-duty plastic bag that can be sealed. Gently sweep up the small pieces and dust using a broom and dustpan. You can use duct tape to pick up fine particles. Seal everything up (including your gloves) in the jar or bag, and take it to a recycling center for disposal.

---

waterborne disease, and provide water without unacceptable color, odor, or taste. However, problems do occur. In 1993, more than 400,000 people became ill and 100 died when Milwaukee's drinking water was contaminated with the bacterium *Cryptosporidium*. The Centers for Disease Control and Prevention (CDC) estimate that 1 million Americans become ill and 900–1000 die each year from microbial illnesses from drinking water. Pollution by hazardous chemicals from manufacturing, agriculture, and household wastes is another concern. (Chemical pollution is discussed later in the chapter.) Worldwide, more than 2 million people, mostly children, die from water-related diseases each year.

## Wellness Tip

Plastic water bottles are a huge source of pollution. The most environmentally friendly way to quench your thirst is by drinking filtered tap water from a reusable, washable bottle. If you buy bottled water, be sure to recycle the bottles.

## Water Shortages

Water shortages are a growing concern in many regions of the world. Some parts of the United States are experiencing rapid population growth that outstrips the ability of local systems to provide adequate water to all. Many proposals are being discussed to relieve these shortages, including long-distance transfers; conservation; the recycling of some water, such as the water in office-building air conditioners; and the sale of water by regions with large supplies to areas with less available water.

According to the World Health Organization (WHO), 1 billion people do not have safe drinking water and 2.6 billion do not have access to basic sanitation. Less than 1% of the world's fresh water—about 0.007% of all the water on Earth—is readily accessible for direct human use.

Groundwater pumping and the diversion of water from lakes and rivers for irrigation are further reducing the amount of water available to local communities. In

---

**fluoridation** The addition of fluoride to the water supply to reduce tooth decay.

some areas, groundwater is being removed at twice the rate at which it is replaced. The Aral Sea, located in Kazakhstan and Uzbekistan, was once one of the world's largest inland seas. Since the 1960s, it has lost two-thirds of its volume to irrigation, and the exposed seabed is now as big as the Netherlands. People living in the area have experienced severe water and food shortages and increased rates of respiratory disease and throat cancer linked to dust storms from the dry seabed. Due to agricultural diversions, the Yellow River ran dry for the first time in China's 3000-year history in 1972, failing to reach the sea for 15 days that year; now, the dry period extends for more than half of each year. In the United States, the Colorado River is now diverted to the extent that it no longer flows into the ocean.

## Sewage

Prior to the mid-nineteenth century, many people contracted diseases such as typhoid, cholera, and hepatitis A by direct contact with human feces, which were disposed of at random. Once the links between sewage and disease were discovered, practices began to change. People learned how to build sanitary outhouses and how to locate them so they would not contaminate water sources.

As plumbing moved indoors, sewage disposal became more complicated. In rural areas, the **septic system,** a self-contained sewage disposal system, worked quite well. Today, many rural homes still rely on septic systems; however, many old tanks are leaking contaminants into the environment.

Different approaches became necessary as urban areas developed. Most cities have sewage-treatment systems that separate fecal matter from water in huge tanks and ponds and stabilize it so that it cannot transmit infectious diseases. Once treated and biologically safe, the water is released back into the environment. The sludge that remains behind is often contaminated with **heavy metals** and is handled as hazardous waste; if not contaminated, sludge may be used as fertilizer, although this practice is being discouraged by scientists and some government agencies and is not permitted in organic agriculture. If incorporated into the food chain, heavy metals, such as lead, cadmium, copper, and tin, can cause illness or death; therefore, these chemicals must not be released into the environment when sludge is burned or buried.

In addition to regulating industrial discharge, many cities have expanded sewage-treatment measures to remove heavy metals and other hazardous chemicals. This action has resulted from many studies linking exposure to chemicals such as mercury, lead, and **polychlorinated biphenyls (PCBs)** with long-term health consequences, including cancer and damage to the central nervous system. The technology to effectively remove heavy metals and chemicals from sewage is still developing, and the costs involved are immense.

## Protecting the Water Supply

By reducing your own water use, you help preserve your community's valuable supply and lower your monthly water bill. By taking steps to keep the water supply clean, you reduce pollution overall and help protect the land, wildlife, and other people from illness. Here are some simple steps you can take to protect your water supply:

- Take showers, not baths, to minimize your water consumption. Don't let water run when you're not actively using it while brushing your teeth, shaving, or hand-washing clothes. Don't run a dishwasher or washing machine until you have a full load.

- Install sink faucet aerators and water-efficient showerheads, which use two to five times less water with no noticeable decrease in performance.

- Purchase a water-saver toilet, or put a displacement device in your toilet tank to reduce the amount of water used with each flush.

- Fix any leaky faucets in your home. Leaks can waste thousands of gallons of water per year.

- Don't pour toxic materials such as cleaning solvents, bleach, or motor oil down the drain. Store them until you can take them to a hazardous waste collection center.

- Don't pour old medicines down the drain or flush them down the toilet. A 2008 report by the Associated Press revealed that the drinking water of some 40 million Americans may be contaminated with prescription and over-the-counter drugs. Some medications enter the water system after human excretion into sewage systems, but many people flush old or unused medicines. The EPA is working on strategies to remove medicines from drinking water, but for now says the drugs appear only in trace amounts and generally are not considered a health hazard.

## SOLID WASTE POLLUTION

Humans generate huge amounts of waste, which must be handled appropriately if the environment is to be kept safe.

### Ask Yourself

**QUESTIONS FOR CRITICAL THINKING AND REFLECTION**

How would you describe the quality of the water where you live? Are there lakes or streams where you can safely swim or fish? What local information sources can you find about water quality in your area?

## Solid Waste

The bulk of the organic food garbage produced in American kitchens is now dumped in the sewage system by way of the mechanical garbage disposal. The garbage that remains is not very hazardous from the standpoint of infectious disease because there is very little food waste in it, but it does represent an enormous disposal and contamination problem.

**What's in Our Garbage?** In 2008, Americans generated about 250 million tons of trash and recycled 83 million tons of materials. The biggest single component of household trash by weight is paper products, including junk mail, glossy mail-order catalogs, and computer printouts (Figure 15.3). Yard waste, plastic, metals, and glass are other significant components. About 1% of the solid waste is toxic; a new source of toxic waste is the disposal of computer components in both household and commercial waste. Burning, as opposed to burial, reduces the bulk of solid waste, but it can release hazardous material into the air, depending on what is being burned.

Solid waste is not limited to household products. Manufacturing, mining, and other industries all produce large amounts of potentially dangerous materials that cannot simply be dumped. At Love Canal (near Buffalo, New York), toxic industrial wastes had been dumped into a waterway for years until, in the 1970s, nearby residents began to suffer from associated birth defects and cancers. The government had to step in, people had to move from their homes, and huge costs were incurred.

**Disposing of Solid Waste** Since the 1960s, billions of tons of solid waste have been buried in **sanitary landfill** disposal sites (Figure 15.4). Careful site selection and daily management are an essential part of this approach to disposal. The site is thoroughly studied to ensure that it is not near groundwater, streams, or any other source of water that could be contaminated by leakage from the landfill. Sometimes protective liners are used around the site, and nearby monitoring wells are now required in most states. Layers of solid waste are regularly covered with thin layers of dirt until the site is filled. Some communities then plant grass and trees and convert the site into a park. Landfill is relatively stable; almost no decomposition occurs in the solidly packed waste.

Burying solid waste in landfills has several disadvantages. Much of this waste contains chemicals, ranging from leftover pesticides to paints and oils, which should not be released into the environment. Despite precautions, buried contaminants sometimes leak into the surrounding soil and groundwater. Burial is also expensive and requires huge amounts of space.

**Biodegradability** *Biodegradation* is the process by which organic substances are broken down naturally by living organisms. Organic materials can be degraded either aerobically (with oxygen) or anaerobically (without oxygen). These organic materials—including plant and animal matter, substances originating from living organisms, or artificial materials similar in nature to plants and animals—are put to use by microorganisms. The term **biodegradable** means that certain products can break down naturally, safely, and quickly into the raw materials of nature, then disappear back into the environment. Table 15.2 shows the amount of time required for different types of material to biodegrade.

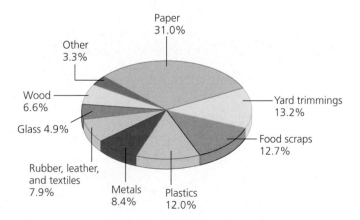

**FIGURE 15.3   Components of municipal solid waste, by weight, before recycling.**

**SOURCE:** Environmental Protection Agency. 2009. *Municipal Solid Waste Generation, Recycling and Disposal in the United States: Facts and Figures for 2008.* Washington, D.C.: Environmental Protection Agency. Pub. No. EPA-530-F-009-021.

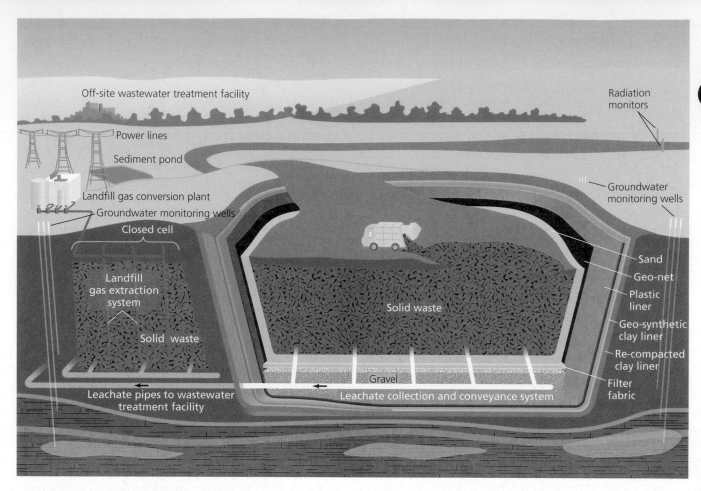

**FIGURE 15.4  A sanitary landfill.**

**Recycling** Because of the expense and potential chemical hazards of any form of solid waste disposal, many communities encourage individuals and businesses to recycle their trash. In **recycling,** many kinds of waste materials are collected and used as raw materials in the production of new products. For example, waste paper can be recycled into new paper products, or an old bicycle frame can be melted down and used in the production of appliances. The number of recycling opportunities is almost limitless. Recycling is a good idea for two reasons. First, it puts unwanted objects back to good use. Second, it reduces the amount of solid waste sitting in landfills, some of which takes decades to decay naturally. Some cities offer curbside pickup of recyclables; others have recycling centers where people can bring their waste. These materials are not limited to paper, glass, and cans but also include things such as discarded tires and used oils.

Even as recycling grows in popularity, however, the total amount of garbage Americans generate will probably continue to rise as the population increases. Researchers estimate that 80% of the nation's landfills will be closed within 20 years.

**Discarded Technology: eWaste** A newer solid waste disposal problem involves the discarding of old computers, televisions, cell phones, MP3 players, and other

> **KEY TERM**
>
> **recycling** The use of waste materials as raw materials in the production of new products.

| Table 15.2 | Biodegrading Times of Different Objects |
| --- | --- |
| **ITEM** | **TIME REQURED TO BIODEGRADE** |
| Banana peel | 2–10 days |
| Paper | 2–5 months |
| Rope | 3–14 months |
| Orange peel | 6 months |
| Wool sock | 1–5 years |
| Cigarette butt | 1–12 years |
| Plastic-coated milk carton | 5 years |
| Aluminum can | 80–100 years |
| Plastic six-pack holder ring | 450 years |
| Glass bottle | 1 million years |
| Plastic bottle | Forever |

# How to Be a Green Consumer

It may seem like a hassle to consider the environmental impact of the things you buy, but a few simple choices can make a big difference without compromising your lifestyle. You can quickly and easily develop habits that direct your consumer dollar toward environmentally friendly products and companies.

- Remember the four Rs of green consumerism:

  - Reduce the amount of trash and pollution you generate by consuming and throwing away less.

  - Reuse as many products as possible—either yourself or by selling them or donating them to charity.

  - Recycle all appropriate materials and buy recycled products whenever possible.

  - Respond by educating others about reducing waste and recycling, by finding creative ways to reduce waste and toxicity, and by making your preferences known.

- Choose products packaged in refillable, recycled, reusable containers or in readily recyclable materials, such as paper, cardboard, aluminum, or glass. Don't buy products that are excessively packaged or wrapped.

- Look for products made with the highest possible content of recycled paper, metal, glass, plastic, and other materials.

- Choose simple products containing the lowest amounts of bleaches, dyes, and fragrances. Look for organically grown foods and clothes made from organically grown cotton, from Fox Fibre, or another naturally colored type of cotton.

- Buy high-quality appliances that have an Energy Star seal from the EPA or some other type of certification indicating that they are energy- and water-efficient.

- Get a reusable cloth shopping bag. Don't bag items that don't need to be bagged. If you forget to bring your bag to the store, it doesn't matter much if you use a paper or plastic bag to carry your purchases home. What's important is that you reuse or recycle whatever bag you get.

- Don't buy what you don't need—borrow, rent, or share. Take good care of the things you own, repair items when they break, and replace them with used rather than new items whenever possible.

- Walk or bike when you can. If you must drive, do several errands at once to save energy and cut down on pollution.

- Look beyond the products to the companies that make them. Support those with good environmental records. If some of your favorite products are overpackaged or contain harmful ingredients, write to the manufacturer.

- Keep in mind that doing something is better than doing nothing. Even if you can't be a perfectly green consumer, doing your best on any purchase will make a difference.

SOURCES: U.S. Environmental Protection Agency. 2010. *The Consumer's Handbook for Reducing Solid Waste* (http://www.epa.gov/osw/wycd/cat book; retrieved June 15, 2011); Natural Resources Defense Council. 2009. *NRDC's Guide to Greener Living* (http://www.nrdc.org/cities/living /gover.asp; retrieved June 15, 2011).

---

electronic devices. Americans scrap about 400 million consumer electronic devices each year. This "e-waste" is the fastest growing portion of our waste stream. Junked electronic devices are toxic because they contain varying amounts of lead, mercury, and other heavy metals. Many components of electronic devices are valuable, however, and can be recycled and reused. Local and state e-waste recycling programs are becoming more common, and private companies are also getting into the e-waste recycling business. If you recycle your electronic devices, look for a "green" program or one that is certified by e-stewards, an organization that advocates for responsible e-waste recycling (www.e-stewards.org).

## Reducing Solid Waste

By recycling more and throwing away less, you can conserve landfill space and put more reusable items back into service. Here are some ideas to help you reduce solid waste:

- Buy products with the least amount of packaging you can, or buy products in bulk (see the box "How to Be a Green Consumer"). For example, buy large jars of juice, not individually packaged juice drinks. Buy products packaged in recyclable containers.

- Buy recycled or recyclable products. Avoid disposables; instead, use long-lasting or reusable products such as refillable pens and rechargeable batteries.

- Avoid using foam or paper cups and plastic stirrers by bringing your own ceramic coffee mug and metal spoon to work or wherever you drink coffee or tea. Pack your lunch in reusable containers, and use a cloth or plastic lunch sack or a lunch box.

- To store food, use glass jars and reusable plastic containers rather than foil and plastic wrap.

- Recycle your newspapers, glass, cans, paper, and other recyclables. If you receive something packaged with foam pellets, take them to a commercial mailing center that accepts them for recycling.

- Do not throw electronic items, batteries, or fluorescent lights into the trash. Take all these to state-approved recycling centers; check with your local disposal service for more information.

- Start a compost pile for your organic garbage (non-animal food and yard waste) if you have a yard. If you live in an apartment, you can create a small composting system using earthworms, or take your organic wastes to a community composting center. Some cities now collect kitchen scraps for recycling into compost, which is sold to farms and wineries.

## CHEMICAL POLLUTION AND HAZARDOUS WASTE

Chemical pollution is by no means a new problem. The ancient Romans were plagued by lead poisoning; industrial chemicals have claimed countless lives over the past few centuries.

Today, new chemical substances are constantly being introduced into the environment—as pesticides, herbicides, solvents, and hundreds of other products. More people and wildlife are exposed and potentially exposed to them than ever before.

The problem of chemical pollution and hazardous waste became so prominent in the 1970s that the EPA established the Superfund program to clean up the nation's uncontrolled hazardous waste sites. A national priorities list determines which locations get cleaned up. To date, the EPA has completed cleanups at hundreds of hazardous waste sites. As the Superfund program matures, so does the size, complexity, and cost of cleanup work. The EPA also pushes industrial polluters to pay the costs of cleanups.

### Asbestos

A mineral-based compound, asbestos was widely used for fire protection and insulation in buildings until the late 1960s. Microscopic asbestos fibers can be released into the air when this material is applied or when it later deteriorates or is damaged. These fibers can lodge in the lungs, causing **asbestosis,** lung cancer, and other serious lung diseases. Similar conditions expose workers to risk in the coal mining industry, from coal and silica dust (black lung disease), and in the textile industry, from cotton fibers (brown lung disease).

Asbestos can pose a danger in homes and apartment buildings, about 25% of which are thought to contain some asbestos. Areas where it is most likely to be found are insulation around water and steam pipes, ducts, and furnaces; boiler wraps; vinyl flooring; floor, wall, and ceiling insulation; roofing and siding; and fireproof board.

### Lead

Thanks to better preventive efforts, lead poisoning is not as serious a problem today as it was in the past. Still, the CDC estimates that about 435,000 children under age 6 may have unsafe lead levels in their blood; the actual number could be much higher. Many of these children live in poor, inner-city areas (see the box "Poverty and Environmental Health"). When lead is ingested or inhaled, it can damage the central nervous system, cause mental impairment, hinder oxygen transport in the blood, and create digestive problems. Severe lead poisoning may cause coma or even death. Neurological damage can be permanent.

Long-term exposure to low levels of lead may cause kidney disease; it can also cause lead to build up in bones, where it may be released into the bloodstream during pregnancy or when bone mass is lost from osteoporosis.

Lead-based paints are the chief culprit in lead poisoning of children. They were banned from residential use in 1978, but as many as 57 million American homes still contain lead paint. In 2006, the EPA proposed new guidelines requiring contractors to take special lead containment measures when doing renovations, repairs, or painting in certain buildings. This became law in April 2008, with full implementation of the law in April 2010. The use of lead in plumbing is now also banned, but some old pipes and faucets contain lead.

### Pesticides

**Pesticides** are used primarily for two purposes: to prevent the spread of insect-borne diseases and to maximize food production by killing insects that eat crops. Both uses have risks as well as benefits. For example, DDT was extremely effective in controlling insect-borne diseases in tropical countries and in increasing crop yields throughout the world, but it was found to disrupt the life cycles of birds, fish, and reptiles and was banned in the United States in 1972. DDT also builds up in the food chain, increasing in concentration as larger animals eat smaller ones, a process known as **biomagnification.**

### Mercury

A naturally occurring metal, mercury is a toxin that affects the nervous system and may damage the brain, kidneys, and gastrointestinal tract; increase blood pressure, heart rate, and heart attack risk; and cause cancer. Mercury slows fetal and child development and causes irreversible

# Poverty and Environmental Health

Residents of poor and minority communities are often exposed to more environmental toxins than residents of wealthier communities, and they are more likely to suffer from health problems caused or aggravated by pollutants.

Poor neighborhoods are often located near highways and industrial areas that have high levels of air and noise pollution; they are also common sites for hazardous waste production and disposal. Residents of substandard housing are more likely to come into contact with lead, asbestos, carbon monoxide, pesticides, and other hazardous pollutants associated with peeling paint, old plumbing, and poorly maintained insulation and heating equipment.

Poor people are more likely to have jobs that expose them to asbestos, silica dust, and pesticides, and they are more likely to catch and consume fish contaminated with PCBs, mercury, and other toxins.

The most thoroughly researched and documented link among poverty, the environment, and health is lead poisoning in children. Many studies have shown that children of low-income black families are much more likely to have elevated levels of lead in their blood than white children. One survey found that two-thirds of urban African American children from families earning less than $6000 a year had elevated lead levels. The CDC and the American Academy of Pediatrics recommend annual testing of blood lead levels for all children under age 6, with more frequent testing for children at special risk.

Asthma is another health threat that appears to be linked with both environmental and socioeconomic factors. The number of Americans with asthma has grown dramatically in the past 20 years; most of the increase has occurred in children, with African Americans and the poor hardest hit. Researchers are not sure what accounts for this increase, but suspects include household pollutants, pesticides, air pollution, cigarette smoke, and allergens like cockroaches. These risk factors are likely to cluster in poor urban areas where inadequate health care may worsen asthma's effects.

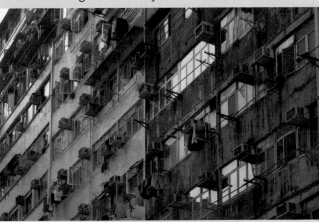

deficits in brain function. As many as 600,000 babies are born each year having been exposed to unsafe levels of mercury. Coal-fired power plants are the largest producers of mercury; other sources include mining and smelting operations and the disposal of consumer products containing mercury.

Mercury persists in the environment, and like pesticides, it is bioaccumulative. In particular, large, long-lived fish may carry high levels of mercury.

## Other Chemical Pollutants

The list of real and potential chemical pollution problems may well be as long as the list of known chemicals. As mentioned earlier, hazardous wastes are commonly found in the home and should be handled and disposed of properly. They include automotive supplies (motor oil, antifreeze, transmission fluid), paint supplies (turpentine, paint thinner, mineral spirits), art and hobby supplies (oil-based paint, solvents, acids and alkalis, aerosol sprays), insecticides, batteries, computer and electronic components, and household cleaners containing sodium hydroxide (lye) or ammonia. These chemicals are dangerous when inhaled or ingested, when they contact the skin or the eyes, or when they are burned or dumped. Many cities provide guidelines about approved disposal methods and have hazardous waste collection days.

## Preventing Chemical Pollution

You can take steps to reduce the chemical pollution in your community. Just as important, by reducing and

### Wellness Tip

Dispose of your household hazardous wastes properly. If you don't know how to dispose of an item, contact your local environmental health office or health department for information.

## Ask Yourself

### QUESTIONS FOR CRITICAL THINKING AND REFLECTION

Are there any hazardous chemicals in your home, such as cleaning products, solvents, paint, or batteries? Would you know what to do if one of these chemicals spilled? How would you clean it up?

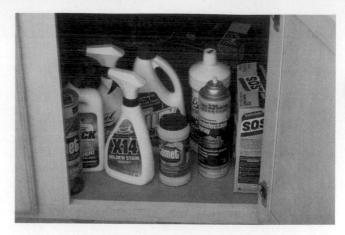

Hazardous chemicals accumulate in many homes, as well as in business and industrial sites.

eliminating the number of chemicals in your home, you may save the life of a child or animal who might encounter one of those chemicals.

- When buying products, read the labels, and try to buy the least toxic ones available. Choose nontoxic, nonpetrochemical cleansers, disinfectants, polishes, and other personal and household products.

- Buy organic produce or produce that has been grown locally.

- If you must use pesticides or toxic household products, store them in a locked place where children and pets can't get to them. Don't measure chemicals with food-preparation utensils, and wear gloves whenever handling them.

- If you have your house fumigated for pest control, be sure to hire a licensed exterminator. Keep everyone, including pets, out of the house while the crew works and, if possible, for a few days after.

## RADIATION POLLUTION

**Radiation** comes in different forms, such as ultraviolet rays, microwaves, or X-rays, and from different sources, such as the sun, uranium, and nuclear weapons

(Figure 15.5). These forms of electromagnetic radiation differ in wavelength and energy, with shorter waves having the highest energy levels.

Of most concern to health are gamma rays produced by radioactive sources such as nuclear weapons, nuclear energy plants, and radon gas. These high-energy waves are powerful enough to penetrate objects and break molecular bonds. Although gamma radiation cannot be seen or felt, its effects at high doses can include **radiation sickness** and death. At lower doses, chromosome damage, sterility, tissue damage, cataracts, and cancer can occur. Other types of radiation can also affect health. For example, exposure to UV radiation from the sun or from tanning salons can increase the risk of skin cancer. The effects of some sources of radiation, such as cell phones, remain controversial.

## Nuclear Weapons and Nuclear Energy

Nuclear weapons pose a health risk of the most serious kind to all species. Public health associations have stated

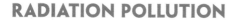

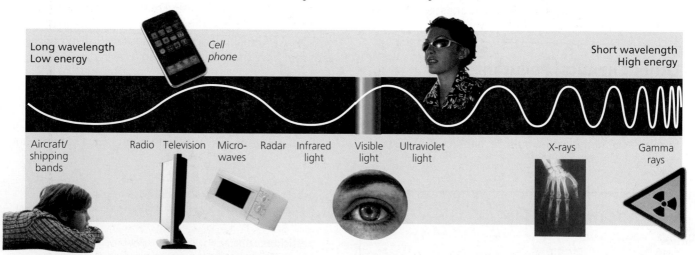

**FIGURE 15.5 Electromagnetic radiation.**
Electromagnetic radiation takes the form of waves that travel through space. The length of the wave determines the type of radiation: The shortest waves are high-energy gamma rays; the longest are radio waves and extremely low frequency waves used for communication between aircraft, ships, and submarines. Different types of electromagnetic radiation have different effects on health.

that in the event of an intentional or unintentional discharge of these weapons, the casualties would run into the hundreds of thousands or millions. Reducing the stockpiles of nuclear weapons is a challenge and a goal for the twenty-first century.

Power-generating plants that use nuclear fuel also pose health problems. When **nuclear power** was first developed as an alternative to oil and coal, it was promoted as clean, efficient, inexpensive, and safe. In general, this has proven to be the case. Power systems in several parts of the world rely on nuclear power plants. However, despite all the built-in safeguards and regulating agencies, accidents in nuclear power plants do happen, many due to human error (as at Three Mile Island in the United States and Tokaimura in Japan), and the consequences of such accidents are far more serious than those of similar accidents in other types of power-generating plants. The 1986 fire and explosion at the Chernobyl nuclear power station in Ukraine caused hundreds of deaths and increased rates of genetic mutation and cancer; the long-term effects are not yet clear. The zone around Chernobyl could be unsafe for the next 24,000 years.

An additional, enormous problem is disposing of the radioactive wastes these plants generate. They cannot be dumped in a sanitary landfill because the amount and type of soil used to cap a sanitary landfill are not sufficient to prevent radiation from escaping. Deposit sites have to be developed that will be secure not just for a few years but for tens of thousands of years—longer than the total recorded history of human beings on this planet. To date, no storage method has been devised that can provide infallible, infinitely durable shielding for nuclear waste. Despite these problems, nuclear power is gaining favor again as an alternative to fossil fuels.

## Medical Uses of Radiation

Another area of concern is the use of radiation in medicine, primarily the X-ray. The development of machines that could produce images of internal bone structures was a major advance in medicine, and applications abounded. Chest X-rays were routinely used to screen for tuberculosis, and children's feet were even X-rayed in shoe stores to make sure their new shoes fit properly. But, as is often the case, this new technology had disadvantages. As time passed, studies revealed that X-ray exposure is cumulative and that no level of exposure is absolutely safe.

Early X-ray machines are no longer used because of the high amounts of radiation they gave off. Each new generation of X-ray machines has used less radiation more effectively. From a personal health point of view, no one should ever have a "routine" X-ray examination; each such exam should have a definite purpose, and its benefits and risks should be carefully weighed.

## Radiation in the Home and Workplace

Recently, there has been concern about electromagnetic radiation associated with common modern devices such as microwave ovens, computer monitors, and even high-voltage power lines. These forms of radiation do have effects on health, but research results are inconclusive.

Another controversial issue today is the effect of radiation from cell phones on health. Cell phones use electromagnetic waves (radio frequency radiation) to send and receive signals. This radiation is not directional, meaning that it travels in all directions equally, including toward the user. Factors such as the type of digital signal coding in the network, the antenna and handset design, and the position of the phone relative to the head all determine how much radiation is absorbed by a user.

Specific absorption rate (SAR) is a way of measuring the quantity of radio frequency energy that is absorbed by the body. If you're concerned about limiting your exposure to possible radiation from your cell phone, look for a phone with a low SAR (some municipalities require phone manufacturers to provide this information on packaging). You can also text instead of calling, use a wired headset or speakerphone whenever possible, and carry your phone at least one inch from your body. Some researchers also caution against using your phone in areas with poor coverage since phones emit more radiation when searching for a signal. Because studies to date have not provided conclusive evidence, the CDC has undertaken a long-term study to determine whether cell phone use actually exposes users to harmful levels of radiation.

Another area of concern is **radon,** a naturally occurring radioactive gas found in certain soils, rocks, and building materials.

## Avoiding Radiation

The following steps can help you avoid unneeded exposure to radiation:

- If your physician orders an X-ray, ask why it is necessary. Only get X-rays that you need, and keep a record of the date and location of every X-ray exam. Don't have a full-body CT scan for routine screening;

# Ask Yourself

QUESTIONS FOR CRITICAL THINKING
AND REFLECTION

Do you live in an area where radon is a problem? If so, has your home been checked for radon?

the radiation dose of one full-body CT scan is nearly 100 times that of a typical mammogram.

- Follow government recommendations for radon testing.
- Find out if there are radioactive sites in your area. If you live or work near such a site, form or join a community action group to get the site cleaned up.

## TIPS FOR TODAY AND THE FUTURE

Environmental health involves protecting ourselves from environmental dangers and protecting the environment from the dangers created by humans.

### RIGHT NOW YOU CAN

- Turn off the lights, televisions, and stereos in any unoccupied rooms.
- Turn off power strips when not in use.
- Turn down the heat a few degrees and put on a sweater, or turn off the air conditioner and change into cooler clothes.
- Check your trash for recyclable items and take them out for recycling. If your town does not provide curbside pickup for recyclable items, find out where the nearest community recycling center is.

### IN THE FUTURE YOU CAN

- As your existing lightbulbs burn out, replace them with compact fluorescent lightbulbs.
- Have your car checked to make sure it runs as well as it can and puts out the lowest amount of polluting emissions possible.
- Go online and find one of the many calculators available that can help you estimate your environmental footprint. After calculating your footprint, figure out ways to reduce it.

## SUMMARY

- Environmental health encompasses all the interactions of humans with their environment and the health consequences of those interactions.

- The world's population is increasing rapidly, especially in the developing world. Factors that may eventually limit human population are food, availability of land and water, energy, and minimum acceptable standard of living.

- Increased amounts of air pollutants are especially dangerous for children, older adults, and people with chronic health problems.

- Factors contributing to the development of smog include heavy motor vehicle traffic, hot weather, and stagnant air.

- Carbon dioxide and other natural gases act as a greenhouse around the earth, increasing the temperature of the atmosphere. Levels of these gases are rising through human activity; as a result, the world's climate could change.

- The ozone layer that shields the earth's surface from the sun's UV rays has thinned and developed holes in certain regions.

- Environmental damage from energy use can be limited through energy conservation and the development of nonpolluting, renewable sources of energy.

- Indoor pollutants can trigger allergies and illness in the short term and cancer in the long term.

- Concerns with water quality focus on pathogenic organisms and hazardous chemicals from industry and households, as well as on water shortages.

- Sewage treatment prevents pathogens from contaminating drinking water; it often must also deal with heavy metals and hazardous chemicals.

- The amount of garbage is growing all the time; paper is the biggest component. Recycling can help reduce solid waste disposal problems.

- Potentially hazardous chemical pollutants include asbestos, lead, pesticides, mercury, and many household products. Proper handling and disposal are critical.

- Radiation can cause radiation sickness, chromosome damage, and cancer, among other health problems.

## FOR FURTHER EXPLORATION

### BOOKS

Ausenda, F. 2009. *Green Volunteers: The World Guide to Voluntary Work in Nature Conservation*, 7th ed. New York: Universe. *Describes a variety of opportunities to volunteer for environmental causes in many different parts of the world.*

Cunningham, W. P., et al. 2009. *Environmental Science: A Global Concern*, 11th ed. New York: McGraw-Hill. *A nontechnical survey of basic environmental science and key concerns.*

Maslin, M., 2009. *Global Warming: A Very Short Introduction*, 2nd ed. New York: Oxford University Press. *A survey of the science and politics of global warming.*

Nadakavukaren, A. 2005. *Our Global Environment: A Health Perspective*, 6th ed. Prospect Heights, Ill.: Waveland Press. *A broad survey of major environmental issues and their effects on personal and community health.*

Wright, R. T. 2010. *Environmental Science: Toward a Sustainable Future*. New York: Pearson. *An easy-to-read introduction to the realm of environmental science and its importance to our future.*

## Q What is renewable energy, and what are its advantages?

**A** With fossil fuels becoming increasingly problematic politically, economically, and environmentally, interest and investment in renewable energy sources have grown in recent years. Renewable energy sources are those sources that are naturally replenished and essentially inexhaustible, such as wind and water. Together with technologies that improve energy efficiency, renewable energy sources contribute to sustainability—the capacity of natural or human systems to endure and maintain well-being over time. A common definition of sustainable development is development that meets society's present needs without compromising the ability of future generations to meet their needs.

Renewable energy sources include wind power, solar power, water and wave power, geothermal power, and biomass and biofuels from renewable sources, among others.

• Wind power uses the energy of the wind to turn blades that run a turbine, which spins a generator, which produces electricity.

• Solar power uses the heat and light of the sun to produce energy via a variety of technologies. One solar technology is the concentrating solar power (CSP) system, which use mirrors, dishes, or towers to reflect and collect solar heat to generate steam, which runs a turbine to produce electricity. Another solar technology is the photovoltaic (solar cell) system, which converts sunlight directly into electricity by means of semiconducting materials.

• Geothermal power taps the heat in the earth's core. It may be in the form of hot water or steam, which can be used to run a turbine to produce electricity. In some geologically unstable parts of the planet, including Yellowstone Park and parts of northern California, geothermal energy is close to the surface.

• Biomass is plant material, including trees. When biomass is burned, it produces energy. If the plants are produced and harvested sustainably, they are a renewable source of energy.

• Biofuels are fuels based on natural materials. Bioethanol is made primarily from sugar and starch crops like corn, although trees and grasses may be used in the future. Ethanol can be used as a fuel for vehicles or added to gasoline. Biodiesel is made from vegetable oils or animal fats and can be used either in a pure form to power vehicles or added to diesel to reduce carbon emissions.

*For more Common Questions Answered about environmental health, visit the Online Learning Center at www.mhhe.com/fahey.*

## ORGANIZATIONS, HOTLINES, AND WEB SITES

*CDC National Center for Environmental Health.* Provides brochures and fact sheets on a variety of environmental issues.
http://www.cdc.gov/nceh/default.htm

*Earth Times.* An international online newspaper devoted to global environmental issues.
http://www.earthtimes.org

*Ecological Footprint.* Calculates your personal ecological footprint based on your diet, transportation patterns, and living arrangements.
http://www.myfootprint.org

*Fuel Economy.* Provides information on the fuel economy of cars made since 1985 and tips on improving gas mileage.
http://www.fueleconomy.gov

*Indoor Air Quality Information Hotline.* Answers questions, provides publications, and makes referrals.
800-438-4318

*National Lead Information Center.* Provides information packets and specialist advice.
http://www.epa.gov/lead/index.html

*National Oceanic and Atmospheric Administration (NOAA): Climate.* Provides information on a variety of issues related to climate, including global warming, drought, and El Niño and La Niña.
http://www.noaa.gov/climate.html

*National Safety Council Environmental Health Center.* Provides information on lead, radon, indoor air quality, hazardous chemicals, and other environmental issues.
http://www.nsc.org/international/env_hth_sty/Pages/EnvironmentalHealthSafety.aspx

*Student Environmental Action Coalition (SEAC).* A coalition of student and youth environmental groups; the Web site has contact information for local groups.
http://www.seac.org

*United Nations.* Several U.N. programs are devoted to environmental problems on a global scale; the Web sites provide information on current and projected trends and on international treaties developed to deal with environmental issues.
http://www.un.org/popin (Population Information Network)
http://www.unep.org (Environment Programme)

*U.S. Department of Energy: Energy Efficiency and Renewable Energy (EERE).* Provides information about alternative fuels and tips for saving energy at home and in your car.
http://www.eere.energy.gov/

*U.S. Environmental Protection Agency (EPA).* Provides information about EPA activities and many consumer-oriented materials. The Web site includes special sites devoted to global warming, ozone loss, pesticides, and other areas of concern.
http://www.epa.gov

*Worldwatch Institute.* A public policy research organization focusing on emerging global environmental problems and the links between the world economy and the environment.
http://www.worldwatch.org

There are many national and international organizations working on environmental health problems. A few of the largest and best known are listed below:

Greenpeace: 800-326-0959; http://www.greenpeace.org

National Audubon Society: 212-979-3000; http://www.audubon
.org
National Wildlife Federation: 800-822-9919; http://www.nwf.org
Nature Conservancy: 800-628-6860; http://www.nature.org
Sierra Club: 415-977-5500; http://www.sierraclub.org
World Wildlife Fund—U.S.: 800-960-0993; http://www
.worldwildlife.org

## SELECTED BIBLIOGRAPHY

CDC National Center for Environmental Health. 2010. *Lead* (http://www
.cdc.gov/nceh/lead/; retrieved October 8, 2010).

Centers for Disease Control and Prevention. 2006. Adult blood lead epidemiology and surveillance—United States, 2003–2004. *Morbidity and
Mortality Weekly Report* 55(32): 876–879.

Centers for Disease Control and Prevention. 2008. Surveillance for waterborne disease and outbreaks associated with drinking water and water
not intended for drinking—United States, 2005–2006. *Morbidity and
Mortality Weekly Report* 55(SS12): 31–58.

Delworth-Bart, J. E., and C. F. Moore. 2006. Mercy mercy me: Social injustice and the prevention of environmental pollutant exposures among
ethnic minority and poor children. *Child Development* 77(2): 247–265.

Dominici, F., et al. 2006. Fine particulate air pollution and hospital admis-
sion for cardiovascular and respiratory diseases. *Journal of the American
Medical Association* 295(10): 1127–1134.

Energy Information Administration. 2005. *Impacts of Modeled Recommendations of the National Commission on Energy Policy.* Washington, D.C.:
U.S. Department of Energy.

Environmental Protection Agency. 2010. *Municipal Solid Waste* (http://
www.epa.gov/waste/nonhaz/municipal/index.htm; retrieved October 8,
2011).

Kunzli, N., et al. 2005. Ambient air pollution and atherosclerosis in Los
Angeles. *Environmental Health Perspectives* 113(2): 201–206.

Laden, F., et al. 2006. Reduction in fine particulate air pollution and mortality: Extended follow-up of the Harvard Six Cities study. *American Journal of Respiratory and Critical Care Medicine* 173(6): 667–672.

The National Academies. 2006. *Surface Temperature Reconstructions for the
Last 2,000 Years.* Washington, D.C.: National Academies Press.

National Oceanic and Atmospheric Administration. 2008. *Billion Dollar
U.S. Weather Disasters, 1980–2007* (http://www.ncdc.noaa.gov/oa
/reports/billionz.html; retrieved October 8, 2010).

Parker, J. D., et al. 2005. Air pollution and birth weight among term infants
in California. *Pediatrics* 115(1): 121–128.

Trasande, L., P. J. Landrigan, and C. Schechter. 2005. Public health and economic consequences of methylmercury toxicity to the developing brain.
*Environmental Health Perspectives* online, 28 February.

United Nations Population Division. 2009. *World Population Prospects: The
2009 Revision.* New York: United Nations.

Virtanen, J. K., et al. 2005. Mercury, fish oils, and risk of acute coronary
events and cardiovascular disease, coronary heart disease, and all-cause
mortality in men in eastern Finland. *Arteriosclerosis, Thrombosis, and
Vascular Biology* 25(1): 228–233.

World Health Organization. 2006. *Fuel for Life: Household Energy and
Health.* Geneva: WHO Press.

World Health Organization. 2010. Cholera, 2010. *Weekly Epidemiological
Record* 85(13): 1177–128.

Worldwatch Institute. 2010. *Vital Signs 2010.* New York: Norton.

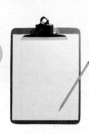

## LAB 15.1  Environmental Health Checklist

The following list of statements relates to your effect on the environment. Put a checkmark next to the statements that are true for you.

_____ I ride my bike, walk, carpool, or use public transportation whenever possible.

_____ I keep my car tuned up and well maintained.

_____ My residence is well insulated.

_____ Where possible, I use compact fluorescent bulbs instead of incandescent bulbs.

_____ I turn off lights and appliances when they are not in use.

_____ I avoid turning on heat or air conditioning whenever possible.

_____ I run the washing machine, dryer, and dishwasher only when they have full loads.

_____ I run the clothes dryer only as long as it takes my clothes to dry.

_____ I dry my hair with a towel rather than a hair dryer.

_____ I keep my car's air conditioner in good working order and have it serviced by a service station that recycles CFCs.

_____ When shopping, I choose products with the least amount of packaging.

_____ I choose recycled and recyclable products.

_____ I avoid products packaged in plastic and unrecycled aluminum.

_____ I store food in glass jars and waxed paper rather than plastic wrap.

_____ I take my own bag along when I go shopping.

_____ I recycle newspapers, glass, cans, and other recyclables.

_____ When shopping, I read labels and try to buy the least toxic products available.

_____ I dispose of household hazardous wastes properly.

_____ I take showers instead of baths.

_____ I take short showers and switch off the water when I'm not actively using it.

_____ I do not run the water while brushing my teeth, shaving, or hand-washing clothes.

_____ My faucets have aerators installed in them.

_____ My shower has a low-flow showerhead.

_____ I have a water-saver toilet or a water displacement device in my toilet.

_____ I snip or rip plastic six-pack rings before I throw them out.

_____ When hiking or camping, I never leave anything behind.

Statements you have not checked can help you identify behaviors you can change to improve environmental health.

connect™  http://www.mcgrawhillconnect.com/
FITNESS AND WELLNESS

# APPENDIXES

**APPENDIX A** Injury Prevention and Personal Safety   A-1

**APPENDIX B** Exercise Guidelines for People with Special Health Concerns   B-1

**APPENDIX C** Monitoring Your Progress   C-1

# NUTRITIONAL CONTENT OF COMMON FOODS

If you are developing a behavior change plan to improve your diet, or if you simply want to choose healthier foods, you may want to know more about the nutritional content of common food items. An appendix with this information is available on the *Fit and Well* Online Learning Center at **www.mhhe.com/fahey.**

You can track your daily food intake, calculate your nutrient intake from foods, and compare your intake with the U.S. Department of Agriculture's recommendations for your age, sex, height, and weight at the MyPlate Web site (**www.choosemyplate.gov**).

You can also look up the nutrient content of the foods you eat in the USDA Agricultural Research Service National Nutrient Database, which lists foods both by description and by nutrient content (**www.ars.usda.gov/Services/docs.htm?docid=17477**). For example, under "protein," you can find out how much protein there is in a chicken pot pie or what foods have the most protein per serving. Although cumbersome, the database is comprehensive.

## Nutritional Content of Popular Items from Fast-Food Restaurants

Although most foods served at fast-food restaurants are high in calories, fat, saturated fat, cholesterol, sodium, and sugar, some items are healthier than others. If you eat at fast-food restaurants, knowing the nutritional content of various items can help you make better choices. Fast-food restaurants provide nutritional information both online and in print brochures available at most restaurant locations. To learn more about the items you order, visit the restaurants' Web sites:

| | | | |
|---|---|---|---|
| Arby's: | www.arbysrestaurant.com | Papa John's Pizza: | http://www.papajohns.com/index.html |
| Burger King: | http://www.bk.com/en/us/index.html | Pizza Hut: | http://www.pizzahut.com |
| Domino's Pizza: | www.dominos.com | Subway: | http://www.subway.com/subwayroot/default.aspx |
| Hardees: | www.hardees.com | | |
| KFC: | www.kfc.com | Taco Bell: | www.tacobell.com |
| McDonald's: | www.mcdonalds.com | Wendy's: | www.wendys.com |
| | | White Castle: | www.whitecastle.com |

Unintentional injuries are the fifth leading cause of death among Americans overall and the leading killer of people under age 35. Injuries affect all segments of the population, but they are particularly common among minorities and people with low incomes, primarily due to social, environmental, and economic factors. The economic cost of injuries in the United States is high, with more than $650 billion spent each year for medical care and rehabilitation of injured people.

Injuries are generally classified into four categories, based on where they occur: motor vehicle injuries, home injuries, leisure injuries, and work injuries.

## MOTOR VEHICLE INJURIES

According to the CDC, more than 36,000 Americans were killed and 2.3 million injured in motor vehicle crashes in 2009. Motor vehicle accidents are a leading cause of paralysis due to spinal injury and the leading cause of severe brain injury.

### Factors in Motor Vehicle Injuries

**Driving Habits**   Nearly 63% of motor vehicle injuries are caused by bad driving, especially speeding. As speed increases, momentum and force of impact increase and the time available for the driver to react decreases. Speed limits are posted to establish the safest *maximum* speed limit for a given area under *ideal* conditions. Aggressive driving—characterized by speeding, frequent and abrupt lane changes, tailgating, and passing on the shoulder—also increases the risk of crashes.

Distracted driving contributes to 8000 crashes every day in the United States. Anything that distracts a driver—sleepiness, bad mood, children or pets in the car, use of a cell phone—can increase the risk of a crash. Sleepiness reduces reaction time, coordination, and speed of information processing and can be as dangerous as drug and alcohol use. Even mild sleep deprivation causes a deterioration in driving ability comparable to that caused by a 0.05% blood alcohol concentration.

Cell phone users respond to hazards about 20% slower than undistracted drivers and are about twice as likely to rear-end a braking car in front of them. According to 2011 statistics from the AAA Foundation for Traffic Safety, drivers who use cell phones are nearly four times as likely to be involved in a crash as drivers who don't. Hands-free devices do not help significantly; the mental distraction of talking is the factor in crashes rather than holding a phone. Newer research shows that text-messaging (texting) on a cell phone while driving is even more dangerous than talking. Several cities and states have outlawed the use of cell phones while driving; similar laws are being considered in many parts of the United States.

**Safety Belts and Air Bags**   A person who doesn't wear a safety belt is twice as likely to be injured in a crash as a person who does wear one. Safety belts not only prevent occupants from being thrown from the car at the time of the crash but also provide protection from the "second collision," which occurs when the occupant of the car hits something inside the car, such as the steering column or windshield. The safety belt also spreads the stopping force of a collision over the body.

Since 1998, all new cars have been equipped with dual air bags—one for the driver and one for the front passenger seat. Air bags provide supplemental protection in a collision but are most useful in head-on collisions. (Many newer vehicles feature side air bags to offer protection in a side-impact crash.) They also deflate immediately after inflating and so do not provide protection in collisions involving multiple impacts. To ensure that air bags work as intended, follow these guidelines:

- Place infants in rear-facing infant seats in the back seat.
- Transport children age 12 and under in the back seat.
- Always use safety belts or appropriate safety seats.
- Keep at least 10 inches between the air bag cover and the breastbone of the driver or passenger.

If you cannot comply with these guidelines, you can apply to the National Highway Traffic Safety Administration for permission to install an on-off switch that temporarily disables the air bag.

**Alcohol and Other Drugs**   Alcohol is involved in about 40% of all fatal crashes. Alcohol-impaired driving, defined by blood alcohol concentration (BAC), is illegal. The legal BAC limit is 0.08% in all states, but driving ability is impaired at much lower BACs. All psychoactive drugs have the potential to impair driving ability.

### Preventing Motor Vehicle Injuries

About 75% of all motor vehicle collisions occur within 25 miles of home and at speeds lower than 40 mph. These crashes often occur because the driver believes safety measures are not necessary for short trips. Clearly, the statistics prove otherwise.

**To prevent motor vehicle injuries:**

- Obey the speed limit. If you have to speed to get to your destination on time, you're not allowing enough time.
- Always wear a safety belt and ask passengers to do the same. Strap infants and toddlers into government-approved

car seats in the back seat. Children who have outgrown child safety seats but who are still too small for adult safety belts alone (usually age 4–8) should be secured using booster seats. All children under 12 should ride in the back seat.

- Never drive under the influence of alcohol or other drugs or with a driver who is.
- Do not drive when you are sleepy or have been awake for 18 or more hours.
- Avoid using your cell phone while driving—your primary obligation is to pay attention to the road. If you do make calls, follow laws set by your city or state. Place calls when you are at a stop, and keep them short. Pull over if the conversation is stressful or emotional.
- Never text while driving.
- Keep your car in good working order. Regularly inspect tires, oil and fluid levels, windshield wipers, spare tire, and so on.
- Always allow enough following distance. Follow the "3-second rule": When the vehicle ahead passes a reference point, count out 3 seconds. If you pass the reference point before you finish counting, drop back and allow more following distance.
- Always increase following distance and slow down if weather or road conditions are poor.
- Choose major highways rather than rural roads. Highways are much safer because of better visibility, wider lanes, fewer surprises, and other factors.
- Always signal before turning or changing lanes.
- Stop completely at stop signs. Follow all traffic laws.
- Take special care at intersections. Always look left, right, and then left again. Make sure you have plenty of time to complete your maneuver in the intersection.
- Don't pass on two-lane roads unless you are in a designated passing area and have a clear view ahead.

## Motorcycles and Scooters

About 1 out of every 10 traffic fatalities among people age 15–34 involves someone riding a motorcycle. Injuries from motorcycle collisions are generally more severe than those involving automobiles because motorcycles provide little, if any, protection. Scooter riders face additional challenges. Motorized scooters usually have a maximum speed of 30–35 mph and have less power for maneuverability.

### To prevent motorcycle and scooter injuries:

- Make yourself easier to see by wearing light-colored clothing, driving with your headlights on, and correctly positioning yourself in traffic.
- Develop the necessary skills. Lack of skill, especially when evasive action is needed to avoid a collision, is a major factor in motorcycle and moped injuries. Skidding from improper braking is the most common cause of loss of control.
- Wear a close-fitting helmet, one marked with the symbol DOT (for Department of Transportation).

- Protect your eyes with goggles, a face shield, or a windshield.
- Drive defensively and never assume that other drivers see you.

## Pedestrians and Bicycles

Injuries to pedestrians and bicyclists are considered motor vehicle–related because they usually involve motor vehicles. About 1 in 8 motor vehicle deaths each year involves a pedestrian; more than 70,000 pedestrians are injured each year.

### To prevent injuries when walking or jogging:

- Walk or jog in daylight.
- Make yourself easier to see by wearing light-colored, reflective clothing.
- Face traffic when walking or jogging along a roadway, and follow traffic laws.
- Avoid busy roads or roads with poor visibility.
- Cross only at marked crosswalks and intersections.
- Don't use headphones while walking or jogging.
- Don't hitchhike. Hitchhiking places you in a potentially dangerous situation.

Bicycle injuries result primarily from not knowing or understanding the rules of the road, failing to follow traffic laws, and not having sufficient skill or experience to handle traffic conditions. Bicycles are considered vehicles; bicycle riders must obey all traffic laws that apply to automobile drivers, including stopping at traffic lights and stop signs.

### To prevent injuries when riding a bike:

- Wear safety equipment, including a helmet, eye protection, gloves, and proper footwear. Secure the bottom of your pant legs with clips and secure your shoelaces so they don't get tangled in the chain.
- Make yourself easier to see by wearing light-colored, reflective clothing. Equip your bike with reflectors and use lights, especially at night or when riding in wooded or other dark areas.
- Ride with the flow of traffic, not against it, and follow traffic laws. Use bike paths when they are available.
- Ride defensively; never assume that drivers can see you. Be especially careful when turning or crossing at corners and intersections. Watch for cars turning right.
- Stop at all traffic lights and stop signs. Know and use hand signals.
- Continue pedaling at all times when moving (don't coast) to help keep the bike stable and to maintain your balance.
- Properly maintain your bike.

## Aggressive Driving

Aggressive driving, known as *road rage,* has increased more than 50% since 1990. Aggressive drivers increase the risk of crashes for themselves and others. They further increase the risk of injuries if they stop their vehicles and confront each other. Even if you are successful at controlling your own aggressive driving impulses, you may still encounter an aggressive driver.

**To avoid being the victim of an aggressive driver:**

- Always keep distance between your car and others. If you are behind a very slow driver and can't pass, slow down to increase distance in case that driver does something unexpected. If you are being tailgated, do not increase your speed; instead, let the other driver pass you. If you are in the left lane when being tailgated, signal and pull over to let the other driver go by, even if you are traveling at the speed limit. When you are merging, make sure you have plenty of room. If you are cut off by a merging driver, slow down to make room.

- Be courteous, even if the other driver is not. Use your horn rarely, if ever. Avoid making gestures of irritation, even shaking your head. When parking, let the other driver have the space that both of you found.

- Refuse to join in a fight. Avoid eye contact with an angry driver. If someone makes a rude gesture, ignore it. If you think another car is following you and you have a cell phone, call the police. Otherwise, drive to a public place and honk your horn to get someone's attention.

- If you make a mistake while driving, apologize. Raise or wave your hand or touch or knock your head with the palm of your hand to indicate "What was I thinking?" You can also mouth the words "I'm sorry."

## HOME INJURIES

Contrary to popular belief, home is one of the most dangerous places to be. The most common fatal home injuries are caused by falls, poisoning, fires, suffocation and choking, and incidents involving firearms.

## Falls

About 90% of fatal falls involve people age 45 and older, but falls are a significant cause of unintentional death for people under age 25. Most deaths occurring from falls involve falling on stairs or steps or from one level to another. Falls also occur on the same level, from tripping, slipping, or stumbling. Alcohol is a contributing factor in many falls.

**To prevent injuries from falls:**

- Install handrails and nonslip surfaces in the shower and bathtub. Place skidproof backing on rugs and carpets.

- Keep floors, stairs, and outside areas clear of objects or conditions that could cause slipping or tripping, such as heavy wax coating, electrical cords, and toys.

- Put a light switch by the door of every room so no one has to walk across a room to turn on a light. Use night lights in bedrooms, halls, stairways, and bathrooms.

- Outside the house, clear dangerous surfaces created by ice, snow, fallen leaves, or rough ground.

- Install handrails on stairs. Keep stairs well lit and clear of objects.

- When climbing a ladder, use both hands. Never stand higher than the third step from the top. When using a stepladder, make sure the spreader brace is in the locked position. With straight ladders, set the base out 1 foot for every 4 feet of height. Don't stand on chairs to reach things.

- If there are small children in the home, place gates at the top and bottom of stairs. Never leave a baby unattended.

## Poisoning

More than 2.4 million poisonings and over 30,000 poison-related deaths occur every year in the United States.

**To prevent poisoning:**

- Store all medicines out of the reach of children. Use medicines only as directed on the label or by a physician.

- Use cleaners, pesticides, and other dangerous substances only in areas with proper ventilation. Store them out of the reach of children.

- Never operate a vehicle in an enclosed space. Have your furnace inspected yearly. Use caution with any substance that produces potentially toxic fumes, such as kerosene. If appropriate, install carbon monoxide detectors.

- Keep poisonous plants out of the reach of children. These include azalea, oleander, rhododendron, wild mushrooms, daffodil and hyacinth bulbs, mistletoe berries, apple seeds, morning glory seeds, wisteria seeds, and the leaves and stems of potato, rhubarb, and tomato plants.

**To be prepared in case of poisoning:**

- Keep the number of the nearest Poison Control Center (or emergency room) in an accessible location. A call to the national poison control hotline (800-222-1222) will be routed to a local center.

**Emergency first aid for poisonings:**

1. Remove the poison from contact with eyes, skin, or mouth, or remove the victim from contact with poisonous fumes or gases.
2. Call the Poison Control Center immediately for instructions. Have the container with you.
3. Do not follow emergency instructions on labels. Some may be out-of-date and carry incorrect treatment information.
4. If you are instructed to go to an emergency room, take the poisonous substance or its container with you.

**Guidelines for specific types of poisons:**

- *Swallowed poisons.* Call the Poison Control Center or a physician for advice. Do not induce vomiting.
- *Poisons on the skin.* Remove any affected clothing. Flood affected parts of the skin with warm water, wash with soap and water, and rinse. Then call for advice.
- *Poisons in the eye.* For children, flood the eye with lukewarm water poured from a pitcher held 3–4 inches above the eye for 15 minutes; alternatively, irrigate the eye under a faucet. For adults, get in the shower and flood the eye with a gentle stream of lukewarm water for 15 minutes. Then call for advice.
- *Inhaled poisons.* Immediately carry or drag the person to fresh air and, if necessary, give rescue breaths (Figure A.1). If the victim is not breathing easily, call 9-1-1 for help. Ventilate the area. Then call the Poison Control Center for advice.

# EMERGENCY CARE FOR CHOKING

- If the victim is coughing, encourage the coughing to clear the object from the airway.
- If the victim is not coughing, follow the steps in "Choking Care for Responsive Adult or Child."

## Choking Care for Responsive Adult or Child

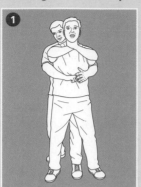

**1** Stand behind an adult victim with one leg forward between the victim's legs. (With a child, kneel behind the victim.) Keep your head slightly to one side. Reach around the abdomen with both arms. Make a fist with one hand and place the thumb side of the fist against the abdomen just above the navel.

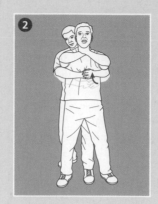

**2** Grasp your fist with your other hand and thrust inward and upward into the victim's abdomen with quick jerks. Continue abdominal thrusts until the victim expels the object or becomes unresponsive. If the victim becomes unresponsive while you are administering abdominal thrusts, lower the victim to the floor onto his or her back, and follow the steps in "Choking Care for Unresponsive Adult or Child."

## Choking Care for Unresponsive Adult or Child: CPR

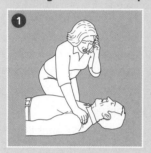

**1** Call 911 and begin CPR.

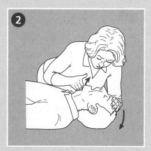

**2** Open the airway to see if the victim is breathing. Use the "head tilt–chin lift" maneuver to open the airway: Push down on the forehead and lift the chin.

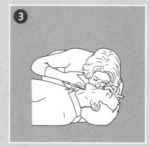

**3** If the victim is not breathing, give two rescue breaths, each lasting 1 second. Pinch the victim's nose shut and blow a normal breath into the victim's mouth. If the first breath does not go in (the chest does not rise), reposition the head to open the airway and try again. Each time you give a rescue breath, look for an object in the victim's mouth and remove it if present.

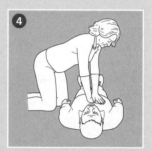

**4** If the obstruction remains, begin chest compressions. Place the heel of one hand in the center of the chest between the nipples and the other hand on top of the first. Position your shoulders over your hands and lock your elbows. Give 30 chest compressions at a rate of 100 per minute. The chest should go down by 1½ to 2 inches. Then give two breaths, looking in the mouth for an expelled object. Continue chest compressions until help arrives. **Remember: Push hard and push fast at a rate of 100 compressions per minute.**

# EMERGENCY CARE FOR CARDIAC ARREST

For cardiac arrest, the American Heart Association's revised (2005) Emergency Cardiac Care guidelines are as follows:

**1** Call 911.

**2** Start CPR (100 compressions per minute, stopping every 30 to 60 seconds to give two rescue breaths).

**3** If an automated external defibrillator (AED) is available, or when one arrives, give one shock to restart the victim's heart.

**4** Go back to CPR immediately after the shock.

## Hands-Only CPR

In 2008, the American Heart Association reported that hands-only (compression-only) CPR can be as effective as conventional CPR. There are only two steps:

**1** Call 911.

**2** Push hard and fast in the center of the chest.

Don't wait for an emergency to learn how to use an AED or perform CPR.
To find a course in your area, contact the American Heart Association (800 242-8721) or the American Red Cross (202 303-4498).

**FIGURE A. 1** Emergency care for choking and for cardiac arrest.

**SOURCES:** Adapted from American Heart Association. 2008. Hands-only (compression-only) cardiopulmonary resuscitation: A call to action for bystander response to adults who experience out-of-hospital sudden cardiac arrest. *Circulation* 117: 2162–2167; National Safety Council. 2007. *First Aid: Taking Action.* New York: McGraw-Hill; American Heart Association. 2005. Adult basic life support. *Circulation* 112: 19–34; New CPR guidelines: Simplicity to the rescue. 2006. *Harvard Health Letter,* March, Streamlined CPR guidelines a life-saving move. 2006. *Harvard Heart Letter,* February.

# Fires

Each year, about 80% of fire deaths and 65% of fire injuries occur in the home. Careless smoking is the leading cause of home fire deaths. Cooking is the leading cause of home fire injuries.

**To prevent fires:**

- Dispose of all cigarettes in ashtrays. Never smoke in bed.
- Do not overload electrical outlets. Do not place extension cords under rugs or where people walk. Replace worn or frayed extension cords.
- Place a wire screen in front of fireplaces and woodstoves. Remove ashes carefully and store them in airtight metal containers, not paper bags.
- Properly maintain electrical appliances, kerosene heaters, and furnaces. Clean flues and chimneys annually.
- Keep portable heaters at least 3 feet away from curtains, bedding, towels, or anything that might catch fire. Never leave operating heaters unattended.

**To be prepared for a fire:**

- Plan at least two escape routes out of each room. Designate a location outside the home as a meeting place. Stage a home fire drill.
- Install a smoke detection device on every level of your home. Clean the detectors and test batteries once a month, and replace the batteries at least once a year.
- Keep a fire extinguisher in your home and know how to use it.

**To prevent injuries from fire:**

- Get out as quickly as possible and go to the designated meeting place. Don't stop for a keepsake or a pet. Never hide in a closet or under a bed. Once outside, count heads to see if everyone is out. If you think someone is still inside the burning building, tell the firefighters. Never go back inside a burning building.
- If you're trapped in a room, feel the door. If it is hot or if smoke is coming in through the cracks, don't open it; use the alternative escape route. If you can't get out of a room, go to the window and shout or wave for help.
- Avoid inhaling smoke. Smoke inhalation is the largest cause of death and injury in fires. To avoid inhaling smoke, crawl along the floor away from the heat and smoke. Cover your mouth and nose, ideally with a wet cloth, and take short, shallow breaths.
- If your clothes catch fire, don't run. Drop to the ground, cover your face, and roll back and forth to smother the flames. Remember: Stop-drop-roll.

## Suffocation and Choking

Suffocation and choking account for about 5000 deaths annually in the United States. Children can suffocate if they put small items in their mouths, get tangled in their crib bedding, or get trapped in airtight appliances like old refrigerators. Keep small objects out of reach of children under age 3, and don't give them raw carrots, hot dogs, popcorn, peanuts, or hard candy. Examine toys carefully for small parts that could come loose; don't give plastic bags or balloons to small children.

Adults can also become choking victims, especially if they fail to chew food properly, eat hurriedly, or try to talk and eat at the same time. Many choking victims can be saved with abdominal thrusts, also called the Heimlich maneuver (see Figure A.1). Infants who are choking can be saved with blows to the upper back, followed by chest thrusts if necessary.

## Incidents Involving Firearms

Firearms pose a significant threat of unintentional injury, especially to people between ages 5 and 29.

**To prevent firearm injuries:**

- Always treat a gun as though it were loaded, even if you know it isn't.
- Never point a gun—loaded or unloaded—at something you do not intend to shoot.
- Always unload a firearm before storing it. Store unloaded firearms under lock and key, away from ammunition.
- Inspect firearms carefully before handling them.
- If you own a gun, buy and use a gun lock designed specifically for that weapon.
- If you ever plan to handle a gun, take a firearms safety course first.

# LEISURE INJURIES

Leisure injuries take place in public places but do not involve motor vehicles. Many injuries in this category involve such recreational activities as boating and swimming, playground activities, in-line skating, and sports.

## Drowning and Boating Injuries

Although most drownings are reported in lakes, ponds, rivers, and oceans, more than half the drownings of young children take place in residential pools. Among adolescents and adults, alcohol plays a significant role in many boating injuries and drownings.

**To prevent drowning and boating injuries:**

- Develop adequate swimming skill and make sure children learn to swim.
- Make sure residential pools are fenced and that children are never allowed to swim without supervision.
- Don't swim alone or in unsupervised places.
- Use caution when swimming in unfamiliar surroundings or for an unusual length of time. To avoid being chilled, don't swim in water colder than 70°F.
- Don't swim or boat under the influence of alcohol or other drugs. Don't chew gum or eat while in the water.
- Check the depth of water before diving.
- When on a boat, use a life jacket (personal flotation device).

## In-Line Skating and Scooter Injuries

Most in-line skating injuries occur because users are not familiar with the equipment and do not wear appropriate safety gear. Injuries to the wrist and head are the most common. To prevent injuries while skating, wear a helmet, elbow and knee pads, wrist guards, a long-sleeved shirt, and long pants.

Wearing a helmet and knee and elbow pads is also important for preventing scooter injuries. The rise in popularity of lightweight scooters has seen a corresponding increase in associated injuries. Scooters should not be viewed as toys, and young children should be closely supervised. Be sure that handlebars, steering column, and all nuts and bolts are securely fastened. Ride on smooth, paved surfaces away from motor vehicle traffic. Avoid streets and surfaces with water, sand, gravel, or dirt.

## Sports Injuries

Since more people have begun exercising to improve their health, there has been an increase in sports-related injuries.

**To prevent sports injuries:**

- Develop the skills required for the activity. Recognize and guard against the hazards associated with it.
- Always warm up and cool down.
- Make sure facilities are safe.
- Follow the rules and practice good sportsmanship.
- Use proper safety equipment, including, where appropriate, helmets, eye protection, knee and elbow pads, and wrist guards. Wear correct footwear.
- When it is excessively hot and humid, avoid heat stress by following the guidelines given in Chapter 3.

## WORK INJURIES

Many aspects of workplace safety are monitored by the Occupational Safety and Health Administration (OSHA), a federal agency. The highest rate of work-related injuries occurs among laborers, whose jobs usually involve extensive manual labor and lifting—two areas not addressed by OSHA safety standards. Back injuries are the most common work injury.

**To protect your back when lifting:**

- Don't try to lift beyond your strength. If you need it, get help.
- Get a firm footing, with your feet shoulder-width apart. Get a firm grip on the object.
- Keep your torso in a relatively upright position and crouch down, bending at the knees and hips. Avoid bending at the waist. To lift, stand up or push up with your leg muscles. Lift gradually, keeping your arms straight. Keep the object close to your body.
- Don't twist. If you have to turn with an object, change the position of your feet.
- Put the object down gently, reversing the rules for lifting.

Another type of work-related injury is damage to the musculoskeletal system from repeated strain on the hand, arm, wrist, or other part of the body. Such repetitive-strain injuries are proliferating due to increased use of computers. One type, carpal tunnel syndrome, is characterized by pain and swelling in the tendons of the wrists and sometimes numbness and weakness.

**To prevent carpal tunnel syndrome:**

- Maintain good posture at the computer. Use a chair that provides back support and place the feet flat on the floor or on a footrest.
- Position the screen at eye level and the keyboard so the hands and wrists are straight.
- Take breaks periodically to stretch and flex your wrists and hands to lessen the cumulative effects of stress.

## VIOLENCE AND INTENTIONAL INJURIES

According to the Federal Bureau of Investigation (FBI), nearly 1.3 million violent crimes occurred in the United States in 2009. Violence includes assault, sexual assault, homicide, domestic violence, suicide, and child abuse. Compared with rates of violence in other industrialized countries, U.S. rates are unusually high in two areas: homicide and firearm-related deaths.

## Assault

Assault is the use of physical force to inflict injury or death on another person. Most assaults occur during arguments or in connection with another crime, such as robbery. Poverty, urban settings, and the use of alcohol and drugs are associated with higher rates of assault. The FBI estimates that about 807,000 aggravated assaults occurred in 2009, and 15,200 Americans were murdered that year. Homicide victims are most likely to be male, between ages 19 and 24, and members of minority groups. Most homicides are committed with a firearm; the murderer and the victim usually know each other.

**To protect yourself at home:**

- Secure your home with good lighting and effective locks, preferably deadbolts. Make sure that all doors and windows are securely locked.
- Get a dog, or post "Beware of Dog" signs.
- Don't hide keys in obvious places, and don't give anyone the chance to duplicate your keys.
- Install a peephole in your front door. Don't open your door to people you don't know.
- If you or a family member owns a weapon, store it securely. Store guns and ammunition separately.
- If you are a woman living alone, use your initials rather than your full name in the phone directory. Don't use a greeting on your answering machine that implies you live alone or are not home.
- Teach everyone in the household how to get emergency assistance.
- Know your neighbors. Work out a system for alerting each other in case of an emergency.
- Establish a neighborhood watch program.

**To protect yourself on the street:**

- Avoid walking alone, especially at night. Stay where people can see and hear you.

- Walk on the outside of the sidewalk, facing traffic. Walk purposefully. Act alert and confident. If possible, keep at least two arm lengths between yourself and a stranger.
- Know where you are going. Appearing to be lost increases your vulnerability.
- Carry valuables in a fanny pack, pants pocket, or shoulder bag strapped diagonally across the chest.
- Always have your keys ready as you approach your vehicle or home.
- Carry a whistle to blow if you are attacked or harassed. If you feel threatened, run and/or yell. Go into a store or knock on the door of a home. If someone grabs you, yell for help.

**To protect yourself in your car:**

- Keep your car in good working condition, carry emergency supplies, and keep the gas tank at least half full.
- When driving, keep doors locked and windows rolled up at least three-quarters of the way.
- Park your car in well-lighted areas or parking garages, preferably those with an attendant or a security guard.
- Lock your car when you leave it, and check the interior before opening the door when you return.
- Don't pick up strangers. Don't stop for vehicles in distress; drive on and call for help.
- Note the location of emergency call boxes along highways and in public facilities. Carry a cell phone.
- If your car breaks down, raise the hood and tie a white cloth to the antenna or door handle. Wait in the car with the doors locked and windows rolled up. If someone approaches to offer help, open a window only a crack and ask the person to call the police or a towing service.
- When you stop at a light or stop sign, leave enough room to maneuver if you need an escape route.
- If you are involved in a minor automobile crash and you think you have been bumped intentionally, don't leave your car. Motion to the other driver to follow you to the nearest police station.
- If confronted by a person with a weapon, give up your car.

**To protect yourself on public transportation:**

- While waiting, stand in a populated, well-lighted area.
- Make sure that the bus, subway, or train is bound for your destination before you board it. Sit near the driver or conductor in a single seat or an outside seat.
- If you flag down a taxi, make sure it's from a legitimate service. When you reach your destination, ask the driver to wait until you are safely inside the building.

**To protect yourself on campus:**

- Make sure that door and window locks are secure and that halls and stairwells have adequate lighting.
- Don't give dorm or residence keys to anybody.
- Don't leave your door unlocked or allow strangers into your room.
- Avoid solitary late-night trips to the library or laundry room. Take advantage of on-campus escort services.
- Don't exercise outside alone at night. Don't take shortcuts across campus that are unfamiliar or seem unsafe.

- If security guards patrol the campus, know the areas they cover and stay where they can see or hear you.

## Sexual Assault—Rape and Date Rape

The use of force and coercion in sexual relationships is one of the most serious problems in human interactions. The most extreme manifestation of sexual coercion—forcing a person to submit to another's sexual desires—is rape. Taking advantage of circumstances that render a person incapable of giving consent (such as when drunk) is also considered sexual assault or rape. Coerced sexual activity in which the victim knows or is dating the rapist is often referred to as date rape.

An estimated 700,000 females are raped annually in the United States, and some males—perhaps 10,000 annually—are raped each year by other males. However, only a fraction of rapes are actually reported to authorities. For example, the FBI states that only 88,000 forcible rapes were reported to authorities in 2009. Rape victims suffer both physical and psychological injury. The psychological pain can be substantial and long-lasting.

**To protect yourself against rape:**

- Follow the guidelines listed earlier for protecting yourself against assault.
- Trust your gut feeling. If you feel you are in danger, don't hesitate to run and scream.
- Think out in advance what you would do if you were threatened with rape. However, no one knows what he or she will do when scared to death. Trust that you will make the best decision at the time—whether to scream, run, fight, or give in to avoid being injured or killed.

**To protect yourself against date rape:**

- Believe in your right to control what you do. Set limits and communicate them clearly, firmly, and early. Be assertive; men often interpret passivity as permission.
- If you are unsure of a new acquaintance, go on a group date or double date. If possible, provide your own transportation.
- Remember that some men think flirtatious behavior or sexy clothing indicates an interest in having sex.
- Remember that alcohol and drugs interfere with judgment, perception, and communication about sex. In a bar or at a party, don't leave your drink unattended, and don't accept opened beverages; watch your drinks being poured. At a party or club, check on friends and ask them to check on you.
- Use the statement that has proved most effective in stopping date rape: "This is rape and I'm calling the cops!"

**If you are raped:**

- Tell what happened to the first friendly person you meet.
- Call the police. Tell them you were raped and give your location.
- Try to remember everything you can about your attacker and write it down.
- Don't wash or douche before the medical exam. Don't change your clothes, but bring a new set with you if you can.
- Be aware that at the hospital you will have a complete exam. Show the physician any bruises or scratches.

- Tell the police exactly what happened. Be honest and stick to your story.
- If you do not want to report the rape to the police, see a physician as soon as possible. Be sure you are checked for pregnancy and STDs.
- Contact an organization with skilled counselors so you can talk about the experience. Look in the telephone directory under "Rape" or "Rape Crisis Center" for a hotline number.

**Guidelines for men:**

- Be aware of social pressure. It's OK not to score.
- Understand that "No" means "No." Stop making advances when your date says to stop. Remember that she has the right to refuse sex.
- Don't assume that flirtatious behavior or sexy clothing means a woman is interested in having sex, that previous permission for sex applies to the current situation, or that your date's relationships with other men constitute sexual permission for you.
- Remember that alcohol and drugs interfere with judgment, perception, and communication about sex.

## Stalking and Cyberstalking

Stalking is characterized by harassing behaviors such as following or spying on a person and making verbal, written, or implied threats. It is estimated that 1 million U.S. women and 400,000 men are stalked each year; nearly 90% of stalkers are men. Cyberstalking, the use of electronic communications devices to stalk another person, is becoming more common. Cyberstalkers may send harassing or threatening e-mails or chat room messages to the victim, or they may encourage others to harass the victim by posting inflammatory messages and personal information on bulletin boards or chat rooms.

**To protect yourself online:**

- Never use your real name as an e-mail user name or chat room nickname. Select an age- and gender-neutral identity.
- Avoid filling out profiles for accounts related to e-mail use or chat room activities with information that could be used to identify you.
- Do not share personal information in public spaces anywhere online or give it to strangers.
- Learn how to filter unwanted e-mail messages.
- If you experience harassment online, do not respond to the harasser. Log off or surf elsewhere. Save all communications for evidence. If harassment continues, report it to the harasser's Internet service provider, your Internet service provider, and the local police.
- Don't agree to meet someone you've met online face-to-face unless you feel completely comfortable about it. Schedule a series of phone conversations first. Meet initially in a very public place and bring along a friend to increase your safety.

## Coping After Terrorism, Mass Violence, or Natural Disasters

Certain areas of the United States are prone to natural disasters like Hurricane Irene, which wreaked havoc along the East Coast in 2011. Other natural disasters include tornadoes, floods, and earthquakes. Less frequent in the United States are episodes of mass violence or terrorist events such as those that occurred in Oklahoma in April 1995 and on September 11, 2001. When such events occur, some people suffer direct physical harm and/or the loss of relatives, friends, or possessions; many others experience emotional distress and are robbed of their sense of security.

Each person reacts differently to traumatic disaster, and it is normal to experience a variety of responses. Reactions may include disbelief and shock, fear, anger and resentment, anxiety about the future, difficulty concentrating or making decisions, mood swings, irritability, sadness and depression, panic, guilt, apathy, feelings of isolation or powerlessness, and many of the behaviorial signs such as headaches or insomnia that are associated with excess stress (see Chapter 10). Reactions may occur immediately or may be delayed until weeks or months after the event.

Taking positive steps can help you cope with powerful emotions. Consider the following strategies:

- Share your experiences and emotions with friends and family members. Be a supportive listener. Reassure children and encourage them to talk about what they are feeling.
- Take care of your mind and body. Choose a healthy diet, exercise regularly, get plenty of sleep, and practice relaxation techniques. Don't turn to unhealthy coping techniques such as using alcohol or other drugs.
- Take a break from media reports and images, and try not to develop nightmare scenarios for possible future events.
- Reestablish your routines at home, school, and work.
- Find ways to help others. Donating money, blood, food, clothes, or time can ease difficult emotions and give you a greater sense of control.

Everyone copes with tragedy in a different way and recovers at a different pace. If you feel overwhelmed by your emotions, seek professional help. Additional information about coping with terrorism and violence is available from the Federal Emergency Management Agency (www.fema.gov), the U.S. Department of Justice (www. usdoj.gov), and the National Mental Health Association (www.nmha.org).

## Emergency Preparedness

Most prevention and coping activities related to terrorism, mass violence, and natural disasters occur at the federal, state, and community levels. However, one step you can take is to put together an emergency plan and kit for your family or household that can serve for any type of emergency or disaster.

**Emergency Supplies**   Your kit of emergency supplies should include everything you'll need to make it on your own for at least 3 days. You'll need nonperishable food, water, first-aid and sanitation supplies, a battery-powered radio, clothing, a flashlight, cash, keys, copies of important documents, and supplies for sleeping outdoors in any weather. Remember special-needs items for infants, seniors, and pets. Supplies for a basic emergency kit are listed in Figure A.2; add to your kit based on your family situation and the type of problems most likely to occur in your area.

## Basic emergency supplies

Map of the area for locating evacuation routes or shelters

Cash, coins, and credit cards

Copies of important documents stored in watertight container

Emergency contact list and phone numbers

Extra sets of house and car keys

Flashlights or lightsticks

Battery- or solar-powered radio

Battery-powered alarm clock

Extra batteries and bulbs

Cell phone or prepaid phone card

Signal flares

Fire extinguisher (small A-B-C type)

Whistle

Ladder

Tube tent and rope

Sleeping bags or warm blankets

Foam pads, pillows, baby bed

Complete change of warm clothing, footwear, outerware (jacket or coat, long pants, long-sleeved shirt, sturdy shoes, hat, gloves, raingear, extra socks and underwear, sunglasses)

Work gloves

Shutoff wrench for gas and water supplies

Shovel, hammer, pliers, screwdriver, and other tools

Compass

Matches in a waterproof container

Aluminum foil

Plastic storage containers, bucket

Duct tape, utility knife, and scissors

Paper, pens, pencils

Needles and thread

## First aid kit

First aid manual

Thermometer

Scissors

Tweezers

Safety pins, safety razor blades

Needle

Latex or other sterile gloves

Sterile gauze pads

Cleansing agents (soap, isopropyl alcohol, antiseptic towelettes)

Sunscreen

Insect repellent

Antibiotic ointment

Burn ointment

Petroleum jelly or another lubricant

Sterile adhesive bandages, several sizes

Sterile rolled bandages and triangular bandages

Cotton balls

Eyewash solution

Chemical heat and cold packs

Aspirin or nonaspirin pain reliever

Anti-diarrhea medication

Laxative

Antacid

Activated charcoal (use if advised by Poison Control Center)

Potassium iodide (use following radiation exposure if advised by local health authorities)

Prescription medications and prescribed medical supplies

List of medications, dosages, and any allergies

Medicine dropper

## Special needs items

Infant care needs (formula, bottles, diapers, powdered milk, diaper rash ointment)

Books or toys

Extra eyeglasses, contact lenses and supplies

Feminine hygiene supplies

Denture needs

Hearing aid or wheelchair batteries; other special equipment

Pet care supplies, including leash, pet carrier, copy of vaccination history, and tie-out stakes

Other (list)

## Food and related supplies

Manual (nonelectric) can opener

Utility knife

Paper towels

Eating utensils: Mess kits, or paper cups and plates and utensils

Plastic garbage bags and resealing bags

Small cooking stove and cooking fuel (if food must be cooked)

Water purification tablets

**Water:** Three-day-supply, at least 1 gallon of water per person per day, stored in plastic containers:

Number of people: _____ x $\underline{\text{1 gallon}}$ x $\underline{\text{3 days}}$ = _____ total minimum gallons of water

Store additional water if you live in a hot climate or if your household includes infants, pregnant women, or people with special health needs. Don't forget to store water for pets. Containers can be sterilized by rinsing them with a diluted bleach solution (one part bleach to ten parts water). Replace your water supply every six months.

**Food:** At least a three-day supply of nonperishable foods—those requiring no refrigeration, preparation, or cooking and little or no water. Choose foods from the following list and add foods that members of your household will eat. Replace items in your food supply every six months.

Ready-to-eat canned meats, fruits, soups, and vegetables

Protein or fruit bars

Dry cereal or granola

Peanut butter

Sugar, salt, pepper

Dried fruit

Nuts

Crackers

Canned, powdered, or boxed juices

Nonperishable pasteurized milk or powered milk

Coffee, tea, sodas

High-energy foods

Comfort/stress foods

MREs (military rations)

Infant formula and baby foods

Pet foods

## Sanitation

Plastic garbage bags (and ties)

Toilet paper

Moist towelettes or hand soap

Washcloth and towel

Personal hygiene items (toothbrush, shampoo, deodorant, comb, shaving cream, and so on)

Plastic bucket with tight lid

Household chlorine bleach, disinfectant

Powdered lime

Small shovel for digging latrine

## For a clean air supply

Face masks or several layers of dense-weave cotton material (handkerchiefs, t-shirts, towels) that fit snugly over your nose and mouth.

Shelter-in-place supplies, to be used in an interior room to create a barrier between you and potentially contaminated air outside: Heavyweight plastic garbage bags or plastic sheeting; duct tape; scissors; and if possible, a portable air purifier with a HEPA filter.

## Family emergency plan

Plan places where your family will meet; choose one location near your home and one outside your neighborhood.

Local _____ Outside neighborhood _____

Have one local and one out-of-state contact person for family members to call if separated during a disaster. (It may be easier to make long-distance calls than local calls.)

Local _____ Out-of state _____

**FIGURE A.2** Sample emergency preparedness kit and plan.

You may want to create several kinds of emergency kits. The primary one would contain supplies for home use. Put together a smaller, lightweight version that you can take with you if you are forced to evacuate your residence. Smaller kits for your car and your workplace are also recommended.

**A Family or Household Plan**   You and your family or household members should have a plan about where to meet and how to communicate. Choose at least two potential meeting places—one in your neighborhood and one or more in other areas. Your community may also have set locations for community shelters. Where you go may depend on the circumstances of the emergency situation. Use your common sense, and listen to the radio or television for instructions from emergency officials about whether to evacuate or stay in place. In addition, know all the transportation options in the vicinity of your home, school, and workplace; roadways and public transit may be affected, so a sturdy pair of walking shoes is a good item to keep in your emergency kit.

Everyone in the family or household should also have the same emergency contact person to call, preferably someone who lives outside the immediate area and won't be affected by the same local disaster. Local phone service may be significantly disrupted, so long-distance calls may be more likely to go through. Everyone should carry the relevant phone numbers and addresses at all times.

It is also important to check into the emergency plans at any location where you or family members spend time, including schools and workplaces. For each location, know the safest place to be for different types of emergencies—for example, near load-bearing interior walls during an earthquake or in the basement during a tornado. Also know how to turn off water, gas, and electricity in case of damaged utility lines; keep the needed tools next to the shutoff valves.

Other steps you can take to help prepare for emergencies include taking a first-aid class and setting up an emergency response group in your neighborhood, residential building, or office. Talk with your neighbors: Who has specialized equipment (for example, a power generator) or expertise that might help in a crisis? Do older or disabled neighbors have someone to help them? More complete information about emergency preparedness is available from local government agencies and from the following:

American Academy of Pediatrics
   (www.aap.org)
American Red Cross
   (www.redcross.org)
Federal Emergency Management Agency
   (www.fema.gov)
U.S. Department of Homeland Security
   (www.ready.gov)

## PROVIDING EMERGENCY CARE

You can improve someone else's chances of surviving if you are prepared to provide emergency help. A course in first aid offered by the American Red Cross and on many college campuses can teach you to respond appropriately when someone needs help. Emergency rescue techniques can save the lives of people who have stopped breathing, who are choking, or whose hearts have stopped beating. Pulmonary resuscitation (also known as rescue breathing, artificial respiration, or mouth-to-mouth resuscitation) is used when a person is not breathing (refer back to Figure A.1). Cardiopulmonary resuscitation (CPR) is used when a pulse can't be found. Training is required before a person can perform CPR. Significant changes were made to the guidelines for lay rescue CPR in 2005. Courses are offered by the American Red Cross and the American Heart Association.

**When You Have to Provide Emergency Care**   Remain calm and act sensibly. The basic pattern for providing emergency care is *check-call-care*:

1. *Check the situation.* Make sure the scene is safe for both you and the injured person. Don't put yourself in danger; if you get hurt too, you will be of little help to the injured person.
2. *Check the victim.* Conduct a quick head-to-toe examination. Assess the victim's signs and symptoms, such as level of responsiveness, pulse, and breathing rate. Look for bleeding and any indications of broken bones or paralysis.
3. *Call for help.* Call 9-1-1 or a local emergency number. Identify yourself and give as much information as you can about the condition of the victim and what happened.
4. *Care for the victim.* If the situation requires immediate action (no pulse, shock, etc.), provide first aid if you are trained to do so (refer back to Figure A.1).

### Selected Bibliography

Bren, L. 2005. Prevent your child from choking. *FDA Consumer,* September/ October.

Central Intelligence Agency. 2011. *The World Factbook.* Washington, D.C.: Central Intelligence Agency.

Federal Bureau of Investigation. 2009. *Hate Crime Statistics,* 2008. Washington, D.C.: U.S. Department of Justice.

Federal Bureau of Investigation. 2010. *Crime in the United States:* 2009. Washington, D.C.: U.S. Department of Justice.

Insurance Information Institute. 2007. *Road Rage* (http://www.iii.org/individuals/auto/lifesaving/roadrage; retrieved August 31, 2011).

Iudice, A., et al. 2005. Effects of prolonged wakefulness combined with alcohol and hands-free cell phone divided attention tasks on simulated driving. *Human Psychopharmacology* 20(2): 125–132.

National Center for Health Statistics. 2011. Deaths: Preliminary Data for 2009. *National Vital Statistics Reports* 59(4).

National Center for Health Statistics. 2011. *Health, United States,* 2010. Hyattsville, Md.: National Center for Health Statistics.

National Safety Council. 2011. *Injury Facts* 2011. Itasca, Ill.: National Safety Council.

U.S. Department of Homeland Security. 2005. *Ready America* (www.ready.gov; retrieved August 31, 2011).

# EXERCISE GUIDELINES FOR PEOPLE WITH SPECIAL HEALTH CONCERNS

As explained in Chapters 2–7, regular, appropriate exercise is safe and beneficial for many people with chronic conditions or other special health concerns. In fact, for many people with special health concerns, the risks associated with not exercising are far greater than those associated with a moderate program of regular exercise.

The fitness recommendations made throughout this book are intended for the general population and can serve as basic guidelines for any exercise program. If you have a chronic health condition, however, you may need to modify your exercise program to accommodate your situation. This appendix presents precautions and specialized recommendations for people with a variety of special health concerns.

These recommendations, however, are not intended to replace a physician's advice. If you have a special health concern, talk to your physician before starting any exercise program.

## ARTHRITIS

- Begin an exercise program as early as possible in the course of the disease.
- Warm up thoroughly before each workout to loosen stiff muscles and lower the risk of injury.
- For cardiorespiratory endurance exercise, avoid high-impact activities that may damage arthritic joints. Consider swimming, water walking, or another type of exercise that can be done in a warm pool.
- Strength train the whole body. Pay special attention to muscles that support and protect affected joints. For example, build the quadriceps, hamstrings, and calf muscles to support and protect arthritic knees. Start with small amounts of weight and gradually increase the intensity of your workouts.
- Perform flexibility exercises daily to maintain joint mobility.

## ASTHMA

- Exercise regularly. Acute attacks are more likely to occur if you exercise only occasionally.
- Carry medication during workouts and avoid exercising alone. Use your inhaler as recommended by your physician.
- Warm up and cool down slowly to reduce the risk of acute attacks.
- When starting an exercise program, choose self-paced endurance activities, especially those involving interval training (short bouts of exercise followed by a rest period). Gradually increase the intensity of your cardiorespiratory endurance workouts.

- Educate yourself about situations that can trigger an asthma attack and act accordingly when exercising. For example, cold, dry air can trigger or worsen an attack. Pollen, dust, and polluted air can also trigger an attack. To avoid attacks in dry air, drink water before, during, and after a workout to moisten your airways. In cold weather, cover your mouth with a mask or scarf to warm and humidify the air you breathe. Also, avoid outdoor activities during pollen season or when the air is polluted or dusty.

## DIABETES

- Don't begin an exercise program unless your diabetes is under control and you have discussed exercise safety with your physician. Because people with diabetes have an increased risk for heart disease, an exercise stress test may be recommended.
- Don't exercise alone. Wear a bracelet that identifies you as someone with diabetes.
- If you take insulin or another medication, adjust the timing and amount of each dose as needed. Work with your physician and check your blood sugar level regularly so you can learn to balance your energy intake and output and your medication dosage.
- To prevent abnormally rapid absorption of injected insulin, inject it over a muscle that will not be exercised, and wait at least an hour before exercising.
- Check your blood sugar before, during, and after exercise. Adjust your diet and insulin dosage as needed. Keep high-carbohydrate foods on hand during a workout. Avoid exercise if your blood sugar level is above 250 mg/dl; if your blood sugar level is below 100 mg/dl, eat some carbohydrate-rich food before exercising.
- If you have poor circulation or numbness in your extremities, check your skin regularly for blisters and abrasions, especially on your feet. Avoid high-impact activities and wear comfortable shoes.
- For maximum benefit and minimum risk, choose moderate-intensity activities.

## HEART DISEASE AND HYPERTENSION

- Check with your physician about exercise safety before increasing your activity level. Your doctor may recommend that you take an exercise stress test before starting your program.

- Exercise at moderate intensity rather than high intensity. Keep your heart rate below the level at which abnormalities appear on an exercise stress test.
- Warm up and cool down gradually. Every warm-up and cool-down session should last at least 10 minutes.
- Monitor your heart rate during exercise, and stop if you experience dizziness or chest pain.
- If your physician prescribes nitroglycerin, carry it with you during exercise. If you take a beta-blocker to manage hypertension, use RPE rather than heart rate to monitor your exercise intensity (beta-blockers reduce heart rate). Exercise at an RPE level of "fairly light" to "somewhat hard." Your breathing should be unlabored, and you should be able to talk during exercise.
- Don't hold your breath when exercising. Doing so can cause sudden, steep increases in blood pressure. Take special care during weight training and do not lift heavy loads. Exhale during the exertion phase of each lift.
- Increase exercise frequency, intensity, and time very gradually.

## OBESITY

- For maximum benefit and minimum risk, begin by choosing low- to moderate-intensity activities. Increase intensity slowly as your fitness improves. Studies of overweight people show that exercising at moderate to high intensities causes more fat loss than training at low intensities.
- People who want to lose weight or maintain weight loss should exercise moderately for 60 minutes or more every day. To get the benefit of 60 minutes of exercise, you can exercise all at once or divide your total activity time into sessions of 10, 20, or 30 minutes.

- Choose non- or low-weight-bearing activities such as swimming, water exercises, cycling, or walking. Low-impact activities are less likely to cause joint problems or injuries.
- Stay alert for symptoms of heat-related problems during exercise (as described in Chapter 3). Obese people are vulnerable to heat intolerance.
- Ease into your exercise program and increase overload gradually. Increase time and frequency of exercise before increasing intensity.
- Include strength training in your fitness program to build or maintain muscle mass.
- Try to include as much lifestyle physical activity in your daily routine as possible.

## OSTEOPOROSIS

- For cardiorespiratory endurance activities, exercise at the maximum intensity that causes no significant discomfort. If possible, choose low-impact, weight-bearing exercises to help safely maintain bone density. (See Chapter 8 for strategies for building and maintaining bone density.)
- To prevent fractures, avoid any activity or movement that stresses the back or carries a risk of falling.
- Include weight training in your exercise program to improve strength and balance and to reduce the risk of falls and fractures. Always use proper exercise technique and avoid lifting heavy loads.
- Include muscle-strengthening exercises 3 days per week.
- Include bone-strengthening exercises, such as jumping, at least 3 days per week.

NAME _____ SECTION _____ DATE _____

As you completed the labs listed below, you entered the results in the Preprogram Assessment column of this appendix. Now that you have been involved in a fitness and wellness program for some time, do the labs again and enter your new results in the Postprogram Assessment column. You will probably notice improvement in several areas. Congratulations! If you are not satisfied with your progress thus far, refer to the tips for successful behavior change in Chapter 1 and throughout this book. Remember—fitness and wellness are forever. The time you invest now in developing a comprehensive, individualized program will pay off in a richer, more vital life in the years to come.

|  | Preprogram Assessment | Postprogram Assessment |
|---|---|---|
| **LAB 2.3** Pedometer | Daily steps: _____ | Daily steps: _____ |
| **LAB 3.1** Cardiorespiratory Endurance | | |
| 1-mile walk test | $\dot{V}O_{2max}$: _____ Rating: _____ | $\dot{V}O_{2max}$: _____ Rating: _____ |
| 3-minute step test | $\dot{V}O_{2max}$: _____ Rating: _____ | $\dot{V}O_{2max}$: _____ Rating: _____ |
| 1.5-mile run-walk test | $\dot{V}O_{2max}$: _____ Rating: _____ | $\dot{V}O_{2max}$: _____ Rating: _____ |
| 12-minute swim test | Rating: _____ | Rating: _____ |
| **LAB 4.1** Muscular Strength | | |
| Maximum bench press test | Weight: _____ lb Rating: _____ | Weight: _____ lb Rating: _____ |
| **LAB 4.2** Muscular Endurance | | |
| Curl-up test | Number: _____ Rating: _____ | Number: _____ Rating: _____ |
| Push-up test | Number: _____ Rating: _____ | Number: _____ Rating: _____ |
| Squat endurance test | Number: _____ Rating: _____ | Number: _____ Rating: _____ |
| **LAB 5.1** Flexibility | | |
| Sit-and-reach test | Score: _____ cm Rating: _____ | Score: _____ cm Rating: _____ |
| **LAB 5.3** Low-Back Muscular Endurance | | |
| Side bridge endurance test | Right: _____ sec. Rating: _____ | Right: _____ sec. Rating: _____ |
|  | Left: _____ sec. Rating: _____ | Left: _____ sec. Rating: _____ |
| Trunk flexors endurance test | Trunk flexors: _____ sec. Rating: _____ | Trunk flexors: _____ sec. Rating: _____ |
| Back extensors endurance test | Back extensors: _____ sec. Rating: _____ | Back extensors: _____ sec. Rating: _____ |

|  | Preprogram Assessment | Postprogram Assessment |
|---|---|---|
| **LAB 6.1** Body Composition | | |
| Body mass index | BMI: _____ kg/m2 Rating: _____ | BMI: _____ kg/m2 Rating: _____ |
| Skinfold measurements (or other methods for determining percent body fat) | Sum of 3 skinfolds: _____ mm | Sum of 3 skinfolds: _____ mm |
|  | % body fat: _____% Rating: _____ | % body fat: _____% Rating: _____ |
| Waist circumference | Circumf.: _____ Rating: _____ | Circumf.: _____ Rating: _____ |
| Waist-to-hip ratio | Ratio: _____ Rating: _____ | Ratio: _____ Rating: _____ |
| **LAB 8.1** Daily Diet | | |
| Number of oz-eq | Grains: _____ | Grains: _____ |
| Number of cups | Vegetables: _____ | Vegetables: _____ |
| Number of cups | Fruits: _____ | Fruits: _____ |
| Number of cups | Milk: _____ | Milk: _____ |
| Number of oz-eq | Meat or beans: _____ | Meat or beans: _____ |
| Number of tsp | Oils: _____ | Oils: _____ |
| Number of g | Solid fats: _____ | Solid fats: _____ |
| Number of g or tsp | Added sugars: _____ | Added sugars: _____ |
| **LAB 8.2** Dietary Analysis | | |
| Percentage of calories | From protein: _____ % | From protein: _____ % |
| Percentage of calories | From fat: _____ % | From fat: _____ % |
| Percentage of calories | From saturated fat: _____ % | From saturated fat: _____ % |
| Percentage of calories | From carbohydrate: _____ % | From carbohydrate: _____ % |
| **LAB 9.1** Daily Energy Needs | Daily energy needs: _____ cal/day | Daily energy needs: _____ cal/day |
| **LAB 10.1** Identifying Stressors | Average weekly stress score: _____ | Average weekly stress score: _____ |
| **LAB 11.1** Cardiovascular Health | | |
| CVD risk assessment | Score: _____ Estimated risk: _____ | Score: _____ Estimated risk: _____ |
| Hostility assessment | Score: _____ Rating: _____ | Score: _____ Rating: _____ |
| **LAB 12.1** Cancer Prevention | | |
| Diet: Number of servings | Fruits/vegetables: _____ | Fruits/vegetables: _____ |
| Skin cancer | Score: _____ Risk: _____ | Score: _____ Risk: _____ |

C

# BEHAVIOR CHANGE WORKBOOK

This workbook is designed to take you step by step through a behavior change program. The first eight activities in the workbook will help you develop a successful plan—beginning with choosing a target behavior, moving through the planning steps described in Chapter 1, and completing and signing a behavior change contract. The final seven activities will help you work through common obstacles to behavior change and maximize your program's chances of success.

**Part 1  Developing a Plan for Behavior Change and Completing a Contract**

1. Choosing a Target Behavior
2. Gathering Information About Your Target Behavior
3. Monitoring Your Current Patterns of Behavior
4. Setting Goals
5. Examining Your Attitudes About Your Target Behavior
6. Choosing Rewards
7. Breaking Behavior Chains
8. Completing a Contract for Behavior Change

**Part 2  Overcoming Obstacles to Behavior Change**

9. Building Motivation and Commitment
10. Managing Your Time Successfully
11. Developing Realistic Self-Talk
12. Involving the People Around You
13. Dealing with Feelings
14. Overcoming Peer Pressure: Communicating Assertively
15. Maintaining Your Program over Time

## ACTIVITY 1   CHOOSING A TARGET BEHAVIOR

Use your knowledge of yourself and the results of Lab 1.2 (Lifestyle Evaluation) to identify five behaviors that you could change to improve your level of wellness. Examples of target behaviors include smoking cigarettes, not exercising regularly, eating candy bars every night, not getting enough sleep, getting drunk frequently on weekends, and not wearing a safety belt when driving or riding in a car. List your five behaviors below.

1. _____
2. _____
3. _____
4. _____
5. _____

For successful behavior change, it's best to focus on one behavior at a time. Review your list of behaviors and select one to start with. Choose a behavior that is important to you and that you are strongly motivated to change. If this will be your first attempt at behavior change, start with a simple change, such as wearing your bicycle helmet regularly, before tackling a more difficult change, such as quitting smoking. Circle the behavior on your list that you've chosen to start with; this will be your target behavior throughout this workbook.

## ACTIVITY 2   GATHERING INFORMATION ABOUT YOUR TARGET BEHAVIOR

Take a close look at what your target behavior means to your health, now and in the future. How is it affecting your level of wellness? What diseases or conditions does this behavior place you at risk for? What will changing this behavior mean to you? To evaluate your behavior, use information from this text, from the resources listed in the For Further Exploration section at the end of each chapter, and from other reliable sources.

Health behaviors have short-term and long-term benefits and costs associated with them. For example, in the short term, an inactive lifestyle allows for more time to watch TV and hang out with friends but leaves a person less able to participate in recreational activities. In the long term, it increases the risk of cardiovascular disease, cancer, and premature death. Fill in the blanks below with the benefits and costs of continuing your current behavior and of changing to a new, healthier behavior. Pay close attention to the short-term benefits of the new behavior—these are an important motivating force behind successful behavior change programs.

**Target (current) behavior** _____

Benefits   *Short-Term*                                            *Long-Term*

_____      _____

_____      _____

_____      _____

Costs       *Short-Term*                                            *Long-Term*

_____      _____

_____      _____

_____      _____

**New behavior** _____

Benefits   *Short-Term*                                            *Long-Term*

_____      _____

_____      _____

_____      _____

Costs       *Short-Term*                                            *Long-Term*

_____      _____

_____      _____

_____      _____

## ACTIVITY 3   MONITORING YOUR CURRENT PATTERNS OF BEHAVIOR

To develop a successful behavior change program, you need detailed information about your current behavior patterns. You can obtain this information by developing a system of record keeping geared toward your target behavior. Depending on your target behavior, you may want to monitor a single behavior, such as your diet, or you may want to keep daily activity records to determine how you could make time for exercise or another new behavior. Consider tracking factors such as the following:

- What the behavior was
- When and for how long it occurred
- Where it occurred
- What else you were doing at the time
- What other people you were with and how they influenced you
- What your thoughts and feelings were
- How strong your urge for the behavior was (for example, how hungry you were or how much you wanted to watch TV)

Figure 1.6 shows a sample log for tracking daily diet. Below, create a format for a sample daily log for monitoring the behavior patterns relating to your target behavior. Then use the log to monitor your behavior for a day. Evaluate your log as you use it. Ask yourself if you are tracking all the key factors that influence your behavior; make any necessary adjustments to the format of your log. Once you've developed an appropriate format, use a separate notebook (your health journal) to keep records of your behavior for a week or two. These records will provide solid information about your behavior that will help you develop a successful behavior change program. Later activities in this workbook will ask you to analyze your records.

## ACTIVITY 4 SETTING GOALS

For your behavior change program to succeed, you must set meaningful, realistic goals. In addition to an ultimate goal, set some intermediate goals—milestones that you can strive for on the way to your final objective. For example, if your overall goal is to run a 5K road race, an intermediate goal might be to successfully complete 2 weeks of your fitness program. If you set a final goal of eating 7 servings of fruits and vegetables every day, an intermediate goal would be to increase your daily intake from 3 to 4 servings. List your intermediate and final goals below. Don't strive for immediate perfection. Allow an adequate amount of time to reach each of your goals.

**Intermediate Goals**                                  **Target Date**

_____        _____

_____        _____

_____        _____

_____        _____

_____        _____

**Final Goals**

_____        _____

## ACTIVITY 5 EXAMINING YOUR ATTITUDES ABOUT YOUR TARGET BEHAVIOR

Your attitudes toward your target behavior can determine whether your behavior change program will be successful. Consider your attitudes carefully by completing the following statements about how you think and feel about your current behavior and your goal.

1. I like _____ because _____
     (current behavior)
_____.

2. I don't like _____ because _____
     (current behavior)
_____.

3. I like _____ because _____
     (behavior goal)
_____.

4. I don't like _____ because _____
     (behavior goal)
_____.

5. I don't _____ now because _____
     (behavior goal)
_____.

6. I would be more likely to _____ if _____
                                    (behavior goal)
_____.

If your statements indicate that you have major reservations about changing your behavior, work to build your motivation and commitment before you begin your program. Look carefully at your objections to changing your behavior. How valid and important are they? What can you do to overcome them? Can you adopt any of the strategies you listed under statement 6? Review the facts about your current behavior and your goals.

### ACTIVITY 6   CHOOSING REWARDS

Make a list of objects, activities, and events you can use as rewards for achieving the goals of your behavior change program. Rewards should be special, relatively inexpensive, and preferably unrelated to food or alcohol—for example, tickets to a ball game, a CD, or a long-distance phone call to a family member or friend—whatever is meaningful for you. Write down a variety of rewards you can use when you reach milestones in your program and your final goal.

_____      _____

_____      _____

_____      _____

_____      _____

Many people also find it helpful to give themselves small rewards daily or weekly for sticking with their behavior change program. These could be things like a study break, a movie, or a Saturday morning bike ride. Make a list of rewards for maintaining your program in the short term.

_____      _____

_____      _____

_____      _____

_____      _____

And don't forget to congratulate yourself regularly during your behavior change program. Notice how much better you feel. Savor how far you've come and how you've gained control of your behavior.

### ACTIVITY 7   BREAKING BEHAVIOR CHAINS

Use the records you collected about your target behavior in Activity 3 and in your health journal to identify what leads up to your target behavior and what follows it. By tracing these chains of events, you'll be able to identify points in the chain where you can make a change that will lead to your new behavior. The sample behavior chain on the next page shows a sequence of events for a person who wants to add exercise to her daily routine—but who winds up snacking and watching TV instead. By examining the chain carefully, you can identify ways to break it at every step. After you review the sample, go through the same process for a typical chain of events involving your target behavior. Use the blank behavior chain on the following page.

Some general strategies for breaking behavior chains include the following:

- **Control or eliminate environmental cues that provoke the behavior.** Stay out of the room where your television is located. Go out for an ice cream cone instead of keeping a half gallon of ice cream in your freezer.
- **Change behaviors or habits that are linked to your target behavior.** If you always smoke in your car when you drive to school, try taking public transportation instead.
- **Add new cues to your environment to trigger your new behavior.** Prepare easy-to-grab healthy snacks and carry them with you to class or work. Keep your exercise clothes and equipment in a visible location.

See also the suggestions in Chapter 1.

| **Chain of Events** | **Strategies for Breaking the Chain** |
|---|---|
| Come home from class | You had planned an afternoon walk as part of your exercise program. |
| Feel tired, not like exercising | Tell yourself you'll feel better and more alert after working out. |
| Look for walking shoes; can't find them | Put shoes and clothes for exercise in an obvious place the night before. |
| Feel annoyed | Remind yourself of your program goals, and tell yourself that you can stick with your program. |
| Go to kitchen, see food | Stay out of the kitchen unless you will be fixing or eating a planned meal or snack. |
| Feel hungry | Look at the picture of a healthy exercise that you've put on the refrigerator to remind you of your goals. |
| Grab a soda and bag of chips | Have a glass of water or a pre-prepared healthy snack. |
| Turn on TV and sit down | Turn on the radio instead; listen to news or music while you get ready to exercise. |
| Eat chips, watch TV | If you really like to watch TV in the afternoon, plan to work out in the morning or exercise on a stationary bike or treadmill in front of the TV. |
| Feel guilty | Even if you do have occasional lapses, don't beat yourself up. Think positively about how you'll resume your program the next day. |

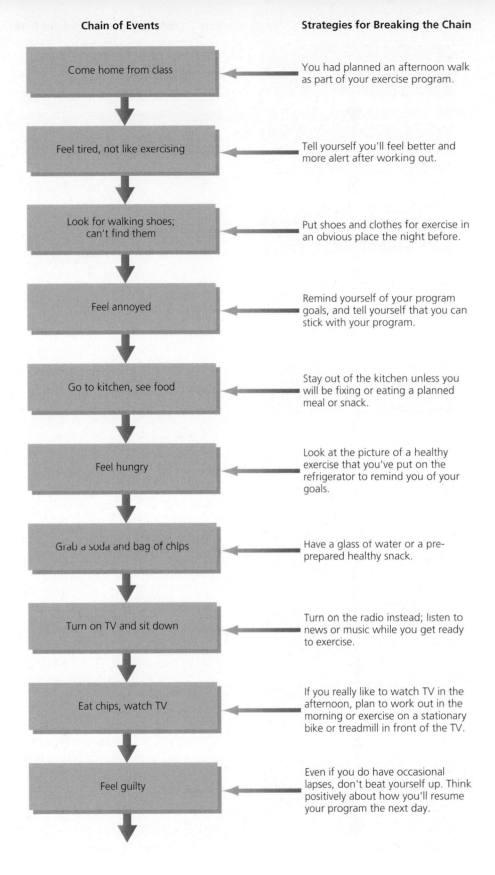

**BEHAVIOR CHANGE WORKBOOK**

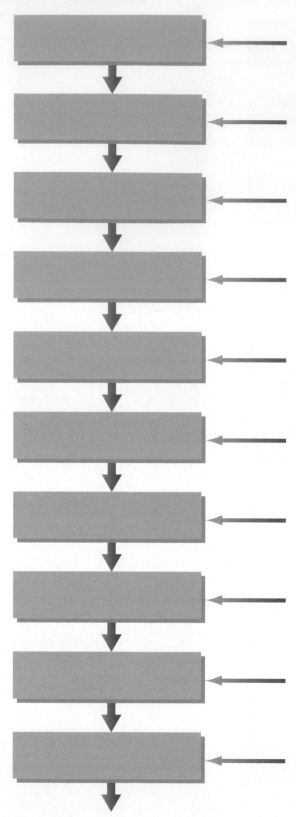

Your next step in creating a successful behavior change program is to complete and sign a behavior change contract. Your contract should include details of your program and indicate your commitment to changing your behavior. Use the information from previous activities in this workbook to complete the following contract. (If your target behavior relates to exercise, you may want to use the program plan and contract for a fitness program in Lab 7.1.)

1. I, _____, agree to _____
   (name)                                  (specify behavior you want to change)

   _____.

2. I will begin on _____ and plan to reach my goal of _____
   (start date)                                        (specify final goal)

   _____ by _____.

3. To reach my final goal, I have devised the following schedule of mini-goals. For each step in my program, I will give myself the reward listed.

   | _____ | _____ | _____ |
   | (mini-goal 1) | (target date) | (reward) |
   | _____ | _____ | _____ |
   | (mini-goal 2) | (target date) | (reward) |
   | _____ | _____ | _____ |
   | (mini-goal 3) | (target date) | (reward) |
   | _____ | _____ | _____ |
   | (mini-goal 4) | (target date) | (reward) |
   | _____ | _____ | _____ |
   | (mini-goal 5) | (target date) | (reward) |

   My overall reward for reaching my final goal will be _____

4. I have gathered and analyzed data on my target behavior and have identified the following strategies for changing my behavior: _____

   _____

   _____

5. I will use the following tools to monitor my progress toward reaching my final goal:

   _____
   (list any charts, graphs, or journals you plan to use)

   _____

   I sign this contract as an indication of my personal commitment to reach my goal.

   _____    _____
   (your signature)                                    (date)

   I have recruited a helper who will witness my contract and _____

   _____
   (list any way in which your helper will participate in your program)

   _____

   _____    _____
   (helper's signature)                                (date)

Describe in detail any special strategies you will use to help change your behavior (refer to Activity 7).

Create a plan for any charts, graphs, or journals you will use to monitor your progress. The log format you developed in Activity 3 may be appropriate, or you may need to develop a more detailed or specific record-keeping system. Examples of journal formats are included in Labs 3.2, 4.3, 5.2, 8.1, and 10.1. You might also want to develop a graph to show your progress; posting such a graph in a prominent location can help keep your motivation strong and your program on track. Depending on your target behavior, you could graph the number of push-ups you can do, the number of servings of vegetables you eat each day, or your average daily stress level.

## ACTIVITY 9   BUILDING MOTIVATION AND COMMITMENT

Complete the following checklist to determine whether you are motivated and committed to changing your behavior. Check the statements that are true for you.

_____ I feel responsible for my own behavior and capable of managing it.

_____ I am not easily discouraged.

_____ I enjoy setting goals and then working to achieve them.

_____ I am good at keeping promises to myself.

_____ I like having a structure and schedule for my activities.

_____ I view my new behavior as a necessity, not an optional activity.

_____ Compared with previous attempts to change my behavior, I am more motivated now.

_____ My goals are realistic.

_____ I have a positive mental picture of the new behavior.

_____ Considering the stresses in my life, I feel confident that I can stick to my program.

_____ I feel prepared for lapses and ups-and-downs in my behavior change program.

_____ I feel that my plan for behavior change is enjoyable.

_____ I feel comfortable telling other people about the change I am making in my behavior.

Did you check most of these statements? If not, you need to boost your motivation and commitment. Consider these strategies:

- Review the potential benefits of changing your behavior and the costs of not changing it (see Activity 2). Pay special attention to the short-term benefits of changing your behavior, including feelings of accomplishment and self-confidence. Post a list of these benefits in a prominent location.

- Visualize yourself achieving your goal and enjoying its benefits. For example, if you want to manage time more effectively, picture yourself as a confident, organized person who systematically tackles important tasks and sets aside time each day for relaxation, exercise, and friends. Practice this type of visualization regularly.

- Put aside obstacles and objections to change. Counter thoughts such as "I'll never have time to exercise" with thoughts like "Lots of other people do it, and so can I."

- Bombard yourself with propaganda. Take a class dealing with the change you want to make. Read books and watch television shows on the subject. Post motivational phrases or pictures on your refrigerator or over your desk. Talk to people who have already made the change.

- Build up your confidence. Remind yourself of other goals you've achieved. At the end of each day, mentally review your good decisions and actions. See yourself as a capable person, as being in charge of your behavior.

List two strategies for boosting your motivation and commitment; choose from the list above, or develop your own. Try each strategy, and then describe how well it worked for you.

BEHAVIOR CHANGE WORKBOOK

W-8

Strategy 1: _____

How well it worked: _____

_____

Strategy 2: _____

How well it worked: _____

_____

## ACTIVITY 10   MANAGING YOUR TIME SUCCESSFULLY

"Too little time" is a common excuse for not exercising or engaging in other healthy behaviors. Learning to manage your time successfully is crucial if you are to maintain a wellness lifestyle. The first step is to examine how you are currently spending your time; use the following grid to track your activities.

| Time | Activity | Time | Activity |
|---|---|---|---|
| 6:00 A.M. | | 6:00 P.M. | |
| 6:30 A.M. | | 6:30 P.M. | |
| 7:00 A.M. | | 7:00 P.M. | |
| 8:00 A.M. | | 8:00 P.M. | |
| 9:00 A.M. | | 9:00 P.M. | |
| 10:00 A.M. | | 10:00 P.M. | |
| 11:00 A.M. | | 11:00 P.M. | |
| 12:00 P.M. | | 12:00 A.M. | |
| 1:00 P.M. | | 1:00 A.M. | |
| 2:00 P.M. | | 2:00 A.M | |
| 3:00 P.M. | | 3:00 A.M. | |
| 4:00 P.M. | | 4:00 A.M. | |
| 5:00 P.M. | | 5:00 A.M. | |

Next, list each type of activity and the total time you engaged in it on a given day in the chart below (for example, sleeping, 7 hours; eating, 1.5 hours; studying, 3 hours; working, 3 hours; and so on). Take a close look at your list of activities. Successful time management is based on prioritization. Assign a priority to each of your activities according to how important it is to you: essential (A), somewhat important (B), or not important (C). Based on these priority rankings, make changes in your schedule by adding and subtracting hours from different categories of activities; enter a duration goal for each activity. Add your new activities to the list and assign a priority and duration goal to each.

| Activity | Current Total Duration | Priority (A, B, or C) | Goal Total Duration |
|---|---|---|---|
| | | | |
| | | | |
| | | | |
| | | | |
| | | | |
| | | | |
| | | | |

Prioritizing in this manner will involve trade-offs. For example, you may choose to reduce the amount of time you spend watching television, listening to music, and chatting on the telephone while you increase the amount of time spent sleeping, studying, and exercising. Don't feel that you have to miss out on anything you enjoy. You can get more from less time by focusing on what you are doing. Strategies for managing time more productively and creatively are described in Chapter 10.

## ACTIVITY 11  DEVELOPING REALISTIC SELF-TALK

Self-talk is the ongoing internal dialogue you have with yourself throughout much of the day. Your thoughts can be accurate, positive, and supportive, or they can be exaggerated and negative. Self-talk is closely related to self-esteem and self-concept. Realistic self-talk can help maintain positive self-esteem, the belief that you are a good and competent person, worthy of friendship and love. A negative internal dialogue can reinforce negative self-esteem and can make behavior change difficult. Substituting realistic self-talk for negative self-talk can help you build and maintain self-esteem and cope better with the challenges in your life.

First, take a closer look at your current pattern of self-talk. Use your health journal to track self-talk, especially as it relates to your target behavior. Does any of your self-talk fall into the common patterns of distorted, negative self-talk shown in Chapter 10? If so, use the examples of realistic self-talk from Chapter 10 to develop more accurate and rational responses. Write your current negative thoughts in the left-hand column, and then record more realistic thoughts in the right-hand column.

**Current Self-Talk About Target Behavior**

_____

_____

_____

_____

_____

_____

**More Realistic Self-Talk**

_____

_____

_____

_____

_____

_____

Your behavior change program will be more successful if the people around you are supportive and involved—or at least are not sabotaging your efforts. Use your health journal to track how other people influence your target behavior and your efforts to change it. For example, do you always skip exercising when you're with certain people? Do you always drink or eat too much when you socialize with certain friends? Are friends and family members offering you enthusiastic support for your efforts to change your behavior, or do they make jokes about your program? Have they even noticed your efforts? Summarize the reactions of those around you in the chart below.

Target behavior _____

| Person | Typical Effect on Target Behavior | Involvement in/Reaction to Program |
|--------|-----------------------------------|-------------------------------------|
|        |                                   |                                     |
|        |                                   |                                     |
|        |                                   |                                     |
|        |                                   |                                     |

It may be difficult to change the actions and reactions of the people who are close to you. For them to be involved in your program, you may need to develop new ways of interacting with them (for example, taking a walk rather than going out to dinner as a means of socializing). Most of your friends and family members will want to help you—if they know how. Ask for exactly the type of help or involvement you want. Do you want feedback, praise, or just cooperation? Would you like someone to witness your contract or to be involved more directly in your program? Do you want someone to stop sabotaging your efforts by inviting you to watch TV, eat rich desserts, and so on? Look for ways that the people who are close to you can share in your behavior change program. They can help to motivate you and to maintain your commitment to your program. Develop a way that each individual you listed above can become involved in your program in a positive way.

| Person | Target Involvement in Behavior Change Program |
|--------|------------------------------------------------|
|        |                                                |
|        |                                                |
|        |                                                |
|        |                                                |

Choose one person on your list to tackle first. Talk to that person about her or his current behavior and how you would like her or him to be involved in your behavior change program. Below, describe this person's reaction to your talk and her or his subsequent behavior. Did this individual become a positive participant in your behavior change program?

_____

_____

_____

_____

_____

**BEHAVIOR CHANGE WORKBOOK**

Long-standing habits are difficult to change in part because many of them represent ways people have developed to cope with certain feelings. For example, people may overeat when bored, skip their exercise sessions when frustrated, or drink alcoholic beverages when anxious. Developing new ways to deal with feelings can help improve the chance that a behavior change program will succeed.

Review the records on your target behavior that you kept in your health journal. Identify the feelings that are interfering with the success of your program, and develop new strategies for coping with them. Some common problematic feelings are listed below, along with one possible coping strategy for each. Put a check mark next to those that are influencing your target behavior, and fill in additional strategies. Add the other feelings that are significant roadblocks in your program to the bottom of the chart, along with coping strategies for each.

| ✔ | Feeling | Coping Strategies |
|---|---------|-------------------|
|   | Stressed out | Go for a 10-minute walk. |
|   | Anxious | Do one of the relaxation exercises described in Chapter 10. |
|   | Bored | Call a friend for a chat. |
|   | Tired | Take a 20-minute nap. |
|   | Frustrated | Identify the source of the feeling and deal with it constructively. |
|   |   |   |
|   |   |   |
|   |   |   |
|   |   |   |
|   |   |   |

Consider the following situations:

- Julia is trying to give up smoking; her friend Marie continues to offer her cigarettes whenever they are together.
- Emilio is planning to exercise in the morning; his roommates tell him he's being antisocial by not having breakfast with them.
- Tracy's boyfriend told her that in high school he once experimented with drugs and shared needles; she wants him to have an HIV test, but he says he's sure the people he shared needles with were not infected.

Peer pressure is the common ingredient in these situations. To successfully maintain your behavior change program, you must develop effective strategies for resisting peer pressure. Assertive communication is one such strategy. By communicating assertively—firmly, but not aggressively—you can stick with your program even in the face of pressure from others.

Review your health journal to determine how other people affect your target behavior. If you find that you often give in to peer pressure, try the following strategies for communicating more assertively:

- Collect your thoughts, and plan in advance what you will say. You might try out your response on a friend to get some feedback.
- State your case—how you feel and what you want—as clearly as you can.
- Use "I" messages—statements about how you feel—rather than "you" statements.
- Focus on the behavior rather than the person. Suggest a solution, such as asking the other person to change his or her behavior toward you. Avoid generalizations. Be specific about what you want.
- Make clear, constructive requests. Focus on your needs ("I would like . . .") rather than the mistakes of others ("You always . . .").
- Avoid blaming, accusing, and belittling. Treat others with the same respect you'd like to receive yourself.
- Ask for action ahead of time. Tell others what you would like to have happen; don't wait for them to do the wrong thing and then get angry at them.
- Ask for a response to what you have proposed. Wait for an answer and listen carefully to it. Try to understand other people's points of view, just as you would hope that others would understand yours.

With these strategies in mind, review your health journal and identify three instances in which peer pressure interfered with your behavior change program. For each instance, write out what you might have said to deal with the situation more assertively. (If you can't think of three situations from your experiences, choose one or more of the three scenarios described at the beginning of this activity.)

1. _____
   _____
2. _____
   _____
3. _____
   _____

Assertive communication can help you achieve your behavior change goals in a direct way by helping you keep your program on track. It can also provide a boost for your self-image and increase your confidence in your ability to successfully manage your behavior.

## ACTIVITY 15  MAINTAINING YOUR PROGRAM OVER TIME

If you maintain your new behavior for at least 6 months, you've reached the maintenance stage, and your chances of lifetime success are greatly increased. However, you may find yourself sliding back into old habits at some point. If this happens, there are some things you can do to help maintain your new behavior.

BEHAVIOR CHANGE WORKBOOK

- Remind yourself of the goals of your program (list them here).

_____

_____

_____

_____

_____

- Pay attention to how your new pattern of behavior has improved your wellness status. List the major benefits of changing your behavior, both now and in the future.

_____

_____

_____

_____

_____

- Consider the things you enjoy most about your new pattern of behavior. List your favorite aspects.

_____

_____

_____

_____

_____

- Think of yourself as a problem solver. If something begins to interfere with your program, devise strategies for dealing with it. Take time out now to list things that have the potential to derail your program and develop possible coping mechanisms.

**Problem**                    **Solution**

_____            _____

_____            _____

_____            _____

_____            _____

_____            _____

- Remember the basics of behavior change. If your program runs into trouble, go back to keeping records of your behavior to pinpoint problem areas. Make adjustments in your program to deal with new disruptions. Don't feel defeated if you lapse. The best thing you can do is renew your commitment and continue with your program.

# CREDITS

**Title page**

Thomas Northcut/Getty Images

**Chapter 1**

p. 1, © Odilon Dimier/PhotoAlto Agency RF Collections/Blend Images; p. 5, Ryan McVay/Getty Images; p. 8, © The McGraw-Hill Companies, Inc./Lars A. Niki, photographer; p. 10, Dynamic Graphics/JupiterImages; p. 12, © Stockdisc/PunchStock; p. 14, Blend Images/Getty Images; p. 19, Photodisc/Getty Images

**Chapter 2**

p. 29, RubberBall Productions/Getty Images; p. 31, © moodboard/Alamy; p. 35, © Erik Isakson/Blend Images/Getty Images; p. 37, © Ezra Shaw/Getty Images; p. 38, © Harold Cunningham/Getty Images; p. 39, Comstock Images/Jupiterimages; p. 42, © Kevin Fleming/Corbis; p. 43, Man in white chair: © Stockbyte/PunchStock, weight lifter arm: Ryan McVay/Getty Images, stretching: The McGraw-Hill Companies, Inc/Ken Karp photographer, bicycling: Joaquin Palting/Getty Images, walking: Doug Menuez/Getty Images, raking: UpperCut Images/Alamy; p. 44, Dancing, RubberBall Productions, Biking, © Royalty-Free/Corbis, weightlifting, © Thinkstock Images/Jupiterimages; p. 47, © IT Stock/PunchStock

**Chapter 3**

p. 61, © Caetano Barreira/X01990/Reuters/Corbis; p. 66, © Bill Varie/Workbook Stock/Getty Images; p. 68, © altrendo images/Stockbyte/Getty Images; p. 69, © Paul Burns/Digital Vision/Getty Images; p. 72, Courtesy Robin Mouat; p. 80, Ingram Publishing; p. 83, © Royalty-Free/Corbis; p. 84, © Siede Preis/PhotoDisc/Getty Images

**Chapter 4**

p. 97, © Paul Bradbury/The Image Bank/Getty Images; p. 100, © Terry Vine/Stone/Getty Images; p. 102, © TMI/Alamy; p. 104, Courtesy Neil A. Tanner; p. 105, © Elie Gardner/MCT /Landov; p. 106L, © The McGraw-Hill Companies, Inc./John Flournoy, photographer; p. 106R, Ingram Publishing; p. 107, © Royalty-Free/Corbis; p. 108, © Comstock Images/Alamy; p. 111, Courtesy Neil A. Tanner; p. 112, © Charles D. Winters/Photo Researchers, Inc.; p. 116T, © Wayne Glusker; p. 116B, © Taylor Robertson Photography; p. 117T, Courtesy Joseph Quever; p. 117M, © Wayne Glusker; p. 117B, Courtesy Joseph Quever; p. 118T, Courtesy Neil A.Tanner; p. 118M, © Taylor Robertson Photography; p. 118B, Courtesy Shirlee Stevens; p. 119T, Courtesy Neil A. Tanner; p. 119B, © Wayne Glusker; p. 120T, Courtesy Joseph Quever; p. 120M, © Taylor Robertson Photography; p. 120B, Courtesy

Neil A. Tanner; p. 121T, © Wayne Glusker; pp. 121M, 121B, Courtesy Joseph Quever; p. 122T, Courtesy Neil A. Tanner; pp. 122M, 122B, Courtesy Joseph Quever; p. 123T, © Taylor Robertson Photography; p. 123M, © Wayne Glusker; p. 123B, Courtesy Joseph Quever; p. 124T, © Wayne Glusker; p. 124B, Courtesy Joseph Quever; p. 129, © Wayne Glusker; p. 131, Courtesy Tom Fahey; pp. 132, 133, © Wayne Glusker; pp. 135, 136, Courtesy Neil A. Tanner; p. 137, © Wayne Glusker

**Chapter 5**

p. 141, © Chris Clinton/Lifesize/Getty Images; p. 144, © Thinkstock Images/Jupiterimages; p. 148, Courtesy Shirlee Stevens; p. 149T, © Taylor Robertson Photography; pp. 149MT, 149MB, © Wayne Glusker; pp. 149B, 150T, © Taylor Robertson Photography; p. 150MT, 150MB, Courtesy Neil A. Tanner; p. 150B, © Taylor Robertson Photography; p. 151T, 151MT, © Wayne Glusker; p. 151MB, Courtesy Shirlee Stevens; p. 151B, Courtesy Neil A. Tanner; p. 158, © Reggie Casagrande/Workbook Stock/Getty Images; p. 159T, © Wayne Glusker; pp. 159B, 160, © Taylor Robertson Photography; p. 161T, Courtesy Neil A. Tanner; pp. 161M, 161B, © Taylor Robertson Photography; p. 165, Courtesy Shirlee Stevens; p. 166, © Wayne Glusker; p. 173T, Courtesy Joseph Quever; p. 173B, © Taylor Robertson Photography; p. 174, © Wayne Glusker

**Chapter 6**

p. 175, © Robin Nelson/Alamy; p. 177, © Ocean/Corbis; p. 181, © EyeWire Collection/Getty Images; p. 183, Courtesy Life Measurement, Inc.; p. 184T, Courtesy Salter Housewares Ltd.; p. 184B, © Julie Brown/Custom Medical Stock Photo; p. 185, © Tony Santo, Ph.D., R.D., CSSD/tonysantophotography.com; p. 192, Courtesy Shirlee Stevens

**Chapter 7**

p. 199, Ingram Publishing; p. 200, © Assembly/Getty Images; p. 203, Comstock Images/Jupiterimages; p. 206, © Thinkstock Images/Jupiterimages; p. 207, © Zia Soleil/Iconica/Getty Images

**Chapter 8**

p. 223, © Valery Rizzo/Botanica/Getty Images; p. 227, © I. Rozenbaum/F. Cirou/Photo Alto; p. 231, © Brand X Pictures/PunchStock; p. 233, © Nathan Benn/Ottochrome/Corbis; p. 235, © Richard Levine/Alamy; p. 240, © Steven Miric/Photodisc/Getty Images; p. 247, ©Stewart Cohen/Blend Images/Getty Images; p. 249, © David Young-Wolff/PhotoEdit; p. 250, © Patrick Murphy-Racey/Sports Illustrated/Getty Images; p. 254, © Dave King/Dorling

Kindersley/Getty Images; p. 255, © Royalty-Free/Corbis

**Chapter 9**

p. 273, Ingram Publishing; p. 276, Scale: Ryan McVay/Getty Images, Orange: © Stockdisc/PunchStock, Cheese: © Photodisc/PunchStock, Beans: C Squared Studios/Getty Images, Cookie: © Brand X Pictures/PunchStock, Broccoli: © Stockdisc/PunchStock, Tomato: © Comstock/Jupiter Images, Bike: © Royalty-Free/Corbis; p. 278, © Rennie Solis/Workbook Stock/Getty Images; p. 281, © David Madison/Stone/Getty Images; p. 282, © Susan Van Etten/PhotoEdit; p. 283, © Fancy Photography/Veer; p. 286, © Tim Boyle/Getty Images; p. 287, © Rick Gomez/Corbis; p. 289, © ZenShui/Alix Minde/PhotoAlto Agency RF Collections/Getty Images; p. 290, © David Oliver/Photographer's Choice/Getty Images

**Chapter 10**

p. 301, © Doug Pensinger/Getty Images; p. 305, © Purestock/PunchStock; p. 309, © Brand X Pictures/PunchStock; p. 310, © Stockbyte/Getty Images; p. 313, Ingram Publishing; p. 317, © Image Source/Getty Images; p. 321, Tetra Images/Getty Images

**Chapter 11**

p. 331, © Stockbroker/Alamy; p. 335, © iStockphoto.com/webphotographeer; p. 336, © David Buffington/Blend Images/Getty Images; p. 338, © Burke/Triolo Productions/Botanica/Getty Images; p. 343L, © Jessica Peterson/Rubberball Productions/Getty Images; p. 343R, © Stockbyte/PunchStock; p. 344, Ingram Publishing

**Chapter 12**

p. 351, © Hollandse Hoogte/Redux; p. 357, © Daniel Simon/Westend61/Corbis; p. 359, © Chuck Franklin/Alamy; p. 361, © Brandi Simons/Getty Images; p. 363, Ed Carey/Cole Group/Getty Images; p. 364, © Andersen Ross/Blend Images LLC; p. 365, Steve Cole/Getty Images

**Chapter 13**

p. 373, © Ingram Publishing/SuperStock; p. 375, © Dex Images/Photolibrary; p. 379, Courtesy DEA; p. 380, © David Young-Wolff/PhotoEdit; p. 384, © Sean Murphy/Stone/Getty Images; p. 388, © Brand X Pictures/PunchStock; p. 392, © Jupiterimages/Brand X Pictures/Getty Images

**Chapter 14**

p. 401, © AP Photo/Tina Fineberg; p. 403, © Erik Isakson/Getty Images; p. 406, © Jenny Matthews/Alamy; p. 407, © Joel Gordon

# INDEX

*Note*: Page references in boldface type indicate pages with definitions.

ABCD test for melanoma, 358
abdominal fat. *See also* waist circumference
  cardiovascular disease and, 336
  defined, 176
  health impacts of, 36, 179
  metabolic syndrome and, 339
absolute risk, 348
abstinence, 408
Academy of Nutrition and Dietetics, 250
Acceptable Macronutrient Distribution Ranges (AMDRs), 228, 230
ACE (American Council on Exercise), 50
acesulfame-K, 279
acetaminophen, 337
acquired immunodeficiency syndrome (AIDS), **402**. *See also* HIV/AIDS
across-the-body stretch, 149
acrylamide, 362
ACS (American Cancer Society), 353, 354, 362, 391
ACSM. *See* American College of Sports Medicine
actin, 98
action stage, 16, 17
active stretching, **148**
acupuncture, 156
ADA (American Dietetic Association). *See* Academy of Nutrition and Dietetics
adaptability, individual limits on, 40
added sugars, 232, 244, 246, 260
addiction. *See also* substance abuse
  alcoholism, 383, 385
  characteristics of addictive behaviors, 374–375
  defined, **374**
  development of, 375
  examples of, 375
  nicotine and, 375, 386
addictive behaviors, **374–375**
adenosine triphosphate (ATP), 64, **65**
Adequate Intake (AI), 238
adipose tissue, 176, **177**. *See also* body fat
adolescents
  body image in, 288
  exercise guidelines for, 207
  nutrition for, 248
  sodas and bone health in, 237
AEDs (automated external defibrillators), 340, 341
aerobic energy system, 64, **65–66**, 98
aerobic exercise. *See* cardiorespiratory endurance exercise
Aerobics and Fitness Association of America (AFAA), 50
aerobic systems, **65**
African Americans. *See also* ethnicity
  asthma in, 437
  body image in, 290
  cancer in, 355, 360, 361
  cardiovascular disease in, 337, 338
  chlamydia in, 408
  disordered eating in, 290
  hypertension in, 8
  leading poisoning in children, 437

obesity in, 274
  sodium recommendations for, 240, 334
aggressive driving, A–3 to A–4
agility, 36
aging. *See also* older adults
  cardiovascular disease and, 337, 338
  chronic stress and, 304
  exercise and, 31
  obesity and, 274
  sarcopenia and, 36
  sexually transmitted diseases and, 417
  strength training and, 36, 68, 101–102, 209
agonist muscles, **109**
AI (Adequate Intake), 238
AIDS (acquired immunodeficiency syndrome), **402**. *See also* HIV/AIDS
air bags, A–2
air quality and pollution
  exercise and, 82, 426
  indoor, 429–430
  preventing, 430
  smog, 425–426, 427
Air Quality Index (AQI), **425**–426
Al-Anon, 394
Alaska Natives, 180, 386. *See also* ethnicity
Alateen, 394
alcohol abuse, **383**
alcohol dependence, **383**
alcoholism, **383**, 385
alcohol poisoning, 382
alcohol-related neurodevelopmental disorder (ARND), 383
alcohol use, 380–385
  alcohol abuse, 383
  alcoholism, 383, 385
  assessment of, 397–398
  binge drinking, 383–384
  bone health and, 237
  calories in alcohol, 224
  cancer and, 362, 383
  cardiovascular disease and, 337, 342–343
  as cause of death, 6–7, 11
  chronic effects of, 381, 383
  coffee drinking and, 394
  dealing with an emergency from, 382
  drinking behavior and responsibility, 381–382, 384, 385
  driving and, 382–383, 385, A–2 to A–3
  immediate effects of, 380–382
  insomnia and, 313
  metabolism of alcohol, 380
  in pregnancy, 383
  standard drink, 380, 384
  stress and, 311
  unintentional injuries and, 11
  unsafe sexual activity and, 416
  withdrawal symptoms, 385
allergens, 261
allostatic load, **307**
alpha-linolenic acid, 227, 228, 229, 265
alternate leg stretcher, 151, 159
alternative fuels, 429, 441
alveoli, **63**
Alzheimer's disease, 31, 246

AMDRs (Acceptable Macronutrient Distribution Ranges), 228, 230
amenorrhea, **181**
American Cancer Society (ACS), 353, 354, 362, 391
American College of Sports Medicine (ACSM)
  on diet for athletes, 250
  on exercise by older adults, 209
  exercise facility certification by, 50
  on exercise frequency, 107
  on exercise in polluted air, 82
  Exercise Is Medicine program, 209
  exercise program guidelines of, 42–44
  exercise recommendations of, 30–32, 43, 74, 144
  on physician involvement, 209
  on stretching exercises, 146
  trainer certifications by, 49, 50
American Council on Exercise (ACE), 50
American Dietetic Association (ADA). *See* Academy of Nutrition and Dietetics
American Heart Association, 228, 332
American Medical Association, 209
American Psychiatric Association (APA), 377
amino acids, 113, 226, **227**
amnesia, anterograde, 379
amphetamines, 376
anabolic steroids, 113
anaerobic energy system, 64, **65**
anaerobic systems, **65**
anal cancer, 411
anal sex, HIV transmission in, 404, 407–408
anaphylaxis, 261
androgens, 113
androstenedione, 113
anemia, **235**–236
anger. *See also* hostility
  cardiovascular disease and, 305, 337, 343, 344
  communication and, 314–315
  conflict resolution and, 315
  dealing with, 316
  eating and, 277, 290
  exercise and, 71
  in nicotine withdrawal, 386
  spirituality and, 33
angina pectoris, 337, **340**
angioplasty, 341
anorexia nervosa, 181, **289**–290
antagonist muscles, **109**, 143
anterograde amnesia, 379
antiangiogenesis agents, 369
antibiotics, 347, 410
antioxidants, **235**, 237–238, 363
antiviral drugs, 406
anxiety, 114, 312
anxiety disorders, 312
aorta, 62, **63**
APA (American Psychiatric Association), 377
appetite suppressants, 114, 287
"apple shape," 179
APR (annual percentage rate), 5
AQI (Air Quality Index), **425**–426
ARND (alcohol-related neurodevelopmental disorder), 383
arrhythmias, **340**, 347

arteries, **63**
arthritis, 144, B–1
artificial sweeteners, 279
*asana*, 158
asbestos, 353, 436, 437
asbestosis, 436, **437**
Asian Americans, 337, 361. *See also* ethnicity
aspartame (NutraSweet), 279
aspirin, 340–341, 354
assault, A–7 to A–9
assessments
  of alcohol use, 397–398
  of body composition, 181–185, 191–196
  of body image, 299–300
  of cardiorespiratory endurance, 89–93
  of cardiorespiratory fitness, 71–72
  of cardiovascular disease risk, 349–350
  of diet, 267–272, 371
  of energy needs, 295–296
  for exercise program design, 41
  of flexibility, 165–170
  of lifestyle, 27–28
  of low-back health, 173–174
  of muscular endurance, 103, 135–138
  of muscular strength, 102–103, 129–134
  preprogram and postprogram, C–1 to C–2
  of safety of exercise participation, 53–54
  of sexually transmitted disease risk, 419–420
  of skin cancer risk, 371–372
  of stress, 325–326
  of swimming fitness, 216
  of tobacco use reasons, 399–400
assisted dip exercise, 123
asthma, 49, 437, B–1
atherosclerosis, 308, **333**, 339
athletes
  body image in, 288
  body mass index calculations for, 182
  diets for, 248, 250
  with disabilities, 38
  female athlete triad, 181
  high-carbohydrate diets and, 232
  immune system in, 403
  older, 68
athletic shoes, 84
ATP (adenosine triphosphate), 64, **65**
atrium, 62, **63**
atrophy, 98, **99**
automated external defibrillators (AEDs), 340, 341
autonomic nervous system, **302**
azithromycin, 410

BAC (blood alcohol concentration), **380**–382, 383
back bridge exercise, 161
back extensors endurance test, 174
back pain. *See* low-back pain and injuries
bacterial vaginosis (BV), **413**
balance, 36, 145
ballistic stretching, **147**
balloon angioplasty, 341
barbiturates, 376
bariatric surgery, 287–288
Bartholin's glands, 410
basal cell carcinomas, **358**
BDD (body dysmorphic disorder), 288
beans, recommended intake of, 244, 245
BeatBum Trainer smartphone application, 206
beer, 380
behavior change
  action plan for, 19–20
  barriers to, 15–16, 17
  defined, **12**
  enhancing readiness for, 16
  gathering data for, 18
  health journals and, 18–19
  help with, 13

  motivation for, 13–16
  personal contract for, 20
  relapse in, 16–17, 206, 207
  self-efficacy and, 15
  small steps in, 12, 17
  SMART goals for, 18–19, 49, 74
  stages of change model of, 16–17
  staying with it, 20–21
  target behaviors for, 12–13, 18
Behavior Change Workbook, W–1 to W–14
  attitudes in, W–3 to W–4
  breaking behavior chains, W–4 to W–6
  contract in, W–7 to W–8
  feelings in, W–12
  goal setting in, W–3
  maintenance in, W–13 to W–14
  monitoring current behavior patterns, W–2 to W–3
  motivation and commitment in, W–8 to W–9
  peer pressure in, W–13
  realistic self-talk in, W–9 to W–10
  rewards in, W–4
  social support in, W–10 to W–11
  target behavior setting in, W–1 to W–2
  time management in, W–9 to W–10
belly breathing, 321
bench press exercises, 116, 120
benign tumors, 352, **353**
benzodiazepines, 376
beta-agonists, 113
beta-hydroxy beta-methylbutyrate (HMB), 114
beverages. *See also* alcohol use; water
  bottled water, 208
  fluid intake for athletes, 80, 250
  nutrient density in, 241
  sugar in, 208, 241
  weight-loss, 285
BIA (bioelectrical impedance analysis), 184, 185
biceps curl exercises, 117, 121
bicycling, 213–215, A–3
bidis, 388. *See also* tobacco use
binge drinking, **383**–384
binge eating, **277**, 290–291, 311
binge-eating disorder, **291**
biodegradability, **433**, 434
biodiesel, 441
bioelectrical impedance analysis (BIA), 184, 185
biofeedback, 320
biofuels, 441
biomagnification, 436, **437**
biomass, energy from, 441
biopsy, **355**, 358, 366, 369
biotechnology, 260–261
biotin, 234, 263
"bird dog" exercise, 119
birth defects, 235, 383
bitter orange extract, 286
black Americans. *See* African Americans
bladder cancer, 360
blaming, 21
blisters, 82
blood alcohol concentration (BAC), **380**–382, 383
blood banks, 404
blood circulation, 62, 63–64
blood pressure. *See also* hypertension
  cardiorespiratory endurance exercise and, 63–64, 67
  defined, 62, **63**
  healthy ranges of, 332–333
  managing, 343
  measurement of, 332, 333
  omega-3 fatty acids and, 228, 229
  potassium and, 242
  sodium and, 240, 250, 338
  stress and, 347
  weight training and, 69, 335
blood vessels, 63, 69

BMI (body mass index), 182–**183**, 191
boating injuries, A–6
Bod Pod, 183
body composition, 176–188
  body fat distribution, 179, 185
  body mass index calculations, 182–183, 191
  defined, 36, **37**
  estimation methods, 183–185
  exercise and, 70, 188
  gender differences in, 176, 179, 183, 193–195
  goals for, 186
  health consequences of, 36
  making changes in, 186
  muscular strength and endurance and, 101
  overweight and obesity defined, 178, 179, 183
  overweight and obesity prevalence, 178, 274
  percent body fat, 176–177, 183–185, 191–196
  physical fitness and, 177, 188
  self-image and, 179
  strength training and, 100, 101, 102
  typical, 176
  very low levels of body fat, 179, 181
  waist circumference and, 179, 182, 195–196, 339
body dysmorphic disorder (BDD), 288
body fat
  abdominal, 36, 176, 179, 336, 339
  calories in, 176, 225
  cardiovascular disease and, 336
  cellulite, 188
  diabetes and, 176, 178–179, 180, 185
  distribution of, 179, 185
  endurance exercise and, 70
  estimation of, 183–185
  factors in excess, 275–277
  hormones and, 176
  lifestyle factors in, 177
  liposuction and, 188, 288
  percent, 176–177, 183–185, 191–196
  strength training and, 101, 102
  types of, 176
  very low levels of, 179, 181
  wellness and, 176, 178–179
body image
  acceptance and change of, 288–289
  assessment of, 299
  avoiding problems in, 290
  defined, 288, **289**
  eating disorders and, 288
  exercise and, 288, 289
  gender, ethnicity and, 290
  "perfect," 293
  severe problems with, 288
body mass index (BMI), 182–**183**, 191
bone density. *See also* osteoporosis
  age and, 237
  in college students, 144
  in female athlete triad, 181
  nutrition and, 236, 237, 242
  in older adults, 68
  physical activity and, 9, 68, 144
  swimming and, 217
  weight-bearing exercise and, 70, 144, 237
bone marrow transplants, 369
borderline disordered eating, 291
boron, 237
bottled water, 208, 431
botulism, 254
brain, exercise and, 31
brain cancer, 360
BRCA1 (breast cancer gene 1), 362
breast cancer
  in African American women, 361
  detection of, 354–355
  exercise and, 354, 364
  obesity and, 354
  prevalence of, 354

prevention of, 70, 354, 355, 356, 367
risk factors for, 11, 354, 362
treatment of, 355
breastfeeding, HIV transmission in, 404
breast self-exam (BSE), 355, 356, 367
breathing
 function of, 63
 for relaxation, 319–320, 321
 in swimming, 216
 in weight training, 111
 in yoga, 158
"broken heart syndrome," 338
bruises, 82
budgeting, wellness and, 5
bulimia nervosa, 181, 290–**291**
bupropion, 388
burnout, 310
butter and margarine, 228, 242, 260
buying, compulsive, 375
BV (bacterial vaginosis), **413**

CAD (coronary artery disease), 42, 339. *See also*
 cardiovascular disease
caffeine
 alcohol and, 394
 insomnia and, 312, 313
 as performance aid, 114
 stress and, 311
 for weight loss, 286
calcium
 bone health and, 236, 237, 242
 Dietary Reference Intake for, 238, 264
 functions of, 236
 high blood pressure and, 346
 in vegetarian diets, 239, 248
calipers, **184**
calisthenics, 105, 107
caloric expenditure. *See* energy expenditure
calories
 athletes and, 250
 in body fat, 176, 225
 calculating daily needs, 246, 295–296
 defined, 224
 in nutrient classes, 224
 in selected activities, 75, 212
 weight management and, 240, 278
*Campylobacter jejuni,* 254
cancer, 352–369
 alcohol and, 362, 383
 anal, 411
 biopsies and, 355, 358, 366, 369
 bladder, 360
 brain, 360
 breast (*See* breast cancer)
 cancer promoters, 362
 carcinogens and, 353, 361–362, 364–365, 386
 cervical (*See* cervical cancer)
 colon (*See* colon cancer)
 cruciferous vegetables and, 238, 239
 defined, 352, **353**
 detecting, 366
 dietary factors and, 233, 246, 362–364, 371
 DNA and, 362
 endometrial, 357, 364, 367
 endurance exercise and, 69–70
 esophageal, 365
 ethnicity, poverty, and, 361
 exercise and, 354, 364
 head and neck, 358
 Hodgkin's disease, 361, 365
 Kaposi's sarcoma, 365, 406
 kidney, 360
 leukemia, 352, 360
 liver, 365, 413
 lung, 11, 353–354, 364
 lymphoma, 360–361, 365

metastasis of, 352, 353
microbes and, 365
non-Hodgkin's lymphoma, 361
nutrition and, 239
obesity and, 179, 354, 364
oral, 362, 388
oropharyngeal, 365, 411
ovarian, 357, 364
pancreatic, 360
penile, 411, 417
prevalence of, 352–353
prostate, 355–356, 361, 367
radiation and, 360, 365
risk factors for, 352
screening guidelines, 367–368
skin (*See* skin cancer)
stomach, 365
testicular, 359–360
tobacco use and, 353, 360, 362
treatment of, 366, 368, 369
tumors in, 352
uterine, 357
whole grains and, 231
cancer promoters, 362
capillaries, **63**, 68
carbohydrates
 added sugars, 232, 244, 246, 260
 athletes and, 250
 calming effect of, 231
 calories in, 224
 defined, 230, **231**
 energy from, 64, 65
 enriched, 239
 glycemic index and glycemic response, 231–232
 low-carbohydrate diets, 284
 recommended intake of, 230, 232, 265
 refined vs. whole grains, 231, 232, 241, 342
 simple vs. complex, 230–231, 293
 weight management and, 293
carbon dioxide, as greenhouse gas, 426–427
carbon monoxide
 in air pollution, 425
 in cigarette smoke, 332, 386, 389
 in indoor air pollution, 429–430
carcinogens, **353**, 362, 364–365, 386
cardiac arrest, 340, 341, A–5
cardiac output, 64, **65**
cardiac risk, exercise and, 42
cardiopulmonary resuscitation (CPR), 341, 345,
 A–5, A–11
cardiorespiratory endurance. *See also*
 cardiorespiratory endurance exercise;
 cardiorespiratory endurance exercise programs
 assessment of, 71–72, 89–93
 benefits of, 35, 66–71
 defined, **35**, 62
 maintaining, 40
 physiology and, 62–66
cardiorespiratory endurance exercise
 air quality and, 82, 426
 benefits of, 66–71, 364
 bicycling as, 214
 body fat and, 70, 188
 cardiorespiratory functioning and, 66–67
 cellular metabolism and, 68
 chronic diseases and, 68–70
 footwear for, 84
 at high altitudes, 85
 immune function and, 70
 interval training, 80, 206
 menstruation and, 85
 obesity and, 281
 older adults and, 209
 in personal fitness plan, 203
 recommendations for, 43, 74, 203
 slow-twitch fibers and, 99

strength training risks and, 69
swimming as, 215
in weather extremes, 79–81
weight management and, 280
well-being and, 70–71
cardiorespiratory endurance exercise programs
 activity selection in, 42
 building fitness in, 77–78
 cross-training and, 79
 diet and, 85
 example of, 79
 FITT equation in, 74–77
 goals for, 73–74
 interval training in, 80, 206
 maintaining fitness, 78–79
 monitoring, 96
 progression in, 77–78, 79
 safety and injury prevention in, 82–83
 staying active between workouts, 78
 warming up and cooling down in, 77
 worksheet for, 95–96
cardiorespiratory fitness, 77–79. *See also*
 cardiorespiratory endurance
cardiorespiratory system, 62–64, **63**
cardiovascular disease (CVD). *See also* heart attacks;
 heart disease; stroke
 alcohol and drug use and, 337, 342–343
 assessment of risk for, 349–350
 atherosclerosis and, 308, 333, 339
 cardiac arrest, 340, 341
 cholesterol levels and, 334, 338, 344
 congestive heart failure, 342
 C-reactive protein and, 337
 defined, **333**
 diabetes and, 336
 diet and, 342–343, 346
 endurance exercise and, 68–69
 ethnicity, gender, and, 337, 338
 exercise and, 334–335, 343, 344, B–1 to B–2
 heredity and, 337
 high blood pressure and, 332–333
 homocysteine and, 337–338
 media reports on, 346
 metabolic syndrome and, 178, 339
 muscular strength and, 102
 nutrition and, 239, 246
 obesity and, 274, 335–336
 prevalence of, 332
 reducing risk factors in, 342–344
 risk factors in, 235, 332–339
 saturated and trans fats and, 228, 229
 stress and, 307, 308, 337–338, 344, 347
 symptoms of, 338, 341
 tobacco use and, 332, 343
 triglyceride levels and, 336
 warning signs of heart attack, stroke, or cardiac
  arrest, 341
carnitine, 285
carotenoids, 238, **363**
carotid pulse, 72
carpal tunnel syndrome, A–7
carrying exercises, 107
car seats, A–2 to A–3
cartilage, **101**
caspase, 369
catecholamine, 287
cat stretch exercise, 159
CD4 T cells, 403, **404**
cell phones
 driving and, A–2, A–3
 exercise applications on, 206
 radiation from, 439
 weight-loss applications for, 284
cellular metabolism, 68
cellulite, 188
Center for Nutrition Policy and Promotion, 246

cephalosporins, 410
cerebrovascular accident (CVA). *See* stroke
Cervarix vaccine, 411
cervical cancer
  ethnicity, poverty, and, 361
  HPV infection and, 357, 365, 411, 417
  prevalence of, 357
  prevention of, 357
  screening guidelines for, 367
cervical cap, STD transmission and, 416
cervical dysplasia, 357
CFCs (chlorofluorocarbons), 426, **428**, 430
CFLs (compact fluorescent lightbulbs), 431
chancres, **413**
Chantix (varinicline), 391
charred foods, 365
CHD (coronary heart disease), 339. *See also*
  cardiovascular disease
check-call-care pattern, in emergency care, A–11
chemical pollution, 436–438
chemotherapy, **353**, 366
chest press exercise, 120
chewing tobacco, 388. *See also* tobacco use
children. *See also* infants
  AIDS orphans, 405
  car seats for, A–2 to A–3
  Dietary Reference Intakes for, 263–265
  emergency care for choking by, A–5
  environmental tobacco smoke and, 390
  exercise guidelines for, 207
  fetal alcohol syndrome in, 383
  fish consumption guidelines for, 256
  heat cramps in, 81
  HIV transmission to, 404, 406
  lead poisoning in, 436, 437
  nutrition for, 248
  type 2 diabetes in, 180
chitosan, 285
chlamydia, 339, 357, 408–410, **409**
*Chlamydia pneumoniae*, 339, 408–410
chloride, 265
chlorofluorocarbons (CFCs), 426, **428**, 430
choking, A–5, A–6
cholesterol. *See also* high-density lipoprotein; low-
  density lipoprotein
  cardiovascular disease and, 334, 338, 344
  defined, 228, **229**, 334
  endurance exercise and, 68–69
  healthy levels of, 334, 336
  managing levels of, 334, 344
  metabolic syndrome and, 339
  pathway through body, 335
  recommended intake of, 342
  soluble fiber and, 233
  types of, 334
choline, 263
ChooseMyPlate.gov, 243, 260, A–1. *See also*
  MyPlate
chromium, 113, 264, 285
chromium picolinate, 113
chromosomes, 362, **363**
chronic diseases. *See also specific diseases*
  death from, 6
  defined, **4**
  endurance exercise and, 68–70
  infectious diseases, 4
  physical activity and, 9–10, 32
chronic inflammation, 178, **179**
cigars, 387–388. *See also* tobacco use
circuit training, 101
circumcision, STD transmission and, 405, 412
cirrhosis, **383**
climate change, 426–428
*Clostridium perfringens*, 254
clothing
  for bike riding, 214

for cold weather, 81
  footwear, 84
  protective, 45–46
  sun protection from, 359
clove cigarettes, 388. *See also* tobacco use
club drugs, 379. *See also* psychoactive drugs
CNS depressants, 376, 379
CNS stimulants, 376, 379
cocaine, 376
cockroaches, 437
codeine, 376
codependency, 394
coffee, alcohol use and, 394
cognitive appraisal, 304
cold weather, 81
collagen, 142, **143**
collars, in strength training, 112
college students
  binge drinking by, 384
  bone density of, 144
  credit cards and, 5
  nutrition for, 248, 249
  obesity and overweight in, 14
  sexually transmitted diseases in, 416
  stress sources in, 309
  weight-loss interventions for, 285
  wellness matters in, 14
colon cancer
  detection and treatment of, 354, 367
  diet and, 354
  exercise and, 354, 364
  obesity and, 354, 364
  risk factors in, 354
  screening guidelines for, 367
colonoscopies, 354, 367
colorectal cancer, 354, 367. *See also* colon cancer
combustion by-products, 429–430
communication
  about sexually transmitted diseases, 414, 420
  guidelines for, 314
  in intimate relationships, 310
  in stress management, 313
  suppressing feelings, 315
compact fluorescent lightbulbs (CFLs), 431
complete proteins, 226
complex carbohydrates, 230–231, 293
compound interest, 5
compulsive behavior, 375
computers, repetitive-stress injuries and, A–7.
  *See also* Internet
concentric muscle contractions, 104, **105**
condoms
  correct use of, 409
  herpes infections and, 412
  HIV transmission and, 405
  in safer sex, 414, 416–417
conflict resolution, 315
congenital syphilis, 413
congestive heart failure, **342**
conjugated linoleic acid, 285
connective tissue, 142–143
constant resistance exercise, 104, **105**
consumer guidelines
  on being a green consumer, 435
  on dietary supplements, 112, 253
  on evaluating health news, 13
  on evaluating mental health professionals, 322
  on exercise footwear, 84
  on fat and sugar substitutes, 279
  on fitness centers, 50
  on food labels, 251, 252, 253
  on heart rate monitors and GPS devices, 73
  on HIV tests, 407
  on smoking cessation products, 391
  on sunscreens and sun-protective clothing, 359
contemplation stage, 16, 17

contract-relax-contract pattern, 148
contract-relax stretching method, 147–148
contracts, in behavior change, 20
controlled studies, 348
cooking temperatures, 255
cooling down, 45, 77, 110
coordination, 36, 125
coping strategies, weight management and,
  281–282
copper, 237, 264
core muscles, **153–154**
core training, 153–154, 203
coronary arteries, **63**
coronary artery disease (CAD), 42, 339. *See also*
  cardiovascular disease
coronary heart disease (CHD), **339**. *See also*
  cardiovascular disease
coronary thrombosis, 340
cortisol
  caffeine and, 311
  defined, **303**
  exercise and, 403
  in stress response, 303, 307
cost-benefit analysis, 17
CPR (cardiopulmonary resuscitation), 341, 345,
  A–5, A–11
crabs (pubic lice), 414
crack cocaine, 376
C-reactive protein (CRP), 337
creatine monohydrate, 113
creatine phosphate, 64, 65, 113
credit cards, 5
cross-training
  defined, **79**
  in fitness programs, 79, 205
  swimming and, 215, 216
cruciferous vegetables, 238, **239**
crunch exercise, 119
*Cryptosporidium*, 431
curl-up exercises, 119, 160
curl-up test, 135–136
CVA (cerebrovascular accident). *See* stroke
CVD. *See* cardiovascular disease
cyberstalking, A–9
cycle training, 205
*cytomegalovirus*, 339

daily hassles, 309
Daily Values, 238–**239**
dairy, 241, 242, 244–245
darbepoetin, 113
DASH eating plan
  healthy eating and, 242, 277–278
  hypertension and, 334
  summary of, 266
date rape, A–8 to A–9
date-rape drugs, 378, 379
DDT, 436
death
  from alcohol use, 382
  from cancer, 352, 353
  eating disorders and, 289–290
  leading causes of, 6–7, 8, 11
  muscular strength and, 100
  obesity and, 7, 10, 179
  physical activity and, 10, 70
  from smoking, 6–7, 11, 386
  sudden, 42, 340
debt, getting out of, 5
deep muscle relaxation, 319, 324
DEET, sunscreen and, 359
defibrillation, 340
deforestation, 427
dehydration, **79–80**. *See also* water
delayed-onset muscle soreness, 125
delirium tremens (DTs), **385**

dental work, antibiotics prior to, 347
depressants, CNS, 376, 379
depression
    cardiorespiratory fitness and, 35
    in college students, 14
    defined, **322**
    eating disorders and, 288, 290, 291
    exercise and, 31, 32, 70, 312
    obesity and, 179
    sleep quality and, 312
    stress and, 306, 308, 309, 321–322
    suicide and, 322
    symptoms of, 321–322
    tobacco use and, 386, 388, 391
DEXA (dual-energy X-ray absorptiometry), 185
DHEA (dehydroepiandrosterone), 113
diabetes mellitus. *See also* type 2 diabetes
    cardiovascular disease and, 336
    defined, 180
    diet and, 250
    excess body fat and, 176, 178–179, 180, 185
    exercise and, 180, B–1
    gestational, 180
    glycemic index and, 231
    overweight and obesity and, 178–179
    pre-diabetes, 180
    strength training and, 180
    treatment and prevention of, 180
    type 1, 180
    warning signs and testing for, 180
*Diagnostic and Statistical Manual of Mental Disorders*
    (APA), 377
diaphragms, STD transmission and, 416
diastole, 62–64, **63**
diastolic blood pressure, 332–333
diet. *See also* nutrition
    for athletes, 248, 250
    body composition and, 177
    cancer and, 354, 355, 362–364, 371
    chronic diseases and, 6
    DASH eating plan, 242, 266, 277–278, 334
    diet books, 283–284
    eating habits, 276–277, 279–280, 298
    endurance exercise programs and, 85
    heart-healthy, 342–343, 346
    high-carbohydrate, 232, 284
    high-fiber, 233
    low-calorie, 282
    low-carbohydrate, 284
    macronutrient intake goals, 230
    Mediterranean, 247
    MyPlate (*See* MyPlate)
    type 2 diabetes and, 233
    vegan, 247
    vegetarian, 226, 239, 242, 247–248
    weight loss books, 283–284
    wellness and, 10
diet aids, 285
dietary fiber. *See* fiber
Dietary Guidelines for Americans, 238, **239**, 240–243
Dietary Reference Intakes (DRIs), 238–240, **239**,
    263–265
dietary supplements. *See* supplements, dietary
diethylproprion, 114, 287
digestion, 224, **225**, 226, 308
digital technology. *See* technology
"dirty dozen" fruits and vegetables, 256
disabilities, physical fitness and, 38
disasters, coping after, A–9
discrimination and prejudice, 338
diseases. *See* chronic diseases; illness; sexually
    transmitted diseases; *specific diseases*
dislocations, 82
disordered eating, 181. *See also* eating disorders
distance measurement, 47, 73
distracted driving, A–2

distress, 306, **307**
diuretics, 113
diversity issues. *See also* ethnicity
    ethnic foods, 257
    ethnicity, poverty, and cancer, 361
    exercise benefits for older adults, 68
    female athlete triad, 181
    fitness and disability, 38
    gender, ethnicity, and body image, 290
    gender, ethnicity, and CVD, 338
    gender and tobacco use, 388
    gender differences in muscular strength, 102
    HIV infection around the world, 405
    poverty and environmental health, 437
    relaxing through meditation, 320
    wellness issues and, 8
DNA, 362, **363**. *See also* genetics
dose-response relationships, 10, 177
double-blind studies, 348
doxycycline, 410
drinking water, 431–432
DRIs (Dietary Reference Intakes), 238–240, **239**,
    263–265
driving
    aggressive, A–3 to A–4
    alcohol and, 382–383, 385, A–2
    distracted, A–2
    injury prevention and, A–2 to A–3
    safety belts and air bags, A–2
drowning injuries, A–6
Drug-Induced Rape Prevention and Punishment
    Act, 379
drugs, **374**. *See also* psychoactive drugs;
    substance abuse
DTs (delirium tremens), **385**
dual-energy X-ray absorptiometry (DEXA), 185
duration of exercise. *See also* FITT principle
    in cardiorespiratory endurance exercise, 76, 77,
        79, 203
    recommendations for, 39–40
    splitting up, 33–34
    in strength training, 108–109
    in stretching programs, 146, 204
    for weight loss, 281
dynamic exercise, 104–**105**
dynamic flexibility, 142
dynamic stretching, **147**

*E. coli (Escherichia coli)*, 254, 255
E85, alternative fuel, 429
eating disorders
    anorexia nervosa, 181, 289–290
    approaching a friend with, 292
    binge eating disorder, 277, 290–291, 311
    body image and, 288
    borderline disordered eating, 291
    bulimia nervosa, 181, 290–291
    checklist for, 299–300
    defined, **289**
    in female athlete triad, 181
    prevalence of, 289
    signs of, 292
    stress and, 311
    treatment for, 291
eating habits, 276–277, 279–280, 298
eccentric loading, 104–**105**
eccentric muscle contractions, 104, **105**
e-cigs, 388–389
ecstasy (MDMA), 376, 379
ectopic pregnancy, **390**
educational attainment
    exercise and, 30
    health disparities and, 8
    smoking and, 386
eggs, 242
elastic elongation, **143**

elastin, 142, **143**
electric vehicles, 429
electromagnetic radiation, 438
electronic cigarettes, 388–389
emergency care. *See* first aid
emergency medical services (EMS), 341
emergency preparedness, A–9 to A–11
emotional wellness, 3, 179
emotions. *See also* anger
    in behavior change, 17
    body image and, 288
    cardiovascular disease and, 308
    eating disorders and, 289, 291
    exercise and, 68, 70–71
    food and, 277
    in health journals, 19
    immune response and, 307–308
    sleep and, 312
    in stress response, 156, 302, 304–305
    weight management and, 179, 281–282
endocrine system, **302**–303
endometrial cancer, 357, 364, 367
endorphins, **303**
endothelial cells, weight training and, 69
endurance training. *See* cardiorespiratory
    endurance exercise
energy-balance equation, 276
energy density, 278–279, 283
energy drinks, 113
energy expenditure
    calculating calorie needs, 246, 295–296
    in selected activities, 75, 212
energy production, in the body, 64
energy sources, global, 424, 428–429, 441
energy systems, in the body, 64–66
enriched foods, 239
entry inhibitors, 406
environment, defined, **422**
environmental contaminants, 256, 258
environmental health, 422–441
    air quality and pollution, 82, 425–426, 428–430
    carcinogens, 353, 361–362, 364–365, 386
    checklist for, 443
    chemical pollution, 436–438
    defined, **422**–423
    energy and, 428–429, 430
    environmental tobacco smoke, 332, 353,
        389–390, 429
    fish consumption guidelines, 228, 241–242,
        256, 258
    green consumers and, 435
    greenhouse effect and global warming, 426–428
    organic foods and, 256
    ozone layer thinning, 428
    plastic water bottles, 208, 431
    population growth, 423–425
    poverty and, 361, 437
    public health systems and, 422
    radiation pollution, 438–440
    solid waste pollution, 432–436
    water quality and pollution, 430–432
environmental stressors, 311
environmental tobacco smoke (ETS)
    avoiding, 390
    children and, 390
    defined, **389**
    heart disease and, 332, 389
    indoor air pollution regulations and, 429
    lung damage and, 353, 389
environmental wellness, 3–4
enzyme activators/blockers, 369
ephedra (*ma huang*), 113, 285
ephedrine, 285
epididymitis, 360
epinephrine, **303**, 307
Epstein-Barr virus, 365

equipment. *See also* technology
  athletic shoes, 84
  for bicycling, 213–214
  for blood pressure monitoring, 333
  for body composition assessment, 183–185
  for rowing, 217
erythromycin, 410
erythropoietin, 113
escalation, 375
*Escherichia coli (E. coli)*, 254, 255
esophageal cancer, 365
essential amino acids, 226
essential fats, 176, **177**, 228
essential nutrients, 224, **225**
estrogen, 338, 354, 362
ethanol fuel, 429, 441
ethnic foods, 257
ethnicity. *See also* diversity issues; *specific ethnic groups*
  body image and, 290
  cancer and, 361
  cardiovascular disease and, 337, 338
  diabetes and, 8, 180
  hypertension and, 8
  obesity and, 274
  poverty, cancer, and, 361
  prejudice and discrimination stressors, 338
  smoking and, 386
  stroke and, 337, 338
  wellness issues, 8
ethyl alcohol, **380**. *See also* alcohol use
ETS. *See* environmental tobacco smoke
eustress, 306, **307**
e-waste, 434–435
exercise. *See also* cardiorespiratory endurance exercise; exercise program design; flexibility exercise; physical activity; strength training
  ACSM recommendations on, 30–32, 43, 74, 107, 144, 209
  advice and help on, 49
  aging and, 31
  air pollution and, 82, 426
  arthritis and, B–1
  asthma and, B–1
  blood pressure and, 63–64, 67, 69, 344
  body composition and, 70, 188
  brain and, 31
  cancer and, 35, 69–70, 354, 364
  cardiac risk and, 42
  cardiorespiratory system during, 63–64
  cardiovascular disease and, 334–335, 343, 344, B–1 to B–2
  children and, 207
  daily, 209
  defined, **31**
  depression and, 31, 32, 70, 312
  diabetes and, 180, B–1
  emotions and, 68, 70–71
  energy systems in, 64–66
  fitness center selection, 50
  hydration during, 208
  hypertension and, 69, 344, B–1 to B–2
  immune function and, 70, 364, 403
  insulin sensitivity and, 339
  low-back pain and, 155, 158, 159–161
  medical clearance for, 40–42
  mental health and, 312
  metabolism and, 276
  obesity and, 177, 179, 180, B–2
  older adults and, 68
  osteoporosis and, B–2
  physicians on, 209
  in pregnancy, 208–209
  quitting smoking and, 393
  sleep and, 71, 206, 312
  special health concerns and, B–1 to B–2

  stress and, 311, 312
  time management for, 49
  weight-bearing, 70, 144, 208, 217, 237
  weight management and, 280–281
  wellness and, 70–71
exercise balls, 106
exercise buddies, 47, 205, 207
Exercise Is Medicine, 209
exercise journals, 207
exercise program design. *See also* cardiorespiratory endurance exercise programs; FITT principle; personal fitness plan; physical training
  activity selection in, 41–44
  cycling volume and intensity in, 46
  fun in, 47, 202
  goals in, 41, 49
  medical clearance in, 40–42
  moderation in, 47–48
  nutrition and, 47
  progression in, 45
  protective equipment and clothing in, 45–46
  rest in, 46
  self-assessment in, 41
  tracking progress in, 47, 59–60
  training guidelines in, 44–47
  training partners in, 46
  varying activities in, 46
  warm-ups and cool-downs in, 45
exercise safety. *See also* injuries; warming up
  air quality and, 82
  in bicycling, 214
  cold weather and, 81
  cooling down, 45, 77, 110
  high altitude and, 85
  hot weather and heat stress, 79–81
  injury prevention guidelines, A–7
  protective equipment and clothing, 45–46
  in strength training, 111–112
  in stretching, 146, 153, 162
exercise stress test, **41**
exercise tests, in heart disease, 340
"explosive" energy system, 64, **65**
external locus of control, 15

falls, injuries from, 68, A–4
families, successful, 313
family planning, 424–425
Family Smoking Prevention and Tobacco Control Act, 390
FAS (fetal alcohol syndrome), **383**
fashion models, 290
fast-food restaurants, 249, 272, A–1
fasting glucose levels, 180, 339
fast-twitch fibers, **99**
fat-free mass, 36, **37**, 176
fats, dietary
  for athletes, 250
  butter and margarine, 228, 242, 260
  calories in, 224, 227
  cancer and, 362
  cholesterol levels and, 228, 344
  energy production and, 64, 65
  essential, 176, 177, 228
  function of, 227
  health effects of, 228, 229
  hydrogenation of, 227–228
  omega-3 fatty acids, 228, 229, 346
  orlistat (Xenical) and, 287
  recommended intake of, 228–229, 230, 242, 244, 265, 342
  reducing saturated and trans fats, 228, 229, 240–242
  SoFAS (solid fats and added sugars), 160, 241, 244, 246
  solid, 241
  types and sources of, 227, 229

fat-soluble vitamins, 233–235
fat substitutes, 279, 287
FDA. *See* Food and Drug Administration
Federal Trade Commission (FTC), 285
feedback, in relationships, 314
female athlete triad, **181**
fetal alcohol syndrome (FAS), **383**
fiber
  benefits of, 232–233
  cancer and, 233, 362–363
  cholesterol and, 233
  defined, **233**
  recommended intake of, 233, 242, 265, 342
  types of, 233
  in weight loss, 285
fight-or-flight reaction, **303–304**, 347
finances, stress from, 309, 310
Financial Literacy and Education Commission, 5
financial wellness, 4, 5
firearm injuries, A–6
fires, A–6
first aid. *See also* injuries
  AEDs (automated external defibrillators) in, 340, 341
  in alcohol emergencies, 382
  American Red Cross courses in, 340, 341, A–11
  calling 911, 341, 382
  for cardiac arrest, A–5
  check-call-care pattern, A–11
  for choking, A–5
  for common exercise injuries, 82
  CPR (cardiopulmonary resuscitation), 341, 345
  R-I-C-E principle in, 83
  for stroke, 341
fish consumption, 228, 241–242, 256, 258
fish farming, 256
fish oils, 228, 229, 346
fitness. *See* physical fitness
fitness centers, 49, 50, 221–222
*Fitness Rx for Women/Fitness Rx for Men,* 49
FITT principle. *See also* duration of exercise; frequency of exercise; intensity of exercise; type of activity
  ACSM exercise recommendations, 43
  in bicycle fitness programs, 214
  in cardiorespiratory endurance programs, 74–77
  in flexibility programs, 146–148
  in personal fitness plans, 202–204, 211
  as progressive overload, 38–40
  in strength training, 107–109
Flagyl (metronidazole), 413
flexibility
  assessment of, 145, 165–170
  benefits of, 143–145
  bicycling and, 214
  joint health and, 144–145
  joint structure and, 142
  low-back pain prevention and, 145
  muscle elasticity and length and, 142–143
  physical training and, 162
  proprioceptors, 143, 147
  range of motion and, 142
  recommendations for, 204
  static and dynamic, 142
flexibility exercise
  amount needed, 162
  benefits of, 36
  defined, 36, **37**
  exercise instructions, 149–151
  FITT principle in, 146–148
  low-back pain prevention and, 145
  muscular strength and, 162
  by older adults, 68, 209
  in personal fitness plan, 171–172

progression in training, 148, 152
recommendations for, 33, 43
safety in, 146, 153, 162
sample program, 146, 148, 152
strength training and, 147
stretches to avoid, 153
stretching types, 146–148
warming up *vs.*, 162
fluid intake. *See* beverages; water
fluoridation, 430, **431**
fluoride, 236, 237, 264, 430
folate (folic acid)
    birth defects and, 235, 248
    cardiovascular disease and, 337, 346
    functions of, 234
    recommended intake of, 239, 241, 248, 263
    supplements, 239, 248
food additives, 252
food allergies, 261
Food and Drug Administration (FDA)
    on dietary supplements, 112, 115, 252, 253
    on e-cigs, 388–389
    on fish consumption, 256
    on food labels, 232, 251, 252, 261
    on HIV tests, 407
    on HPV vaccines, 357, 411
    on nonnutritive sweeteners, 279
    on performance aids, 113
    on smoking cessation products, 391
    on sunscreens, 359
    on tobacco product control, 390
    on weight-loss products, 285, 287
foodborne illness, 252, 254
food handling safety, 255
food intolerances, 261
food irradiation, 254–256, **255**
food labels
    on dietary supplements, 252, 253
    evaluating foods by, 251, 252, 271
    finding whole grains on, 232
    genetic modification and, 261
    reading, 251
    trans fats on, 228
food security, 243
food storage, 255
food supply, 423
footwear, 84
formaldehyde gas, 430
fossil fuels, **425**, 428, 441
fractures, 82, 144
free radicals, 68, **237**–238
freestyle swim stroke, 215–216
free weights, 106, 111–112, 116–120
frequency of exercise. *See also* FITT principle
    in cardiorespiratory endurance exercise, 79,
      203–204
    cardiorespiratory fitness and, 77, 79
    in FITT principle, 39, 74
    in strength training, 107, 125, 203
    in stretching programs, 146, 204
fried foods, cancer and, 362
friendships, 310, 313
frostbite, **81**
fruits
    cancer and, 363
    "dirty dozen," 256
    intake recommendations, 241, 244, 245, 260
    low energy density in, 278–279
    pesticide residues on, 256
    serving sizes of, 245
FTC (Federal Trade Commission), 285
full squat with bent back, 153
fun, in exercise program design, 47, 202
functional fiber, **233**
functional stretching, **147**
"Fu" series of smartphone applications, 206

gambling, compulsive, 375
gamma hydroxy butyrate (GHB), 376, 379
gamma rays, 438
garbage. *See* solid waste
*Garcinia cambogia,* 286
Gardasil vaccine, 411
GAS (general adaptation syndrome),
    306–**307**
gastric bypass surgery, 287–288
gender differences. *See also* men; women
    in alcohol effects, 380
    in body fat, 176, 179, 183, 193–195
    in body image, 290
    in body mass index, 182
    in cardiovascular disease, 337, 338
    in muscular strength, 102
    in obesity prevalence, 274
    in physical activity levels, 8
    in recommended fat intake, 228
    in stress response, 305–306
    in tobacco use, 386, 388
gender roles, stress from, 306
general adaptation syndrome (GAS), 306–**307**
genes, 362, **363**
genetically modified (GM) foods, 260–261
genetics
    body composition and, 185
    cancer and, 354, 362
    cardiovascular disease and, 337
    excess body fat and, 275
    flexibility and, 142
    lifestyle and, 11
    metabolic rate and, 276
genital herpes, 412, **413**
genital warts, **411**–412
geothermal power, 441
gestational diabetes, 180
GHB (gamma hydroxy butyrate), 376, 379
ghrelin, 177
ginseng, 114
global warming, 426–428, **427**
glucose
    defined, **65, 231**
    diabetes and, 180
    in digestion, 230–231
    in energy production, 64, 65
    in fight-or-flight response, 347
glycemic index, **231**–232
glycemic response, 231–232
glycogen
    defined, **65, 231**
    in energy production, 64, 65
    use of, in exercise, 68, 231
GM (genetically modified) foods,
    260–261
"Go, Slow, and Whoa," 260
gonococcal conjunctivitis, 410
gonorrhea, 410, **411**
GPS (global positioning system) monitors,
    73, 213
grace period, for credit cards, 5
graded exercise test (GXT), **41**
grains
    digestion of, 230–231
    food labels and, 232
    glycemic response and, 231–232
    intake recommendations for, 244, 342
    refined *vs.* whole, 231, 232, 241, 342
    serving sizes, 244
greenhouse effect, 426, **427**
greenhouse gases, 426, **427**
green tea extract, 114, 286
grilling meats, 365
growth hormone, 114
guarana, 286
guns, injuries from, A–6

*H. pylori,* 339, 365
hallucinogens, 376, 379
hardiness, 305
hashish, 376
hats, 359
HBV (hepatitis B virus), 365, 412–413
HCG (human chorionic gonadotropin), 114
HDL. *See* high-density lipoprotein
headaches, 324
head and neck cancers, 358, 365
head turns and tilts, 149
health, defined, **2**
health disparities, 7, 8, 361
health information, evaluating, 13, 348
health insurance, 361
health journals, 18–19
health-related fitness, 34–37, **35**
Healthy Eating Pyramid, 266
*Healthy People 2020,* 6–7, 8
Healthy People Initiative, 6–7
heart, 62, 67. *See also* heart rate
heart attacks. *See also* cardiovascular disease
    defined, **340**
    during exercise, 42
    prevalence of, 339–340
    smoking and, 332
    symptoms of, 340, 341
    what to do in, 340, 341
    in women, 338
heart disease, 6–7, 340–341. *See also* cardiovascular
    disease
heart murmurs, 346–347
heart rate
    arrhythmias in, 340, 347
    heart rate reserve, 74–75
    maximum, 74, 76
    monitoring, 72, 73, 333
    physical fitness and, 67, 72
    at rest and during exercise, 63
    resting, 67, 73
    swimming and, 217
    target heart rate zone, 74–75, 217, 218
    in weight loss, 281
heart rate monitors, 73, 333
heart rate reserve, 74–**75**, 76
heat cramps, **81**
heat exhaustion, **81**
heat stress, 79–81
heatstroke, **81**
heavy metals, 432, **433**, 436–437
heel raise exercises, 118, 124
height/weight tables, 176
*Helicobacter pylori,* 339, 365
hemorrhagic stroke, 342. *See also* stroke
hepatitis, 365, **412**–413
hepatitis B virus (HBV), 365, 412–413
herbal supplements, 285
herbicide resistance, in plants, 261
heredity. *See* genetics
heroin, 376
herpes simplex viruses, 357, 412
high altitude, exercise in, 85
high blood pressure. *See* blood pressure;
    hypertension
high-density lipoprotein (HDL)
    cholesterol transport and, 334–335
    defined, 228, **229, 335**
    functions of, 334
    metabolic syndrome and, 339
    recommended levels of, 334, 336
    tobacco use and, 332
high-fructose corn syrup, 246
high-intensity interval training (HIT), 80
hip and trunk stretch, 151
Hispanic Americans, 8, 337, 361. *See also*
    ethnicity

HIV/AIDS
  consequences to women, 417
  global prevalence of, 402–403, 405, 417
  HIV infection, 402, 403–404
  prevention of, 407–408
  symptoms of, 406
  testing for, 406, 407
  transmission of, 404, 406, 417
  treatment for, 406–407, 416
  vaccine development for, 406–407
HIV infection, **402**–404
HIV-positive, **406**
HIV Replication Capacity, 406
HMB (beta-hydroxy beta-methylbutyrate), 114
Hodgkin's disease, 361, 365
Home Access, 407
home injuries, A–4 to A–6. *See also* injuries
homeostasis, 304, **305**
home test kits, for HIV, 407
homocysteine, 337–338
hormone replacement therapy (HT), 338
hormones. *See also specific hormones*
  body fat and, 276
  defined, 302, **303**
  sleep deprivation and, 312
  in stress response, 302–303, 307
hostility. *See also* anger
  assessment of, 350
  cardiovascular disease and, 344
  in dealing with anger, 316
hot weather, 79–81
household hazardous wastes, 437
human chorionic gonadotropin (HCG), 114
human herpesvirus, 365
human immunodeficiency virus (HIV), **402**. *See also* HIV/AIDS
human papillomavirus (HPV), 357, 365, **411**–412, 417
humidity, heat stress and, 79
humor, in stress management, 318
hurdler stretch, 151, 153
hybrid electric vehicles (HEVs), 429
hydration, 208, 237
hydrocodone, 376
hydrogenation, **227**–228
hyperplasia, 98, **99**
hypertension. *See also* blood pressure
  in African Americans, 8, 337, 338
  atherosclerosis and, 333
  blood pressure ranges in, 332–333, 334, 338
  cardiovascular disease and, 332–333
  DASH eating plan and, 266
  defined, 332, **333**
  endurance exercise and, 69, 344
  exercise guidelines for, B–1 to B–2
  metabolic syndrome and, 339
  obesity and, 179
  omega-3 fatty acids and, 228, 229
  physical activity and, 344
  sodium and, 240, 250
  stress and, 308
  symptoms of, 334
  weight training and, 69
hypertrophy, 98, **99**
hyponatremia, 80
hypothermia, **81**

ibuprofen, 143, 354
ice, in injury treatment, 83
IGF (insulin-like growth factor), 114
IHRSA (International Health, Racquet, and Sports Club Association), 50
illness. *See also* chronic diseases; sexually transmitted diseases; *specific illnesses*
  exercise programs and, 49
  water contamination and, 431

immediate energy system, 64, **65**
immune function
  in athletes, 403
  exercise and, 70, 364, 403
  genetically modified immune cells, 369
  in HIV/AIDS, 403–404
  obesity and, 179
  psychoneuroimmunology and, 307–308
  stress and, 307–308
income. *See* socioeconomic status
incomplete proteins, 226
indoor air pollution, 429–430
infants
  car seats for, A–2 to A–3
  dietary reference intakes for, 263–265
  environmental tobacco smoke and, 390
  fetal alcohol syndrome in, 383
  herpes infections in, 412
  maternal smoking and, 388, 390
  syphilis infections in, 413
  vitamin K and, 264
infectious diseases, **4**. *See also* sexually transmitted diseases
inflammation
  alcohol use and, 342–343
  of blood vessels, 36
  cancer and, 364
  cardiorespiratory endurance exercise and, 69
  cardiovascular disease and, 337
  chronic, 178, 179
  C-reactive protein and, 337
  exercise and, 364, 403
  in muscle soreness, 85, 125
  omega-3 fatty acids and, 228, 229, 346
  R-I-C-E principle for, 83
  saturated fats and, 228
  stress and, 307
In Focus reports
  on benefits of quitting smoking, 389
  on breathing for relaxation, 321
  on classifying activity levels, 33
  on club drugs, 379
  on counterproductive strategies for stress, 311
  on diabetes, 180
  on exercise and cardiac risk, 42
  on financial wellness, 5
  on healthy beverages, 208
  on interval training, 80
  on wellness for college students, 14
  on yoga and pain relief, 158
inhalants, 376
injection drug use, HIV and, 404
injuries. *See also* exercise safety; low-back pain and injuries
  assault, A–7 to A–8
  in bicycling, 214
  care of, 82–83
  choking, A–5, A–6
  coping after terrorism or disasters, A–9
  drowning and boating, A–6
  falls, 68, A–4
  from firearms, A–6
  from fires, A–6
  flexibility and, 145
  fractures, 144, 181
  guidelines for, 83
  at high altitude, 85
  in interval training, 80
  lifting technique and, 110–111, 157, A–7
  motor vehicle, 382–383, A–2 to A–4
  muscular strength and endurance and, 101
  poisoning, A–4
  rehabilitation after, 83, 104
  R-I-C-E treatment for, 83
  sexual assault, A–8 to A–9
  skating and scooter, A–6 to A–7

  sports, A–7
  stalking and cyberstalking, A–9
  strength training and, 101, 102, 104, 111–112
  stretches to avoid, 153
  in stretching, 147, 153
  suffocation, A–6
  unintentional, 11, A–2 to A–7
  when to call a physician, 82
  work, A–7
injury prevention, A–2 to A–11
in-line skating injuries, A–6 to A–7
inner thigh stretch, 150
insoluble fiber, **233**
insomnia, 308, 313
instability training, 203
insulin, 114, 180, 231
insulin-like growth factor (IGF), 114
insulin resistance
  body composition and, 36
  calcium and, 346
  diabetes and, 180
  physical activity and, 177
  prostate cancer and, 355
insulin resistance syndrome. *See* metabolic syndrome
intellectual wellness, 3
intensity of exercise. *See also* FITT principle
  in cardiorespiratory endurance exercise, 74–76, 77, 79, 203
  examples of, 32, 75, 202
  METs, 75
  periodization of, 46
  ratings of perceived exertion, **76**
  recommendations for, 31–32, 33, 43–44
  in strength training, 107–108, 203–204
  in stretching programs, 146
  talk test, 76
  target heart rate zone and, 74–75, 76
  weight loss and, 281
intermittent explosive disorder, 316
internal locus of control, 15
International Health, Racquet, and Sports Club Association (IHRSA), 50
International Sports Sciences Association (ISSA), 49, 50
Internet
  addiction to, 375
  ChooseMyPlate.gov website, 243, 260, A–1
  cyberstalking, A–9
  evaluating health information on, 13
  fast-food restaurant websites, A–1
  weight-loss programs on, 284
interpersonal wellness, 3
interval training
  in bicycling, 214
  pros and cons of, 80, 206
  in rowing, 218
  in swimming, 215, 216
intervertebral disks, 152–**153**
intoxication, **374**. *See also* alcohol use
intra-abdominal fat
  cardiovascular disease and, 336
  defined, 176, **177**
  health impacts of, 36, 179
  metabolic syndrome and, 339
iodine, 236, 264
iPhones, exercise applications on, 206
iron, 236, 239, 248, 264
irradiation, food, 254–256, **255**
ischemic stroke, 342
isokinetic exercise, **105**
isometric exercise, **103**–104, 160
isometric side bridge exercise, 160
isotonic exercise, 104–**105**
"I" statements, 314

job-related stressors, 310
jogging, 42, 211–213
jogging exercise plan, 211–213
joint capsules, 142, **143**
joints, 82, 142, 144–145
journals
   in behavior change, 17–19
   exercise, 207
   health, 18–19
   stress logs, 315, 326
   in weight-management, 282

Kaposi's sarcoma, 365, 406
Kegel exercises, 209
ketamine, 376, 379
kettlebells, **105**
kidney cancer, 360
kilocalories, 224, **225**. *See also* calories
kissing, HIV transmission and, 408
*Kitchen Companion* (USDA), 255
knee extension exercise, 123
kreteks, 388
K-Y jelly, 409
kyphosis, 145

labels. *See* food labels
laboratory activities
   alcohol problem assessment, 397–398
   body image problems and eating disorders,
     299–300
   body mass index and composition, 191
   cancer prevention, 371–372
   cardiorespiratory endurance assessment, 89–93
   cardiorespiratory endurance program
     development, 95–96
   CVD risk assessment, 349–350
   dietary analysis, 269–270
   energy needs calculation, 295–296
   environmental health checklist, 443
   fitness facilities, 221–222
   flexibility assessment, 165–170
   flexibility program creation, 171–172
   food choices, 271–272
   lifestyle evaluation, 27–28
   low-back health assessment, 173–174
   muscular endurance assessment, 135–138,
     173–174
   muscular strength assessment, 129–134
   MyPyramid *vs.* your daily diet, 267–268
   PAR-Q (Physical Activity Readiness
     Questionnaire), 53–54
   pedometer use, 59–60
   personal fitness program plan and contract,
     219–220
   physical activity barriers, 55–58
   safety of exercise participation, 53–54
   smoking, reasons for, 399–400
   spiritual wellness, 329–330
   STD behaviors and attitudes, 419–420
   strength training program design, 139–140
   stress levels and key stressors, 325–326
   stress-management techniques, 327–328
   target body weight, 197–198
   weight loss goals, 297–298
   wellness profile, 25–26
lactate threshold, 65
lactic acid, **65**
lacto-ovo-vegetarians, 247
lacto-vegetarians, 247
laparoscopy, **411**
Lap-Band/VGB surgery, 287–288
lapses, in exercise programs, 206, 207
lateral raise exercises, 118, 122
lateral stretch, 150
late syphilis, 413
latex allergies, 409

Latino/Latina Americans. *See* Hispanic Americans
lat pull exercise, 120
LDL (low-density lipoprotein). *See* low-density
   lipoprotein
lead contamination, 436, 437
leanness, extreme, 179, 181
leg extension exercise, 123
leg press exercise, 123
legumes, 226, **227**
leisure injuries, A–6 to A–7
leptin, 276
leukemia, 352, 360
life changes, stress from, 309
life expectancy
   gender and, 8
   historical trends in, 4
   marriage and, 313
   muscular strength and, 100
   obesity and, 274
   physical activity and, 10
   quality of life and, 4
   smoking and, 387
lifestyle choices. *See also* behavior change
   body fat and, 186, 276–277
   death rates and, 6–7
   defined, **6**
   diabetes and, 180
   evaluation of, 12
   laboratory activity on, 27–28
   physical activity in, 7–8, 9
   self-efficacy and, 15
   stress management and, 327
   target behavior and, 12–13, 18
   weight management and, 283
   wellness and, 6, 11–21
lifting technique, 111–112, 157, A–7
ligaments, **101**, 142
light activity, 33
linoleic acid, 227, 228, 230, 265
lipids. *See* fats, dietary
lipoprotein(a), 338–339
lipoproteins, 334, **335**, 338–339. *See also* high-
   density lipoprotein; low-density lipoprotein
liposuction, 188, 288
liquor, 380. *See also* alcohol use
listening skills, 314
*Listeria monocytogenes*, 254, 255
liver, 380, 383, 413
liver cancer, 365, 413
locus of control, **15**
low-back pain and injuries
   bed rest and, 155
   causes of, 154–155
   core muscle fitness and, 155, 203
   exercises for, 156, 159–161
   muscular endurance assessment for, 173–174
   pain management for, 155–156, 158
   posture and, 157
   prevalence of, 152
   prevention of, 145, 155
   spine function and structure, 152–153
   yoga and, 156, 158
low-carbohydrate diets, 284
low-density lipoprotein (LDL)
   cardiovascular disease and, 334, 339
   defined, **229**, 235, **335**
   functions of, 334–335
   pattern B, 339
   recommended levels of, 334, 336
   smoking and, 332
lower-leg stretch, 151
Lp(a), 338–339
LSD, 376, 379
lumpectomy, 355
lung cancer
   detection of, 353–354

   environmental tobacco smoke and, 353
   exercise and, 364
   gender and, 353
   prevalence of, 353
   risk factors for, 11
lunge walk, 147
lying down, 157
lymphatic system, 352, **353**
lymphocytes, 307, 403
lymphoma, 360–361, 365

macronutrients, 224, **225**. *See also* carbohydrates;
   fats, dietary; protein, dietary
macrophages, 403
magnesium, 236, 237, 264
mainstream smoke, **389**
maintenance stage, 16, 17
malignant tumors, 352, **353**
mammograms, 354–**355**, 367
manganese, 237, 264
margarine, 228, 242, 260
marijuana, 311, 376, 394
mass violence, coping after, A–9
mastectomy, 355
maximal oxygen consumption
   benefits of increasing, 68
   defined, 66, **67**
   in fitness assessment, 71
   limits to improvement of, 40
maximum heart rate (MHR), 74, 76
maximum swimming heart rate (MSHR), 217
mazindol (Sanorex), 287
MDMA (ecstasy), 376, 379
meat, 245, 354, 362, 365
media
   body image and, 293
   evaluating health information in, 346, 348
   television viewing and weight gain, 277,
     280, 287
medical clearance for exercise, 40–42
medical marijuana, 394
medications, disposing of, 432, 433
medicine balls, 107
meditation, 4, 320
Mediterranean diet, 247
melanoma, **357**, 358
men. *See also* gender differences
   cardiovascular disease and, 337
   circumcision of, 405
   Dietary Reference Intakes for, 263–265
   HIV infection in, 404, 406
   muscular strength in, 102
   nutrition for, 230
   prostate cancer in, 355–356, 361, 367
   sexual anatomy of, 408
   strength training by, 102
   testicular cancer in, 359–360
   tobacco use by, 388
menstruation, exercise and, 85, 181
mental health, exercise and, 312
mental health professionals, 322
men who have sex with men (MSM), HIV and,
   404, 406
mercury contamination, 256, 431,
   436–437
mescaline (peyote), 376
"metabolic-optimizing" meals, 114
metabolic rate, 64, **65**
metabolic syndrome
   cardiovascular disease and, 178, 339
   characteristics of, 339
   defined, 178, **179**
   excess body fat and, 339
   exercise and, 344
   muscular strength and, 100
   prevalence of, 339

metabolism
  of alcohol, 380
  cellular, 68
  defined, 36, **37**, 64
  exercise and, 276, 344
  metabolic rate, 75, 275–276
  muscle mass and, 36, 101
  resting metabolic rate, 75, 275–276
  treatment of, 339
metastasis, 352, **353**
methamphetamine, 376, 379
methane, as greenhouse gas, 426
methaqualone, 376
metronidazole (Flagyl), 413
METs, **75**
Mexican Americans, cardiovascular disease in, 337.
    *See also* Hispanic Americans
MHR (maximum heart rate), 74, 76
MI (myocardial infarction). *See* heart attacks
microbes
  cancer and, 365
  as pollutants, 430
micronutrients, 224, **225**
migraine headaches, 324
military press exercise, 117
milk. *See* dairy
minerals, **235**–236. *See also specific minerals*
minimum monthly payment, 5
Miss America pageant winners, 290
mitochondria, 36, **65**, 68
mitral valve prolapse (MVP), 347
mode of exercise. *See* FITT principle
moderate-intensity physical activity. *See also*
    intensity of exercise
  benefits of, 44
  examples of, 32–33, 39, 202
  recommendations for, 43
mold, indoor, 430
molybdenum, 264
money, stress from, 309, 310
monitoring progress, 204–205, C–1 to C–2
monosodium glutamate (MSG), 252, 261
monounsaturated fatty acids, 227, 228, 229
morphine, 376
motorcycle injuries, A–3
motor units, **99**
motor vehicle injuries, 382–383, A–2 to A–4
MP3 players, exercise applications on, 206
MSG (monosodium glutamate), 252, 261
MSHR (maximum swimming heart rate), 217
MSM (men who have sex with men), HIV and,
    404, 406
multicenter studies, 348
multiple sclerosis, 307
muscle cramps, 82, 145
muscle dysmorphia, 288
muscle fibers, 98–**99**
muscle learning, **99**
muscle mass, 36, 99, 102, 276
muscles
  after stopping strength training, 125
  agonist *vs.* antagonist, 109, 143
  cellular metabolism in, 68
  components of, 98
  concentric *vs.* eccentric contractions in, 104
  core, 153–154
  elasticity and length of, 142–143
  fatigue in, 65
  fiber types in, 98–99
  motor units and, 99
  nervous system regulation and, 143
  soreness in, 82, 85, 125
  strains in, 82
muscular endurance
  assessment of, 103, 173–174
  benefits of, 36, 100–102

defined, 36, **37**
  low-back health and, 173–174
muscular strength. *See also* strength training
  aging and, 101–102
  assessment of, 102–103, 129–134
  benefits of, 35–36, 100–102
  defined, **35**
  flexibility and, 162
  gender differences in, 102
  intensity of exercise and, 203–204
  metabolism and, 36, 101
  premature death and, 100
  reversibility of, 40
music, in relaxation, 320
mutations, 362
MVP (mitral valve prolapse), 347
myocardial infarction (MI). *See* heart attacks
myofibrils, 98, **99**
myosin, 98
MyPlate (formerly MyPyramid)
  alternative food-group plans, 246–247
  ChooseMyPlate.gov website, 243, 260, A–1
  comparing your diet to, 267–268
  defined, 238, **239**
  key messages of, 243
  on physical activity, 246
  portion sizes in, 245
  recommendations of, 244–246
  vegetables and fruits in, 244, 260
  weight management and, 277–278
MyPyramid, 246. *See also* MyPlate

nasopharynx cancer, 365
National Cholesterol Education Program (NCEP),
    334, 342
National Nutrient Database, A–1
National Nutritional Foods Association, 253
National Strength and Conditioning Association
    (NSCA), 49, 50
National Suicide Prevention Lifeline, 322
National Weight Control Registry, 284
Native Americans, 8. *See also* ethnicity
natural disasters, coping after, 422, A–9
natural killer cells, 403
natural resources, population and, 423–424
NCEP (National Cholesterol Education Program),
    334, 342
neck cancer, 358
neck circles, 153
negatives, 105
negotiating, 315
*Neisseria gonorrhoeae*, 410
neoplasms, 352
neotame, 279
nerve roots, 152, **153**
nervous system, 143, 302–303, 305
neural tube defects, 235
neurogenesis, exercise and, 31
neuromuscular training, 33, 36–37
neuropeptides, 307
neurotransmitters, 302
newborns. *See* infants
NHL (non-Hodgkin's lymphoma), 361
niacin, 234, 263
nicotine, 375, **386**
nicotine replacement therapy, 388, 391
911, calling, 341, 382
nitrates and nitrites, 364–365
nitric oxide, 69
nitrogen dioxide, 425
nitrosamines, 364–365
nitrous oxide, as greenhouse gas, 426
non-comedogenic sunscreens, 359
non-Hodgkin's lymphoma (NHL), 361
nonnutritive sweeteners, 279
nonoxidative energy system, 64, **65**

nonoxynol-9, 408, 409
nonsteroidal anti-inflammatory drugs (NSAIDs),
    82, 155, 354
norepinephrine, **302**
nuclear power, **439**
nuclear weapons, 438–439
nuclei, of muscle cells, 98, **99**
nutrient density, 241, 242, 283
nutrition, 224–261. *See also* diet;
    supplements, dietary
  alcoholic beverages and, 224
  antioxidants, 235, 237–238
  assessing and changing your diet, 258
  for athletes, 248, 250
  for bone health, 236, 237, 242
  calories and, 240, 246
  cancer and, 233, 246, 362–364, 371
  carbohydrates (*See* carbohydrates)
  cardiovascular disease and, 239, 246
  for children and teenagers, 248
  for college students, 248, 249
  Daily Values, 238–239
  DASH eating plan, 242, 266, 277–278, 334
  defined, **225**
  dietary analysis, 260, 269–270
  Dietary Guidelines for Americans, 238, 239,
    240–243
  Dietary Reference Intakes, 238–240,
    263–265
  environmental contamination and, 256
  essential nutrient classes, 224
  ethnic foods, 257
  fast-food restaurants and, 249, 272, A–1
  fats (*See* fats, dietary)
  fiber (*See* fiber)
  fish consumption guidelines, 228, 241–242,
    256, 258
  food additives, 252
  food allergies, 261
  foodborne illness and, 252, 254
  food irradiation and, 254–256
  food labels and, 228, 232, 251, 252,
    261, 271
  foods to increase, 241–242
  foods to reduce, 228, 240–241
  genetically modified foods, 260–261
  global food supply, 423
  glycemic index and glycemic response,
    231–232
  Healthy Eating Pyramid, 266
  intake goals for, 230
  for men, 228
  minerals, 235–236
  MyPlate (*See* MyPlate)
  nutritional content of common foods, A–1
  for older adults, 248
  organic foods, 256
  phytochemicals, 238, 239, 363
  portion sizes, 242, 244–246, 251
  protein (*See* protein, dietary)
  safe food handling, 255
  Social Ecological Model, 243
  sodium and potassium, 240
  SoFAS (solid fats and added sugars), 241, 244,
    246, 260
  special health concerns and, 248, 250
  strategies for, 258
  in stress management, 311
  supplements (*See* supplements, dietary)
  trans fatty acids, 227–229, 240–242, 260
  in vegetarian diets, 226, 239, 242, 247–248
  vitamins, 233–235
  water and, 236–237, 265
  weight management and, 240, 277–280
  for women, 228, 248
Nutrition Facts, on food labels, 251, 280

oatmeal, 343
obesity. *See also* weight management
  back pain and, 155
  body fat percentage and, 183
  Body Mass Index and, 191
  cancer and, 179, 354, 364
  cardiovascular disease and, 274, 335–336
  in college students, 14
  defined, 178, **179**
  diabetes and, 178–179, 180
  ethnicity and, 274
  exercise and, 177, 179, 180, B–2
  factors contributing to, 240
  gender and, 274
  health implications of, 10–11, 178–179, 274
  metabolic syndrome and, 339
  mortality and, 7, 10, 179
  physical activity and, 177
  prevalence of, 178, 274
  socioeconomic status and, 361
"obesogenic food environment," 240
occupational exposure, 365
occupational wellness, 4
oils
  cholesterol and, 228
  intake recommendations, 244, 245–246
  serving sizes of, 246
older adults. *See also* aging
  cardiovascular disease in, 337
  exercise and, 68, 209
  falls by, 68, A–4
  flexibility in, 144–145
  muscular strength and, 36, 101–102
  nutrition for, 248
  strength training and, 36, 68, 108, 209
  swimming and, 185
  vitamin B-12 and, 239
  vitamin D and, 239
omega-3 fatty acids, 228, 229, 346
omega-6 fatty acids, 228, 229, 362
oncogenes, 362, **363**
one drink, defined, **380**
1-mile walk test, 71, 89–90
1.5-mile run-walk test, 71, 91–92
one-repetition maximum (1 RM) test, 102–103
opium, 376
optimism, 305
oral cancer, 362, 388
oral contraceptives, 416–417
oral-genital sex, STD transmission in, 404, 408,
  410, 412
orange juice, 241
Orasure test, 407
organic foods, **256**
orlistat (Xenical), 287
oropharyngeal cancer, 365, 411
osteoarthritis, 144
osteoporosis
  calcium intake and, 236, 237
  defined, **237**
  exercise guidelines in, B–2
  in female athlete triad, 181
  lead exposure and, 436
  nutrition and, 237
  physical activity and, 70, 144
  prevalence of, 237
  smoking and, 387
  weight training and, 36, 70, 102
ovarian cancer, 357, 364
Overeaters Anonymous (OA), 286
overhead press exercises, 117, 121
overhead stretch, 149
overload, 38–40, 77–78
over-the-counter (OTC) medications, 377, 432, 433
overtraining
  defined, **45**

immune function and, 70, 403
  in strength training, 109, 125
overweight, 178, **179**. *See also* obesity
oxidative energy system, 64, **65–66**
oxycodone, 376
oxygen consumption, maximal. *See* maximal
  oxygen consumption
oxygen exchange, 63
ozone, in air pollution, 425–426
ozone layer, **428**

pacemakers, 62
pain management, 155–156, 158. *See also*
  low-back pain and injuries
pancreas, diabetes and, 180
pancreatic cancer, 360
pantothenic acid, 234, 263
Pap test, **357**, 367
Paralympics, 38
parasympathetic division, **302**, 304
Parkinson's disease, 246
PAR-Q (Physical Activity Readiness Questionnaire),
  41, 53–54
partially hydrogenated oil, 228, 240
partial vegetarians, 247
particulate matter (PM), 425
passive stretching, **148**, 162
pathogens, **252**, 254
PCBs (polychlorinated biphenyls), 432, **433**
PCP, 376
"pear shape," 179
pedestrians, motor vehicle injuries to, A–3
pedometers, 47, 59–60, 85, 213
peer counseling, 320–321
pelvic inflammatory disease (PID), 408, 410–**411**
pelvic tilt exercise, 161
penile cancer, 411, 417
percent body fat
  defined, 176–**177**
  estimating, 183–185, 191–196
  gender and, 176
  setting goals for, 197–198
percutaneous electrical nerve stimulation
  (PENS), 156
performance. *See* sports performance
performance aids, 112–115
perinatal transmission, 404
perineum, 411
periodization of training, 46, 110
Personal Challenges
  on activity level, 9
  on barriers to exercise, 32
  on cancer risk factors, 366
  on current health status, 41
  on current strength, 103
  on drinking behavior, 384
  on eating habits, 225
  on environmental requirements of lifestyles, 424
  on heart rate monitoring, 345
  on keeping your back pain-free, 156
  on problem solving, 319
  on staying active between workouts, 78
  on target behaviors, 18
  on weight management, 275, 282
  on weight tracking, 186
personal fitness plan, 200–209
  activity selection in, 200, 202
  bicycling sample program, 213–215
  cardiorespiratory endurance exercise in, 203
  for children and adolescents, 207
  contract in, 20, 201, 204
  digital motivation for, 206
  fitness facilities in, 221–222
  FITT principle in, 202–204, 205, 211
  general guidelines for, 211
  goals in, 49, 200, 204

  implementing, 205–206
  lapses in, 206, 207
  lifestyle physical activity in, 204
  mini-goals and rewards in, 204, 207
  monitoring progress in, 204–205, C–1 to C–2
  for older adults, 209
  in pregnancy, 208–209
  rowing machine sample program, 217–218
  sample plan and contract, 201, 219–220
  stability balls in, 203
  strength and endurance training in, 203–204
  swimming sample program, 215–217
  variety in, 205
  walking/jogging/running sample program,
    211–213
personality, **305**
personal trainers, 49, 50
pescovegetarians, 247
pesticides, 256, 436, **437**
peyote, 376
phantom chair exercise, 161
phenolphthalein, 285
phentermine, 114, 287
phenylpropanolamine (PPA), 114, 285
phenytoin, 285
phosphorus, 236, 237, 264
photovoltaic systems, 441
physical activity. *See also* exercise
  aging and, 31
  barriers to, 30, 55–58
  body composition and, 177, 179
  bone and joint disease and, 144
  brain and, 31
  caloric expenditure in, 75, 295
  cancer and, 364
  cardiovascular disease and, 334–335, 343, 344
  classifying levels of, 33
  defined, **31**
  immediate and long-term benefits of, 7–10, 66–71
  life expectancy and, 10
  lifestyle, 44, 204
  moderate-intensity, 32–33, 39, 43–44, 202
  MyPlate recommendations on, 246
  physical fitness and, 177
  questionnaire on, 9, 32
  recommendations for, 32–34
  sleep and, 312
  statistics on, 9, 30, 277
  stress and, 311, 312
  in weight management, 280 281, 283
  between workouts, 78
*Physical Activity Guidelines for Americans*, 10, 30
physical activity pyramid, 42–44
Physical Activity Readiness Questionnaire
  (PAR-Q), 41
physical dependence, **377**
physical fitness, 30–50. *See also* personal
  fitness plan
  adaptability limits in, 40
  assessing, 71–72
  benefits of, 30–34
  body composition and, 36
  cardiorespiratory endurance, 35, 62–85
  defined, **7**
  disability and, 38
  energy production and, 66
  exercise and, 34
  flexibility and, 36
  goals for, 49
  health-related, 34–37
  interval training and, 80
  life expectancy and, 10
  monitoring progress in, 204–205, C–1 to C–2
  muscular endurance and strength, 35–36
  physical activity vs., 177
  skill-related, 36–37

physical training. *See also* exercise program design
　adaptability limits in, 40
　basic principles of, 37
　defined, **37**
　guidelines for, 44–47
　overtraining, 45, 70, 109, 125, 403
　progressive overload, 38–40
　reversibility, 40
　specificity principle, 38, 39
physical wellness, 3
physicians, 82, 209
phytochemicals, 238, **239**, **363**
PID (pelvic inflammatory disease), 408
Pilates, 106–107
pipes, 387–388. *See also* tobacco use
Planned Parenthood, 407, 414
plantar fasciitis, 82
plantar flexion, 169
plant stanols and sterols, 346
plaques, **339**
plastic elongation, **143**
plasticity, exercise and, 31
plastic water bottles, 208, 431
platelets, 332, **333**, 347
plethysmography, 183
pliometric contractions, 104
pliometric loading, 104–**105**
plyometrics, **105**, 143
PM (particulate matter), 425
pneumatic strength training machines, 104
*Pneumocystis* pneumonia, 406
PNF (proprioceptive neuromuscular facilitation),
　143, 147–148
PNI (psychoneuroimmunology), **307**–308
poisoning, A–4
pollution
　air, 82, 425–426, 428–430
　cancer and, 365
　chemical, 436–438
　indoor air, 429–430
　radiation, 438–440
　solid waste, 432–436
　water, 430–432
polychlorinated biphenyls (PCBs), 432, **433**
polypeptide supplements, 114
polyps, 354
polyunsaturated fatty acids, 227–228, 229
population growth, 423–425
portion sizes
　estimating, 245
　on food labels, 251
　in MyPlate, 244–246
　underestimating, 276–277, 278
post-traumatic stress disorder (PTSD), 309
posture, 145, 155, 157
potassium
　blood pressure and, 242
　bone health and, 237
　Dietary Reference Intake for, 265
　functions of, 236
poverty. *See* socioeconomic status
power activities, fast-twitch fibers and, **99**
PPA (phenylpropanolamine), 114, 285
precontemplation stage, 16, 17
pre-diabetes, 180
pregnancy
　alcohol use during, 383
　Dietary Reference Intakes for, 263–265
　dietary supplements in, 248, 250
　ectopic, 390
　exercise during, 208–209
　fish consumption guidelines, 256
　folate and, 235, 239, 248, 263
　genital herpes and, 412
　gestational diabetes in, 180
　HIV transmission in, 404, 406

　nutrition in, 248
　psychoactive drugs during, 379
　smoking during, 388, 390
　syphilis in, 413
prehypertension, 334
preparation stage, 16, 17
prescription drugs. *See also specific drugs*
　disposing of, 432, 433
　in weight loss, 287
primary HIV infection, 406
primary syphilis, 413
primary tumor, 352
processed foods, 279
procrastination, 21
program logs, 204–205
progress charts, 204–205
progressive overload, 38–40, **39**
progressive relaxation, 319, 324
prone arch, 153
proof value, **380**
proprioceptive neuromuscular facilitation (PNF),
　143, 147–148
proprioceptors, **143**, 147
prostate cancer, 355–356, 361, 367
prostate-specific antigen (PSA) blood test, **355**, 367
protease inhibitors, 406
proteasome inhibitors, 369
protein, dietary
　amino acids in, 113, 226
　for athletes, 250
　bone health and, 237
　calories in, 224
　complete *vs.* incomplete, 226
　content in common foods, 226
　defined, **225**
　energy from, 64, 224, 226
　mental boost from, 226
　in MyPlate, 245
　recommended intake, 226, 230, 241–242,
　　244–245, 265
　serving sizes, 245
　strength training and, 114, 125
PSA (prostate-specific antigen) blood test,
　**355**, 367
psilocybin, 376
psychoactive drugs, 375–385
　cardiovascular disease and, 337
　characteristics of users of, 377–378
　club drugs, 379
　considerations before using, 379
　date-rape, 378, 379
　defined, **374**
　drug abuse, use, and dependence, 377
　effects of, 376
　helping someone with a problem with, 394
　injection drug use and HIV, 404
　intoxication from, 374
　over-the-counter medications as, 377
　potential of, for dependence, 378
　statistics on use of, 374
　treatment for abuse and dependence, 378
　unsafe sexual behavior and, 416
psychoneuroimmunology (PNI), **307**–308
psyllium, 233
PTSD (post-traumatic stress disorder), 309
pubic lice, **414**
pullover exercise, 122
pull-up exercises, 116, 121
pulmonary circulation, 62, **63**
pulmonary edema, 342
pulmonary resuscitation, A–11
pulse, taking one's, 72
purging, 290, **291**
push-ups, 109, 136–137
push-up test, 136–137
pyruvate, 285

quality of life, 4, 6, 101. *See also* wellness

race. *See* ethnicity
radial pulse, 72
radiation
　avoiding, 439–440
　cancer from, 360, 365
　in cancer therapy, 366, 368
　defined, 438, **439**
　electromagnetic spectrum and, 438
　in the home and workplace, 439
　medical uses of, 439
　ultraviolet, 357–358, 371–372, 428
radiation sickness, 437, **438**
radon, **439**
RAE (retinol activity equivalents), 264
raloxifene, 355
randomized studies, 348
range of motion, 142, **143**, 166–169
range-of-motion assessment, 166–169
rape, 382, A–8 to A–9
ratings of perceived exertion (RPE), 76
rationalizing, 21
reaction time, 36
rebaudioside-A, 279
Recommended Dietary Allowances (RDAs), 238
recovery time, 39
rectal cancer, 354, 367
recycling, **434**, 435
red meat consumption, colon cancer and, 354
reflex actions, 143, 302–304
rehabilitation after injuries, 83
reinforcement, 374
relapse, in behavior change, 16–17, 391
relationships, interpersonal, 310
relative risk, 348
relaxation, 145, 318–320, 321, 324
relaxation response, 318, **319**
religion. *See* spiritual wellness
renewable energy, 429, 441
repetition maximum (RM), 102–**103**
repetitions, **103**
repetitive-strain injuries, A–7
rescue breathing, A–11
resistance bands, 106, 107
resistance training. *See* strength training
respiratory system, **63**
rest, in exercise programs, 46
resting heart rate, 67, 73, 74
resting metabolic rate (RMR), 75, **275**–276
retinol, 237
retinol activity equivalents (RAE), 264
reversibility principle, 40, **41**
riboflavin, 234, 263
R-I-C-E principle, 83
rimonabant (Acomplia), 114, 285
risk factors, defined, 2, **3**
ritalin, 376
RM (repetition maximum), 102–**103**
RMR (resting metabolic rate), 75, **275**–276
road rage, A–3 to A–4
Rohypnol, 379
role models, 15, 17
Roux-en-Y gastric bypass, 287–288
rowing machine sample fitness program, 217–218
RPE (ratings of perceived exertion), 76
RunKeeper smartphone application, 206
run-walk test, 1.5-mile, 71, 91–92

saccharin (Sweet 'N Low), 279
safer sex, 14, 414, 416–417
safety. *See* exercise safety
safety belts, A–2
*Salmonella*, 254, 255
salt intake, 240, 338. *See also* sodium
sanitary landfills, **433**, 434

SAR (specific absorption rate), 439
sarcomeres, 98, 143
sarcopenia, 36, 101
saturated fats
    health effects of, 228, 229
    recommended intake of, 228–229, 240, 342
    reducing intake of, 242
scabies, **414**
scooter injuries, A–3, A–6 to A–7
screening tests, cancer, 367–368
seated leg curl exercise, 124
seated single-leg hamstring, 151
secondary syphilis, 413
secondary tumors, 352
secondhand smoke. *See* environmental
    tobacco smoke
sedatives, 374, 379
sedentary lifestyle
    defined, **9**
    longevity and, 10
    obesity and, 277
    in physical activity pyramid, 43
    physical activity *vs.*, 10, 177
    prevalence of, 9, 334–335
selective estrogen-receptor modulators (SERMs), 355
selenium, 236, 238, 264
self-concept, 25, 322
self-disclosure, 314
self-efficacy, **15**
self-esteem, 101, 179, 277, 281
self-image, 17, 101, 179
self-talk
    defined, **15**
    lifestyle changes and, 15, 17
    in stress management, 318, 324
    in weight management, 281
semivegetarians, 247. *See also* vegetarian diets
septic systems, 432, **433**
SERMs (selective estrogen-receptor modulators), 355
seropositive diagnosis, 406
serotonin, 287
serving sizes. *See* portion sizes
SES. *See* socioeconomic status
sets, in weight training, 108, **109**
sewage, 432
sexual anatomy, 408, 410
sexual assault, 382, A–8 to A–9
sexually transmitted diseases (STDs), 402–417
    bacterial vaginosis, 413
    behaviors and attitudes and, 419–420
    cervical cancer, 357 (*See also* cervical cancer)
    chlamydia, 339, 357, 408–410
    college students and, 416
    condoms and, 405, 409, 412, 414, 416–417
    defined, **402**
    diagnosis and treatment of, 414
    education on, 414
    genital herpes, 412, 413
    gonorrhea, 410, 411
    hepatitis B, 365, 412–413
    HIV/AIDS, 402–408, 417
    human papillomavirus and, 357, 365,
        411–412, 417
    pelvic inflammatory disease, 408, 410–411
    prevalence of, 402
    prevention of, 414–415, 416
    pubic lice, 414
    risk assessment of, 419
    safer sex, 14, 414, 416
    scabies, 414
    syphilis, 413
    trichomoniasis, 413
    women and, 417
sexually transmitted infections (STIs). *See* sexually
    transmitted diseases
Shape Up America!, 213

shin splints, 82
shoes for exercise, 84
shopping, compulsive, 375
shoulder press exercises, 117, 121
sibutramine (Meridia), 114, 285
side bridge endurance test, 173
side bridge exercise, 120
side lunge stretch, 150
side stitch, 82
sidestream smoke, **389**. *See also* environmental
    tobacco smoke
sidestroke, 216
SIDS (sudden infant death syndrome), 390
simple carbohydrates, 230–231. *See also* sugars
sinoatrial (SA) node, 62
sit-and-reach test, 145, 165
sitting at a computer, 157
skating injuries, A–6 to A–7
skill-related fitness, 36–**37**
skin cancer
    ABCD test for melanoma, 358
    ozone layer thinning and, 428
    prevalence of, 352–353
    prevention of, 358, 359, 371–372
    risk factors for, 357–358, 371–372
    types of, 358
skinfold measurements, 183–185, 191–192
sleep
    college students and, 14
    deprivation symptoms, 312
    disorders, 312–313
    exercise and, 71, 206, 312
    insomnia, 308
    obesity and, 177
    posture during, 155, 157
    stress management and, 312–313
sleep apnea, 313
sleep disorders, 312–313
slipped disks, 155
slow-twitch fibers, 98–**99**
Small Steps, 283
SMART goals, 18–19, 49, 74
smart phones, exercise applications on, 206
smog, 425–426, **427**
smokeless tobacco, 388. *See also* tobacco use
smoking. *See* tobacco use
snuff, 388
Social Ecological Model, **243**
social support
    in behavior change, 15, 17, 20–21
    breast cancer and, 355
    cardiovascular disease and, 337, 344
    drug abuse treatment and, 378
    exercise buddies, 47, 205, 207
    in stress management, 306, 313
socioeconomic status (SES)
    cancer and, 361
    cardiovascular disease and, 338
    environmental exposures and, 361, 437
    health disparities and, 8, 361
    obesity and, 361
sodas
    added sugars in, 241
    diet, 277
    health impacts of, 208, 237
    underestimating calories from, 208
sodium
    blood pressure and, 240, 250, 338
    bone health and, 237
    Dietary Reference Intake for, 265
    functions of, 236
    recommended intake, 240, 265, 342
SoFAS (solid fats and added sugars)
    added sugars in beverages, 241
    limiting the amount of, 232, 241, 246, 260
    MyPlate limits on, 244

soft tissues, 142, **143**. *See also* muscles
solar power, 441
solid waste
    biodegradability and, 433, 434
    components of, 433
    disposing of, 433, 434
    eWaste, 434–435
    recycling, 434
    reducing, 435–436
soluble fiber, **233**
somatic nervous system, **305**
soy foods, cholesterol and, 346
specific absorption rate (SAR), 439
specificity of training, 38, **39**
speed, 36
speed loading, **105**
sphygmomanometers, 332, 333
spine, structure and function of, 152–153
spine extension exercises, 119, 160
spiritual wellness, 3, 4, 315, 329–330
spit tobacco, 388. *See also* tobacco use
split routine, 107
sports. *See also* athletes; sports performance
    disabilities and, 38
    flexibility and, 145
    injuries from, A–7
    skill-related fitness and, 36–37
sports drinks, 80, 250
sports performance
    air pollution and, 82
    in athletes with disabilities, 38
    core muscles and, 203
    dehydration and, 79
    dietary fats and, 250
    genetics and, 40
    menstruation and, 85
    muscular endurance and, 36
    overtraining and, 45, 109, 311
    strength training and, 101, 125
    stretching and, 77, 146
    supplements and, 112, 113–114, 250
    visualization and, 15, 319
spot reducing, 188
spotters, 46, 106, **107**, 111–112
sprains, 82
sprinting, 99, 105, 145
sprouts, 254, 255
squamous cell carcinomas, **358**
squat endurance test, 137–138
squats, 118, 153
St. John's wort, 252
stability (exercise) balls, 106, 154, 203
stages of change model, 16–17
stalking, A–9
standard drink, defined, 380, 384
standard of living, 424
standing, posture in, 157
standing ankle-to-buttocks quadriceps stretch, 153
standing hamstring stretch, 153
standing toe touch, 153
static exercise, **103**–104
static stretching, 142, **147**
statin drugs, 337
statistics
    on cancer deaths, 7
    evaluating, 348
    on leading causes of death, 6, 7
    on nonmedical drug use, 374
    on obesity and overweight, 274
    on physical activity and exercise, 30
    on sexually transmitted diseases, 402
    on smoking, 386
STDs. *See* sexually transmitted diseases
stents, coronary, 341
step stretch exercises, 150, 159
step test, 3-minute, 71, 90

stevia, 279
stimulants, CNS, 376, 379. *See also* caffeine
stomach cancer, 365
stones, in strength training, 107
strength. *See* muscular strength
strength training
    advanced, 110–111
    agonist *vs.* antagonist muscles in, 109
    benefits of, 99
    bicycling as, 214–215
    blood pressure and, 69, 335
    body composition and, 100, 101, 102
    body weight and, 125
    cardiorespiratory endurance training and, 69
    cardiovascular risk and, 69
    constant *vs.* variable resistance, 104
    diabetes and, 180
    dynamic stretches and, 147
    equipment for, 105–106, 125
    FITT principle in, 107–109, 203–204
    flexibility exercise and, 147
    free weights in, 106, 111–112, 116–120
    gender and, 102
    lifting technique in, 111–112
    metabolism and, 101
    muscle physiology and, 98–99
    muscle soreness and, 125
    by older adults, 36, 68, 209
    order of exercises in, 109
    osteoporosis and, 36, 70, 102
    overtraining in, 109, 125
    Pilates, 106–107
    program design activity, 139–140
    progression in, 110
    protein intake and, 125
    recommendations for, 33, 40, 43, 107–109
    safety guidelines, 111–112
    sample programs, 109, 110
    sports performance and, 125
    static *vs.* dynamic exercises, 103–105
    stopping, 125
    supplements and drugs in, 112–115
    videos of, 108
    warm-up and cool-down in, 109–110
    weight machine exercises, 120–124
    weight machines *vs.* free weights, 105–106
    weight management and, 125, 280
    workout cards for, 110
stress, 302–324. *See also* stress management
    aging and, 304
    alcohol use and, 311
    allostatic load, 307
    assessment of, 325–326
    behavior change and, 21
    blood pressure and, 347
    carbohydrates and, 231
    cardiovascular disease and, 307, 308, 337–338, 344, 347
    chronic, 307–308
    in college students, 14
    defined, **302**
    depression and, 306, 308, 309, 321–322
    emotions and, 156, 302, 304–306
    exercise and, 311, 312
    fight-or-flight reaction, 303–304, 347
    finances and, 309, 310
    gender and, 305–306
    general adaptation syndrome, 306–307
    headaches from, 324
    hormones in, 302–303, 307, 403
    immune function and, 307–308
    nervous tension *vs.*, 302
    overload as, 38–40, 77–78
    past experiences and, 306
    performance and, 304
    personality and, 305

    physical responses to, 302–304
    post-traumatic stress disorder, 309
    psychoneuroimmunology and, 307–308
    sources of, 309–311
    symptoms of excess, 306, 325
    wellness and, 11, 306–309
stress cardiomyopathy, 338
stress fractures, 181
stress logs, 315, 326
stress management
    biofeedback, 320
    cognitive techniques, 318
    by college students, 14
    communication, 314–315
    conflict resolution, 315
    counterproductive strategies for, 311
    counting to ten, 315
    exercise in, 311, 312
    getting help in, 320–322
    humor in, 318
    identifying stress level and stressors, 325–326
    lifestyle changes in, 327
    meditation, 320
    mental health professionals in, 321, 322
    nutrition in, 311
    realistic self-talk, 318
    relaxation techniques, 318–320, 321, 324, 328
    sleep in, 312–313
    social support and, 313
    spiritual wellness in, 315, 329–330
    stress logs, 315, 326
    time management, 315, 317–318
    weight management, 283
    wellness and, 11, 306–309
stressors, **302**
stress response, **302**
stress tests, **41**, 340
stretching. *See also* flexibility
    ballistic, 147
    dynamic, 147
    frequency of exercises, 146
    intensity and duration of, 146, 200
    passive *vs.* active, 148
    proprioceptive neuromuscular facilitation, 143, 147–148
    for relaxation, 324
    safe, 146, 153, 162
    sample program, 146, 148–152
    static, 142, 147
    stretches to avoid, 153
    stretching exercises, 149–151
    stretching too far, 162
    warming up *vs.*, 45, 162
stroke. *See also* cardiovascular disease
    African Americans and, 337, 338
    aging and, 337
    alcohol consumption and, 342–343
    aspirin therapy and, 341
    blood pressure and, 333, 334, 337
    cardiorespiratory fitness and, 335
    defined, **340**, 341–342
    exercise and, 335, 344
    first aid for, 341
    gender and, 337
    ischemic *vs.* hemorrhagic, 342
    plaque buildup and, 334, 339
    silent, 342
    smoking and, 332
    treatment for, 342
    warning signs of, 341
    whole grains and, 342
stroke volume, **63**, 67
subcutaneous fat, 176, **177**
substance abuse, 374–394. *See also* alcohol use; psychoactive drugs; tobacco use
    addictive behaviors, 374–375

    characteristics of abusers, 377–378
    club drugs, 379
    defined, **377**
    drug effects, 376
    drug use, abuse, and dependence, 377, 383
    helping someone with, 394
    prevalence of, 374
    prevention of, 378
    role of drugs, 379
    signals of dependence, 378
    treatments for, 378
substance dependence, **377**
sucralose (Splenda), 279
suction lipectomy, 188, 288
sudden cardiac death, 42, **340**
sudden infant death syndrome (SIDS), 390
suffocation, A–6
sugar alcohols, 279
sugars
    added, 232, 241, 244, 246
    in American diets, 246
    in beverages, 208, 241
    energy from, 230
    reducing intake of, 241
sugar substitutes, 277, 279
suicide, 322
sulforaphane, 238, 363
sulfur dioxide, 425
sunburns/suntans, 358, 359
sunscreens, 359
Superfund program, 436
supplements, dietary
    adverse reactions to, 253
    cancer and, 362
    Food and Drug Administration on, 112, 115, 252, 253
    herbal, 285
    in pregnancy, 248
    reading labels on, 252, 253
    recommendations for, 239–240
    regulation of, 252
    sports performance and, 112, 113–114, 250
    in strength training, 112–115
    tips for choosing, 239–240, 253
    vegetarian diets and, 239
    vitamins in, 235, 239
    weight loss and, 285, 286
support groups, 320–321
*The Surgeon General's Vision for a Healthy and Fit Nation,* 30
surgery
    for cancer, 366
    for weight loss, 287–288
suspension training, 107
sustainable development, 441
sweating, 79
swimming, 92, 215–217
swim test, 92
sympathetic division, **302**
synovial fluid, 142
syphilis, **413**
systemic circulation, 62, **63**
systole, 62, **63**, 64
systolic blood pressure, 332–333

t'ai chi, 319
Take Charge strategies
    in alcohol emergencies, 382
    in behavior change, 17
    breast self-exam, 356
    in building social support, 313
    in choosing more whole-grain foods, 232
    compact fluorescent lightbulbs, 431
    in dealing with anger, 316
    in drinking behavior and responsibility, 385
    in eating for strong bones, 237

in eating strategies for college students, 249
effective communication guidelines, 314
in getting fitness programs back on track, 207
in good posture and low-back health, 157
in heart attack, stroke, or cardiac arrest, 341
if someone you know has an eating disorder, 292
in insomnia, 308
intake goals for protein, fat, and carbohydrate, 230
in judging portion sizes, 245
lifestyle strategies for weight management, 283
in male condom use, 409
in realistic self-talk, 318
in reducing saturated and trans fats, 242
in rehabilitation after a minor injury, 83
in safe food handling, 255
in safe stretching, 146, 153
in safe weight training, 111
in STD protection, 414
testicle self-examination, 360
in varying your activities, 46
talk test, 76
tamoxifen, 355
tanning salons, 359
target behavior, **12–13**, 18
target body weight, 197–198
target heart rate zone, 74–**75**, 217, 281
target rate reserve, 74–**75**
technology. *See also* equipment
    bicycling computers, 214
    bioelectrical impedance analyzers, 184, 185
    biotechnology, 260–261
    blood pressure monitors, 333
    for body composition assessment, 183–185
    cell phones, 206, 284, 439
    digital workout aids, 47
    GPS devices, 73
    heart rate monitors, 73, 333
    in mammography, 355
    motivational applications, 206
    pedometers, 47, 59–60, 85, 213
    videos for improving technique, 108
    videos of weight-training movements, 108
    in weight management, 284
    workout aids, 47
teenagers. *See* adolescents
television viewing, weight gain and, 277, 280, 287
telomerase, 369
"tend-and-befriend," 306
tendinitis, 82
tendons, **101**
tension-release breathing, 321
10,000 Steps program, 213
termination stage, 16, 17
terrorism, coping after, A–9
tertiary syphilis, 413
testicle self-examination, 360
testicular cancer, 359–360
testosterone, muscular strength and, **101**, 102
therapists, choosing and evaluating, 322
thiamin, 234, 263
3-minute step test, 71, 90
throat cancer, 358, 365
time, in FITT equation. *See* duration of exercise
time management, 49, 315, 317–318
Tips for Today guidelines
    on body composition changes, 187
    on cancer prevention, 368
    on cardiorespiratory fitness, 84
    on cardiovascular disease, 345
    on diet improvements, 258
    on environmental health, 440
    on flexibility, 162
    on personal fitness programs, 209
    on physical activity and exercise, 48
    on sexually transmitted diseases, 415
    on strength training, 115

on stress management, 323
on substance dependence, 392
on weight management, 292
on wellness, 21
tissue plasminogen activator (tPA), 341
titin, 142
tobacco use, 386–391
    action against, 390
    assessment of reasons for, 399–400
    back pain and, 155
    cancer and, 353, 360, 362
    cardiovascular disease and, 332, 343
    as cause of death, 6–7, 11, 386
    cigars and pipes, 387–388
    clove cigarettes and bidis, 388
    depression and, 386, 388, 391
    electronic cigarettes, 388–389
    environmental tobacco smoke, 332, 353,
        389–390, 429
    exercise and, 393
    gender and, 386, 388
    health hazards of cigarettes, 386–387
    "light" and "low-tar" products, 390
    nicotine addiction, 386
    in pregnancy, 388, 390
    quitting, 388, 389, 391
    smoking statistics, 11, 386
    spit tobacco, 388
    stress and, 311
    vitamin C and, 239
Tolerable Upper Intake Level (UL), 238
tolerance, **377**
TOPS (Take Off Pounds Sensibly), 286
total body electrical conductivity (TOBEC), 185
total fiber, **233**
towel stretch, 149
*Toxoplasma,* 254
tPA (tissue plasminogen activator), 341
trace minerals, 235–236
training. *See* physical training
training threshold, 74, 75
training volume, 108–109
transcriptase inhibitors, 406
trans fatty acids (trans fats)
    in butter and margarine, 228, 242, 260
    defined, **227**
    health effects of, 228, 229
    reducing in the diet, 228, 240–242
    restrictions on use of, 241
    sources of, 227
transtheoretic model, 16–17
trash. *See* solid waste
trastuzumab (Herceptin), 355
*Treponema pallidum,* 413
triceps extension exercise, 122
trichomoniasis ("trich"), **413**
triglycerides
    cardiovascular disease and, 336
    healthy levels of, 334, 336
    metabolic syndrome and, 339
    structure of, 227
    tobacco use and, 332
trunk flexors endurance test, 173
trunk twist exercise, 159
tuberculosis, 406
tumors, 352, **353**
tumor suppressor genes, 362
12-minute swim test, 92
"two-for-two" rule, 110
Type A/TypeB/TypeC personality, 305
type 1 diabetes, 180. *See also* diabetes mellitus
type 2 diabetes. *See also* diabetes mellitus
    body fat and, 176, 178–179, 180, 185
    endurance exercise and, 70
    insulin and, 180
    obesity and, 178–179

prevalence of, 274
stress and, 307
type of activity, in FITT equation. *See also*
        FITT principle
    in cardiorespiratory endurance exercise, 76–77
    in program design, 40
    in strength training, 109
    in stretching programs, 146–148

UL (Tolerable Upper Intake Level), 238
ultrasonography, **355**
ultraviolet protection factor (UPF), 359
ultraviolet (UV) radiation, **357**–358, 371–372, 428
underwater weighing, 183
underweight, 290. *See also* eating disorders
unintentional injuries, **11**, A–2 to A–7
United States Department of Agriculture (USDA),
        243–247, 256, A–1
UPF ratings, 359
upper-back stretch, 149
upright rowing exercise, 117
urethritis, 409, 410
USP (United States Pharmacopeia), 253
uterine cancer, 357
UVA/UVB radiation, 358, 359
UV index, 359
UV (ultraviolet) radiation, **357**–359, 371–372, 428

vaccines
    for cancers, 357, 369, 411
    for hepatitis B, 413
    for human papillomavirus, 357, 411
vaginal intercourse, HIV transmission in, 404,
        407–408
variable resistance exercise, 104, **105**
vegans, 247
vegetables
    calories and, 260
    cancer and, 363
    cooking, 242
    cruciferous, 238, 239
    "dirty dozen," 256
    intake recommendations for, 238, 241,
        244–245, 260
    low energy density in, 278–279
    pesticide residues on, 256
    serving sizes of, 245
vegetarian diets
    defined, **247**
    food plans for, 247–248
    protein combinations in, 226
    recommendations for, 242
    supplements in, 239
    types of, 247
veins, **63**
venae cavae, 62, **63**
venereal diseases. *See* sexually transmitted diseases
ventricles, 62, **63**
ventricular fibrillation, 340
vertebrae, 152–**153**, 154
vertical banded gastroplasty (VGB/LapBand), 287–288
vertical press exercise, 120
vertical transmission, 404
videos, in strength training, 108
vigorous exercise. *See also* intensity of exercise
    benefits of, 44
    definitions of, 33, 75, 76
    examples of, 202
    immune function and, 403
    joint damage and, 144
    recommendations for, 34, 39
violence
    assault, A–7 to A–8
    firearms injuries, A–6
    mass, coping after, A–9
    sexual assault, A–8 to A–9

visceral fat, 176, **177**
viscous fiber, **233**
visualization, 15, 17, 207, 319
vitality, increasing, 11
vital statistics. *See* statistics
vitamin(s), **233**–235. *See also specific vitamins*
vitamin A, 234, 235, 263
vitamin B-6
   cardiovascular disease and, 337, 346
   Dietary Reference Intake for, 263
   functions of, 234, 235
vitamin B-12
   cardiovascular disease and, 235, 337, 346
   Dietary Reference Intake for, 263
   functions of, 234
   for older adults, 239
   supplements, 239
   in vegetarian diets, 239, 247–248
vitamin C
   bone health and, 237
   Dietary Reference Intake for, 263
   functions of, 234, 238
   smoking and, 239
vitamin D
   bone health and, 237, 242
   cancer and, 235, 354
   cardiovascular disease and, 235, 338
   cholesterol and, 334
   Dietary Reference Intake for, 263
   functions of, 234
   in older adults, 239
   sources of, 235, 241, 242, 248
   supplements, 235
   in vegetarian diets, 248
vitamin E, 234, 238, 263
vitamin K, 234, 237, 264

waist circumference
   assessment of, 195–196
   health risks and, 179
   in metabolic syndrome, 339
   WHO and NIH classifications, 182
waist-to-hip ratio, 185, 195–196
walking
   exercise plan for, 211–213
   posture in, 157
   stress and, 307, 312
   weight loss and, 281
walk tests, 71, 89–90
wall squat exercise, 161
warming up
   for cardiorespiratory endurance exercise, 77
   function of, 45
   for interval training, 80
   for strength training, 109–110
   stretching and, 45, 147, 162
   for swimming, 216
warning signs
   of alcohol dependence, 383
   of cardiac arrest, 341
   of diabetes, 180
   of drunk driving, 383
   of eating disorders, 292

   of heart attack, 341
   of stroke, 341
water
   for athletes, 250
   bottled water, 208, 431
   contamination and treatment of, 430–431
   importance of, 236–237
   protecting, 432
   recommended intake of, 237, 265
   sewage, 432
   shortages of, 431–432
water quality and pollution, 430–432
water-soluble vitamins, 233–234
Web sites. *See* Internet
weight-bearing exercise
   bone mass and, 70, 144, 237
   in pregnancy, 208
   swimming and, 217
weight belts, 125
weight gain, 125, 293
weight-loss products, 285, 286
weight-loss programs, 285–287
weight machines, 105–106, 120–124
weight management, 274–293. *See also* obesity
   bariatric surgery, 287–288
   body image and, 288–289
   calories and, 240, 278
   cancer and, 179
   cardiovascular disease and, 274
   by college students, 285
   coping strategies and, 281–282
   daily food journals in, 282
   diabetes and, 180
   diet and eating habits, 240, 277–280
   dietary supplements and diet aids, 285, 286
   diet books for, 283–284
   emotions and, 179, 281–282
   energy need calculation, 295–296
   exercise in, 33–34, 280–281, 283
   fat and sugar substitutes in, 277, 279
   hormones and, 276
   independent weight loss, 282–283
   lifestyle strategies for, 283
   maintenance in, 283
   metabolism and energy balance, 275–276
   National Weight Control Registry, 284
   portion sizes and, 276–277, 278
   prescription drugs for weight loss, 287
   reasonable goals in, 293
   smoking and, 393
   spot reducing and, 188
   strength training and, 125
   stress management and, 283
   target body weight in, 197–198
   technology for, 284
   thoughts and emotions and, 281–282
   underestimating food intake and, 276–277, 278
   weight gain, 125, 293
   weight-loss goals, 297–298
   weight-loss programs, 285–287
weight training. *See* strength training
Wellbutrin (bupropion), 388
wellness, 2–21. *See also* behavior change

behaviors contributing to, 7–11
body fat and, 176, 178–179
body weight and, 10–11
college students and, 14
continuum of, 2
defined, **2**
diet and, 10
diverse populations and, 8
emotional, 3, 179
environmental, 3–4
exercise and, 70–71
financial, 4, 5
intellectual, 3
interpersonal, 3
life expectancy and, 4
lifestyle management and, 6, 11–21
occupational, 4
physical, 3
physical activity and, 7–10, 30–33
spiritual, 3, 4, 315, 329–330
stress and, 11, 306–309
target behavior, 12–13, 18
types of, 2–4
wellness profile, 25–26
whole grains, 230–**231**, 232, 241, 342
wind chill, **81**
wind power, 441
wines, 380
withdrawal symptoms, **377**
women. *See also* gender differences; pregnancy
   breast self-exam, 355, 356
   cardiovascular disease in, 338
   cervical cancer in, 357
   date-rape drugs and, 378, 379
   Dietary Reference Intakes for, 263–265
   female athlete triad, 181
   folic acid for, 235, 239, 263
   lung cancer in, 353
   menstruation and exercise, 85, 181
   muscular strength in, 102
   nutrition for, 230, 239, 248
   osteoporosis in, 102
   pelvic inflammatory disease in, 410–411
   sexual anatomy of, 410
   sexually transmitted diseases and, 417
   social power of, HIV and, 405
   strength training by, 102
   tobacco use by, 386, 388
work injuries, A–7
workout cards, 110
World Health Organization, 182

X-rays, 360, 365, 439

yerba mate, 286
yoga, 158, 319
yoga plow, 153

zinc
   Dietary Reference Intake for, 264
   functions of, 236, 237
   in vegetarian diets, 239, 248
Zyban (bupropion), 391